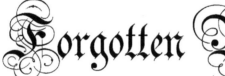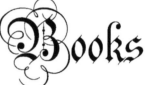

ISBN 978-1-5278-9493-8
PIBN 10926341

1 MONTH OF
FREE
READING

at

www.ForgottenBooks.com

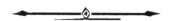

By purchasing this book you are
eligible for one month membership to
ForgottenBooks.com, giving you
unlimited access to our entire
collection of over 1,000,000 titles via
our web site and mobile apps.

To claim your free month visit:

www.forgottenbooks.com/free926341

English
Français
Deutsche
Italiano
Español
Português

www.forgottenbooks.com

Mythology Photography **Fiction**
Fishing Christianity **Art** Cooking
Essays Buddhism Freemasonry
Medicine **Biology** Music **Ancient**
Egypt Evolution Carpentry Physics
Dance Geology **Mathematics** Fitness
Shakespeare **Folklore** Yoga Marketing
Confidence Immortality Biographies
Poetry **Psychology** Witchcraft
Electronics Chemistry History **Law**
Accounting **Philosophy** Anthropology
Alchemy Drama Quantum Mechanics
Atheism Sexual Health **Ancient History**
Entrepreneurship Languages Sport
Paleontology Needlework Islam
Metaphysics Investment Archaeology
Parenting Statistics Criminology
Motivational

A

PRACTICAL TREATI

ON

DISEASES OF THE

BY

J. MOORE NELIGAN, M.D., M.R.I

FIFTH AMERICAN FROM THE SECOND REVISED AND ENLARGED

BY

T. W. BELCHER, M.A., M.D., D

B. M , M. A., OXON. ;

FELLOW, CENSOR, EXAMINER IN MATERIA MEDICA AND MEDICAI
AND IN ARTS, AND HON. LIBRARIAN, KING AND QUEEN'S C
PHYSICIANS IN IRELAND ;
HONORARY MEMBER OF THE CORK MEDICAL SOCIE'
PHYSICIAN TO THE DUBLIN DISPENSARY FOR SKIN DIS
AND SOMETIME ONE OF THE PHYSICIANS TO THE CORK FEVE

RATIONE ET EXPERIENTIA.

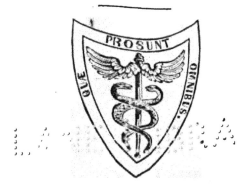

PHILADELPHIA:
HENRY C. LEA
1866.

WR

LAME LIBRARY

PHILADELPHIA:
4 PRINTER, 705 JAYNE STREET.

TO

THOMAS EDWARD BEATTY, Esq.

DOCTOR IN PHYSIC;

PRESIDENT OF THE KING AND QUEEN'S COLLEGE OF PHYSICIANS
IN IRELAND.

SIR,

To none can this Volume with more propriety be dedicated than to you, who preside over the College of which the late Dr. Neligan was sometime Vice-President, and long a distinguished Member. Allow me, in some small degree, to acknowledge that high personal and professional worth, and that exemplary regard for the honor and usefulness of what you yourself have called "our God-like profession," which have placed you in the highest seat of our ancient and learned Society, and added your name to the long and honorable roll of Presidents of the College of "the beloved Physician."

Believe me to be, SIR,

Your faithful Servant,

T. W. BELCHER.

23226

EDITOR'S PREFACE

TO THE

SECOND EDITION.

THE first edition of the late Dr. Neligan's *Practical Treatise on Diseases of the Skin* having been exhausted, I was requested by the publishers of that work to undertake the editing of a second edition. This responsibility I accepted, not without misgivings as to my ability to perform such a task; but on consideration that I had the advantage of having been Dr. Neligan's pupil at Jervis-street Hospital, and of having subsequently devoted much attention to the study and treatment of this class of diseases, I determined to undertake the task, the result of which I now beg to set before the Profession, for whom alone this work is designed.

It might perhaps be expected that a memorial notice of Dr. Neligan should be appended to this volume. I thought of doing this; but on re-reading the admirably written obituary memoir of him which appeared in the *Dublin Quarterly Journal of Medical Science*, for August, 1863, from the pen of its talented editor, Dr. Kidd, I arrived at the conclusion that what was there said was well and wisely said, and that I should best show my respect for Dr. Neligan's reputation by directing the attention of the readers of this volume to that memoir.

Since the appearance of the first edition of this work in 1852 a great change has taken place in the relation of

1*

Dermatology to Medicine. Numerous works of value have been published; important discoveries have been made, and papers without number, on isolated cases or classes of skin disease, have continually issued from the medical press. Thus the subject has taken a high professional rank, and has been completely rescued from the shade under which it had fallen, from its having been made a ready means of ill-gotten gain by the quack and the impostor.

The present edition contains the substance, in most cases the very words, of the edition of 1852, and from it no opinion, statement, recommendation, or fact, recorded by Dr. Neligan, has been omitted. The whole has undergone a careful revision, and has been enlarged by the addition of 100 pages. The discoveries of medical science, and the opinions of the best authorities, from 1852 to the present month, have been added under their several heads; and the result of the Editor's experience has also been inserted where it particularly confirmed or differed from that of Dr. Neligan.

The phraseology employed requires explanation. Wherever the first person singular is employed the reader will understand that Dr. Neligan speaks, and that I agree with, or, unless otherwise expressed in the text or in a note, see no reason to differ from him. Editorial remarks are given in the third person singular, while facts and the opinions of others are simply given as such. Wherever I have been able to trace an authority for a statement of Dr. Neligan's I have inserted it; and, as far as lay in my power, I have invariably done so with my own records of facts, and of the opinions of others.

The following additions are now made to this work:—

1. A copious Table of Contents.

2. Considerable additions to Chapter I, on Classifica-

tion; chiefly as regards the modern nosologies of Hardy, Hebra, Buchanan, and others.

3. Derivations and meanings of technical terms; and their synonyms.

4. References to Dr. Neligan's *Atlas of Cutaneous Diseases*, as also to the plates of Cazenave and Hebra.

5. References to Professor Macnamara's Sixth Edition of Dr. Neligan's *Materia Medica*.

6. Quotations from, and references to authorities in every case, particularly where the full description of the subject is excluded by reason of the practical nature of the work.

7. Explanations of the peculiar modes of treatment, and in some cases the prescriptions, of the best home and foreign dermatologists.

8. An entire translation of the numerous prescriptious in the first edition, with those now added, into the technical language of the *British Pharmacopœia*.

9. A Posological Table of the most important, and mostly poisonous, medicines used in the treatment of cutaneous diseases.

10. A copious Bibliographical Index of the chief authorities quoted.

Notices of the following, among other diseases, are now for the first time added: Rubeola, Scarlatina, Variola and its allies, Furunculus, Anthrax, Pustula Maligna, Lepra Hebræorum; a full account of Elephantiasis, Morphie, Frambœsia, Morbus Tauricus, Aleppo Evil, Ngerengere, Pellagra, Morbus Addisonii.

The Chapter on Parasitic Diseases, or Dermatophytæ, has been revised, and considerably added to, as also that on Diseases of the Hair and Nails, and that on Therapeutics.

The General Index has been enlarged and re-written.

A prominent feature in the enlargement is the addition of the cutaneo-nosological synonyms used by ancient and modern writers in our own and in foreign countries.

The chief aim throughout has been to make this book thoroughly fit for the practical man. This has led to necessary retrenchment in the scientific departments, and some will, doubtless, consider this a defect; but I have endeavored to compensate for it by the additions just enumerated, particularly by the fair and honest system of quoting authorities, and giving numerous references for minute information. In this way I trust the work will not only suit the busy practitioner, the man of one book (on this subject), for whom this volume is primarily designed, but also the industrious medical student, the practitioner "getting up" a paper for a medical society, and the Lecturer, for ready reference and saving of valuable time. Most of the books and papers quoted will be found in our public libraries.

My best acknowledgments are due, and are hereby given, to the hundreds of writers of whose works I have availed myself. Many of these cannot be here particularized, but I cannot omit to note specially the admirable works of Mr. Erasmus Wilson and Dr. Tilbury Fox, and the elaborate and learned reviews which appeared in the *Medical Times and Gazette*, and in the *British and Foreign Medical and Chirurgical Review* for the present year, which are respectively entitled *Dermatology*, and *Recent Re-* on *Scabies*.

further thank Messrs. Fannin & Co., the pub-
their compliance with my suggestions about
n, and Mr. J. B. Falconer, B. A., for his careful
arly revision of the proof sheets.

                                        T. W. B.

DR. NELIGAN'S

PREFACE TO THE FIRST EDITION.

In submitting the observations contained in the following pages to the Profession, the Author has been influenced chiefly by a desire to offer, as an aid to the diagnosis and treatment of an important class of diseases, the results of an experience acquired during several years' special attention to the study of cutaneous eruptions. Of late years the British Medical press has abounded with monographs on other special affections, but few have been published on those of the skin; he has, therefore, thought that a concise practical Treatise on them might find favor with the Profession.

As regards the plan adopted in the construction of the work, the only points requiring notice are the omission of the details of cases which might be cited to prove the correctness of the views propounded, and the slight reference to other writers on the same subject: for both the only apology he has to offer is his anxious desire to condense the inquiry he proposed to himself within as narrow limits as possible, being fully aware "how great an evil a great book" is to the physician busily engaged in practice.

17 Merrion Square, East, Dublin,
June 1, 1852.

TABLE OF CONTENTS.

CHAPTER I.

CLASSIFICATION.—Importance of the Study of the Diseases of the Skin—Antiquity of Jewish, Egyptian, Arabian, Greek, and Latin Classifications—Important Changes caused in Cutaneous Nosology by Microscopic Discoveries—Classifications: Artificial, Natural, and Regional—Systems of Riolanus, Plenck, Willan, Lorry, Mercurialis, Turner, Alibert, Cazenave, Wilson, Hardy, Hebra, Buchanan, Fox, Bennett, and Neligan—pp. 25-45.

CHAPTER II.

EXANTHEMATA.—General Definition. *Erythema*—Varieties of—Hebra's Division of—E. Simplex—E. Intertrigo—E. Circinatum—E. Marginatum—E. Papulatum—E. Nodosum—E. Tuberculatum et Œdematosum—E. resembling Superficial Acrodynia—Diagnosis of Erythema—Prognosis—Treatment—pp. 48-56. *Erysipelas*—E. Iodiopathicum—E. Traumaticum—E. Phlegmonodes—Causes—Contagious Properties — Diagnosis—Prognosis—Pathology— Treatment—Authorities on—pp. 56-72. *Urticaria*—Febrilis, Evanida, Tuberosa, Conferta, Intermittens, Subcutanea—Diagnosis — Prognosis—Pathology — Treatment—pp. 72-80. *Roseola*—Idiopathica, Symptomatica, Æstiva, Autumnalis, Annulata, Punctata—Cause—Diagnosis — Prognosis— Treatment—pp. 80-85. *Rubeola*—Vulgaris—Maligna—Nigra—Sine Catarrho—Sine Exanthemate—Notha—Camp Measles—Exciting Causes—Sequelæ—Diagnosis—Treatment—Authorities on—pp. 85-89. *Scarlatina*—Simplex—Anginosa—Maligna—Sine Exanthemate—Papulosa vel Milliformis—Vesicularis—vel Phlyctænosa vel Pustulosa— Prognosis—Diagnosis—Treatment—Sequelæ—Authorities on — Rosalia—pp. 89-92. *Variola*—Discreta—Confluens, Varioloid, Sine Eruptione—Diagnosis—Treatment—Prevention of Pitting in—Plan of a . for Use in cases of—Varicella—Vaccinia—Vaccinella—Maculæ of Typhus and Typhoid—Hillier's Table for Diagnosing between various Exanthemata—List of Authorities—pp. 92-100.

Pilaris, Circumscriptus, Solitarius, Gyratus, Umbratus—Strophulus Confertus, Volaticus, Candidus, Albidus—Lichen Tropicus—L. Urematosus, Papulatus, Sudativus, Scrofulosus, Ruber—Causes—Diagnosis—Prognosis — Treatment — pp. 202-217. Prurigo — Synonyms—Prurigo Mitis, Formicans, Senilis, Vulgaris. Pedicularis—Phthiriasis Corporis—Phth. Pubis—Phth. Capitis—Prurigo Scroti, Pudendi, Podicis, Præputialis, Palmaris—Causes—Diagnosis—Pathology—Treatment—pp. 217-227.

CHAPTER VI.

Squamæ.—General Description of the class. *Psoriasis*—Derivation and Synonyms—Identity of with Lepra—Nature of the Disease—Ps. Guttata, Aggregata, Lepræformis, Diffusa, Confluens, Vulgaris, Inveterata, Labialis, Palpebrarum, Capitis, Scrotalis, Præputialis, Pudendalis, Palmaris, Unguium, Alphoïdes, Annulata, Rupioides, Nummularis—Causes—Diagnosis—Prognosis—Pathology—Treatment—Use of Arsenic and Hydropathy in—Plans of Hunt, Milton, Hebra, Hardy, Bazin, Cazenave, Biett, &c.—pp. 228-253. *Pityriasis*—Derivation and Synonyms—P. Diffusa, Localis—Chloasma of Rayer—Melasma of Wilson—P. Palpebrarum, Oris et Labiorum, Præputialis et Pudendalis, Palmaris et Plantaris, Capitis—Causes—Diagnosis—Prognosis—Treatment·· pp. 53-262.

CHAPTER VII.

Hypertrophiæ.—*Ichthyosis*—Derivation and Synonyms—Wilson, mson, Hebra, and Gustav Simon on its Classification—Ichthyosis plex, Cornea, Squamosa, Spinosa, Hysterix, Scutellata—Seborrhœa t, Acné Cebacée Cornée—Papillary Ichthyosis—Porcupine Men and maids—Case of the Lamberts—Causes of Ichthyosis—Diagnosis—Treatment—Remarkable Cases of—pp. 263-273. *Mollus*-ing of the term—Synonyms—Molluscum Contagiosum—giosum—Acne Molluscoides—Acne Varioliformis—Molluscutum, Chronicum—Contagious Nature of Molluscum—Causesis—Prognosis—Treatment—pp. 274-278. *Stearrhœa*—Deri-of the term—S. Simplex, Flavescens, Nigricans—Inflammatio orum - Remarkable Case of S. Nigricans—Causes of Stearrhœa .s-—Prognosis—Treatment—pp. 278-283. *Elephantiasis*—of the term—Synonyms—E. Græcorum—Description of—and Lucretius on—Identical with Mediæval Leprosy—Hospitals, particularly in Great Britain and Ireland—

CHAPTER XI.

DERMATOPHYTÆ.—Derivation and Definition—Parasites, Animal and Vegetable—Treatment of Guinea-worm Disease—Authorities on Parasites and Parasitic Skin Diseases—pp. 358–360. *Porrigo*—Synonyms, Description, Parasitic Nature of—Causes—Contagious Nature of—Diagnosis — Prognosis—Treatment — Authorities on — pp. 360–371. *Sycosis*—Derivation, Definition, Description, and Parasitic Nature of—Causes—Diagnosis—Prognosis—Treatment—pp. 371–376. *Madura Foot*—Propagation of Epiphytic Disease by Contagion, and from man to lower animals, and *vice versâ*—Authorities on—pp. 376–377.

CHAPTER XII.

THE SYPHILIDES.—Common features of. *Syphilitic exanthemata*—Erythema, Urticaria, Roseola—pp. 378–384. *Syphilitic Vesiculæ*—Eczema, Pemphigus, Rupia—pp. 384–386. *Syphilitic Pustulæ*—Acne, Impetigo, Ecthyma—pp. 386–389. *Syphilitic Papulæ*—Lichen—pp. 389–390. *Syphilitic Squamæ*—Psoriasis—pp. 390–392. *Syphilitic Hypertrophiæ*—Tubercles—pp. 392–394. *Syphilitic Maculæ*—Roseola —pp. 394–395. Diagnosis, Prognosis, General, Specific, and Topical Treatment of Syphilides—pp. 395–404.

CHAPTER XIII.

DISEASES OF THE APPENDAGES OF THE SKIN.—*Diseases of the Hair*—Change of Color from a Light to a Dark Hue—Canities—Case of Queen Marie Antoinette—Case of an Aged Female, in which Canities was Absent—Canities of the Beard—Its Connection with the Use of the Razor—Treatment of Canities ; *Plica Polonica*—Nature and Description of—Authorities on ; *Alopecia*—Its Derivation, Meaning, and Causes—Porrigo Decalvans of Willan—Comparative Rareness of Alopecia in Ireland, as compared with England—Alopecia from Mental Anxiety, Stearne's Case of—Treatment—Symptomatic Alopecia of Hardy—Alopecia Areata of Wilson—Authorities on Alopecia—pp. 405–411. *Diseases of the Nails*—Alopecia Unguale—Onychomycosis Description—Microscopic Examination—Treatment—Authorities on— pp. 411–414.

CHAPTER XIV.

THERAPEUTICS OF DISEASES OF THE SKIN.—General Review of Remedies Used, and the Mode of their Administration—Topical and Con-

Elephantiasis in Northern Europe, Spain, and Morocco—E. Tuberculosa, Anæsthetica—Treatment, Danielssen and Böeck on—Elephantiasis in India—Dr. Carter on Nature of the Disease—*Morphic* of Brazil
—*Frambœsia*, or *Radesyge*, Treatment of—*Morbus Tauricus*, the Aleppo
Evil—*Ngerengere* of New Zealand—*Cacubay* of Jamaica—*Pellagra*, or
Elephantiasis Italica—Treatment—Authorities—pp. 284-294. *Elephantiasis Arabum*—Causes—Pathology—Treatment—Authorities on—
pp. 294-297. *The Leprosy of the Hebrews*—What was the disease?
Accounts of the Levitical Canon and Ancient Historians—Technical
terms employed in the Hebrew, Greek, Latin, and English Versions of
the Mosaic Law—Celsus, Galen, Rhenferdius, Schilling, Mead, Mason
Good and others on—Jewish Leprosy not Elephantiasis, but rather
Psoriasis—Authorities on—pp. 297-305. *Verrucœ*, Nature and Treatment of—*Clavus*, Nature and Treatment of—*Callositates, Condylomata,*
and *Nævus*, Nature and Treatment of—pp. 305-311.

CHAPTER VIII.

HÆMORRHAGIÆ.—Rashes of Fevers—*Purpura*, Simplex, Hæmorrhagica, Cachectica, Contagiosa—Causes—Diagnosis—Prognosis—Pathology—Treatment—Neligan's Treatment by Turpentine—*Scorbutus*, the
Plague at Athens, as described by Thucydides—pp. 312-324.

CHAPTER IX.

MACULÆ.—*Vitiligo*—Derivation and Meaning of the term—Its Na-
ture, Causes, Diagnosis, Prognosis, Treatment—pp. 325-329. *Ephelis*
—Derivation and Meaning—Ephelis Lenticularis, Hepatica—Ephélides
Ignéales — Diagnosis — Treatment — Ephelis Violacea, Cyanopathis,
American Carate—Treatment of E. Violacea—E. Melasma, or Mor-
bus Addisonii, Black Jaundice of Hippocrates, Galen, and Aretœus;
Melanopathia and Melasma Universum of Wilson—Authorities on
Morbus Addisonii—pp. 329-338.

CHAPTER X.

CANCROIDES.—Lupus—Synonyms and Description of—L. Exedens,
Non-exedens, Superficialis, Serpiginosus, Devorans, Esthiomenos—L.
Vorax, Jacob's Ulcer—Prognosis of Lupus—Pathology—Treatment,
Local, and by Cod-liver Oil, Arsenic, and Mercury—Authorities on—
pp. 339-354. *Keloïs*—Derivation, Synonyms, and Description-
Nature, Causes, Diagnosis, Prognosis, Treatment, and Authorities
pp. 354-357.

agrees, in many of its functions and properties, with the mucous membrane of which it is manifestly a continuation—the mucous membrane protecting the internal parts of the body, while the skin protects those that are external: there is consequently a remarkable agreement between them. In deranged conditions of the skin, the mucous membrane becomes more or less engaged; and, in diseases which affect the mucous membrane, the functions of the skin, as regards absorption and excretion, are also affected to a greater or less degree.

Owing to the great obscurity which so long enveloped the study of this class of diseases, and the late period in the history of medicine at which any attempt was made to classify them at all regularly, a great deal is left for the inquirer, even of the present day, to clear up. Yet we have abundant evidence, in the writings of the Jewish, the Egyptian, the Arabian, the Greek, and the Roman legislators and physicians, of their existence from the remotest antiquity; and that they were very numerous, often occurring as scourges of mankind, is easily proved by a reference to the Leprosy of the Jews, and the Elephantiasis of the Greeks and of the Arabians. Of late, much has been expected from the employment of the microscope in discovering the exact nature of diseases of the skin, but in this expectation we have, as yet, been to some extent disappointed. It is true, that by its aid much valuable information has been gained, as to the normal structure of the skin, yet but little addition has been hitherto made thereby to our knowledge of its diseased conditions, more particularly with reference to their diagnosis and treatment, as based on minute anatomy. There is one important fact, however, which has been attained by the use of the microscope in the investigation of the nature of diseases of the skin, namely, the discovery that, in certain affections, a vegetable production—a cryptogamic plant—is present on the cutaneous surface, and is evidently intimately connected with their true pathology. A difference of opinion exists as to whether these vegetable growths are the cause or the consequence of the disease in which they have been found to occur; but there can be no doubt—now that nearly all dermatologists admit the truth of the discovery, and consequently believe in the existence of these vegetable growths—that a new classification, containing a group or order, of which the presence of these fungi will form the essential character, must be constructed.

An important point of view in which diseases of the skin must be regarded, and one that adds much to their interest, is the effect they produce upon the system generally. We sometimes find that in persons who have labored even for a long time under these affections, but little constitutional derangement is, in many cases, caused by them—so little, indeed, that it has often been doubted whether the existence of an affection of the skin, in a chronic form, tends to shorten life, or should be taken into account in coming to a conclusion as to eligibility, in a medical examination, for assurance. For my own part, I believe that as long as the individual remains unaffected with any acute or inflammatory affection, the existence of a skin disease will not, in any respect, diminish the average chances of longevity; yet I have no doubt but that a person laboring under any general cutaneous affection, the existence of which unquestionably deranges the functions of this extensive membrane, must be more or less liable to have the symptoms of an ordinary acute disease, such as fever or any of the internal inflammations, aggravated, and the treatment rendered more difficult and complicated by its presence. Thus, although a chronic affection of the skin may not directly tend to shorten life, yet it may do so indirectly. As, however, these various points will be more fully considered in speaking of each eruption individually, I shall not dwell on them at present, but proceed to describe the classification of diseases of the skin which I propose to adopt.

No subject in the study of medicine has created more difficulty, or for a longer period tended to retard its advancement, than that of nosological arrangements. It was at one time believed to be impossible to understand the nature of diseases, or their proper treatment, without an intimate knowledge having been previously acquired of their classification, and we therefore find that all the writers on medicine of the last, and of the commencement of the present century, sedulously devoted themselves to devise new systems, each more complicated than the other. As regards diseases generally, it is now agreed by all that the less complicated and more simple the classification under which they are arranged, for the purpose of description or of teaching, the more advantageous is it for the acquirement of a knowledge of them; and few, therefore, take the trouble of making themselves acquainted with the labored systems of Cullen, Sauvages, Mason Good, or the many nosologists of their day. Simplicity, I need scarcely say, is of equal advantage in classifying any special set of diseases, as those of the skin; yet even in our own time it seems to me to be strangely overlooked by dermatologists; writer after writer, impelled, as it were, by an ambition to devise something novel, propounds a new classification, careless how complicated and difficult of being comprehended it may be, provided only it differs from those which preceded.

As in the arrangement of objects of natural history, so in that of diseases, a classification may be either *artificial* or *natural;* the former being based on external appearances, or those which come directly under the cognizance of our senses, without any respect to intimate nature, structure, or properties; while the latter has especial regard to natural qualities, as a bond of affinity. In addition to these two, a third has been adopted by some writers on diseases of the skin, which may be called a *local* or *regional* arrangement—that is, one in which they are placed in groups, dependent on the part of the body upon which they are seated; but, of course, in this system, regard must also be had to the individual character and form of the various eruptions.

Of the many systems of classification of diseases of the skin which have been, from time to time, proposed, two especially of those of the earlier writers are worthy of notice, not alone as being the first which had any pretentions to accuracy or completeness, but as forming, to a certain extent, the basis of most of those which have been since propounded—I allude to the *artificial* system of

Willan, and the *natural* one of Alibert. Although Willan adopted, as the groundwork of his classification, an arrangement originally proposed by Plenck—following out the idea of Riolanus put forth nearly a century previously—of placing diseases of the skin in groups, according to their form and appearances, yet, from the accuracy and appropriateness of his nomenclature, which is that now almost universally employed, and the clearness with which he defined the leading features of his general divisions or orders, it is correctly regarded as being the first important step made to the correct understanding of diseases of the skin. Alibert, in the first instance, following Turner, an Englishman, who was himself preceded by Mercurialis, adopted a *regional* classification, dividing all eruptions into two classes, as they were situated on the head or on the trunk of the body; but this he soon abandoned for a *natural* system, which, though grandly conceived, did not survive its author, being found too complicated and difficult of application when attempted to be reduced to practice.[1]

In Willan's system, cutaneous diseases are divided into eight orders, characterized by the form of the eruption, viz:—

Papulæ.	Vesiculæ.
Squamæ.	Pustulæ.
Exanthemata.	Tubercula.
Bullæ.	Maculæ.

The distinctive features of the eruptions, by which these orders are characterized, be defined as follows; and here I may again remark that his nomenclature and definitions are still in use, and generally recognized as correct:—

1. *Papula* (Pimple).—A very small and acuminated

---

[1] Lorry's classification of 1777 was based on the presumed nature of the affections, and was primarily divided into maladies arising from *external* and from *internal causes.* Respecting the *natural* and *artificial* systems, M. Hardy observes: "De même que la classification de Plenck est le point de départ des classifications basées sur les lésions anatomiques, de même Lorry doit être regardé comme le premier auteur des classifications basées sur la nature des maladies." —*Leçons sur les Maladies de la Peau.* Partie I. (1860) p. 9.

elevation of the cuticle, with an inflamed base, not containing a fluid, nor tending to suppuration.

2. *Squama* (Scale).—A lamina of morbid cuticle, hard, thickened, whitish, and opaque.

3. *Exanthema* (Rash).—Red patches on the skin, variously figured, in general confluent, and diffused irregularly over the body, leaving interstices of a natural color.

4. *Bulla* (Bleb).—A large portion of the cuticle detached from the skin by the interposition of a transparent, watery fluid.

5. *Vesicula* (Vesicle).—A small, orbicular elevation of the cuticle, containing lymph, which is sometimes clear and colorless, but often opaque and whitish, or pearl-colored.

6. *Pustula* (Pustule)—An elevation of the cuticle, with an inflamed base, containing pus.

7. *Tuberculum* (Tubercle).—A small, hard, superficial tumor, circumscribed and permanent, or proceeding very slowly to suppuration.

8. *Macula* (Stain).—A permanent discoloration of some portion of the skin, often with a change of its texture, but not connected with any disorder of the constitution.

As already noted, this classification, first published in 1798, will be seen to have been a modification of that of Plenck, first published in 1776, as follows:—

1. Maculæ.
2. Pustulæ.
3. Vesiculæ.
4. Bullæ.
5. Papulæ.
6. Crustæ.
7. Squamæ.
8. Callositates.
9. Excrescentiæ Cutaneæ.
10. Ulcera Cutanea.
11. Vulnera Cutanea.
12. Insecta Cutanea.
13. Morbi Unguium.
14. Morbi Pilorum.

Alibert, in his natural arrangement, considers cutaneous diseases to resemble a tree which he terms *l'arbre des dermatoses*, and the branches of which constitute the various divisions or groups, which are subdivided into genera. His primary groups, which are twelve in number, he designates as follows :—

Dermatoses Eczemateuses.	Dermatoses Véroleuses.
" Exanthema-	" Strumeuses.
" teuses.	" Scabieuses.
" Teigneuses.	·· Hémateuses.
" Dartreuses.	" Dyschroma-
" Cancéreuses.	teuses.
" Lépreuses.	Hétéromorphes.

Biett, the immediate and most celebrated pupil of Alibert, soon perceiving the difficulties which the complicated system of his master, though based on the natural affinities of the various eruptions of the skin, threw in the way of their successful diagnosis, forsook it for that of Willan, which he modified and so far improved that all the artificial systems of classification which have been proposed since his time include the changes made by him.

Viewed abstractedly, it is manifest that a classification of diseases of the skin which, as a natural system is supposed to do, takes into account not merely the form but the essential nature and pathological characters of a cutaneous eruption, should possess many advantages, both practical and theoretical, over an artificial arrangement which takes cognizance merely of the alterations of the skin which cause the eruption, or, in other words, regards solely the apparent changes in the cutaneous structure of the part affected. Consequently, we find that most modern writers on the subject have bestowed their attention on the construction of a perfect *natural* system, but hitherto, in the Editor's opinion, without success; amongst them all Dr. Neligan considered two only at all deserving of notice, that of Erasmus Wilson in England, and of Cazenave in France.

Wilson formerly adopted, as the basis of his arrangement above referred to, the anatomy and physiology of the skin, a groundwork which, owing to the modern additions made to our knowledge of this structure by microscopic investigation, and the degree of certainty which extended observation has stamped upon it, has been well employed by him, and has rendered this system of classification justly entitled to be designated a *natural* one. He constituted four *primary* divisions of the subject, viz:—

1. Diseases of the Derma.
2. Diseases of the Sudoriparous Glands.
3. Diseases of the Sebiparous Glands.
4. Diseases of the Hairs and Hair Follicles.

Of the first, five *secondary* divisions were made: 1. *Inflammation* of the Derma; 2. *Hypertrophy of the Papillæ* of the Derma; 3. *Disorders of the Vascular Tissue* of the Derma; 4. *Disorders of the Sensibility* of the Derma; 5. *Disorders of the Chromatogenous Function* of the Derma. The first of these subdivisions constituted six groups, viz: *a. Congestive* Inflammation, divided into two subgroups; the first including those affections in which both the mucous membranes and the derma are inflamed, and which are *attended with* constitutional symptoms of a specific kind; and the second, those in which the derma alone is engaged, and in which there are *no* specific constitutional symptoms; *b. Effusive* Inflammation; *c. Suppurative* Inflammation; *d. Depositive* Inflammation; *e. Squamous* Inflammation; *f.* Inflammation from *the presence of Acari.*

Of the second primary division, three *secondary* were constituted, as the diseases are attended with, 1. *Augmentation;* 2. *Diminution;* 3. *Alteration* of Secretion.

Of the third, five *secondary* divisions were made, as the diseases of the sebiparous glands are dependent on, 1. *Augmentation;* 2. *Diminution;* 3. *Alteration;* 4. *Retention, of Secretion;* and 5. In which the *Glands and adjacent Tissues are inflamed.*

And the fourth constituted six *secondary* divisions: 1. *Augmented Formation;* 2. *Diminished Formation;* 3. *Abnormal Direction,* of the Hair; *Alteration of Color;* 5. Diseases of the *Hairs;* and 6. Diseases of the *Hair Follicles.*

In consequence of a more extended experience, Mr. Wilson abandoned this classification, and in the *fourth* edition of his work, published in 1857, substituted for it what he terms an *Etiological* classification, as compared with the first, or *Physiological*.

In this Etiological arrangement he divides all cutaneous diseases into *two primary groups:* 1. Diseases affecting the general structure; and, 2. Diseases affecting the special structure of the Skin.

The diseases of the first class are such as implicate at once all the tissues entering into the composition of the skin; while diseases of the second class are those which select the separate components of the skin, *e. g.*, vessels, nerves, papillæ, and pigment; or its special organs, *e. g.*, sudoriparous glands, sebiparous glands, hair follicles, and hairs, and nail follicles and nails.

Under Class I. are five *secondary* groups:—

1. Diseases arising from general causes.
2.   "   special external causes.
3.   "   special internal causes.
4.   the syphilitic poison.
5.   animal poisons of unknown origin, and giving rise to eruptive fevers.

Under Class II. are eight *secondary* groups:—

1. Diseases of the vascular system.
2.   "   nervous structure.
3.   "   papillary structure.
4.   pigmentary structure.
5.   sudoriparous organs.
6.   sebiparous organs.
7.   hair follicles and hair.
8.   nail follicles and nails.

The elaborate details of this classification would fill several pages, and the curious must refer to Mr. Wilson's large work for them. In the latest systematic treatise of that veteran (*Student's Book, &c.*, 1864–65), this etiological classification is in turn set aside in favor of a *Clinical* arrangement in twenty-two groups, thus:—

1. Eczematous affections.
2. Erythematous   "

   3. Bullous affections
   4. Furuncular "
   5. Nervous   "
   6. Vascular   "
   7. Hæmodyscrasic affections.
   8. Developmental and nutritive affections.
   9. Hypertrophic and atrophic   "
 10. Zymotic   "
 11. Alphous
 12. Strumous
 13. Syphilitic
 14. Carcinomatous
 15. Leprous   "
 16. Affections of the hair and hair follicles.
 17.   "   sebiparous apparatus.
 18.   "   chromatogenous "
 19.   sudoriparous "
 20.   "   nails.
 21. Traumatic affections.
 22. Phytodermic "

M. Cazenave, adopting likewise an anatomical basis for his *natural* system, arranged diseases of the skin in eight groups :—

1. Inflammations.
2. Lesions of Secretion.
3. Hypertrophies.
4. Deteriorations.
5. Hemorrhages.
6. Lesions of Sensibility.
7. Foreign Bodies.
8. Diseases of the Appendages.

The first group contains four Orders : 1. Non-specific Eruptions, which may exist in an acute or chronic state ; 2. Non-specific Eruptions, existing always in a chronic state ; 3. Acute Specific Eruptions ; 4. Chronic Specific Eruptions.

The second group is divided into three Orders : 1. Lesions of the Follicular Secretion ; 2. Lesions of the Epidermic Secretion ; 3. Lesions of the Coloring Secretion.

The third group, which constitutes but a single Order, is defined to consist in an abnormal development of the parts affected.

The fourth group contains those diseases which have a tendency to destroy the parts attacked.

The fifth group is characterized by the presence of blood, more or less altered, without its proper vessels.

The sixth group is divided into two orders: 1. General or Local Hyperæsthesia; 2. Anæsthesia.

In the seventh group are placed those diseases which seem to depend on the presence of parasitical insects or animalcules.

The eighth consists of two orders: 1. Diseases of the Hair; 2. Diseases of the Nails.

Several other modern classifications may be briefly noted. The latest adopted by M. Hardy, of Paris, consists of eleven primary groups:—

    1. Deformities.
    2. Inflammatory affections.
    3. Artificial   "
    4. Parasitic   "
    5. Gangrenous
    6. Congestions.
    7. Hemorrhages.
    8. Fluxes.
    9. Neuroses.
    10. Febrile affections.
    11. Constitutional affections.[1]

The Primary groups of Professor Hebra's (of Vienna) arrangement are as follows:—

1. Hyperæmias.   7. Atrophies.
2. Anæmias.   8. Neoplasmata.
3. Anomalies of secretion.   9. Pseudoplasmata.
4. Exudative.   10. Ulceration.
5. Hemorrhages.   11. Parasitic.
6. Hypertrophies.   12. Neuroses.

The late Dr. A. B. Buchanan, of Glasgow, published in

---

[1] This is taken from his latest work, *Leçons sur la Scrofule et les Scrofulides, et sur la Syphilis et les Syphilides.* Paris: 1864. And it is a slight modification of the arrangements given in Part I. of his *Leçons sur les Maladies de la Peau.* Second Edition. 1860.

the *Edinburgh Medical Journal* for January, 1863,[1] an excellent natural classification, one of the best yet invented. Without entering into its minute details, it may be here given as follows:—

Class I.—Inflammations.
- 1. Erythematous.
- 2. Eczematous.
- 3. Phlegmonous.

Class II.—New formations:

A. Homologous.
- 1. Epidermic.
- 2. Pigmentary.
- 3. Dermic.

B. Heterologous.
- 1. Pseudoplasms.
- 2. Neoplasms.

Class III. Hemorrhages.
" IV. Diseases of accessory organs.
" V. Diseases defined by uniform causes:—
    - A. Parasitic Diseases.
    - B. Syphilitic Eruptions.
    - C. Febrile Eruptions.

Beside these there are several other good arrangements, to which even a passing reference cannot here be made. So extended, indeed, has the subject of cutaneous nosology become, and so numerous have been the proposed classifications, that it would require a volume in itself to do justice to the entire question.

In Dr. Tilbury Fox's treatise *On the Classification of Skin Diseases* the student or the critic will find ample information and a series of comparative tables illustrating the systems already noted, and some others.

These *natural* systems, among the most perfect that have yet been proposed, present, in some respects, great advantages over *artificial* classifications, yet, I think, for many reasons, are not to be preferred. Could we, for example, predicate that the various eruptive diseases, placed by Wilson[2] or Cazenave in the group of *inflam-*

---

[1] "The Theory and Classification of Diseases of the Skin." Also, "Synopsis of the Diseases of the Skin." Glasgow. 1863.
[2] It is Mr. Wilson's first or *physiological* classification, to which reference is here made.

mations, were invariably characterized by inflammatory action, we should receive an important aid, not alone in diagnosis, but in treatment. But such is not the case in the classification of either. Both place scaly diseases of the skin in the same natural group, though in a different subdivision, with the eruptive fevers; yet can any two classes of diseases be more different in their nature? The former characterized by a chronic inflammation of so low a form that it is very doubtful whether it should be designated as inflammation at all; while the latter are especially marked by high inflammatory action: the former, tedious and slow in their progress, often lasting for years; the latter, acute and rapid, running their course in a few days: the former requiring a prolonged constitutional treatment, and the latter demanding immediate and active remedies. Thus an erroneous impression, acquired from a supposed natural affinity between two eruptive diseases, may lead to error, both in diagnosis and treatment.

Another important objection to the employment of a *natural* system of classification in the study of diseases of the skin is, that, being more complicated, and not so easy of comprehension, it is more difficult to be borne in mind than an artificial arrangement, and thus great obstacles are, by its adoption, thrown in the way of the student at the very threshold of his inquiry. No *artificial* classification of diseases of the skin can possibly be perfect, for different persons will, of course, form different ideas of the external characteristics and features of individual eruptions: yet it is an arrangement which seems to be better adapted for attaining a knowledge of the subject; and this, after all, is the only important use of any system of classification. It is especially one more easy to be remembered. It is one which aids us considerably at the bedside, for it requires a less complex process of reasoning than a natural classification, to discover by its agency what may be the disease in any special case. It is, therefore, this which I purpose to adopt.

A *regional* classification of eruptive diseases, although it is not adapted for a general inquiry into affections of

4

the skin, possesses much value in their individual study, as they often present great differences in character and even in form, and frequently require peculiar modifications in treatment, dependent on the region on which they may occur. I have thus adopted it in a small work which I published a few years since on Eruptive Diseases of the Scalp, and also in an Essay on those which affect the face, which appeared in the eleventh volume of the New Series of the *Dublin Quarterly Journal of Medical Science*. Were I to propose a *regional* system of classification, I would suggest that cutaneous eruptions should be divided into three groups: 1. Those which occur on parts of the body constantly exposed to the air; 2. Those which appear on parts that are protected from the atmosphere by clothing; and, 3. Those which affect the hairy scalp. The first group should be subdivided into those which occur on the face (and neck in females), and on the hands; for as the latter, especially in several trades and occupations, are exposed to various matters which cause irritation, and as the skin there differs anatomically, in some respects, from that on the face, eruptive diseases which affect them often present different appearances, as they are seated on either. Vesicular eruptions, in especial, present a peculiar character when they occur upon parts of the body covered with hair—as, for example, on the scalp. If a blister be applied to the surface of the scalp, deprived of the hair, the blister, in common language, is said not to rise; the epidermis upon this part of the body being not only somewhat thicker than elsewhere, except on the soles of the feet and palms of the hands, but being bound down by the numerous involutions which constitute the hair follicles. When, therefore, a vesicular eruption occurs upon the scalp there is no apparent vesicle; and this, I believe, will account for that great difference of opinion which exists amongst writers as to the nomenclature of certain eruptive diseases of the scalp—I allude especially to the forms of Herpes.

The chief improvements which have been made on Willan's original classification are contained in the systems of Biett, of Cazenave, and Schedel, in their joint work,[1] in that of Dr. Tilbury Fox, in his recent learned treatise on skin diseases, and in that of Dr. Hughes Bennett, of Edinburgh. Dr. Bennett's modification of Biett's arrangement was first published in the *Edinburgh Monthly Journal of Medical Science* for April, 1850, and is, in many respects, deserving of commendation.—See his large-work on Clinical Medicine.

The great difficulty in devising an *artificial* system of classification of cutaneous diseases depends upon the changes which, in the progress of the disease, all eruptions undergo with respect to their characteristic form and appearance. These changes are often so great that it is sometimes almost impossible to diagnose to what order a special eruption may belong in its advanced stage, and it is therefore made to occupy a different place in different systems. For example, observers differ as to whether scabies, common itch, is a vesicular, a pustular, or a papular eruption. It certainly changes rapidly, in most cases, from vesicular to pustular, or the vesicles become mixed up with pustules; but, in my opinion, it is always, in its primary stage, a vesicular eruption. In most diseases of the skin, we are, however, by careful observation, able to discover the elementary form of the eruption in the early stage of the disease: and from experience we shall always be able to diagnose, even in its most extreme changes, what the primary form was. This, of course, can only be learned by prolonged practical experience.

In proceeding to describe the system of classification of diseases of the skin which I intend to adopt, I wish, *in limine*, to disclaim any pretensions to originality. My chief object is to endeavor to simplify a subject which has often not received from the student and practitioner the attention it merits, owing to the difficulties with which complicated arrangements and ever-changing nomenclature have invested it. I shall therefore take advantage of the labors of those who have preceded me and endeavor to reduce the grouping together of

[1] See also the English edition of it by Dr. Burgess.

cutaneous eruptions to as few subdivision as attention to accuracy will admit.

In the first edition of this work Dr. Neligan followed the example of Mr. Plumbe, Dr. Hughes Bennett, and M. Fabre (*Bibliothèque du Médecin Pratique*) in omitting any notice of the eruptive fevers, in which the skin affection plays so prominent a part; and also some constitutional affections which are specially characterized by a cutaneous eruption. The one class he excluded, because he considered, as we all do, eruptive fevers not to be skin diseases in a pathological sense. The other he excluded because the skin affection was secondary to the constitutional. That his reasons were weighty cannot be denied; but all things considered, and following the best home and foreign cutaneous nosologists of the present day, it has been thought best to remedy what many considered a defect in the first edition, by introducing short notices of the eruptive fevers *with special reference to their cutaneous eruptions*, referring the reader to authorities on general medicine for more full information; and also descriptions of those diseases, chiefly to be met with abroad, in which the eruption plays a secondary but a very important part. While thus including several diseases not treated of in the first edition, certain affections excluded by Dr. Neligan continue to be excluded: for example—ulcers, injuries caused by heat—as burns and scalds; and those caused by cold—as chilblains and frostbite. These are traumatic, and therefore should be considered as surgical affections.

I propose to divide cutaneous diseases into ten Groups or Orders, as follow:—

1. EXANTHEMATA.	6. HYPERTROPHIÆ.
2. VESICULÆ.	7. HÆMORRHAGIÆ.
3. PUSTULÆ.	8. MACULÆ.
4. PAPULÆ.	9. CANCROÏDES.
5. SQUAMÆ.	10. DERMATOPHYTÆ.

Adding two supplementary groups, SYPHILIDES and DISEASES OF THE APPENDAGES OF THE SKIN.

The diseases contained in the Order EXANTHEMATA

are characterized by the occurrence, on a greater or less extended surface of the skin, of a blush of inflammatory redness, usually more or less elevated, which mostly terminates in epidermic desquamation, in the form of fine mealy scales. The most essential character of the Order is, that, as a general rule, the redness momentarily disappears on pressure with the finger. In one form of eruption, classed amongst the exanthemata, namely, erysipelas, the epidermis is very commonly raised in large blebs by serous effusion; but this is evidently caused by the intensity of the inflammation which is present, takes place in the progress of the disease, and is not a constant or essential symptom. In general, the redness is in large uncircumscribed patches, or uninterruptedly diffused over the surface; but in some forms it occurs in well-defined regular spots. The essential nature of the exanthemata is, that they are inflammatory, and they seem to have their seat in the vascular rete of the derma. This Order to some extent corresponds with the second sub-group of the first group of the first secondary division of Wilson's Natural System, defined by him as "Inflammation of the derma, without constitutional symptoms of a specific kind." It contains seven genera: ERYTHEMA, ERYSIPELAS, URTICARIA, ROSEOLA, RUBEOLA, SCARLATINA, VARIOLA and its allies.

The VESICULÆ are characterized by an eruption of vesicles or blebs, which consist in an elevation of the epidermis, varying in size, in some forms minute (vesicles), and in some of tolerable magnitude (bullæ or blebs), containing a transparent, serous fluid, which, with the progress of the disease, becomes opaque, and dries into thin scales or hard crusts. The fluid by which the elevation of the epidermis is caused in the vesiculæ is at first transparent and albuminous, but after a short time becomes opaque, and often puriform. This order nearly corresponds with the second group of the first secondary division of Wilson, which he defines as "Effusive Inflammation of the Derma." It contains five genera: ECZEMA, HERPES, PEMPHIGUS, RUPIA, SCABIES. Wilson places scabies in a distinct sub-group, defining it to be "Inflammation of the derma, from the presence of acari."

4*

The third Order, PUSTULÆ, is characterized by the eruption of *Pustules*—rounded elevations of the epidermis containing pus, which, bursting, form scabs or thick crusts. The pustules may be of small size, and closely aggregated together, or large and isolated; the former constituting the *Psydracia*, the latter, the *Phlyzacia* of Willan; a psydracious pustule being defined by him to be "a minute pustule, irregularly circumscribed producing but a slight elevation of the cuticle, and terminating in a laminated scab," and a phlyzaceous one "of a larger size, raised on a hard, circular base of a vivid red color, and succeeded by a thick, hard, dark-colored scab." The epidermic covering of a pustule is much thicker than that of a vesicle, consequently it takes a longer time to maturate, or, in other words, to burst and form a scab or crust; but in their advanced stage the diagnosis between the two is sometimes not unattended with difficulty. The eruptions placed in this order correspond with those classed by Wilson in the third group of his first secondary division: "Suppurative Inflammation of the Derma." The genera are four in number: ACNE, IMPETIGO, ECTHYMA, and FURUNCULI. Wilson, however, puts acne in a group, the definition of which that he gives being, "Inflammation of the glands and adjacent textures."

The PAPULÆ are characterized by an eruption of minute, solid elevations—*pimples*, generally reddish, but sometimes of the natural color of the skin, containing neither serum nor pus, terminating in the desquamation of fine scales, and almost invariably attended with intolerable itching. In some forms, the top of the pimple is of a reddish-brown or black color, but this merely depends on the accidental presence of a small, dried crust of blood, usually effused by scratching. This Order contains two genera: LICHEN, PRURIGO. It corresponds with the fourth group of Wilson's first secondary division, which he defines: "Depositive inflammation of the derma."

The eruptive diseases contained in the Order SQUAMÆ are characterized by the secretion of dry, laminated, whitish scales on the cutaneous surface, usually occurring in patches, often of a circular form. The scales, which are somewhat elevated above the level of the skin, readily fall off, to be again rapidly renewed; the part which they cover is of a smooth, glistening aspect, reddish, and dry. The Order corresponds with the fifth group of the first secondary division of Wilson's classification: "Squamous inflammation of the derma." It contains two genera: PSORIASIS, PITYRIASIS.

In the Order HYPERTROPHIÆ I include those diseases which are characterized by an hypertrophied condition of the derma or epidermis, or of both, or of the hair follicles. The term has been used much in this sense by Simon, in his *Anatomical Description of Diseases of the Skin;* and from him I have adopted it. In its application it is nearly synonymous with the TUBERCULA of former artificial systems of classification. The latter term, although probably not so faulty, when first employed to designate a group of cutaneous diseases, is, I think, highly objectionable at present, when it is invariably understood to designate a peculiar morbid deposit, and its application in any other sense must tend to cause confusion. Wilson, in his Natural System, has a group in which are placed those affections that consist in an "hypertrophied state of the papillæ of the derma;" but I propose to extend the application of the term, and to include in the Order those diseases in which the hypertrophy affects the other cutaneous structures. I shall place in it nine genera: ICHTHYOSIS, MOLLUSCUM, STEARRHŒA, ELEPHANTIASIS, and its allies, VERRUCÆ, CLAVUS, CALLOSITATES, CONDYLOMATA, NÆVI.

The characteristics of the seventh Order, HÆMORRHAGIÆ, scarcely require to be defined. In it there is a morbid alteration of the capillary circulation, accompanied by a changed or diseased condition of the blood, in which this fluid, escaping from its proper vessels, is extravasated in rounded spots or patches beneath the epidermis, and also beneath the epithelium of the mucous and serous membranes. Bursting through the latter finer structure, more or less bleeding usually takes place from the surfaces of both these membranes. It contains but one genus, PURPURA.

The Order MACULÆ is characterized by an alteration in the color of the skin, occurring usually in large patches, and unattended with any eruption. The natural color may be deepened, diminished, or altered in hue, and the affection has its seat evidently in the apparatus of the skin which secretes the pigmentary matter. The Order corresponds with the fifth secondary division of Wilson: "Disorders of the Chromatogenous Function of the Derma." It contains two genera, VITILIGO, which includes *albinoismus*, and EPHELIS, which includes Morbus Addisonii.

The Order CANCROÏDES contains those diseases of the skin which in many of their features resemble cancerous affections. They are characterized by a degree of semi-malignancy, usually attended with foul ulceration of a slow and insidious nature, often with severe stinging pain, and a marked tendency to return after apparent cure, or after excision, in the same or in remote parts of the cutaneous surface. It contains two genera: LUPUS, KELOÏS.

The tenth Order, DERMATOPHYTÆ, I have adopted from Bennett. It includes those diseases of the skin which depend on, or are characterized by the presence of, parasitic plants. It contains two genera: PORRIGO, SYCOSIS.

Of the two supplementary Orders, the first—the SYPHILIDES—contains those eruptions of the skin which are ordinarily termed *secondary*, being caused by, or consequent on, the introduction of the venereal virus or poison into the system: and the second includes diseased conditions of the *hair* and *nails*.

This classification, in the drawing up of which I have had chiefly in view an attempt to simplify what is admittedly a difficult study, may be tabulated as follows:—

ORDER.	GENERA.
1. EXANTHEMATA, .	Erythema, Erysipelas, Urticaria, Roseola, Rubeola, Scarlatina, Variola and its allies.[1]
2. VESICULÆ, . .	Eczema, Herpes, Pemphigus, Rupia, Scabies.
3. PUSTULÆ, . . .	Acne, Impetigo, Ecthyma, Furunculi.
4. PAPULÆ, . . .	Lichen, Prurigo.
5. SQUAMÆ, . . .	Psoriasis, Pityriasis.
6. HYPERTROPHIÆ,	Ichthyosis, Molluscum, Stearrhœa, Elephantiasis and its allies, Verruca, Clavus, Callositates, Condylomata, Nævus.
7. HEMORRHAGIÆ, .	Purpura.
8. MACULÆ, . . .	Vitiligo, Ephelis.
9. CANCROÏDES, . .	Lupus, Keloïs.
10. DERMATOPHYTÆ, .	Porrigo, Sycosis.

Supplementary Groups:

SYPHILIDES.

DISEASES OF THE APPENDAGES OF THE SKIN.

[1] The following additions are now made to Dr. Neligan's Classification:—

1. EXANTHEMATA, . . .	Rubeola, Scarlatina, Variola, and its allies.
3. PUSTULÆ, . . .	Furunculi.
6. HYPERTROPHIÆ, . .	Elephantiasis—its allies.

CHAPTER II.

EXANTHEMATA.

The term "Exanthemata" (literally "eruptions,"from ἰξάνϑημα) was employed by the ancient writers on medicine to designate every variety of eruption of the skin; but in modern days, and more especially since the time of Willan, it has been restricted to denominate a peculiar group of cutaneous diseases—one so well defined by external appearances, that there is no difficulty in diagnosing any of its forms during all their stages. They are characterized by the sudden appearance, on a greater or less extended portion of the skin, of an inflammatory redness in variously shaped patches, which momentarily disappear on pressure, are usually attended with a slight elevation of the surface, and terminate in exfoliation of the epidermis. The diseases belonging to this Order are almost invariably accompanied by more or less inflammatory fever, and they thus constitute a *natural* group. In the treatment of them, however, we should be careful not to let this idea of inflammation being one of their marked characters, lead us to take too exclusive a view as to the remedial measures indicated; for the attendant inflammation may be either of a low asthenic form, as it frequently is, or it may assume a highly sthenic type.

The eruptive fevers, rubeola, scarlatina, variola and its allies, should be properly included in this order, as they are in the Exanthemata of Cullen.

The definition already given applies pretty closely, though not absolutely, to them all. They are quite as entitled to be considered skin diseases as erysipelas, for example; and it would be hard to show why they should be excluded, if other symptomatic diseases be admitted into a cutaneous nosology. In the nosology of Willan and Bateman rubeola and scarlatina are classed as *Exanthemata;* variola is classed among *Pustulæ,* and varicella, and vaccinia among *Vesiculæ.* As already observed, however, they constitute a natural group, and are here classed together.

These eruptive fevers are now commonly termed *Zymotic* diseases, from ζύμη, leaven, in accordance with the revived ancient doctrine which considers their origin due to fermented leaven acting as a poison or poisons on the blood. The revival of this ancient doctrine of the humoral pathology is but one of many instances in which the wisdom of the ancient observers is apparent. Mr. Wilson, who has elaborately treated of these diseases, is of opinion that their pathology consists in active congestion of the capillaries of the skin, and he believes rubeola, scarlatina, and variola to be successive stages, each of the other, and all due to the same poison. The identity of the poison in these diseases is, however, strongly disputed.

In a strict pathological sense these affections are fevers, not local diseases; and for a full account of them resort must be had to works on general medicine. The appearances on the skin will be chiefly noted in this chapter, but full references to books containing everything known on the subject will supply the want of matter outside the scope of this volume.

In Erysipelas, one of the diseases included amongst the Exanthemata, the epidermis is often elevated by serous effusion into bullæ or even large blisters, which has induced some writers to describe it as a vesicular eruption;[1] but these vesications are not a constant or necessary feature of erysipelas, and when they do occur are evidently dependent on the high degree of local inflammation which may be present.

The seven genera belonging to the order are: Erythema, Erysipelas, Urticaria, Roseola, Rubeola, Scarlatina, Variola and its allies.

---

[1] It is placed in Willan's order " Bullæ."

ERYTHEMA.

Erythema: ἐρύθημα, of Hippocrates (from ἐρυθαίνω, to redden; or from ἐρυθρός, red). Erysipelas, of Celsus and Galen; Phlogosis Erythema of Cullen; Dartre Erythemoide, Herpes Erythemoide of Alibert.—See Atlas, Plate I.

ERYTHEMA (*Inflammatory blush*) consists in an eruption of superficial, deep red stains or patches, more or less circumscribed, and slightly elevated, attended with heat and tingling, and terminating either in resolution, or with slight furfuraceous desquamation. It is non-contagious, of a mildly febrile character, and rarely a disease of much importance; most forms of it terminating in a few days, and seldom becoming chronic.

The erythematous eruption very frequently appears on the skin in the course of many acute affections, especially fevers and inflammatory diseases; often occurs in dropsies, when it affects the depending parts of the body or those exposed to pressure; may be produced by irritation of the cutaneous surface, as by the friction of the clothes or of the exposed surfaces of the skin, as when it appears in the axillæ or in the groins; and is likewise caused on the uncovered parts of the body by exposure to harsh winds, or to the sun in travelling. The eruption may appear on any part of the cutaneous surface, but some of its forms occur with great regularity in certain regions of the skin.

Several varieties of erythema have been noticed by dermatologists, particularly by Willan and Bateman, whose nomenclature is in the main adopted by all writers. Dr. Tilbury Fox, following Hardy, arranges them in three groups:—

1. Those purely local: Varieties—E. simplex; E. intertrigo.

2. Those accompanied by general symptoms simulating acute febrile diseases: Varieties—E. papulatum; E. tuberculatum; E. nodosum; E. fugax; E. scarlatinaforme: E. marginatum; E. circinatum.

3. Those secondary to or symptomatic of other diseases, *e. g.*, the exanthem of cholera; Erythema leve.

Hebra divides the forms of Erythema into *congestive* and *exudative;* including under the first head the idiopathic or local; and the constitutional or symptomatic; but all of them may, I think, be described under three heads :—

Erythema simplex.
"   papulatum.
"   nodosum.

Erythema simplex (Plate I, Fig. 1), under which I include the E. fugax, E. leve, E. intertrigo, E. marginatum, and E. circinatum of other writers, is generally a very mild form of eruption of the skin, requiring but little attention, unless when it assumes a chronic character —as intertrigo, when neglected, or when the causes by which it is produced are continued, not unfrequently does. It appears in the form of uncircumscribed red patches, seldom exceeding the size of the palm of the hand, and scarcely elevated above the surrounding skin; it generally occurs in the course of some inflammatory disease, when, owing to the patches suddenly disappearing, and again as suddenly reappearing on some other part of the body, it has been termed erythema *fugax;* it also assumes the same character as indicative of or connected with derangements of the digestive organs, or obstructed menstruation. The usual seat of this sub-variety is on the face, the neck, the trunk, or the under extremities; there is no constitutional disturbance marking its occurrence, and the only local symptom is a slight degree of heat in the part attacked. Thus, then, it would appear to be a very unimportant disease, were it not for a remark of Hippocrates, the truth of which has been confirmed by most modern observers, that the occurrence of erythema fugax in fevers or acute diseases is an unfavorable sign.

Mr. Erasmus Wilson observes, that this affection, by him termed E. fugax, is sometimes chiefly remarkable for a tendency to swell; and relates two cases in point. In one, the subject, a military officer, when on parade was occasionally seized with so sudden a swelling of the face that he had to be led to his quarters completely blinded.

5

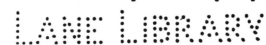

toms of which it usually disappears; and the latter seems to be a form which erythema simplex frequently assumes in the old.

Erythema papulatum (Plate I, Fig. 3) is of frequent occurrence, especially in young persons about the age of puberty, and in females in whom the menstrual functions may have been obstructed. It is said to be a common form of disease amongst the Turkish soldiers (*vide Hubsch. Gaz. Méd. d'Orient*, II, 11th February, 1859; and Schmidt's *Jahrb.* Vol. CI, p. 180—quoted by Dr. Tilbury Fox, *Skin Diseases*, p. 51). It appears most generally on the backs of the hands and fingers, but also occurs on the face, the neck, and other parts of the body. It is characterized by an erythematous blush on an uncircumscribed surface of skin, on which there are numerous small, round elevations, about the size of a pea, of a deeper red hue, the portions of the skin between the elevations being always of a paler or less bright color. The commencement of an attack of this variety is attended with some fever, headache, and slight nausea, and there are heat and a disagreeable sensation of tingling in the affected parts, which are also slightly sore to the touch. This form of the eruption is of no great importance, lasting usually for only a few days, and very rarely assuming a chronic character. Sometimes rather larger elevations are intermixed with the others, or they may all, from the commencement, assume the size of a nut or a large marble, when the variety has been named *tuberculatum;* it presents this character most frequently on the extremities; the raised spots are there harder to the touch, attended with more local annoyance, and the eruption more frequently becomes chronic.

Erythema nodosum (Plate I, Fig. 4) is so called from the appearance which the eruption presents. It usually occurs on the anterior aspect of the lower extremities, generally from the knee to the ankle. I have seen a few cases in which it was situated on the back of the arms, and I have occasionally seen a few spots on the anterior surface of the body. It appears in distinct rounded or oblong red patches, from half an inch to even two inches in diameter, with a well-defined border, circumscribed, and slightly elevated in the centre—but the elevation is more apparent to the eye than to the finger when passed over the part. The centres of the patches or *knots* are of a somewhat brighter color than the borders, which have a dark red blush; the general redness fades but slightly on pressure, which, however, causes pain, and on the pressure being removed the color immediately reappears. This form of erythema is most generally met with in young girls from the age of 14 to 19 or 20, rarely appearing in males. Dr. Tilbury Fox (*op. cit.*, p. 52) believes it to be sometimes associated with chorea and rheumatism; and Hardy states that it may become chronic in persons of a scrofulous habit, producing sores like syphilitic ones. It has been described by some as being connected with a deranged state of the menstrual functions, but in my experience I have rarely seen it produced by such a cause. It is attended with more fever than any of the other forms of erythema, being generally ushered in with nausea, sometimes even vomiting, pains in the back, loins, and head, together with loss of appetite and slight shivering. This state may continue for from twelve to twenty-four hours. The patient then feels a sensation of heat and tingling on the fronts of the legs, and on examination the characteristic eruption is seen. The *knots* or patches appear simultaneously over the surface, not coming out in succession, increase in size, and become harder and more painful for three or four days, then deepen in color until the eighth or tenth day, when they begin to fade, and passing often through the green and yellow stages of a bruise, disappear with slight desquamation of the epidermis in about a fortnight or three weeks from the commencement of the attack.

Under the title E. tuberculatum et œdematosum, Dr. Durkee has described a disease consisting of small tubercular elevations, vesicating at their apices, then flattening; the skin showing a shrivelled or collapsed condition of cuticle.—*Boston Med. and Surg. Journal*, 17th April, 1856, p. 189.

The seat of erythema is manifestly in the vascular structure of the derma, the nervous functions being but little affected; the causes by which it is produced have been already adverted to. An *epidemic* of erythema has been described as having occurred in Paris in 1828–29, as a complication of a painful affection of the extremities, thence termed Acrodynia, which raged there at that period. M. Cazenave, who witnessed it in the Hôpital St. Louis, describes its characters as consisting in "an erythematous circle of a crimson color appearing on the soles of the feet and on the palms of the hands, covering a space of from one-third to two-thirds of an inch, and disappearing under the pressure of the finger; it presented the peculiarity that the portion of the skin which surrounded it was generally of a yellowish color, swollen, and very hard, while the affected patch was manifestly depressed and very painful to the touch. These spots of erythema also appeared occasionally on the thighs, the scrotum, and in the axilla."

Dr. Tilbury Fox (*op. cit.*, p. 55) describes the following form of erythema not before remarked on, so far as I know, by any writer: "It occurs especially about the back and sides of the hands and fingers in those out of health. The skin becomes red, in little circular spots, from which the epidermis peels off by a centrifugal death, as it were, leaving behind a red dry surface marked by circular ridges of what appear to be normal papillæ. The places are many, the disease is chronic, and requires no treatment. It looks simply like the death of the epidermis, beneath which is seen the reddened derma marked by circular ridges of prominent papillæ. It is not erythema circinatum; it is more like a superficial acrodynia."

The *diagnosis* of any of the forms of erythema is in very few instances attended with much difficulty. It may be mistaken for the milder forms of erysipelas, especially in their early stage, but the blush of erythema is of a deeper red, and less livid than that of erysipelas, is not attended with the same amount of local tumefaction, burning heat, and pain, and is marked by much less disturbance of the system generally, and much less fever. That form of erythema simplex which has been named fugax has sometimes been mistaken for urticaria evanescens; they are both exanthematous eruptions; but in the latter the eruption disappears and reappears with constant rapidity, generally in the same places; while erythema fugax, though nearly equally evanescent, does not return to the same parts; it is, too, unattended with the acute itching and annoying tingling so characteristic of urticaria, and moreover occurs in the course of some disease of the general system, while urticaria evanescens is an idiopathic affection. Erythema papulatum has sometimes been mistaken for some of the eruptive fevers, as for measles or scarlatina; but its local character, its appearance upon the hands, and its papular elevation, serve to distinguish it from measles, in which the eruption is of a crescentic form, of a duller red color, and attended with a catarrhal fever. As regards scarlatina, the bright redness of the efflorescence and the acute inflammatory fever, together with the sore throat of that disease, should suffice to render the diagnosis easy. Intertrigo may be confounded with chronic eczema, occurring behind the ears, in the axillæ, or in the groins; the latter, however, is a vesicular eruption in its primary stage, and, as it advances, is marked by the copious serous discharge, tumefaction, and deep red fissures, which so remarkably characterize the disease.

The *prognosis* in any form of erythema is, of course, very favorable; all the varieties being of a slight character, lasting but for a short time, and the patient recovering without any detriment to the general health.

Treatment.—In the very common form of erythema simplex caused by exposure to the heat of the sun or harsh winds in travelling, nothing further is required than anointing the parts affected with some mild oleaginous application, such as cold cream or fresh olive oil: a common domestic remedy, but not so efficacious, is the cream of cow's milk. When the eruption occurs in the course of any acute disease, no local application should be used except the warm bath, if it is not otherwise contraindicated; and where it is symptomatic of any derangement of the digestive organs or of any other part or function of the general system, the constitutional, not the local, affection should be treated. In erythema leve the parts should be carefully protected from pressure, gently sponged with the dilute solution of subacetate of lead warmed, then well dried, dusted over with flour, and enveloped in raw cotton. When the disease appears inclined to spread, I have found lint wet with the lead-wash, and covered with oil silk, the best application.

Erythema intertrigo is sometimes very obstinate, especially in children, when it occurs behind the ears, as it very frequently does. As a preventive, and in the early stages, dusting the parts with very finely powdered lapis calaminaris is often useful; but when it becomes at all chronic, an ointment, consisting of two grains of the carbonate of lead, half an ounce of white wax ointment, and half a drachm of glycerine, is better adapted. With some very chronic cases, all greasy applications seem to aggravate the disease, when I have seen it rapidly get well from the use of a lotion containing three grains of the sulphate of copper in an ounce of elder-flower water, applied on lint, kept constantly wet with it. In adults, intertrigo of the groins is occasionally very troublesome and sometimes obstinate, especially when the irritation is kept up by walking; the cucumber ointment of the French pharmaceutists has proved more successful in my hands in these cases than any other application: in the commencement of the eruption it generally effects a cure in a few days, the affected parts having been each time previously cleansed with a moist towel, and then dried; it should be rather thickly smeared over them three times a day. If the cucumber ointment cannot be obtained, an ointment prepared by rubbing together two grains of acetate of zinc dissolved in a drachm of rose-water, and an ounce of cold cream, may be substituted for it. Juniper tar soap has also been used with the addendum of applying zinc ointment to the part after each application of the tarry preparation. Erythema papulatum is best treated in young persons by mild antiphlogistics, especially the saline cathartics, or emeto-cathartics. When the accompanying fever is at all well marked, and the disease occurs in robust constitutions, the use of a mixture containing two grains of tartar emetic and two ounces of sulphate of magnesia in a pint of water, of which a wineglassful is taken every second hour until vomiting or

When the erysipelatous inflammation extends to the subcutaneous tissues and deeper seated structures, the disease is denominated erysipelas *phlegmonodes.* This form appears more frequently on the extremities than on the head and trunk of the body. The constitutional symptoms by which it is ushered in, and which accompany it, are of a more severe character, and very frequently assume a typhoid type. As regards the local characteristics, the portion of the integuments affected presents a dull red or livid color, is intensely painful, hot, and tense, pits more deeply on pressure, and is more tumefied. The inflammation here very seldom terminates in resolution, suppuration usually occurring in the areolar tissue, with death and sloughing to a greater or less extent of this structure, occasionally ending in mortification of the part attacked.

Erysipelas spreads over the cutaneous surface often with great rapidity, yet assuming a regularly progressive course, the parts on which it first appeared being those, when the disease ends in resolution, which first desquamate. Thus it sometimes occurs that the eruption is fading from the face and the swelling disappearing there, while the disease is beginning to show itself on the side of the head or the neck. Erysipelas is in an occasional case seen to assume a singularly erratic course, fading rapidly from the part on which it appeared, and suddenly attacking another portion of the skin at some distance, not spreading to it by contiguity. This, as already noted, has been made a distinct variety by some writers under the name of erysipelas *erraticum.* Dr. Graves was the first to notice a singular fact as regards the mode of spreading of erysipelas, that when it commences at any point of the mesial line of the body it is very apt to spread in a symmetrical manner;[1] that is to say, corresponding portions of the integuments are simultaneously attacked on both sides.

In the course of erysipelas, the inflammation sometimes attacks **one** or more of the internal organs, as the

---

ne. **Second Edition,** Vol. ii, p. 327; or Reprint of 4), p. 690.

membranes of the brain, the larynx, and trachea, or the gastro-intestinal mucous membrane. By some this is considered to be a metastasis; and on this supposition it has been described as a distinct variety of the eruption under the name of erysipelas *metastaticum*; but in all the cases that I have seen in which any internal part of the body became thus affected, the local erysipelatous inflammation still remained unchanged, and therefore it could not be correctly termed metastatic.

Traumatic erysipelas has its origin in some local injury which may or may not have caused breach of the surface; it more usually, however, succeeds the former: when it spreads from an ulcerated surface it is also said to be traumatic. In its local characteristics it corresponds in most cases with the phlegmonous form of the disease, presenting, however, more effusion of the liquor sanguinis into the deep-seated tissues, in consequence, seemingly, of which vesications rarely appear on the surface. The inflammation is also more diffuse, spreading rapidly from the wound, and, unless checked by treatment, rarely becoming circumscribed. The parts affected, too, are more apt to become gangrenous, a not uncommon result in bad constitutions. The general symptoms of traumatic erysipelas most frequently assume a typhoid-type, and are attendant on, not antecedent to, the local inflammation. In some few rare cases of this form both the local and constitutional symptoms are very mild, and do not last for a longer period than a week or ten days; in general, however, their duration is prolonged to from a fortnight to three weeks, if death does not take place at an earlier date.

In idiopathic erysipelas death most usually occurs from the result of inflammation attacking some internal organ; but patients occasionally sink under this disease with the ordinary fatal symptoms of asthenic or typhus fever. The traumatic form often terminates in gangrene, or, the veins becoming inflamed, purulent deposits take place in the lungs or liver, and the individual dies of phlebitic pneumonia or hepatitis.

Erysipelas may occur at any age, even in new-born children, in whom it attacks the umbilical region, from whence spreading rapidly, it almost invariably proves fatal. General experience seems to prove that it is more frequent in females than in males, and in adult life than in the very young or the aged.

The *causes* of erysipelas are at times very obscure, yet in many cases its origin can be distinctly ascribed either to some local action, as in the traumatic form or when it is produced by some direct irritant, or to some general constitutional disturbance; indeed, the latter may be said to be always requisite as a predisposing cause. Thus it is often seen to arise from the same causes as those which under other circumstances produce fever: it follows exposure to cold or wet, especially when the persons so exposed are deprived of their usual food or stimulants; I saw several cases of erysipelas of the face and head occurring in car-drivers and others, who, from their occupation, were much exposed to the weather, at the time when the total abstinence movement first occurred in Ireland, and in whom the disease was evidently traceable to the want of the stimulants which they had been previously in the habit of using freely. On the other hand, it must be observed that "good livers" are more liable to bad attacks of it than those who are "temperate in all things."

· A very fatal form of erysipelas is caused by the introduction of an animal poison into the system, as by the inoculation of morbid matter arising from wounds received during dissection, from persons laboring under phlebitis, &c. Erysipelas may be produced by a sudden violent mental emotion, as a fit of passion—such cases are on record—in which the local determination of blood probably aids in the production of this disease. In young children vaccinating is sometimes the exciting cause of erysipelas, when it usually presents an œdematous character. I witnessed a case lately which thus arose, and in which the inflammation spread from the vaccine pustule on the left arm to the fingers, thence proceeded up along the fingers of the opposite arm, and stopped when it reached the same height on this arm that it originated from on the other: the child recovered.

As to whether erysipelas is contagious or not a singular difference of opinion has always existed, and still

6

exists, between the practitioners of the French and
English school; the former laying it down as one of the
characteristic definitions of the disease that it is *non-
contagious*, and the latter with almost universal consent
asserting that it is *markedly contagious*. The simultaneous occurrence of the disease amongst a number of
persons is attempted to be explained away by the French
writers on the principle that such p s ns were predisposed to it, or that an epidemic influence, or a peculiar
atmospheric condition reigned at the time. It is
unquestionable that at certain seasons or during certain
years the contagiousness of erysipelas is more manifested
than at other times, but this is equally true of all other
contagious diseases. The direct proofs now accumulated
are too numerous and too certain, I think, for the question to be any longer one of doubt, and no British
surgeon would, I feel confident, undertake an operation
in an hospital in which erysipelas was present. The
form of erysipelas arising from an animal poison is
decidedly the most contagious; the medical attendants
and nurses are in such cases generally infected, and they
convey the disease even to others. It has been often
remarked that when puerperal fever—which is manifestly
due to the presence of a morbid poison in the system—
prevails, wounds are very apt to take on erysipelatous
inflammation, and the disease spreads rapidly by contagion; and likewise when erysipelas occurs epidemically,
that puerperal fever is apt to arise. The truth of these
observations has been several times confirmed in the
Rotunda Lying-in Hospital and large surgical hospitals
of this city.

Persons who have had an attack of erysipelas are very
liable to be again affected with it, a distinguishing
feature between it and the eruptive fevers.

The *diagnosis* of erysipelas is rarely attended with any
difficulty. From erythema, which, however, some dermatologists regard as merely a mild form of erysipelas,
it is distinguished by the attendant constitutional
symptoms, the smoothness of the tumefied surface, the
greater degree of swelling, and the burning pain and
tension. It differs from the eruptive fevers in the

uniform redness which the inflamed surface exhibits; from phlebitis, in the absence of the cord-like feeling which the inflamed veins present, and in the inflammation not spreading in lines over the track of the large vessels; and from synovitis in the inflammation not being confined to, or taking its origin from, the integuments covering the synovial membranes; but in many cases synovitis terminates in true erysipelas.

The *prognosis* in idiopathic erysipelas is in general favorable, unless when the disease occurs in the very old, in broken-down habits of body, or in extreme infancy. The chief indications of danger are, the attendant fever assuming a low typhoid type, or some internal organ becoming affected. When the erysipelatous inflammation attacks the larynx and glottis, which may always be apprehended when it is seated on the integuments covering these parts, it usually proves rapidly fatal, owing to the tumefaction which ensues, closing up the respiratory tube. Erysipelas of the phlegmonous character is always more dangerous than when the inflammation is superficial; and in the traumatic form, unless the local symptoms are very mild, the prognosis is always grave.

With reference to the *pathology* of erysipelas, it is evidently an acute inflammation of all the structures of the skin, the vascular rete being chiefly affected. M. Blandin has propounded the theory that the seat of the inflammation is in the capillary lymphatics, and MM. Cruveilhier and Ribes that it is situated in the capillary veins of the integuments.

The *treatment* of idiopathic erysipelas may be conveniently considered under two heads—the constitutional and the local. As regards the former, many different views have been propounded, the supposed indications depending on the idea formed as to the essential nature of the disease. Thus those who believe it to depend on some deranged condition of the hepatic secretion—the prevalent opinion among them being that it is caused by a deficient secretion of bile and a consequent accumulation of it in the system—treat all forms of erysipelas, no matter what may be the age or condition of the patient, by the administration of remedies calculated to promote a copious evacuation of that fluid by the alimentary canal. Others, regarding it as a highly inflammatory disease, employ depletion, and other active antiphlogistics; but this plan of treatment, although it may succeed in the robust dwellers in country districts [? ED.], is not at all suited for the inhabitants of towns or large cities. With some, the affection being viewed as one of asthenia, being attended with or dependent on diminished vital power, the use of tonics or stimulants is relied upon; while again, others, finding that the urine is highly acid in the early stages of the disease, as it is in all febrile affections, recommend an alkaline treatment.

Seeing that these so opposite plans of treating erysipelas are reported by those who have proposed or adopted them as being attended with almost invariable success, we are forced to the conclusion that in the ordinary run of cases constitutional treatment is of little importance. Unquestionably cases occur in which there are extreme inflammatory action and high fever, apparently demanding the use of bleeding and antiphlogistics; and others in which the vital power is so low and the accompanying fever assumes from the onset so marked a typhoid type, that the most powerful tonics, stimulants, and nutrients are clearly indicated. My own experience, which, however, it is right to say, has been chiefly acquired in this large and crowded city, is decidedly in favor of the tonic and stimulant plan of treatment. I ordinarily rely on the use of bark, which I give from the very commencement of the disease—in the very old or debilitated combining it with tincture of serpentaria, as in the following form :—

R. Tincturæ Cinchonæ Flavæ,   drachmas quatuor.
   Tincturæ Serpentariæ, . .   drachmas tres.
   Tincturæ Croci, ... drachmam.
   Decocti Cinchonæ Flavæ, .   uncias undecim. Misce.
           Sumat unciam horis sextis.

at the same time giving wine and nourishing diet according to the circumstances of each case.

Treatment by bark has been recommended by Dr

Fordyce, Dr. Wells, and Dr. Heberden. Dr. Jackson, an American physician, has used it in large doses, and Dr. Todd has given it in comparatively small doses. It is not a favorite remedy with Dr. Watson, nor does the Editor recommend its use in these cases. Without going the length to which Dr. Todd advanced, he fully adheres, from experience, to the main principle of the supporting plan advocated by that eminent authority.—See *Clinical Lectures*, Beale's edit., p. 167. This consists in the precise and regular administration of beef-tea, and, *if necessary*, of some alcoholic stimulant in moderate doses. His views on this subject were fully stated in a paper in *The Dublin Quarterly Journal of Medical Science*,[1] and from an earnest conviction of its worth he can endorse the view of Dr. Todd, who said of the supporting plan in the treatment of erysipelas: "It is the best adapted to save life, and check the progress of the disease; and . . under it, if begun early and with decision, you will seldom have to deal with the secondary phenomena of the malady."

The preparations of iron are by many preferred to those of bark in the treatment of this disease; their mode of action would appear to be similar: the tincture of the sesquichloride, in the dose of from twenty to twenty-five drops every second or third hour, has been especially recommended by Dr. and Mr. Bell, of Edinburgh;[2] and Dr. George W. Balfour, of Cramond, after using it much in the same way in twenty cases,[3] believes that we now have "a certain and unfailing remedy, whether the erysipelas be infantile or adult, idiopathic or traumatic."[3] It must, however, be remembered that the tincture of the perchloride of iron which in the *British Pharmacopœia* represents the tincture of the sesquichloride of the last *Dublin Pharmacopœia*, is only one*fourth* of the strength of the latter.

I consider the use of purgatives in the early stages of erysipelas as decidedly objectionable: they tend to in-

[1] "Notes on the Treatment of Continued Fevers and other Acute Diseases."—*D. Q. J. Med. Sci.*, Vol. **xxxv.** p. 200.
[2] *Monthly Journal of Medical Science*, June, 1851.
[3] *Monthly Journal of Medical Science*, May, 1853, p. 428.

crease the debility, usually so important a characteristic feature of danger, and determining to the mucous membrane of the alimentary canal and to the abdominal viscera, their action prevents the full development of the eruption on the cutaneous surface—a circumstance to be especially avoided in the treatment of all inflammatory diseases of the skin—and thus gives rise to local congestions and transference of the inflammation to some internal organ.

The use of biliary evacuants has been very strongly supported in an excellent practical essay published by Dr. Albert Walsh;[1] the remedy he recommends being tartar emetic, in rather minute doses—one grain dissolved in a quart of some emollient drink, as whey or barley-water, in the twenty-four hours; he continues its use until the eruption begins to fade, when he administers sulphate of quinia and other tonics.

Mr. Lawrence is the chief advocate in the present day for bloodletting and active antiphlogistics; but in his views, as regards the constitutional treatment of the disease, he has very few followers. Dr. Watson, who may be regarded as the most able and moderate exponent of the antiphlogistic school of our day, only advises bloodletting under exceptional circumstances, and then in "the smallest available quantity."—*Lectures*, Vol. II, p. 919, 4th edit.

If any internal organ be attacked during erysipelas, the most active derivatives to the surface should be employed. Thus, when the membranes of the brain are engaged, sinapisms and blisters should be applied to the legs, and warm stupes to the head; active purgatives also are now indicated, and of these the most valuable is the turpentine enema. When the inflammation seizes on the larynx, leeches, even although great debility be present, should be applied beneath the angles of the jaws, and hot stuping to the throat, with relays of sponges assiduously employed; a blister to the nape of the neck is also here a valuable remedy. The operation of tracheotomy

[1] *Dublin Quarterly Journal of Medical Science*, New Series, August, 1850.

is not applicable in such cases, for the erysipelatous inflammation spreads rapidly downwards through the respiratory tubes, causing copious effusion into their submucous areolar tissue.

When erysipelas affects the scalp, the hair should be immediately cut as close as possible, with the view of keeping the surface cool, and of permitting local remedies to be more easily applied. The local remedy which the Editor has always found most useful and very comfortable to the patient is constant fomentation with flannels first saturated with, and then wrung out of, a hot decoction of poppy heads and chamomiles, or of poppy heads only. Dr. Watson speaks very highly of the latter use, and urges a point respecting it which is frequently overlooked—the necessity for its continuous application, so long as it is soothing to the patient.

In the milder forms of idiopathic erysipelas, the best and only local treatment requisite consists in dusting the inflamed parts freely with wheaten flour or finely powdered starch, which may be conveniently applied from an ordinary dredging-box; the dredging should be repeated several times in the twenty-four hours. It allays the burning pain and irritation, and always proves highly grateful to the patient; therapeutically it appears to act by protecting the surface from the air, and by drying up the discharge as fast as it exudes from any vesications which may have formed. When the vesications are numerous, and the discharge excessive, I have found the addition of a drachm of oxide of zinc and twenty grains of finely powdered carbonate of lead to half a pound of starch, of much advantage. In using this combination the mixed powders should be well shaken each time before the parts are dusted with them, as, in consequence of their specific gravity, the zinc and lead soon sink to the bottom of the vessel in which they are kept. The Editor recommends the daily application of mucilage of starch. Each morning the parts should be sponged with tepid water, and the mucilage applied afresh. He has found this the best local application of many others, and has fully described the results of its use.—See *Dub. Hosp. Gaz.,* Vol. III, 2d Series, p. 72; *Ranking's Abstract, &c.,*

Vol. XXXVII, p. 131; *Dub. Qu. Journ.*, Vol. XXXV, p. 204; and *Med. Times and Gaz.*, Vol. I, 1863, p. 526.

Anointing the inflamed surface with melted lard is by some preferred to the use of dusting powders. Mr. Wilson speaks highly of his experience of it, having first, he says, employed it on the recommendation of Mr. Grantham, whose method is, "to relax the skin with hot water or steam fomentations, and after each fomentation to saturate the inflamed surface with hot lard, which is afterwards covered with wool."

When erysipelas is spreading rapidly, although superficially, over the cutaneous surface, the inflammation still persisting in the parts where it first appeared, inunction with mercurial ointment has in my experience more effect than any other local application in checking its progress. The ordinary mercurial ointment, to every ounce of which a drachm of glycerine has been added, should be smeared thickly over the inflamed surface, and on the sound skin for a considerable distance beyond; it need be applied only twice in the twenty-four hours, and if any symptoms of salivation be produced, its employment should be at once stopped.

Acting as an impermeable varnish, and probably producing some effect also by the compression it causes, collodion has been successfully employed by Spengler and Rapp as a local application in erysipelas; the parts are thickly coated with it by means of a camel-hair pencil, and it is renewed, as often as may be required in consequence of its cracking and peeling off when dry. When the disease affects one of the extremities, bandaging the limb has been used with very favorable results: this practice originated with the Continental School; its action seems to depend chiefly on the equable compression exercised on the congested capillaries and cutaneous veins, whereby they are emptied of the excess of blood contained in them; but some of the good effect produced is also probably due to the protection from the action of the air thereby given.

M. Guernsaut applies once daily, for three days, a preparation composed of 30 parts of collodion to 2 parts of castor oil. The proposal to mix these substances originated with M. Robert Latour.—*Med. Times and Gaz.*, 27th Nov., 1852, p. 549. M. Aran also applies collodion, but in a ferruginous form, described as made of equal parts of collodion and of ethereal ticture of perchloride of iron.—*Brit. and For. Med.-Chir. Rev.*, July, 1853, p. 277. Mr. Hugh Norris looks on the application of tincture of iodine as a specific; its use was first urged by Dr. Davies, of Hartford.—*Med. Times and Gaz.*, 11th December, 1852, p. 590.

Dr. Goolden, of St. Thomas's Hospital, advises wrapping the parts in a thick sheet of cotton wool, and then smearing with a thick coat of white paint (*Med. Times and Gazette*, 12th November, 1853, p. 502); and Dr. G. Hamilton, of Falkirk, applies a solution of gutta percha in naphtha, and over this he puts thin gutta percha tissue.[1]—ED. *Med. Jour.*, Dec. 1857, p. 512.

Dr. Livezay, an American physician, recommends the application of muslin saturated with strong tincture of lobelia.—*Med. Times and Gaz.*, 14th March, 1857, p. 269.

Phlegmonous and traumatic erysipelas demand more active local medication than when the inflammation affects the superficial layers of the integuments merely. In these forms of the disease many rely on topical depletion by leeches, by punctures, or by deep incisions. While leeches may produce a good effect by withdrawing blood from the inflamed superficial vessels, the determination caused to parts on which their suction power is exerted is to a certain extent productive of mischief. The same objection does not hold with regard to punctures; their employment has been highly advocated, amongst others, by Sir Richard Dobson, by Liston, and by Wilson; they should be made with a lancet, all over the inflamed part, at distances of from a quarter of an inch to an inch, according to the extent of the surface engaged, and penetrate to the depth of a quarter of an inch. As soon as they have nearly ceased to bleed, a warm bran poultice may be applied. Mr. Copland Hutchinson strongly recommended free incisions, and his practice has been

---

[1] See remarks on Dr. Graves's solution of gutta percha in chloroform, in Chap. XIV. of this work.

adopted by Lawrence, Guthrie, and others;[1] they should be made down to the subcutaneous fascia, and be several inches in length. When there is much deep-seated effusion of the liquor sanguinis, as is so frequently the case in traumatic erysipelas, they are decidedly productive of the best effect, and they should never be omitted when matter has formed.

Nitrate of silver is used in the treatment of erysipelas with two intentions—to check the spread of the inflammation superficially, and to promote resolution in the parts which have been attacked. With the former view a broad line or *cordon* is made on the sound skin, at a short distance from the margin of the inflamed surface, by the application of a solid stick of the nitrate on the part, previously wet with pure water; when the disease is situated on one of the extremities, this line is made to surround the limb completely. Mr. Higginbottom, who amongst English surgeons is the chief advocate for the use of this agent, at first recommended the employment of the solid nitrate to the inflamed surface; but in his observations recently published, and which contain the results of his accumulated experience, he states that he prefers a solution containing a scruple of the salt to a drachm of distilled water. He gives the following direction for its application: "The affected part should be washed well with soap and water, then with water alone, to remove every particle of soap, as the soap would decompose the nitrate of silver, then to be wiped dry with a soft cloth. The *concentrated* solution of the nitrate of silver is then to be applied two or three times on the whole of the inflamed surface, and *beyond it* on the surrounding healthy skin, to the extent of two or three inches."[2] In twelve hours, should the erysipelatous inflammation be unaffected, it is to be again applied; when vesications exist, they should be opened previously to the application. I prefer to use the nitrate of silver in the form of ointment, a drachm to the ounce of lard; it thus comes more completely into

[1] See *Med. Chir. Trans.*, Vol. xiv.
[2] *On the Use of the Nitrate of Silver*, Third Edition, 1865, p. 33.

contact with the inflamed surface, does not dry up so rapidly, and is more easy of application to some parts of the body, as to the scalp.

Sulphate of iron, both in solution and in ointment, has been recommended as a most valuable local application in erysipelas by Velpeau,[1] but I have not seen it prove so useful as nitrate of silver; the solution which he uses contains one part of the salt dissolved in fifteen parts of water, and the ointment consists of one part of the sulphate to three or four of lard. M. Debout (see *Braithwaite's Retrospect*, Vol. XXXI, p. 275) uses from 10 to 20 or 40 parts of sulphate of iron dissolved in 120 to 110 or 90 parts of water, or in 70 parts of glycerine.

Blisters are sometimes employed with success to prevent the spread of erysipelatous inflammation; they are applied at the margin of the affected surface: their effect appears to depend on a new action being excited in the parts, and their use seems to prove especially of service in the erratic form of the disease. The only other local remedies requiring notice are, creasote, which, painted over the surface, has recently proved successful in the hands of some practitioners; and congelation of the surface by means of pounded ice and salt mixed in a bladder, which has been proposed by Dr. Arnott: from the use of the latter it may be apprehended that some internal organ might be attacked. Dr. Delarue (*Med. Times and Gazette*, 4th April, 1857, p. 344) looks upon creasote as a *specific*, and uses this formula: "Creasote, 8 parts; lard, 30 parts; apply every two hours." With reference to Dr. Arnott's proposition the reader may consult, with advantage, Esmarch *On the Uses of Cold in Surgical Practice*. It forms one of the "selected monographs," edited, in 1861, by the New Sydenham Society, and it has been reviewed at length in the *Dublin Quarterly Journal* for Nov. 1862.

Should erysipelas assume a gangrenous tendency, in addition to the internal administration of the most powerful tonics, as wine, bark, and quinia, the parts

---

[1] See *Med. Times and Gaz.*, Vol. i, 1855, pp. 239, 289, and *Braithwaite*, Vol. xxxi, p. 275.

ought to be enveloped with a charcoal poultice, and afterwards dressed with lint soaked in a lotion containing from one to two ounces of the solution of chlorinated soda or chlorinated lime to the pint of distilled water.

URTICARIA (from Urtica).—See Plate II.

URTICARIA (*Nettle Rash*) may be defined to consist in an eruption of irregularly-shaped prominent patches, or wheal-like elevations of the skin, of a yellowish-white or reddish-yellow color, which are surrounded by a diffuse redness, are often evanescent, and are attended with a burning sensation, tingling, and extreme itching. It is non-contagious, and is usually accompanied by a greater or less degree of fever; and it may be either acute or chronic, in the former case lasting for a few weeks, in the latter for months or even years. The name of this disease is derived from the resemblance which the eruption bears, both in appearance and symptoms, to that occasioned by the sting of the common nettle—*Urtica urens.* Willan describes several varieties of urticaria, and numerous subdivisions of it have also been made by other dermatologists; but I think they may all be conveniently classed under three heads:—

Urticaria febrilis.
"   evanida.
"   tuberosa.

An attack of *Urticaria febrilis* (Plate II, Fig. 1) is ushered in with the ordinary symptoms of mild fever—shivering, headache, hot skin, thirst, loss of appetite, pains in the limbs, and in many cases vomiting. In from twelve to twenty-four hours the cutaneous surface becomes covered with numerous patches of the characteristic eruption, the parts on which it appears having been for a short time previously the seat of a burning sensation, attended with tingling and itching. The wheal-like elevations generally appear simultaneously on various portions of the body—on the face, the neck, over the back, and on the anterior aspect of the arms and legs; they often disappear suddenly, and as suddenly reappear on some other part of the skin. They bear much resemblance to the sting of a nettle, being slightly elevated, of a bright red color, with raised yellowish spots or lines; in most cases the itching which attends them is very intense, and accompanied by a burning sensation, and additional patches are produced on the apparently unaffected surface by the patient rubbing or scratching the part. The eruption runs its course generally in from six to eight hours, but to be succeeded by a fresh crop on the same or on different parts of the body—in most cases appearing in the evening—and the outbreak of which is attended, as before, with tingling and itching. Febrile urticaria is thus prolonged for a week or ten days, the eruption being less extensive and the constitutional symptoms less marked with each successive crop; the general febrile symptoms subside to a certain extent when the rash comes fully out, but are usually again somewhat aggravated each time the eruption disappears. The epidermis of the parts which have been affected desquamates in fine mealy scales after the disease has subsided, but no stain or mark is left behind.

When the eruption does not recede and again reappear, as now described, but remains permanently on the surface on which it first presents itself, it assumes somewhat of a more chronic character, lasting for three or four weeks, and is termed urticaria *perstans*. This subvariety is attended with milder constitutional symptoms, and with less local irritation and itching. In the variety named *conferta* (Plate II, Fig. 2), the local and general symptoms are precisely similar to those of urticaria febrilis, but in general more severe; the patches of eruption are numerous, and, coalescing, cover a much more extensive surface of the skin. (A form of urticaria has been described under the appellation of *intermittens*, in which the appearance of successive crops of the eruption assumes a regular intermittent type, usually quotidian, sometimes, however, more prolonged, being tertian or quartan, or the rash may not reappear until the end of every seventh, eighth, or ninth day—coming out in the evening, attaining its greatest intensity during the night, and disappearing almost entirely before morning. Willan mentioned

7

as a variety of this disease, under the name *subcutanea*, what was manifestly chiefly a nervous irritation, there being constant and violent itching of the cutaneous surface, commencing on some spot of one of the extremities, thence extending to the entire limb, to the trunk, and finally over the whole body, with only an occasional eruption of urticaria at distant intervals.

Urticaria evanida (Plate II, Fig. 3) is a chronic form of the disease, which not unfrequently lasts for years : and, although unattended with fever, renders the life of the person who suffers from it almost intolerable, from the unceasingly painful itching by which it is characterized. The eruption appears in small, rounded, reddish-yellow elevations—often two, three, or more such, closely set together, forming a wheal like that caused by the lash of a whip—with little, if any, surrounding redness of the skin; they may appear on any part of the body, but are usually developed by scratching, or by friction of the clothes; in females they are most frequently seated around the neck, where the upper part of the dress rubs the surface, and on the arms, where they are likewise caused by the friction of the sleeves of the dress. The rash generally begins to appear before evening, and is fully developed during the night, fading away before morning. The itching it occasions is most intense, causing absolute suffering, and persons even of the utmost fortitude cannot refrain from scratching violently the parts affected, by which an additional eruption is caused. The wheals do not remain longer on the surface than five or six hours, but they are renewed by the least local irritation, and the disease thus continues for months with occasional intermissions, being always most severe during the summer and autumn. After it has lasted for some time the general health becomes more or less affected, both from the constant irritation it occasions and the derangement of the natural functions of the skin.

Urticaria tuberosa (Plate II, Fig. 4), which is a very rare variety of the eruption, occurs in the form of distinct rounded elevations, about the size of a small walnut, hard and firm, extending evidently into the subcutaneous areolar tissue, of a livid red color, with a yellowish raised centre. The portion of the integuments affected is stiff, tense, and painful to the touch, or on motion. The tumors generally appear on the extremities, coming out during the night, with pain, much itching, and some fever, and nearly disappearing before morning, leaving the patient weak, tired, and sick. It is essentially chronic in its course, and very obstinate in its duration, sometimes extending to two or three years, or even longer, with short intervals of remission.

Urticaria is of more frequent occurrence in females than in males, which may be accounted for by its seldom attacking any but those whose skin is fine and delicate; for the same reason, while it appears not uncommonly in infants and children, it is not a disease of advanced life. The *causes* by which the febrile form is produced are, in most cases, well marked, but those on which urticaria evanida and urticaria tuberosa depend are not so manifest. A marked connection exists between the appearance of this eruption on the cutaneous surface and derangements of the digestive organs, or rather the irritation caused in some persons by certain indigestible articles of food. Shell-fish, especially mussels, oysters, crabs, cockles, periwinkles, and shrimps, have been long noted as producing urticaria in many individuals, the eruption appearing in a few hours after any of them may have been eaten. Similarly it has been seen to arise after the ingestion of pork, veal, or goose, of salted, spiced, or dried meats or fish, of cheese, of honey, of many fruits and vegetables, particularly gooseberries, cucumbers, melons, mushrooms, pickles, &c. I know two persons in both of whom urticaria appears in half an hour after they have eaten almonds or nuts, if the brown skins had not been previously removed. In all these cases the occurrence of the eruption must be due to some individual idiosyncrasy, with the nature of which we are unacquainted. The use of certain medicines, especially of copaiba or valerian, sometimes gives rise to this disease; in one instance which I witnessed, copaiba was given to a woman who was at the time suckling her infant, and urticaria appeared both on herself and on her child. Frank mentions his having seen it occur from drinking Seltzer water. In the case of a boy, aged 15, who was admitted into Jervis Street Hospital in the month of December, 1851, for acute pleuritis, a copious eruption of urticaria appeared over the face, the upper extremities, and the trunk, on the third day after his admission; the feverish symptoms had commenced to subside, and his system had been brought under the influence of mercury the day previously.

Urticaria has been often noticed as occurring in connection with other febrile diseases, especially with rheumatism; and Dr. Graves has pointed out the connection which exists between rheumatism, deranged conditions of the liver, and this eruption.[1] In children it frequently appears at the periods of dentition, being evidently associated with the gastric irritation which then occurs. Many have described some of the forms of this disease as being caused in the female sex by deranged states of the menstrual function; but my experience is quite opposed to this view.

Urticaria occasionally appears as a complication of other cutaneous eruptions, more particularly eczema, impetigo, prurigo, and lichen; and Mr. Balmanno Squire believes that acute cases are sometimes occasioned solely by the presence of the Acarus Scabiei in the epidermis.

The *diagnosis* of urticaria cannot be attended with any difficulty, its local characteristics are so well marked. From erythema it is well distinguished by the absence of the diffuse redness of the cutaneous surface, and by the intense itching which accompanies it. Erythema nodosum might be mistaken for urticaria tuberosa, but the evanescent character of the latter, even in its most chronic form, suffices to diagnose it; the former also is marked by the presence of acute febrile symptoms. Roseola, the only other of the exanthemata which might be confounded with febrile urticaria, is not attended with the intense itching of this disease, and also differs considerably in the color and appearance of the eruption. One of the varieties of lichen has been termed urticatus, in

---

[1] *Clinical Medicine*, Second Edition, Vol. I, p. 446, and Reprint of Second Edition, 1864, p. 339.

consequence of the troublesome stinging by which it is accompanied, owing to which symptom it has been occasionally mistaken for and described as a form of urticaria, but it is a distinctly papular eruption.

The *prognosis* in any of the forms of urticaria must be favorable, as may be understood from what has been already said. A few fatal cases of the disease, it is true, have been recorded by some of the older writers, but that they were instances of this eruption uncomplicated with an internal organic affection may well be doubted. We have, however, the testimony of Willan that a case fell under his observation in which death occurred from the *sudden* retrocession of the eruption about the fifth day; but the patient was a very intemperate man, and had suffered from great pain in the stomach, and nausea, which were much relieved when the cutaneous eruption came out, and delirium and high fever followed its sudden disappearance.

The seat of urticaria is in the superficial layers of the derma and the epidermis; as regards its *pathology*, it seems to be chiefly an affection of the nerves of the skin. Dr. Gull supposes the wheals to be caused by a contraction of the muscular tissues of the skin; and he grounds this idea on the fact that if two scratches be made side by side the wheals produced by them approximate, while "by stretching the skin the wheal could be obliterated apparently by overcoming the contraction of the muscular tissue."— See *Guy's Hosp. Rep.*, V, p. 88 (1859). From an analysis of the urine by Dr. Douglas Maclagan, of Edinburgh, he came to the conclusion that urticaria is intimately connected with a deficiency of the organic salts of the urine—urea and uric acid—and their probable retention in the system; and the correctness of this opinion is favored by the connection, already adverted to, which exists between this disease and rheumatism.

Treatment.—The febrile form of urticaria requires the employment of antiphlogistic purgatives, and diaphoretics, or, should the fever run very high in full habits, local or general bleeding [? ED.] may even be requisite. The best purgative is the sulphate of magnesia, given in the acid infusion of roses, with an excess of acid; thus

an ounce of the salt may be dissolved in twelve fluid
ounces of the acid infusion, and to it two fluidrachms of
dilute sulphuric acid should be added; of this the dose
is a sixth part every third hour until the bowels are
freely moved: the purgatives should be repeated every
second day as long as the feverish symptoms have not
subsided. Nitre whey, given at bedtime, forms a good
diaphoretic, or two drachms of the water of the acetate
of ammonia may be added to the whey instead of nitre.
Acting on his view of the pathology of the disease, Dr.
Maclagan has treated it with colchicum;[1] and this medicine is certainly indicated when the eruption is complicated with rheumatism.

When urticaria is produced by eating any particular
article of food, an active and immediate emetic, such as
the sulphate of zinc, or ipecacuanha, should be at once
administered, and its action followed by the exhibition
of a mercurial cathartic; if the subsequent fever be well
marked, bleeding may be required, but only a small
quantity of blood should in any case be withdrawn, as
general symptoms of poisoning, with much depression,
not unfrequently follow.[2] The intermittent form of the
disease requires to be treated constitutionally with tonics
and antiperiodics, especially the preparations of bark,
the bowels having been first freely acted on by a saline
cathartic; this variety of urticaria may occasionally be
cut short by the administration of an emetic a few hours
previously to the expected reappearance of the eruption.

In urticaria evanida, a lowering plan of treatment is
decidedly contraindicated, as the disease invariably assumes a chronic form. I have derived especial benefit
in it from the use of preparations of iron, and from the
administration of Dover's powder; of the former the
compound iron mixture may be generally prescribed in
doses of from one to two ounces every morning, or from
twenty to sixty minims of the tincture of the perchloride,
three times a day, in an ounce of the infusion of quassia

---

[1] *Monthly Journal of Medical Science*, Jan. 1852, p. 57.
[2] The Editor cannot coincide in Dr. Nelligan's recommendation to

or calumba, or two ounces, twice daily, of Bewley's *aqua chalybeata;* of the latter, from eight to twelve grains every night at bedtime. Under the administration of these combined remedies I have seen most obstinate chronic cases of the disease yield in a few weeks; while administering them, the bowels should be kept freely open by mild saline purgatives. Urticaria tuberosa should be treated similarly; but in cases in which the disease has been of very long standing, it will occasionally only yield to the prolonged administration of arsenic. When any of the forms are connected with or complicated by the presence of any other disease, the treatment ought to be modified accordingly.

The itching and tingling of urticaria are somewhat allayed by the use of the warm bath; but as soon as the skin is dried afterwards, these painful sensations are augmented in consequence of the friction of the surface requisite to remove the moisture. In febrile urticaria I have employed, as a local application, with much effect, the following alkaline spirituous wash:—

R. Carbonatis Potassæ,   . . grana triginta.
   Aquæ Sambuci,   . . . uncias undecim cum semisse.
   Spiritus Vini Rectificati,   . semi-unciam. Misce.

Pieces of lint saturated with lotion should be laid on the parts where the itching is most troublesome. In the chronic forms of the disease, chloroform is an excellent topical remedy for the same purpose; an ointment of it, prepared by rubbing together half a drachm of chloroform and an ounce of cold cream, should be smeared rather thickly over the affected surface. Lotions and ointments, containing prussic acid, opiates, and other narcotics, have proved successful in the hands of others.

In urticaria occurring in infants and children, the state of the digestive organs demands especial attention, and in all cases, whether the teeth are appearing or not, the gums should be lanced; in infants at the breast, the health of the nurse is in particular to be attended to; the local irritation, at this early age, may be allayed by sponging the surface of the body with a warm infusion of chamomile.

Whenever the sudden retrocession of the eruption in urticaria is attended with evidences of derangement of any internal organ, the hot bath should be used, with friction over the surface, and blisters applied to the epigastrium and nape of the neck.

As regards the diet in urticaria, the chief point to be attended to is the avoidance of the use of any food which, from individual experience, has been found to produce the eruption. In the acute forms of the disease the patient should live low; but when it becomes chronic, the food should be nourishing, yet not rich or heating.

ROSEOLA.—(Plate II.)

ROSEOLA (*Rose-rash*[1]) is by many dermatologists regarded as being merely a variety of erythema, erysipelas, or measles, and its existence is a distinct eruption not admitted; but I fully agree with Willan that its local characteristics are sufficiently well defined to separate it from any of these diseases, and to require a special description. The name, which has been applied to it in consequence of the peculiar rose-color which it usually presents, is to a certain extent objectionable, as this color varies much in the different stages and forms of the eruption. It consists in the appearance of very slightly elevated rose-red patches, of irregular shape, transient, fading at times, and again reappearing; non-contagious, and attended with some degree of fever. The various forms of Roseola may be classed under two heads:—

Roseola idiopathica.
      "   symptomatica.

An attack of *Roseola idiopathica* (Plate II, Fig. 5) is usually attended with slight fever, which, however, in children is sometimes well marked and severe; the febrile symptoms subsiding to a great extent when the eruption appears freely on the skin. It comes out in numerous reddish-yellow patches, which soon assume a

---

[1] In Scotland erysipelas is commonly termed "The Rose," which has caused this eruption to be occasionally confounded with it.

roseate hue and are irregularly distributed over the cutaneous surface; generally appearing first on the face and
neck, and spreading quickly thence to the trunk and the
upper and lower extremities; occasionally the eruption
is confined to the face, neck, and trunk, and at times it
occurs on the extremities only. The rash is often very
transient, disappearing completely in from twenty-four
to forty-eight hours—when the feverish symptoms become aggravated, and reappearing again within the next
twelve hours, it usually runs its course in from five to
seven days, terminating with slight epidermic desquamation. When roseola occurs in infants and children, it is
not unfrequently attended with more or less tumefaction
of the integuments, which precedes the appearance of
the eruption, being most marked in those places where
the rash is to come out.

Two forms of the disease have been described under
the names *æstiva* and *autumnalis*, from their appearing at
these seasons of the year: in the former, the feverish
symptoms sometimes run high, and are attended with
more or less sore throat, which, on inspection, is seen to
be somewhat swollen and of a bright rose-red color—the
rash, too, is very generally distributed over the cutaneous surface; in the latter, the eruption is of a duller hue,
in smaller-sized patches, and attended with very slight
fever or sore throat—this symptom, however, being often
absent. When the disease attacks infants, it has by some
dermatologists been described as a distinct form, and
termed roseola *infantilis;* it is in them usually very mild,
and disappears in a few days; but in some cases is
marked by itching, as would appear from the annoyance
it seems to give the little patient; it is then also more
prolonged.

The eruption in idiopathic roseola not unfrequently
appears in the form of rings or circles, of a bright rosy
hue, surrounding a healthy portion of the skin which is
unaltered in color; it is then termed roseola *annulata.*
(Plate II, Fig. 6.) This is a more aggravated form of
the disease, setting in with well-marked symptoms of
fever, a distinct shivering fit, followed by sickness of the
stomach, headache, pains in the limbs, and hot skin, pre-

ceding the appearance of the eruption for from twenty-
four to forty-eight hours; œdema of the integuments is
also not uncommon in this form, particularly in children,
in whom the disease usually occurs, appearing especially
should the eruption suddenly retrocede. In one case
which I attended in 1849, that of a boy aged six years,
the entire body became enormously swollen on the sudden disappearance of the rash, so much so that both eyes
were closed, and there was great difficulty of breathing
and of swallowing, owing to the tumefaction of the fauces.
This variety of roseola may appear on any part of the
cutaneous surface, but is most frequently seen on the
lower extremities, and the trunk of the body. It comes
out in the form of numerous small, round, reddish patches,
which, rapidly spreading by their circumference, assume
the character of rings, some being quite circular, and
others irregularly so; the central portion of healthy skin,
which at first is only a few lines in diameter, gradually
extends to half an inch, or even two inches, the surrounding rose-red eruption being from a quarter to half
an inch in width; sometimes two or three of the rings,
meeting, coalesce, and may thus extend beyond one of
the joints, or nearly round a limb. Heat of the skin and
itching generally accompany this form of roseola.

Mr. Erasmus Wilson describes a variety of roseola
under the name of *punctata*, in which the eruption, attended with fever of a subacute type, appears on the
mucous membrane and skin, "on the latter, in the form
of small red spots around the mouths of the follicles,
then becoming diffused so as to cover the greater part of
the body, reaching its height on the third day; at first
of a bright raspberry-red color, afterwards acquiring a
dull roseate hue, the dulness increasing with the progress
of the decline." The disease lasts for ten days. He
speaks of it as a rare disease, having seen only a few examples; I never met with it as an idiopathic affection,
but I have seen syphilitic roseola present these characteristics. Dr. Tilbury Fox (*op. cit.*, p. 64) suggests the
question: Is it a form of measles?

Roseola symptomatica occurs in the course of, or as an
accompaniment to, many febrile diseases, but its charac-

ters are so similar to those of the idiopathic form as not to require a distinct description. It is thus witnessed in smallpox—the eruption of which it usually precedes by about twenty-four hours—cow-pock, fevers, acute rheumatism, epidemic cholera, &c.; and as it may attend any of these diseases, it has been named by dermatologists R. variolosa, R. vaccina, R. miliaris vel febrilis, R. cholerica, &c. When the practice of inoculation prevailed, roseola is described as appearing very regularly on the second or third day of the fever incubation, and was regarded as a favorable sign, indicating that the variolous eruption would be mild. In cow-pock it occurs about the period of maturation of the vaccine pustule, spreading from it along the arm, and often appearing also on the trunk; it is not of very frequent occurrence, is of a very mild character, and fades away in two or three days. Its appearance during either fever or acute rheumatism is rather a favorable sign than otherwise; it does not require any special treatment, nor does it interfere with that of either of these diseases. The cholera exanthem has been described by Kier, Babington, and Rayer, all of whom witnessed it in the epidemic of 1832; it accompanied the fever of reaction, and its appearance does not seem to have in any way influenced the progress of the disease.

Roseola may occur at any age, but is more frequent in the young than in the old. It may be *caused* by any local irritation of the skin, or by any circumstance acting on the system generally, which gives rise to determination of blood to the cutaneous capillaries; the latter is evidently the cause of the symptomatic form of the eruption. In summer it is occasioned by exposure to a hot sun when the digestive organs are deranged, or by the perspiration being suddenly checked; its frequent occurrence in autumn is traceable to the gastric irritation which is at that season of the year so frequently caused by the too free use of fruit and new vegetables. In children it commonly appears about the periods of first and second dentition, and is manifestly connected with the derangements of the system which then so commonly

... ... by the
... ...

... ...
... ... to be mistaken for either measles
... of ... ... distinguished by
... ... different ... ... fully
... ... of measles, it is not
... ... and by the
... ... From scarlatina, with
... ... of the sore throat, it is in its early
... ... the ... of the rash, its
... ... and not being generally
... ... the comparatively mild charac-
... ... of the attendant sore throat, and the
... ... of the skin, are sufficient to
... ... characteristics between
... ... roseola ... are, the elevation, the
... ... shape of the latter; and the chief
... ... between it and urticaria are, the
... ... itching and of the wheal-like
... ...

The *prognosis* in roseola is always favorable: the
eruption being attended with but slight annoyance,
disappearing generally in the course of ten days, though
occasionally prolonged for three or four weeks: but in
all cases it is a simple affection, and one attended with
little or no danger, and in many febrile diseases its occurrence is manifestly salutary.

The *treatment* of the disease is simple: rest in bed, or
even confinement to the house, with low diet, the use of
diluent drinks, and, when the eruption is well out, mild
purgatives, being sufficient in most cases to effect a cure.
Mercurial seem better adapted than saline purgatives for
the treatment of roseola; with infants and children the
... ... magnesia appears especially to agree.
... ... run high, and the eruption be slow ...
... the warm bath will prove of service ...
... ... used with children. When there is ...
... surface, small doses of the spirit of ...
the water of the acetate of ammonia are ...
... benefit. In chronic cases, or in weak ...

habits of body, should the disease become chronic, vegetable tonics and the mineral acids are indicated. If much itching or heat of surface attends the eruption, it will be allayed by a weak alkaline spirituous wash, such as the following:—

R. Boracis, ... grana triginta.
    Aquæ Sambuci, ... uncias undecim cum semisse.
    Spiritus Rosmarini, . . . semi-unciam. Misce.

In most cases, however, no local application, except the general warm bath, or sponging the skin with warm water, will be needed. Symptomatic roseola requires no special treatment apart from the disease which it accompanies, and the employment of any which might repel the eruption from the surface should be especially guarded against.

RUBEOLA.

RUBEOLA, or Measles (from *Rubeo*); also called Morbilli; Rougeole of the French; Masern of the Germans.

Measles is a contagious affection, occurring once during life; and is characterized primarily by acute catarrhal fever, and secondarily by the appearance, on or about the *fourth* day, of a peculiar exanthem or cutaneous eruption, followed by desquamation. This eruption appears in the form of small red spots, frequently arranged in the figure of segments of circles, and occurs first on the face and neck, and upper extremities; next on the body, and lastly on the lower extremities. The rash is punctiform, sometimes papular, and about the sixth day becomes vesicular. It begins to fade generally about the seventh day, and about the tenth is followed by desquamation, which usually begins on the face and neck, and thence extends over the body. This desquamation occurs in the form of small scales, or of large flakes; and not uncommonly the cuticle of the hands and feet comes off in the shape of gloves and socks.

The time which elapses between the appearance of the disease and the exposure to contagion is about twelve days, and is called *the period of incubation.* Dr. Watson very forcibly observes that "the eruption is the *distin-*

8

RUBEOLA. 87

seed meal suddenly thrown into the eyes and throat. He
also remarks that Dr. Kidd, of this cit , made some flax-
seed meal mouldy, and then, by the aid of the microscope,
detected in it fungi " very like, if not identical with, some
of those figured in the plate of Dr. Salisbury."

Measles may occur at any age, but is most common in
infancy and childhood; as a general rule it does not
attack the same person twice, but the Editor knows the
exceptions to this rule to be frequent enough. It is most
to be apprehended in winter and spring. As already
suggested by the papers of Drs. Salisbury and Henry
Kennedy, its *exciting cause* is believed to be due to a specific contagion, and it is one of the *zymotic* diseases of
some modern writers.

The *sequelæ* of Rubeola are most important to the
practitioner; among these have been enumerated—pneumonia, œdema of the lungs, bronchitis, pleuritis, tracheitis
or croup, phthisis, diarrhœa; aphthæ and gangrene of the
mucous membrane of the mouth; and in those of a strumous diathesis, affections of the mesenteric glands, of the
eyes, the ears, and the parotid glands. Many cases of
phthisis may be traced to a strumous habit which was
first developed after an attack of measles, in previously
healthy children; and many suffer from delicate health
through life from the results of the sequelæ of measles.
The *prognosis* is in general favorable, but it depends largely
on the nature of the sequelæ.

Diagnosis.—The catarrhal fever, the characteristic
eruption, and the day on which that eruption appears,
sufficiently distinguish it from scarlatina on the one hand,
and from variola on the other.

The treatment of measles resolves itself, for the most
part, into the treatment of febrile catarrh or of bronchitis.
The latter frequently becomes pneumonia, and so causes
death. In cases which recover, spontaneous diarrhœa,
if not excessive, is a favorable symptom and should be
looked for. If it has not supervened, it may be induced
by mild laxatives; but should it prove excessive, the
    of pulvis cretæ aromaticus cum opio will be found
beneficial.

In the severe or malignant cases in which the eruption

modern knowledge of the subject. That much of our knowledge is not *new* the reader of the Arabian Rhazes on the smallpox and measles will very soon perceive.

SCARLATINA.

Scarlatina; Scarlatine of the French; Scharlachfieber of the Germans; *Anglicè* Scarlet Fever.

SCARLATINA is a contagious affection, occurring once during life; and is characterized primarily by general febrile symptoms and sore throat, and secondarily by the appearance, on or about the *second* day, of a scarlet cutaneous eruption, followed by desquamation. The *period of incubation* is from two to ten days.

In England there is a popular difference, unknown in this country, drawn between *Scarlet Fever* and *Scarlatina;* the latter being the name applied to the milder forms of the disease.

There are four varieties of scarlatina usually described: S. *simplex;* S. *anginosa;* S. *maligna;* and S. *sine exanthemate.*

S. simplex, which is characterized by a slight inflammation of the fauces, sets in with febrile symptoms, and generally on the *second* day a brilliant scarlet efflorescence is observable on the face and neck and upper extremities; extending thence all over the body. This rash is brightest in the evening when the fever is highest. The skin is rendered pale by pressure, on the removal of which the color immediately returns; and when the eruption is at its height it may be likened to the color of a boiled lobster. In a day, or two days, the efflorescence becomes partial, is seen in patches, and does *not* disappear under pressure. The skin is mostly rough to the touch, and is sometimes studded with miliary vesicles; this is called S. *papulosa vel milliformis.* When the eruption is smooth, from œdema of the skin, the affection is termed S. *plana vel levigata.* When vesicles and pustules coexist, it is termed S. *vesicularis, vel phlyctænosa, vel pustulosa.* The rash of S. simplex generally declines on the *fifth* day, and does so gradually until the *eighth,* when it disappears.

Desquamation generally begins on the *fifth* or *sixth*

day. The cuticle peels off in flakes from the body and limbs, and in large scales, sometimes in shape like gloves or socks, from the hands and feet. Great itching and tenderness of the skin frequently accompany this process.

The *prognosis* in S. simplex is generally favorable, especially if the throat affection be slight, if hemorrhage from the nose or a critical diarrhœa occur.

Scarlatina anginosa, or Fothergill's sore throat, is an aggravated form of S. simplex in which the throat and adjacent parts are severely affected, while the skin eruption is more deeply colored and spreads over the surface in a very rapid manner. Externally the submaxillary glands are enlarged and painful to the touch. Internally the fauces and adjacent parts are of a florid color, while the tonsils are soft and the palate and uvula enlarged. The tongue is coated with white mucus, and studded with red papillæ. Thick mucus collects at the back of the throat, and sometimes almost suffocates the patient, whose deglutition is rendered very difficult. Sometimes gangrenous sloughs take place, and a purulent discharge issues from the nostrils and ears. Besides general debility and languor, acceleration of pulse, loss of sleep and failure of appetite, and sometimes delirium, the secretion of urine is very scanty; and anasarca, either alone or with ascites or hydrothorax, speedily makes its appearance.

The *prognosis* in S. anginosa is not by any means so favorable as in S. simplex.

Scarlatina maligna, or putrid sore throat, may be described as S. anginosa very much aggravated; and is characterized by grave typhoid symptoms, with extensive ulceration of the fauces and parts adjacent, while the exanthem is imperfectly developed. The *prognosis* is very unfavorable, as the disease, often the typical scarlatina of an epidemic, is highly fatal.

Scarlatina sine exanthemate is, simply, a mild form of sore throat with febrile symptoms, but without the characteristic eruption of the typical forms. It occurs mostly in persons who have previously had scarlatina: and the Editor's experience leads him to believe it to be most frequent in adults during the prevalence of an epidemic; while few can doubt its property of communicating the typical disease to the " unprotected."

Diagnosis.—Scarlatina is distinguished from Rubeola by the absence of catarrhal symptoms, by the different color of the exanthem, and by the time at which the eruption appears. It is distinguished from Variola by the character and time of appearance of the eruption, and by the absence of angina in the latter disease.

Treatment.—S. simplex and S. sine exanthemate may be treated by keeping the patients cool and quiet; using light diet, acidulated and saline drinks, preceded, in some cases, by an emetic and a gentle purgative. S. anginosa must be treated on the general principle of endeavoring to reduce the inflammation of the throat and general febrile action without unduly lowering the strength of the patient. The best *local* applications, according to the Editor's experience, are—cold affusion, poultices, ice, and a strong solution of nitrate of silver. In the type of Scarlatina which has prevailed of late years in this country, constant support with beef-tea, and in some cases with wine, is necessary, if the patient is ever to reach the stage when tonics may be given with advantage. *Scarlatina maligna* must be treated on the general principles adopted in cases of typhoid fever. Locally the throat must be treated by the use of strong astringent and stimulating gargles, or by the application of nitrate of silver. Dr. Watson recommends a drink of chlorate of potash, and the Editor has always found this to be most useful. Two drachms of the salt are dissolved in two ounces of hydrochloric acid, diluted with two ounces of water. The mixture must be kept in a stoppered bottle and in a dark place: of it two drachms may be added to a pint of water, and a dose of half an ounce or one ounce given every hour or two hours. The use of carbonate of ammonia is very popular with some in this disease. The plan has been already described when treating of Rubeola.

The *sequelæ* of scarlatina are much to be dreaded, leading, as they often do, to diseases of the kidneys, eyes, ears, and chest. For full information as to all these, and as to the question of contagion, the reader must refer to the works on general medicine already noted, and to the following among many monographs:—

Hood, Peter. *The Successful Treatment of Scarlet Fever and Affections of the Throat, &c.,* Lond. 1857; Kennedy, Henry. *Some Account of the Epidemic of Scarlatina which Prevailed in Dublin from 1834 to 1842, &c.,* Dublin, 1843; Cremen, David. "Report on the Epidemic Scarlatina which visited Cork in 1862, &c."—(*Dub. Quar. Jour. Med. Sci.,* May, 1863): the works of Drs. Witt and Graham, noted under Rubeola: Cummings, W. J., "Remarks on Scarlatina"—(*Dub. Quar. Jour.,* Feb., 1865); and O'Connor, Professor (Queen's Coll., Cork), "On Contagion Viewed Practically"—(*Dub. Quar. Jour.,* Feb., 1864).

Roseola is a disease which, according to Dr. Tilbury Fox (*op. cit.,* p. 67), "stands midway between roseola and scarlatina." Dr. Copland included it under the term *Roseola,* and Dr. Richardson gave a description of it to the Epidemiological Society, on the 3d of Nov., 1862.

It differs from scarlatina by reason of the non-affection of the throat, the absence of kidney disease, and desquamation; from Rubeola by the absence of its peculiar eruption, and of coryza, &c. It resembles scarlatina in its pyrexia, followed by a rash somewhat resembling the eruption of that disease; and it is not unlike Rubeola in having the mucous surfaces affected, and the conjunctivæ suffused. Dr. Richardson considers the alimentary canal its prime seat, and supposes the efficient agency to be a non-volatile acid in the blood. In the Cork Fever Hospital the Editor has frequently seen this affection, which was popularly considered to be a mild mixture of measles and scarlatina when both were simultaneously prevalent, just as he has frequently observed fever cases which could be said to be neither typhus nor typhoid, but to have prominent symptoms of both, without the distinctive features of either.

VARIOLA.

VARIOLA (from *varus,* a pimple), Petite Vérole of the French; Blattern of the Germans; *Anglicè, Smallpox.*

Smallpox is a contagious affection, occurring once during life; and is characterized primarily by an acute febrile attack, and secondarily by the appearance on the *third* day of a peculiar exanthem or cutaneous eruption, frequently, if not generally, preceded by slight erythema. The following species are generally enumerated : Variola *discreta*, V. *confluens, varioloid,* and Variola *sine eruptione.*

Variola discreta, or distinct smallpox, is ushered in by general febrile symptoms, in which pain in the back and loins, and nausea are very prominent. On the *third* day the face and neck become more or less studded with minute scattered papulæ, which during that and the *fourth* day extend all over the body. On the *fifth* day the papules become vesicles, and the eruptive fever abates. On the *sixth* day the mucous membranes generally become affected, and on them (*e. g.* in the mouth) may be seen minute white spots. On the *eighth* day the vesicles become pustules; and the face becomes so swollen as sometimes to close the eyes, giving the patient a horrible and revolting appearance. By the *eleventh* day the pustules have attained their full size the swelling abates in the face, but travels to the hands and feet. The pustules soon discharge, leaving crusts on the face; the places of these are often occupied by seams and "pits;" while the face for some time after retains a semi-purple dusky appearance.

The *period of maturation,* technically so called, is the time occupied by the change of vesicles into pustules. The *secondary fever,* a set of symptoms marked by sleeplessness, quick pulse, unhealthy urine, and mostly by delirium, sets in on or about the *eighth* day.

Variola Confluens.—Confluent smallpox is ushered in by a more intense fever than V. *discreta.* The fever increases up to the period of maturation; the *secondary* fever is more severe, sometimes typhoid, and accompanied with coma and delirium; diarrhœa and salivation also occasionally occur.

The eruption is commonly preceded by erythma of the face : the pustules coalesce; maturation occurs early; and instead of pus a fluid called "brownish ichor" is sometimes discharged from them. The pustules also are flattened and irregularly formed; severe inflammation and sloughing sometimes attack the surrounding parts; the fever becomes more typhoid in character; the eruption becomes livid; the patient dies about the eleventh day; or recovers, deeply and permanently pitted and scarred.

The period of *incubation* in variola is reckoned at from five to twenty days.

Varioloid, or modified smallpox, occurs in cases where the patient has had the more severe form previously, or has been vaccinated; it is also caused by *inoculation*.

Variola sine eruptione.—The variolous' fever of Frank and Sydenham consists of the fever and mucous congestion of variola without the vari. Mr. Wilson thinks its occurrence is "rare," and the Editor believes it to be so rare that it may be reckoned a mythical disease.

The *cause* of variola, as shown in works on general medicine, is clearly *contagion*.

The *prognosis* is generally favorable in the *discrete* variety, but unfavorable in the *confluent*.

The *sequelæ* are abscesses, ulcers, boils, sloughing, blindness, deafness, and many acute diseases.

Diagnosis.—In the Editor's experience there is scarcely any use in attempting a differential diagnosis of variola from rubeola and scarlatina at the commencement of the attack; but the character of the eruption, and the time at which it appears, will sufficiently distinguish it from rubeola on the one hand, and from scarlatina on the other.

Treatment.—The general treatment must be conducted on the principles acted on in febrile affections. The Editor's experience, however, has led him to reject the lowering plan, and to adopt that of a fair and moderate support, avoiding alike the opposed extremes of depressants and undue stimulants. Each symptom must be met as it appears, and be treated accordingly; due regard being had to the special nature of the disease. Beyond the general line of treatment above indicated little can be said in so brief a notice as this. Yet one point must not be omitted—a notice of the *secondary fever*. This must be treated by full doses of opium, where any degree of irritation is present; and the value of the drug is so widely acknowledged under these circumstances that it may be almost termed a *specific*.

The *local treatment* of variola is a subject on which
many write, and about which perhaps there is more
variety than difference of opinion. During the eruptive
fever, cold or tepid sponging is grateful to the patient,
who, so far as the Editor's experience goes, generally prefers the tepid to the cold application. When the face
swells, blisters are sometimes placed behind the ears, and
leeches applied to the temples; blisters are also applied
to the throat, which is gargled where there is difficulty
of swallowing. When the eruption recedes, counter-
irritants are employed as in typhus fever. During convalescence, which begins about the twentieth day, warm
baths should be repeatedly used. To *prevent pitting*
numerous plans have been suggested. They have been
concisely classed by Dr. Guy, as: 1. Those which consist in protecting the parts from the air; 2. Those which
let out the contents of the vesicles before they have
changed from lymph to pus; and 3. Those which excite
common in lieu of specific inflammation. The last-named
plan consists in applying nitrate of silver or tincture of
iodine to the pustules. The second consists in puncturing
the fully-developed vesicles, and absorbing their contents
with soft cotton. The first is that most generally followed.
Mercurial ointment, powdered starch, collodion, glycerine,
a mixture of lapis calaminaris and sweet oil, and many
other like applications, have been recommended. Dr.
Hughes Bennett uses a mixture of powdered starch with
mercurial ointment. Dr. Stokes recommends a solution
of gutta percha in chloroform.—See *Braithwaite*, XXVI,
374. Others advise a solution of India-rubber in chloroform; while M. Trousseau uses a preparation called *elastic
collodion*, composed of 30 parts of collodion, 1½ of Venice
turpentine, and ⅓ of castor oil.—*Braithwaite*, XXXII,
257. The Editor, when one of the physicians to the Cork
Fever Hospital, had the advantage of seeing different
local applications used by his colleagues, and a comparison of the results from them with his own cases,
leads him to strongly recommend the use of mucilage of
starch applied as described when treating of erysipelas.—
(See p. 67). An experience of several years has convinced him that the patients so treated will rarely become

pock-pitted. For a full account of this plan, and cases
in point, see the following papers by him: "On the
External Use of Starch in Cases of Smallpox and other
Skin Diseases of an Inflammatory Nature."—*Dub. Hosp.
Gaz.*, 1856, p. 72. "Notes on the Treatment of Continued Fevers and other Acute Diseases."—*Dub. Quar.
Jour.*, Feb., 1863 (Vol. 35). In bad cases of smallpox,
and of the exanthemata, in which bed-sores or other
troublesome sequelæ result. it is of importance for the
patient to have a bed specially suited for these cases. A
bed designed by Dr. Corrigan, and described in his Lectures on Fever (p. 85), has been long known to the profession. In the *Dublin Quart. Journal* for February,
1864. the Editor published "A Description of a Bed intended to be Used in Protracted Fever Cases." This bed,
which adopts the essential principle of Dr. Corrigan's,
has the advantage over his of free access to air and light
underneath. is very inexpensive, and can be made in a
few hours by any carpenter or amateur mechanic. Its
dimensions are: Length. *six feet six inches:* breadth,
two feet six inches; height from the ground, *one foot six
inches.*

The annexed diagram shows it as it may be used for a
case of bed-sores: the uppermost third forming an angle
of about 135° with the other two-thirds. This, or any
amount or variety of inclination. may be obtained by
shortening or lengthening the leather straps, A A, and
so working the hinges. B B. The action of the hinges,
F F, is reversed. to enable the lowest and middle thirds
to form any angle, in the opposite direction to B B, that
may be desired to ease the lower extremities: in which
latter case the patient would assume the posture usual
with persons in the dressing-rooms of Turkish bath esta-
blishments. These hinges being under the frame cannot
be shown in the drawing. The leather straps. A A. are
attached at C C, and like those of girt-web. D D D D D,
&c.. are fastened at one end on brass buttons like the
window straps of a railway carriage, while they are fixed
at the other extremities. At E E E E are four holes for
the insertion of the attaching portions of head and foot-
boards, if such should be deemed desirable, while the bed

is in a horizontal position. It is not necessary that there should be any mattress, for the surface forms an even

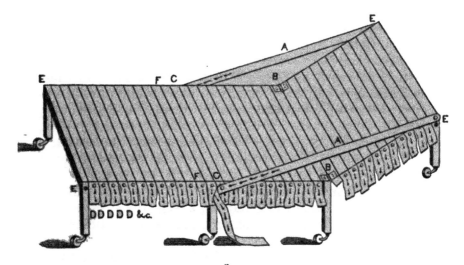

plane; blankets folded from above and below, leaving a gap for the sore, as recommended by Dr. Corrigan, will answer every purpose. If, however, a mattress should be required, it ought to be made in several parts, each capable of being temporarily joined to the others, so that one part might be withdrawn while the others are kept in use. Any one or more of the girth-web straps may be loosened to admit of the use of the bed-pan, which can be readily introduced at any part of the bed; and, of course, the strap or straps immediately under the sore parts should be loosened, *while all the rest are kept perfectly tight.* In this last direction, as to the tightening and loosening of the straps, the entire principle of the bed is contained. It can be easily moved from one apartment to another, without causing any disturbance to the patient, who may remain on it throughout; while its capability of elevation at the head, combined with its portability, would give the patient most of the advantages of being out of bed without any of the risk incurred by rising prematurely.

Connected with, or analogous to, variola are varicella, or chicken-pock, and vaccinia, or cow-pock.

Varicella is by some supposed to be a modified small-

9

... or varioloid. Its general features may be said to resemble those of variola in a mild and slight degree. Dr. Fox states that, generally speaking, it is distinguished from small-pox by—

1. Less severity of general symptoms; 2. The shortness of the course of the eruption; 3. The absence of secondary fever; 4. The characters of the eruption: often oval, non-umbilicated, areola and induration less, thin scabs, and absence of pitting; 5. Appearance often on the back first; 6. Eruption successive, and thus prolonged a good time.

Unless when confluent, this disease is free from danger; it is communicable by contagion, affects the system, as a rule only once, and seldom requires any medicine beyond gentle saline aperients.

Dr. Fox has constructed the following table to assist in the diagnosis of some of the eruptive diseases already noticed:—

MEASLES.	SCARLATINA.
Rash appears on fourth day: begins near	Rash on second day: begins on neck and face.
... ... in the ... th week	Colour rose-red or crimson. Punctiform, uniform.
... ...	Copious desquamation.
Accompanying symptoms: ... ... and cough. Heat of skin moderate.	Accompanying symptoms: sore throat, strawberry tongue, great heat of skin, rapid pulse.

VARIOLA.	VARIOLOID.	VARICELLA.
Rash on third day: first	Rash on second or third day: first	Rash on first or second day: first on back.
... ... papules going on ... ... vesicles, ... pustules, with much ... ... when confluent	... ... papules same: becoming vesicular, ... pustular ... ... and not confluent	Papules some not advancing, others vesicular, a few pustular without umbilication: eruption irregular in progress.
Thick scabbing and scars	Scabs ... ... leaving scars.	Usually no scars.
Accompanying symptoms: ... ... fever, secondary fever.	Symptoms as in variola, but milder at first: no secondary fever.	Constitutional symptoms insignificant.

Vaccinia, or cow-pock (from *Vacca,* a cow), is a disease communicated to the human hand from an eruption on the teats and udder of the cow. The eruption is seen about the seventh day after inoculation, and consists (as Dr. Fox concisely puts it) "of red   papulæ, which go through the usual smallpox stages of vesiculation, pustulation, umbilication, and desiccation, leaving behind pitting of the surface."

Vaccination, as all the world knows, is inoculation of the human subject by scratching or puncturing into the skin the morbid matter taken either from the teats of the cow, or, secondarily, from the vaccinated subject.

If the operation has been successfully performed, the following appearances may be looked for:—

2d day.—Small, red, hard spots.

5th day.—Pearly circular vesicles.

8th day.—Matured vesicles, with depressed surface and raised edge, surrounded by an erythematous areola of the skin, which is painful, and accompanied with slight febrile disturbance.

11th day.—The areola having increased during the 9th and 10th days, the vesicles now burst, if not previously opened; the areola begins to fade, the vesicle becomes a brown scab, and falls off about *the 20th day*, leaving a cicatrix with pits proportioned in size and number to the cells in the vesicles. Dr. Fox's "rules" to be observed in performing vaccination are most clear and concise, and are here given:—

1.—Get lymph from a perfectly formed vesicle; and

2.—Obtain it on the eighth day, before the areola is formed; and

3.—From a healthy child.

4.—Vaccinate in several distinct places; the more vesicles produced by vaccination the greater is the protective power.

5.—Use scarification with a lancet as the method.

6.—Do not vaccinate "too many from the same arm."

7.—Do not use matter taken from the adult, or from one who has been vaccinated before.

8.—Two months is the most suitable age for operation.

9.—The desirability of re-vaccination depends upon the degree of exposure (probable), the existence of an epidemic, the number of cicatrices, and their degree of visibility and extent.

10.—Be very careful not to use the vaccine matter

which has been taken from any member of a family in
which syphilis has occurred.

11.—The lymph pretty recently taken.

As to the alleged diminished efficacy of vaccination,
in the present day, see Mr. Thomas Vasser Harding's
papers on Smallpox and Vaccination, in the *Medical
Times and Gazette* for Sept. 1868.

Varicella is a name given to those secondary eruptions which, in various irregular vesicular forms, follow
the operation of vaccination—they occur over the body
generally. For a full history of cow-pock, see Mr.
Ceeley's account in the tenth volume of the *Transactions
of the Provincial Medical Association*, and Dr. Watson's
account in his lectures, in which will also be found a
history of the inoculation of smallpox, formerly practised universally in this country.

The maculæ of typhus fever and the rose rash of *typhoid*
are eruptions of the skin, but are only secondary to the
graver symptoms of these diseases in which they are not
invariably present. For a full description and plates of
them reference may be made to Murchison's *Treatise on
Continued Fevers*, to Tweedie's *Lectures on Fever*; and they
will also be found fully treated of in the works of two
Dublin physicians—Dr. Corrigan, in his *Lectures on the
Nature and Treatment of Fever*, and Dr. Lyons, in his
Treatise on Fever.

CHAPTER III.

VESICULÆ (Vesicles).

THE term VESICULÆ, formerly employed to designate any cutaneous eruption in which *matter* was effused beneath the cuticle, was restricted by Willan to those forms in which the effusion is a transparent fluid, contained in minute, orbicular, epidermic elevations, corresponding to his definition of a vesicle; when these elevations were of larger size, the diseases in which they occurred were placed in a distinct class, denominated by him *Bullæ;* but with respect to their visible phenomena, as they differ only in magnitude, I shall include all in one class. The Order Vesiculæ, then, may be defined to be characterized by an eruption of vesicles or blebs, which consist in an elevation of the epidermis varying in size, sometimes minute (vesicles), sometimes of tolerable magnitude (bullæ or blebs), containing a transparent, serous fluid, which, with the progress of the disease, becomes opaque, and dries into thin scales or crusts. There are five genera contained in the Order: Eczema, Herpes, Pemphigus, Rupia, Scabies. Of these the first two are attended usually with acute symptoms; pemphigus and rupia with fever of a low type; and scabies with local inflammatory action, but very rarely with constitutional derangement. In all, the fluid contained in the vesicles becomes opaque and sero-purulent with the progress of the disease, and they are then often diagnosed with difficulty from pustular eruptions.

ECZEMA.

Eczema, ἰκζεμα, from ἰκζίω, effervesco, included by Moses under the Hebrew term *Seeth*, and rendered "a rising" in Leviticus xiii, 2; translated by the LXX ὀυλή

9*

a scar or mark. Dartre Vive of Sauvages: Dartre Squamm-me se Humide of Alibert.—See Plate III.

Eczema (*Scall* or *Humid Tetter*) is a most important and interesting disease of the skin, being of extremely frequent occurrence,[1] at times very difficult of diagnosis —particularly in its advanced stages—and *usually most rebellious to treatment*. It is characterized by the eruption of numerous minute transparent vesicles, closely set and irregularly aggregated on an uncircumscribed inflamed surface, and attended generally with burning pain and intense itching. It is highly inflammatory, but non-contagious. The vesicles, which are at first perfectly transparent, become opaque on the second or third day after their appearance—the contained fluid assuming a semi-purulent character—and either dry up with a fine furfuraceous desquamation, or bursting, become covered with thin, yellow crusts, from beneath which an acrid, watery exudation takes place. Eczema differs much in appearance, as it occurs on the parts of the cutaneous surface which are ordinarily covered or exposed, or on which hair grows, and therefore must be described more or less with reference to a regional system of classifica-tion. The forms of the disease, according to the course which they run, are naturally divided into two groups, the acute and chronic: and as regards external charac-teristics, two varieties are well marked:—

Eczema simplex.
" rubrum.

But it is also requisite to consider it specially, as it may be seated on the face or on the scalp:—

Eczema faciei.
" capitis.

Eczema simplex (Plate III, Fig. 1) is attended with scarcely any fever, slight nausea and headache occa-sionally preceding its eruption, which is accompanied by

[1] Mr. Erasmus Wilson states that Eczema occurs in the proportion of 30 cases out of every 100.—*Inquiry into Relative Frequency, Duration, and Causes of Diseases of the Skin* (1864), p. 4. Devergie's cases give an average of one-third—600 in 1,800.

some heat and tingling of the surface. It consists in the appearance of numerous minute shining vesicles, not exceeding in size the head of a small pin, which are closely aggregated, and irregularly distributed on apparently healthy skin of the natural color; but with a magnifying glass each vesicle may be seen to be surrounded by a narrow red areola; in forty-eight hours the fluid contained in them becomes opaque, and on the third or fourth day they dry up, and are followed by a fine mealy desquamation of the epidermis, and thus the disease may run its course in from four to six days. In most cases, however, a fresh crop of vesicles appears as soon as the first has matured, and by successive crops its duration may be prolonged for as many weeks; under such circumstances, thin yellowish crusts or scabs are formed, and a serous exudation continues to flow from the surface while the disease lasts, often in large quantity. The heat and itching are then also troublesome; and if the part be scratched or irritated, the eruption may become chronic, or may change into the second form. For a long time after the disappearance of the disease the epidermis continues to desquamate, but it leaves no stain on the skin, or other trace of its existence.

This form of eczema usually appears on the backs of the hands and arms, sometimes on the scalp, but rarely on the lower extremities, on the trunk, or on the face.

Eczema rubrum (Plate III, Fig. 2) is an acutely inflammatory disease, an attack of it being ushered in generally with sharp fever, and always with much local pain, heat, and swelling of the portions of the integuments about to be affected. Numerous pellucid, small vesicles are rapidly developed on a highly inflamed, uncircumscribed surface, of a bright red color, and tumefied, over which they are irregularly distributed, but crowded together in patches; the parts feel painfully tense, and cause a continued tingling rather than itching. The vesicles, becoming opaque, enlarge somewhat, look fuller, and, bursting, form yellowish crusts; in a few rare cases the disease terminates in from a fortnight to three weeks with the falling off of these crusts and subsequent epidermic desquamation. But in most instances, and invariably when the parts have been torn by scratching or otherwise irritated, a serous discharge of an acrid, thin, serous fluid continues to flow from the inflamed surface, apparently without the formation of new vesicles: the inflammation spreads to the adjoining portions of the skin, often seemingly caused by this discharge flowing over them: bright red cracks and fissures form in the integuments, which are excoriated, thickened, much swollen, and attended with intense pain and itching, and blood flows freely should they be scratched. The serous exudation is usually in very large quantity so great as at times to require to be continually wiped away, that from even a limited surface *wetting completely* a large handkerchief in a few moments: when it is not so copious it dries quickly into thin lamellar scales, a constant desquamation of which takes place. The aspect of this form of the disease, *when fully developed, is highly* characteristic: the shining crimson or bright red surface, covered in parts with the serous discharge, and in parts with the thin film of desquamating epidermic secretion, the deeper-colored fissures and cracks, from which blood occasionally flows, and the *tensely* tumefied appearance of the whole. This cracked or fissured aspect of the disease, described as above in the former edition of this work, is looked on as a variety in itself by some writers. It is called "Eczema *fendillé*" by the French, and "Eczema rimosum" by Dr. McCall Anderson.—*Practical Treatise on Eczema* (London, 1863), p. 28. The Editor finds it to be a very common secondary condition among the mechanics who chiefly resort to the Dispensary for Skin Diseases in Bishop Street.

Eczema rubrum, when it presents the aggravated characters now described, seldom gets well in a shorter space of time than two or three months, and occasionally, becoming chronic, lasts for years. In some cases the local inflammation is still more acute, the discharge becomes more purulent or purulent, concreting into thick yellowish scabs, and scattered pustules form on the surface; it is then termed eczema *impetiginodes* (Plate III, Fig. 3), from the resemblance which it presents to impetigo. This variety of the eruption is generally met with in infants and children, is attended with well-marked febrile symptoms and much local pain and itching, and lasts for from three to six weeks, or occasionally, becoming chronic, for as many months; its duration being kept up by the successive eruption of semi-purulent vesicles.

When any of the forms of eczema become chronic they are usually described as a distinct variety, under the name of eczema *chronicum* (Plate III, Fig. 4); the disease then loses its vesicular character, the integuments which are swollen, thickened, and elevated above the surrounding portion of the skin that may remain unaffected, assume a permanently dark crimson hue, with numerous deep fissures which discharge a bloody ichor, and, taking on an inflammatory action from the least constitutional excitement or local irritation, are painful to the touch, tense, and attended with an acrid watery discharge and extreme itching. The constitution also, after a time, becomes affected, the digestive organs being deranged, and general debility ensuing.

Eczema rubrum may be seated on any part of the body, *but generally attacks a large extent of the cutaneous surface,* spreading rapidly from the place where it first appears. It thus occurs on the face, the scalp, the trunk, the arms and hands, and the thighs, rarely extending to the legs or feet except in very extreme cases. It also not unfrequently is local, appearing merely on the scalp, the face, the fingers, the backs of the hands, the ears, around the nipples in females, or in a single patch on the lower extremities, or in the pudendal region, being in all these cases very obstinate to treatment, and apt to become chronic. Each of these local forms of the disease has been constituted by some dermatologists into a distinct variety—an unnecessary refinement, as, with the exception of the first two, they present no essential differences, whether as regards diagnosis or treatment.

The outbreak of *Eczema faciei* (Plate III, Fig. 5) is preceded in young persons by a sharp attack of fever, attended with burning heat and soreness of the part about to be affected, which lasts for two or three days: in adults these symptoms are very trifling. Numerous minute vesicles then appear, closely crowded together, on a highly inflamed patch of the cuticular surface, characterized by acute burning pain and intense itching. These vesicles do not maturate, but burst usually on the day or day but one after their first appearance, giving exit to an abundant irritating serous fluid, which dries into soft thin scales. In some few instances the disease does not proceed beyond this stage, the cuticle of the part affected gradually exfoliates, and recovery takes place; but more generally the inflammation of the surface goes on increasing, fresh crops of vesicles continuously appear, the discharge becomes more copious and of a more acrid character, exciting irritation of those portions of the neighboring healthy skin over which it may flow, and the itching and painful tingling are most intense, scarcely allowing the patient a moment's rest, night or day. The skin which is the seat of the eruption becomes swollen as the disease advances, the epidermis exfoliates with the soft scabs, or is torn off by scratching, and deep bright red cracks appear all over the surface, from which a sanious, often bloody, discharge exudes. The sufferings caused by eczema when it reaches this stage can scarcely be described; suffice it to say, that they totally incapacitate adults affected with the disease from following any trade or employment.

Whether eczema rubrum attacks young or old persons, when it assumes a chronic character, *it is the most intractable of the eruptions which appear on the face.* It not unfrequently lasts for years (in one case, regarding which I was lately consulted, it had been of upwards of twenty-five years' duration), and is rarely cured in less than several months' treatment.

The most usual part of the face on which it appears in infants and young children is the forehead, to which it ordinarily spreads from the scalp, and, unlike most of the other eruptive diseases, is much more obstinate there than on its primary situation. This seems to depend on the greater delicacy of the skin of the face permitting those cracks and fissures, to which the rebellious nature of the disease appears to be chiefly due, to form more easily. In adults it occurs with greater frequency on the nose and lips, but in many cases spreads also to the forehead and cheeks.

Eczema capitis (Plate III, Fig. 6) soon loses its vesicular character, and in its various stages presents so much diversity of appearance that its diagnosis is not always unattended with difficulty. The eruption is preceded by heat, tingling, and itching, which are rapidly followed by the appearance of minute vesicles, crowded together in irregular-shaped patches, or scattered over a large surface. The interspaces between the vesicles and the whole of the scalp on which they are seated are red and inflamed; in most cases the vesicles are so minute as to be scarcely recognizable, or at least are not seen by the physician until they have burst and given exit to a copious exudation of a serous fluid, by which the roots of the hair are accreted together. In the acute forms of the disease this serous exudation continues for a long time, and is a most troublesome symptom; but in the chronic forms—and some cases assume a chronic character almost from the first—it rapidly dries into furfuraceous scales, which are pushed forward by the hair as it grows.

The vesicles of eczema capitis usually appear first behind the ear, close to the edge of the hairy scalp, from whence the disease spreads rapidly, very generally attacking the ear itself; in some cases the entire of the scalp will be covered with the eruption in a week or ten days, but in others the disease spreads very slowly.

With the progress of the affection, the appearance of the diseased surface varies much; sometimes it is scarcely, if at all, elevated above the healthy parts, and the eruption is only to be recognized by the watery exudation which keeps the hairs in a constantly moist state. In other cases the scalp is raw or excoriated, and secretes a thin, whitish pus, which dries into grayish-brown scabs, presenting cracks or fissures, through which the inflamed surface is seen. In a third form of the disease the serous exudation dries rapidly into extremely thin membranaceous scales, which are readily removable by the slightest friction, but cause much itching. And a fourth variety is characterized by a repeated eruption of minute patches of vesicles—the patches rarely exceeding the size of a small bean—all over the scalp, which pass through the stages of eczema as witnessed on other parts of the cutaneous surface, and disappear in seven or eight days, but to be rapidly succeeded by a fresh outbreak of the disease.

The hair in eczema, no matter how long the disease may have existed, remains unaltered. When in the acute forms, attended with much inflammation, ulceration of the scalp occurs, the hair, of course, falls off: but in the progress of cure it grows again in a perfectly healthy state, except that in individuals past the age of puberty the new growth of hair is often gray.

Eczema occurs at all ages, from the infant at the breast to the very aged: in new-born children it not uncommonly appears on the umbilical region—eczema umbilicale—evidently arising from the local inflammation attendant on the separation of the remains of the funis, or from a want of due attention to cleanliness.

The *causes* of the disease are often sufficiently apparent, but equally often it is not to be accounted for: thus, as regards the head and face, the eruption occurs on the scrofulous and non-scrofulous child, on the healthy and the delicate, on the ill-fed, ill-housed, deficiently-clothed children of the poor, and the highly-nurtured, well-housed, warmly-clad children of the rich: in short, frequently the only cause that can be plausibly assigned for its outbreak is that scarcely understood one, *constitutional*. The French would refer an attack of eczema, under most of these circumstances, to what they call the "Dartrous diathesis," a phrase which is as highly convenient to our Gallican neighbors as the word *constitutional* is among ourselves. Mr. Erasmus Wilson thinks that the essence of the disease is "debility."—*Inquiry into the Relative Frequency, the Duration, and Causes of Diseases of the Skin*, 1864. It certainly affects females more frequently than males, for the same reason that those of all ages, whose skin is fine and delicate, are more liable to the disease than those in whom the skin is coarse and hard; in many families, too, a peculiar predisposition to diseases of the skin exists, and this predisposition, which appears to be hereditary, is well marked, as regards the causation of eczema.

Exposure to the direct rays of the sun often produces the disease in summer, so commonly that Bateman made a distinct variety of eczema when so caused, naming it eczema *solare;* a numerous class of causes, amongst which this must be included as one, is the action of local irritants, as of blisters, of Burgundy pitch plasters, of croton oil and turpentine liniments, &c.; thus, too, in washer-women, the eruption is produced by the irritation of the alkali of the soda or soap which they use, and in house-scourers and char-women, of the potash—in both cases the disease is termed *washer-women's itch;* in grocers and makers of confectionery, of the sugar, in them it is named *grocers' itch;* in bricklayers it is produced by the irritation of brick-dust, and is accordingly called *brick-layers' itch;* Hebra describes a variety (E. marginatum) as occurring on the inside of the thighs in the case of riders on horseback, shoemakers, and others; in glove and clothes-cleaners it is a very usual disease, arising from the irritation of the oil of turpentine or resin which they employ; and in the higher walks of life a not unfrequent cause of the eruption is the too frequent use of stimulating soaps and cosmetic washes to the face and hands, and also the habit of washing the face, when heated, in cold water, or of not drying it sufficiently after it has been washed. Sitting in close, heated rooms, engaged in any occupation in which the face is constantly kept stooped, as in that of writing, is also a common cause of eczema faciei. An eruption of eczema is of very frequent occurrence on the legs of old persons in whom the small superficial veins are in a varicose condition; and in them, if irritated, it is apt to degenerate into troublesome ulceration.

The constitutional irritation caused by the action of mercury on the system produces in some cases—now more rare than formerly, when the employment of the preparation of this metal was so much abused—a very grave form of eczema; it is usually termed eczema *mercuriale,* but was described as a distinct affection, under the name of *Hydrargyria,* by the late Mr. Alley of this city, in an original and highly valuable essay on the disease, published by him in the year 1810. In the majority of cases it seems to have occurred when only a very small quantity of a mercurial preparation had been

10

taken. In its milder forms it resembles the acute *****
of eczema rubrum, arising from other causes; *** *
more frequently assumes a much more severe char****
when it is ushered in by fever, difficult respiration; ***
cough, and tightness across the chest, with a ****
smarting and burning feel of the skin over the w****
body. These symptoms are soon followed by an ***
tion of minute vesicles, which break and discharge **
very fetid fluid. As the disease increases in severity ***
eruption extends over the face and the whole of ***
body, which become covered with incrustations; ***
fever assumes a typhoid type, the difficulty of breath***
increases and is accompanied by bloody expectoration,
spots of purpura appear, and death ensues, preceded **
delirium or convulsions. On the first appearance of **
eruption the use of mercury ought to be immediately
relinquished, and the accompanying symptoms treated
by the means appropriate for the individual case.

The *diagnosis* of eczema in its advanced stages, and in
some of its local forms, is not unattended with difficulty.
Eczema simplex may at its origin be mistaken for *herpes*;
but the vesicles in the latter are larger, more distinct
from each other, and occur in patches always well defined, and often of small extent. When it appears on
the fingers the serious mistake of confounding it with
scabies is not unfrequently made, and thus much mental
annoyance may be caused not alone to individuals but
to families, owing to the dread and anxiety with which
that eruption is viewed by all; even at their commencement they are, however, readily to be distinguished, the
vesicles in itch being solitary, large, and conical, and becoming rapidly purulent; the tingling, burning heat of
eczema is also very different from the intense itching of
scabies, and by careful examination the itch insect, the
existence of which is an unfailing diagnostic sign, may
be discovered in the latter. In fevers and other diseases,
in which profuse sweating occurs, a vesicular eruption
which, from the cause by which it is produced, is termed
sudamina, appears not unfrequently on the cutaneous
surface, and might be mistaken for eczema simplex; but
in it the vesicles, though of a small size, are few in num-

ber, perfectly distinct, and separated from each other, and, drying up in a few days, disappear without any serous exudation or local irritation.

Eczema *impetiginodes*, as its name indicates, very closely resembles impetigo; in both there is a purulent discharge, but the crusts or scabs which form on the affected part are always of a greenish hue, and the discharge purulent in the latter, while they are yellowish or yellowish-brown, and the discharge sero-purulent in the former. The chronic forms of the disease are liable to be mistaken for chronic lichen, especially for lichen agrius when seated on the hands, a serous exudation being then usually present; but the latter eruption never loses its papular character, the portion of the integuments which is affected being raised unevenly, rough, and not marked by the cracks and fissures so characteristic of chronic eczema; and the serous exudation is small in quantity, is evidently caused by the local irritation to which the eruption gives rise, and only occurs occasionally. With psoriasis, too, chronic eczema may be confounded by the superficial observer, in consequence of the epidermic desquamation by which it is attended; but the formation of true scales never takes place in the latter, nor the copious serous exudation in the former. The diagnostic marks between intertrigo and eczema have been noticed when describing that eruption. Eczema faciei is distinguished from herpes, in addition to the difference in the character of the eruptions already mentioned, by the latter affecting the mouth or lips alone, while the former is not confined to any special locality.

Eczema *capitis* may be confounded with impetigo or herpes of the scalp; it is diagnosed from either by the copious serous exudation, which dries rapidly into yellowish, not greenish crusts, by the rapid and excessive formation of soft furfuraceous scales, and by the hair not being affected. For porrigo capitis it can scarcely be mistaken, but the characteristic differences between the two eruptions will be more easily understood by deferring the mention of them until describing that disease.

In point of fact the difficulty of diagnosis in eczema

depends very much on the complications commonly occurring in cases of it. In the Editor's experience complicated cases are more frequent than the typical ones,
which are to be met with for the most part in books.
This difficulty of diagnosis arises not only from the complications already referred to, but also from the general
custom in this country of not consulting a physician
until the early stage of the disease has passed away, when
the medical attendant will in vain look for any trace of
a vesicle. It is no uncommon thing to see a case of eczema which simultaneously presents the appearance of
two or three different diseases, or stages of the one disease, in different parts of the body.   The Editor has detailed at length an important instance of this kind in
The Dublin Quarterly Journal of Medical Science for August, 1865 (p. 254). In this case, on admission to the
Dispensary for Skin Diseases, the disease exhibited on
the right arm a vesicular eruption with acrid watery exudation; on the left arm an impetiginous eruption with
purulent discharge ; and on the left cheek a circular
erythematous blush. Further, in about a fortnight, the
disease on the left arm became rimous (E. rimosum).

This part of the subject opens another matter to which
reference here must be made—the modern difference of
opinion as to the *elementary lesion* in eczema.

The Willanist theory, that eczema is essentially a vesicular disease, was accepted, as above laid down, by Dr.
Neligan.   Mr. Erasmus Wilson, the *facil princeps* of the
English School, believes elementary lesions to be mu-
tually convertible: "that an erythema, for example, may
become a lichen by the development of pimples, or an
impetigo by the production of pustules. In the same
manner, the pimples of lichen having subsided, the lymph
or ichor of eczema being dried up, and the pus of impetigo exfoliated in crusts, there may remain behind a
chronic erythema to which another term, namely, *psoriasis*, has been applied. Therefore, in essential nature,
erythema, lichen, eczema, impetigo, and psoriasis are
simply modified manifestations of inflammation of the
skin, corresponding with recognized stages of common
inflammation."—*Diseases of the Skin*, fifth edition, p. 71.

Mention has been already made of the *Dartrous* dia-thesis of the French School. M. Hardy includes under that head pityriasis, lichen, eczema, and psoriasis, affections of different elementary lesions, and defines the chief features of this diathesis to be as follows: that it is non-contagious; often of hereditary transmission; of almost constant recurrence; is accompanied by an itching which has a tendency to spread from one part to another; is chronic; recovers without scars, though often accompanied with ulcerations.—*Leçons sur les Maladies de la Peau.* Partie I, 2ième Edition. Paris: 1860, p. 19.

Some writers, and particularly Hardy and De Vergie, divide eczema into three stages: 1, inflammatory; 2, secretory; and 3, scaly. These divisions the Editor knows to be really useful and practical, and the recognition of them will furnish a solution to many difficulties in diagnosis.

Having given the opinions of Wilson of the English and of Hardy of the French School, it will be necessary to state concisely those of the modern German School, as represented by Hebra, of Vienna.

Hebra makes pityriasis, lichen, eczema, and impetigo all stages, the one of the other; and, with Hardy, he states that the elementary lesion of eczema is not exclusively vesicular, but may be an erythema, a papule, a vesicle, a pustule, or a fissure. A full exposition of this theory will be found in Dr. McCall Anderson's work on eczema. In this book Hebra's theory is advocated, and the received meaning of the term eczema is sought to be so extended as to upset *in toto* the time-honored theory of Wilan. The late Dr. A. B. Buchanan founded a classification of eczema on this theory.—See *Edin. Med. Journ.*, Jan. 1863. Dr. McCall Anderson gives four features as characteristic of eczema: 1, infiltration; 2, exudation; 3, formation of crusts; and 4, itching. Here Dr. Tilbury Fox observes (*op. cit.*, p. 96): "these are surely not peculiar to eczema; herpes and ecthi instance, possess them;" and he adds:—"In sp that has been said or written, it appears to me t is essentially and entirely vesicular." In th of a scholarly and unprejudiced reviewer

down at length the arguments for and against the distinct nature of eczema; and having well 'weighed the whole question, he says: "The real conclusion seems to be this, that eczema is distinguished from its supposed allies essentially by its being a secretory disease; that the secretion is peculiar in its character, best described as stiffening linen, and drying into light yellow crusts; that the outpouring of this secretion in the first instance is connected with the formation of vesicles; but that the latter may be rapidly produced, or imperfectly developed, or may quickly burst after their appearance; and hence, also, be overlooked. But we cannot refuse to admit that the tendency in all cases of eczema is the formation of vesicles and the production of a *peculiar* secretion. Eczema is of all diseases most prone to complication, *e. g.*, by lichen. Again, eczema may be modified by treatment; it becomes chronic, or puts on special aspects, *e. g.*, it may fissure; hence eczema is modified by three great causes: (*a*) arrest of development, so that the disease assumes the aspect of an erythema; (*b*) free secretion or fissuring; (*c*) by complications, *e. g.*, as by lichen."
—*Op. cit.*, p. 99.

The Editor candidly confesses that he regards this question—as to the nature of the elementary lesion in eczema—as yet *sub judice.* He feels that much can be said on both sides, and that the clear arguments advanced by Dr. McCall Anderson on the one hand, and by Dr. Tilbury Fox on the other, cannot be lightly overlooked by practical men.

In eczema the *prognosis* varies as regards the duration of the disease with the different forms, but in very few instances can the affection be said to be dangerous to life; yet some do occur; these are cases of debilitated old persons in whom it becomes complicated with pemphigus; and whenever such a complication takes place the prognosis should be most grave. Eczema simplex, when submitted to treatment at an early stage of the eruption, very seldom becomes chronic, but it is very apt to return on exposure to any local cause, and especially when it has been originally produced by the direct action of irritant substances. Eczema rubrum is always an ob-

stinate and severe affection of the skin, and most rebellious to treatment, years sometimes elapsing before it can
be subdued; in such cases the general health sympathizes
more or less, from the continued annoyance caused by
the local irritation, the individual affected being not unfrequently altogether incapacitated from mental or other
occupation. When the disease affects the scalp or face,
it is also one of the most obstinate of the eruptions which
appear on these parts. The occurrence of a general attack of eczema in the course of some chronic constitutional affection, particularly of the nervous system, is
often not incorrectly regarded as a favorable sign.

With reference to the precise anatomical *seat* of eczema
dermatologists are not agreed: Cazenave adopts Biett's
view, that it is an inflammatory affection of the sudoriparous glands, but it is evident that other structures of
the derma are also equally engaged. "It seems to be in
the Malpighian layer of the epidermis, not unfrequently
close round the orifices of the hair follicles."—Hillier,
Handbook of Skin Diseases (Lond., 1865), p. 121.

Treatment.—Eczema is essentially an inflammatory
eruption, even in its most chronic stages, and this fact
should always influence our choice of remedies, whether
topical or constitutional, for its treatment. In eczema
simplex occurring in adults, mild saline antiphlogistics
with alkalies, as in the following form, are prescribed
with advantage at its commencement:—

R. Sodæ et Potassæ Tartratis, . . . unciam.
    Solutionis Alkalinæ (Brandish), . drachmas quatuor.
    Aquæ destillatæ, ... uncias novendecim.
                                              Misce.
        Sumat uncias duas ter indies.

For children, gentle mercurial purgatives are better
adapted, combined with antimonials such as James's
powder if the febrile symptoms are well marked. In the
mild forms of the disease the best local treatment in the
acute stage is the use of the general tepid bath, or of
warm water sponging, the parts being thoroughly but
gently dried afterwards. Dr. Goolden, physician to St.
Thomas's Hospital, has recommended the use of what is
popularly termed the "Turkish bath."—See *Braithwaite's*

Retrospect, Vol. XLIII, p. 371. When the local affection is more severe, the weak lead-wash—a drachm of the solution of subacetate of lead to twelve fluidounces of rose or elder-flower water—applied on old linen wet well with it, is an excellent application: if the eruption is seated on any part of the extremities, it is best and most efficiently applied by means of bandages evenly put on, and kept constantly moist with the wash. In some cases of eczema moisture appears to disagree singularly, always aggravating the local symptoms; under such circumstances an ointment containing four grains of the carbonate of lead or of the acetate of zinc, to an ounce of cold cream, may be used; and if there is much tingling or itching in the part, two minims of dilute hydrocyanic acid should be added to the latter, or six minims of chloroform to the former ointment. If simple eczema occurs, as is not unfrequently the case, in children of a scrofulous diathesis, it is very apt to become chronic; when it does so, local remedies seem to have little effect on the eruption, but it yields rapidly to the internal administration of cod-liver oil, and the daily use of the tepid fresh-water bath.

In the early stages of eczema rubrum general antiphlogistic treatment, proportionately active according to the inflammatory character of the constitutional and local symptoms, is requisite; in persons of full habit of body bleeding from the arm even may be indicated,[1] and in most cases topical bleeding by leeches from the neighborhood of the affected parts is attended with much benefit; active saline cathartics should be administered and repeated at short intervals until the febrile symptoms are subdued. The local heat, swelling, and tingling are best alleviated by gelatine baths, and at night the application of poultices, prepared by first steeping the best white bread in boiling water, squeezing it out as dry as possible, and then moistening the pulp with the weak lead-wash above mentioned.

The Editor is in the habit of prescribing a decoction of bran for local application. One pound of bran is put into

---

[1] If the essence of the disease be *debility* it is obvious that this recommendation of Dr. Neligan cannot be coincided in.—ED.

a quart of water, and boiled down to a pint. The residue of bran is also useful as a poultice.

When this form of eczema becomes chronic, it is usually most rebellious to treatment, and requires the employment of internal specific or alterative medicines to produce a change in the state of the constitution with which it is combined or on which it may depend, and this is requisite even though the eruption is of small extent and local. In many cases the preparations of iodine prove most efficacious, but sometimes it is requisite to combine them with arsenic, or to give that medicine alone; in delicate constitutions, or if debility be present, the iodide of potassium is the best form; it may be given in some tonic decoction, as follows :—

R̟. Potassii Iodidi, ... grana octo.
Decocti Ulmi (cortices recentis), uncias duodecim.
Infusi Dulcamaræ, ... uncias quatnor.
Misce.
Sumat uncias duas omni nocte horâ decubitûs,

When thus given it is not liable to sicken the stomach; and in my experience small doses of iodine or its preparations act most efficaciously in the treatment of diseases of the skin. Dr. Neligan was of opinion that where the use of arsenic is indicated, either from the obstinacy of the affection or the failure of other remedies, five minims, very gradually increased to eight, of the liquor arsenicalis, or of the liquor arsenici chloridi (De Valangin's solution), may be added to each dose of the above mixture; but that whether iodine or arsenic be administered alone or in combination, their use must be continued for a long time, at least for two or three months, and that beneficial results are always most effectually derived from the system being brought very gradually under their influence. The Editor cannot coincide in Dr. Neligan's recommendation—to give gradually increasing doses of an arsenical preparation. His practice is to give three minims thrice daily of the liquor arsenicalis, or of the liquor sodæ arseniatis, at or after meals; to intermit its use on the supervention of arsenical symptoms; to administer a purgative at least once weekly, but to persevere steadily in the use of the arsenical preparation except when contraindicated as above mentioned. He has found the joint exhibition of quinia with arsenic very useful in some cases; but as the mode of administering this drug, and the question of its cumulative property, cannot be hastily discussed, he must refer the reader to an able paper on the subject, in *The Dublin Quarterly Journal* for November, 1864, by Dr. Cummins, of Cork. The Editor has also published in the same Journal, during this year, several cases in point.—See "Clinical Records" in Nos. for February, May, and August, 1865. Numerous internal medicines, as well as local applications, have been recommended by different writers for the treatment of chronic eczema; of the former the most generally employed are the tincture of cantharides, antimonials, sulphur, especially in the form of the sulphurous mineral waters, mercurials, and various vegetable tonics; but my own experience leads me to rely on either or both of the powerful alteratives above recommended; even in the most chronic cases I have seen the sulphurous waters—so valuable in other diseases of the skin— prove injurious, and mercurials generally disagree except with children, in whom the green iodide of mercury combined with the hydrargyrum cum cretâ often acts as a most valuable alterative.

The itching and copious secretion attendant on chronic eczema demand the employment of local sedatives and astringents. The unguentum plumbi subacetatis, to every ounce of which two drachms of glycerine and eight minims of chloroform have been added, constitutes a most useful ointment, no matter on what part of the surface the eruption may be seated; or the carbonate of lead or acetate of zinc ointment already described may be substituted for it should there be much tendency to local inflammatory action. Tannic acid, in the proportion of from four to twelve grains to the ounce of cold cream, with or without the addition of chloroform, is also an excellent application. Some recommend highly stimulating compounds for the local treatment of chronic eczema, such as anthrakokali or fuligokali (forms of carburet of potassium, which, when introduced into the practice of medicine a few years since, were highly

vaunted for their remedial powers, but have now fallen
into disuse), tar, pitch, sulphurous preparations, &c. By
distilling tar with water, a mixture of impure oil of turpentine, a pyrogenous oil, and some pyrentine is procured; this liquid has been recently used and highly
praised by some French dermatologists, under the name
of *huile de cade*, as a local application, inunctions being
made with it twice daily. By the term *huile de cade*,
however, most of the French pharmacologists understand
a tarry oil obtained by the dry distillation of the wood
of the juniperus oxycedrus. This *huile de cade* is manu-
factured at Aix-la-Chapelle, and those who desire it
should be certain that it is the proper article, and not
one prepared from common tar. On the recommendation of Dr. McCall Anderson, at the Glasgow Dispensary
for Skin Diseases, during the past year, the Editor
adopted, at the dispensary in this city, a preparation of
Hebra's, known as "Tinctura saponis vindis cum pice."
This consists of equal parts of tar, soft soap, and methylated spirit. It should be applied twice daily, suffered
to dry on the skin, and washed off with soft soap or petroleum soap. From experience he can highly commend
its use; and in *The Dublin Quarterly Jour.* for this year
he has given cases illustrative of it.—See "Clinical Records" in May number. Dr. M'Call Anderson gives essentially the same thing to the "better classes," in this
form: Soft soap, rectified spirit, oil of cade, of each one
ounce; oil of lavender, one drachm and a half; mix.—
See his work, p. 80. The Editor has also used with
good effect the local application of tincture of iodine
made with *methylated* spirit.—See cases in *Dublin Quarterly Journal,* 1865. Professor Malmsten, of Stockholm,
uses cod-liver oil externally, along with alkaline baths
twice weekly.—*Medical Times and Gazette,* 7th July,
1855, p. 8. No matter what local remedy is employed,
it will be found of advantage to sponge the affected parts
carefully with a *weak* alkaline wash—ten grains of the
carbonate of soda to a pint of distilled water—each time
previously to its fresh application. M. N. Guillot, of the
Necker, recommends an ointment composed of thirty
parts of lard, and of from two to four parts each of sub-

carbonate of soda, oil of cade, and tar.—See *Medical Times and Gazette*, 24th March, 1860, p. 229. Dr. Routh uses this formula: Oil of juniper, an ounce and a half; suet, half an ounce; lard, an ounce and a half; mix.— *Lancet*, 22d October, 1853, p. 397.[1]

When eczema occurs on the face or hands, the treatment as above described for its different forms is equally applicable, but in either situation, in consequence of the exposure to atmospheric vicissitudes and to various local irritants, it is usually more obstinate, and when the disease is general over the body the face is, for the same reasons, the last part to get well. The use of soap in washing should be interdicted, the weak carbonate of soda lotion warmed to blood heat being substituted for it; and especial care should be taken not to expose the surface to the action of harsh winds, the sun, the heat of the fire, or any cause which might produce determination of blood to the affected parts.

In eczema capitis the hair should be cut close to the scalp with a sharp pair of scissors—not *shaved* off—and kept as short as possible while the disease lasts, and for a short time after it is apparently cured. The crusts and scabs should be removed by poulticing with linseed meal, and sponging with the weak carbonate of soda solution mixed with an equal quantity of new milk, the surface being carefully dried afterwards. When the scalp is thus cleaned, in the milder and less inflammatory forms of the eruption an alkaline ointment, containing twelve grains of the bicarbonate of soda to the ounce of cold cream, may be applied morning and evening, the surface having been previously sponged as above directed; but if there be any tendency to inflammatory action the carbonate of lead or the tannic acid ointment, and the sub-acetate of lead wash, prove more beneficial. The scalp should be kept cool, very lightly covered or exposed to the air when in the house. As regards constitutional treatment, in scrofulous habits of body either cod-liver oil or iodide of potassium, with tonics, should be admin-

---

[1] See also Dr. Moore's paper "On the Nature and Treatment of some of the more ordinary Diseases of the Skin."—*Dub. Hosp. Gaz.*, 1859, p. 117.

istered; but the best alterative for children who are not scrofulous is the green iodide of mercury, as before men tioned.

In all forms of eczema, when the origin of the disease can be traced to any local irritant, this of course should be carefully guarded against, both during the progress of treatment and when a cure is effected; in the case of persóns engaged in trades, and others who cannot abandon the occupation by which the eruption was caused, the cutaneous surface should be protected as much as possible by the use of wash-leather gloves. The diet of persons affected with eczema should be regulated according to the constitutional circumstances, but in children much benefit will be derived from placing them on a strictly milk and farinaceous diet. In both adults and children the bowels require to be carefully attended to, the use of mild saline purgatives, if possible the natural mineral waters, of which probably the Pullna is the best, being employed with excellent effects.[1] In children the process of teething must be watched and the gums lanced when necessary; and the eruption on the scalp should not be dried up too suddenly if there exists a tendency to disease of the brain or of any other internal organ.

From the number and variety of the medical agents recommended for the treatment of eczema it will be readily seen how very tedious and intractable this disease frequently is. What will prove most useful in one case will not be of the slightest advantage in another, and the same drug will often disagree at one time with the person who takes it beneficially at another. On the other hand, steady and constant perseverance in the use of some one or more of the chief remedies already noted rarely fails to bring a success, which, however, must be earned by the joint patience of patient and physician.

[1] Dr. Fox (op. cit., p. 109) advises the use of the sulphureous mineral waters of Luchon, d'Enghein, Barèges, and St. Gervais.

11

HERPES.

Herpes—Greek, from ἕρπω, serpo. I creep: Ignis sacer of Latin authors: Erysipelas Phlyctenodes of Cullen; Dartre-dartre of the French.—See Plate IV.

HERPES (Tetter).—This term, though very generally used in the nomenclature of cutaneous diseases by the older medical writers, had with them no special reference: it is now employed to designate an eruption of small globular vesicles clustered together, and often regularly grouped, on inflamed patches of the skin usually of small extent and distinctly separated. The eruption is preceded by heat, tingling, and some degree of swelling and redness in the parts on which it is about to appear, but there is no antecedent or accompanying fever unless, which is rarely the case, it is developed simultaneously over an extended surface, and even then the febrile symptoms are but slight. It is described by most English dermatologists as being *non-contagious:* but an accumulation of direct evidence has convinced me that one form of the eruption is propagated by contagion, *no matter on what part of the cutaneous surface it may be situated.* The vesicles, which on their first appearance are globular and transparent, on the second or third day become somewhat flattened, opaque, and semi-confluent; they then burst and give exit to a trifling serous discharge, which, concreting into a soft, thin, yellowish-brown crust, falls off and leaves a superficial ulceration that heals rapidly. The causes of herpes, when it affects the body generally, cannot be traced with certainty, but in some of its local varieties are often sufficiently manifest.

The forms of this eruption present great variety, and have been differently named with reference both to their external phenomena and the parts on which they may appear: this has led to numerous subdivisions of the disease in classifying it for the purposes of description, thereby tending to complicate the inquiry. I shall describe them all under the three following heads:—

Herpes phlyctenodes.
  "   zoster.
  "   circinatus.

Herpes phlyctenodes (*Nirles*), Herpes *miliaris* of various authors, Dartre phlyctenoide of Alibert (Plate IV, Fig. 1), is occasionally, more particularly when it occurs in adults, attended with slight fever, foul tongue, loss of appetite, nausea, and thirst, but the pulse is rarely quickened; there is a deep-seated pain in the part on which the eruption is about to appear, and superficial heat and tingling. Small, irregularly-shaped patches of the skin become slightly swollen and red, and in about twenty-four hours afterwards an eruption of vesicles appears on them. The majority of these vesicles are of small size, but a few of them obtain the magnitude of a pea; they are distinct from each other, rounded, and contain a transparent serous fluid; they occur in groups, varying in size from one to three or four inches in length or breadth, but rarely exceeding that of the palm of the hand; usually, when of large extent, constituting but a single group, which, however, is often made up of three or more smaller, by the eruption spreading over the intermediate sound skin. On the second day after their appearance, the fluid in the vesicles becomes opaque or sero-purulent, and they burst on the third or fourth day; those that were closely aggregated together having previously become confluent, forming soft crusts or brown scabs, from beneath which a thin sero-purulent matter exudes in small quantity. These scabs, falling off on or about the tenth day, leave small superficial ulcers which heal in three or four days, so that the disease rarely lasts longer than a fortnight. But it is sometimes prolonged by the eruption of a distant patch of vesicles on the third or fourth day after the appearance of the first, and in their neighborhood; they unite with the former, and the entire thus cover a rather extended surface; requiring, however, the same time for maturation and healing, the duration extends to three or four days more. Should there be any attendant fever, it abates or disappears with the outbreak of the eruption, but the local symptoms increase until the vesicles burst, when some slight itching only remains.

The local pain, which is often severe previously to the appearance of the eruption, is usually much alleviated then, but sometimes returns with greater intensity after its surface is healed and presenting somewhat of a ... character ... with great obstinacy frequently be ... Occasionally in old persons or in bad constitutions an herpetic eruption terminates in troublesome ulceration.

The ... form of herpes may appear on any part of the body ... its most usual seat is on the trunk, the neck and the arms rarely occurring on the lower extremities. It attacks some special portions of the integuments with great regularity and its occurrence there requires to be seriously ... these are the lips and the prepuce. Herpes ... is a slight form of the disease ... and is merely in consequence of the local irritation which is produced by its situation; the eruption which is preceded by a certain degree of irritation dryness of the skin heat tingling, and redness appears in the angles of the mouth or on the upper or lower lip more easily or the lower* being of small extent rarely exceeding the size of a shilling. The vesicles which are in ... closely aggregated and covering the surface of the inflamed surface, are at first globular, transparent and shining; within forty-eight hours the contained serum grows ... and the vesicles become opaque forming bulae of the size of a pea, and on the fourth or fifth day soft brown ... crusts appear on their surface, with ... fall off in two or three days more, leaving a slight degree of redness and swelling of the part, that lasts for about a week. Should the crusts however, be torn off by scratching or irritated from their situation at the commissures or on the vascular portion of the lips, the surface bleeds and a hard dark brown scab is formed, which is slow in separation. Sometimes the herpetic eruption on the lips extends completely round the mouth, when it is a troublesome and obstinate affection; but unless under these circumstances it runs usually a rapid course, its duration seldom exceeding a week or ten days. A variety of herpes, similar in all respects to this, occasionally appears on the ears: it is then termed herpes *auricularis*.

* The Editor has seen it more frequently on the upper lip.

Herpes præputialis has been so named from its appearing on the prepuce, being situated either upon the external cuticular surface or on the mucous membrane. It was first described by Dr. Bateman, and is delineated by him in Plate LI of his well-known *Delineations of Cutaneous Diseases.* The eruption is preceded by heat and tingling in the part, and some degree of soreness; and when it occurs on the internal aspect of the prepuce there is also more or less tumefaction; the transparent orbicular vesicles soon appear in a small group, but distinct from each other, on a somewhat circular inflamed patch of the integument, rarely exceeding the size of a sixpence; when they occur on the external surface they maturate quickly, becoming opaque, and forming brownish crusts, which fall off on the fifth or sixth day, leaving the part on which they had been seated slightly tender and red; but when the eruption is situated on the mucous membrane the vesicles are larger, become sero-purulent, and from the confluence of two or three attain the size of a split pea;' the scabs which form are softer, and of a yellowish color, and, being easily rubbed off, leave a small ulcerated surface, which, from the swelling of the surrounding mucous membrane, occasionally presents a slightly excavated character, in consequence of which it is likely to be mistaken for a chancre. Herpes præputialis sometimes becomes chronic when the disease spreads, by the appearance of successive crops of the eruption, over the entire of the prepuce, especially affecting the part where the mucous membrane and the skin meet; there is much thickening from the effusion into the submucous areolar tissue, caused by the repeated attacks of inflammation; the surface becomes hard, rugose, fissured in parts, and in parts covered with brownish crusts, from between and beneath which an unhealthy, fetid, sero-purulent discharge takes place, and as the glans penis cannot be uncovered, foul ulceration of it not unfrequently occurs to complicate the original disease. When the eruption is of this chronic character, it often lasts for months, and the general health becomes affected in consequence of the anxiety and distress of mind' it occasions.

In females herpes phlyctenodes sometimes appears on the pudendal region, being situated at the vaginal orifice on both the skin and mucous membrane; its characters correspond precisely with those of the disease of the prepuce in males, but in consequence of the parts being more exposed to the irritation arising from local discharges and from the urine, it is generally more chronic and rebellious to treatment. By some writers it is made a distinct variety, and termed herpes *pudendalis*.

Herpes Zoster—Ζωστήρ of Greek authors—from ζώννυμι, to gird; one of the species of Ignis sacer, described by Celsus (Lib. V, cap. 28); called, simply, *Zoster*, by Pliny (*Nat. Hist.*, Lib. XXVI, cap. 11), and *Zona*, or *Zona ignea*, by other Latin writers.—See Plate IV, Fig. 2.

This disease, vernacularly termed "the shingles" (probably from *cingulum*, a belt), has derived its specific name from the peculiar form which the eruption assumes, extending in the course of the anterior branch of the spinal nerves, and resembling, as it were, a girdle or sword-belt. The constitutional and local symptoms are more severe than in the variety last described, the former often amounting to a well-marked fever preceding the outbreak of the disease, attended with a distinct shivering fit and vomiting. Locally there are sharp stinging pains, burning heat, redness, and some tumefaction of the integuments in the part on which the vesicles are about to appear; these occur of tolerable magnitude, and closely grouped together in three or four distinct but neighboring patches, each surrounded by an inflammatory areola, which gradually spreads, new vesicles appearing on it, and the entire constitutes a crescentic or oblique demi-zone from half an inch to one or two inches in breadth, seated on one side of the neck or trunk, often extending from mesial line to mesial line, by which it seems to be distinctly bounded, very rarely passing its limits. The eruption runs the same course as in herpes phlyctenodes, but the vesicles become more confluent, thus often attaining the magnitude of bullæ, those which first appear being always the largest; and it is somewhat more chronic in all its stages, the scabs being often particularly slow in separating.

Most authorities are now agreed that this disease is due to a nervous origin. Von Bärensprung believes that it proceeds from an irritation of the spinal ganglia, and that the posterior roots are implicated.—See *Ranking's Abstract*, XLI, 123. Heller states that the urine is alkaline, and has chlorides, phosphates, and ammonia in excess, sulphates and uric acid in diminished quantity, together with the presence of fat and oxalate of lime.

The local pain which precedes the appearance of the eruption in herpes zoster is not unfrequently very severe and apparently deep-seated, seeming to shoot through the chest or abdomen if the disease is about to occur on the integuments of either of these regions. This pain, which to a great extent disappears when the vesicles are developed, usually returns with greater or less intensity, especially in adults or old people, when the crust falls off, sometimes lasting even for years, and causing great suffering. At times chronic ulceration succeeds this form of herpes in bad constitutions, and this may terminate even in gangrene, and thus prove fatal. Mr. Hutchinson, in his observations before the Hunterian Medical Society, on 25th February, 1863, has concluded that it rarely occurs twice in a lifetime.

The usual seat of herpes zoster is on the thorax or abdomen; it also appears occasionally on the neck; when the eruption commences over the scapula, or in the neighborhood of the hip, it may extend to the shoulder or thigh, including either in the semicircle which it forms, but it very rarely originates on the extremities. By Franck and Cazenave the disease is stated to appear more frequently on the right side of the body, but Dr. Neligan's experience agrees with that of Reil and Wilson, that it is situated on the left in the greater number of cases. Dr. Tilbury Fox (*op. cit.*, p. 110) says, that "of 178 cases collected by Bärensprung, in 101 the herpes was on the right side, in 77 on the left. Mr. Hutchinson's observations are confirmatory." It is so extremely rare for the demi-zone of herpes to pass the median line, that among the ancients, particularly among the Greeks and Arabians, it was popularly believed, and the fact is mentioned by Pliny, that if the eruption surrounded the body it should prove necessarily fatal;[1] yet ~~cases are~~ corded by modern writers—Franck and others—in wl such took place by the simultaneous development of eruption on both sides and their extremities meeting, the patients recovered. In Lorry's quarto volume, *Morbis Cutaneis*, published at Paris, in 1777, the aut says (p. 405) he never saw it to be fatal (eam nunqi lethalem vidi), save in phthisical persons.

Herpes *circinatus*.—From *circino*, I go round (and from Κίρκινος, a pair of compasses), circular tetter, *An*, RINGWORM—Formica ambulatoria of Celsus, Ann herpétique of the French.—Plate IV, Fig. 3.

Herpes circinatus (*Ringworm*), like the last descri variety, derives its name from the shape of the gro in which the eruption appears, namely, distinct ring circles, inclosing healthy skin in the centre. Sli pricking sensation or tingling accompanies the outbr of the disease, but it is not attended with any consi tional symptoms. At first one or more small, red, ci lar patches, from half an inch to an inch in diame appear apart from each other on some portion of integuments, on the outer border of which numer minute, globular, transparent vesicles are developed the second or third day; the redness then fades from centre of each circle, which remains unaffected afterwi during the progress of the disease, but the ring of v cles has an inflammatory border both external and in nal. The vesicles, which are closely aggregated, bec more or less confluent within forty-eight hours after t appearance, assume a pearly aspect, and then burst discharge a small quantity of a serous fluid, which d into thin brownish crusts that fall off on the eightl ninth day, to be succeeded by a fine epidermic desc mation that lasts for some time. The disease, howe rarely terminates thus, but is prolonged by the repei eruption of fresh crops of vesicles on the outer infl matory border, each set running an independent cou but one similar to the first; spreading in this man from the circumference, the rings at times attain the

---

[1] "Zoster appellatur, ut enecat, si cinxerit."—*Nat. Hist.*, supra.

of the palm of the hand, which they rarely exceed. The
circles may be few or many in number, rarely, however,
more than four or five, and when of larger size there is
usually but one; they may appear simultaneously on
the surface or in succession: in the latter case the disease
often becomes chronic, lasting for months.

Occasionally it occurs that the vesicles, instead of bursting and forming crusts, dry up, and are succeeded by a
secretion of fine, soft scales, which continue to be exfoliated, not alone from the circumference, but from the
centre of the circles. This form has been specially described by Cazenave, who denominates it herpes *squamosus* (Plate IV, Fig. 5); it is always chronic, and very
obstinate to treatment.

Herpes circinatus occurs with greatest frequency on
the face, neck, and scalp, being, however, occasionally
situated on the chest, the shoulders, the arms, and the
hands. When it appears on the face its most usual
situations are the cheeks and the forehead; as the circles
spread from their circumference they often extend from
the former to the nose, but do not pass the mesial line,
and from the latter into the scalp. In its milder forms
ringworm disappears in eight or ten days, but its duration is more usually prolonged for three or four weeks,
either by the spreading of the circles or by the successive
development of fresh patches of the eruption; occasionally, as above remarked, it becomes chronic, and lasts
for months, producing annoyance more from the unsightliness of its appearance, when it is situated on any of the
exposed regions of the skin, than from any local uneasiness.

This form of herpes, otherwise known and described
as Porrigo scutulata, Tinea tonsurans, Tinea capitis, and
Trichosis capitis, when it occurs on the scalp, requires to
be specially described, as it constitutes almost a distinct
variety, which might be termed herpes *capitis;* it resembles in many of its characteristics the herpes squamosus
of Cazenave; but that distinguished dermatologist, in
consequence of the effect its presence exerts on the hair,
proposes to term it herpes *tonsurans.* Its occurrence on
the scalp at all is denied by many of the celebrated Eng

...with writers on diseases of the skin, who regard the eruption about to be described as a species of porrigo; but prolonged... observation, independent of their corroboration by so deservedly high an authority as M. Cazenave, has satisfied... to convince me of the correctness of the views I propounded some years since.[2]

Herpes ... *Plate IV. Fig. 6* ... usually attacks children from the age of 8 to 12. It is very rare in early infancy, and I have never met with it after the age of puberty, except in the instance in which it had commenced at the age of 18, and had lasted for more than five years before I saw the case. It is very rarely witnessed in its first stage—that of vesicle—as it then produces but little annoyance, and advice is consequently not sought for until it becomes more developed. When seen, however, at its commencement it presents the appearance of a small ring of minute vesicles, not more than an eighth of an inch in diameter, without any redness or other mark of inflammation beyond a slight tinging—not itching. These vesicles are attended with scarcely any discharge, soon drying up and desquamating; but as they dry up in the centre they spread from the circumference, and the diseased spots, in the course of a few days, attain the size of a shilling. When we examine them in this stage, the centre, the part where the eruption first appeared, is thickened, elevated above the surface of the surrounding scalp, and covered with fine scales, which are renewed rapidly on being removed. As the disease proceeds, the patches extend from their periphery, still retaining a perfectly circular shape, and, finally, after some weeks, attain the size of a crown-piece, which they rarely exceed, no matter how chronic the case may have been. Having attained this size, and ceased to spread, the entire of the diseased surface is thickened, elevated, and covered with fine, soft scales, which the

---

[1] It is called Porrigo scutulata by Bateman, and after him by Thomson, Burgess, and others. It is called Trichosis tonsurans by Wilson, and Tinea tonsurans by Fox, and most of the moderns, who regard it as a parasitic affection. See also Dr. Moore's Papers in *Dub. Hosp. Gaz.*, 1859, pp. 35 and 117.

[2] *Dublin Quarterly Journal of Medical Science*, N. S., Vol. vi. p. 33.

least touch removes: this, the advanced stage of the disease, is usually attended with much itching. Sometimes but one patch of herpes is found on the scalp, but more generally there are three, four, or more circles, distinct, and at some distance from each other.

As the disease advances, the hair assumes a very peculiar appearance, almost pathognomonic of this form of eruption of the scalp. In the early stage each hair appears to be slightly bent on itself, and turned against the grain, obstinately refusing to lie smooth; the roots are also somewhat matted together by the scaly crusts of the eruption. After some time it presents a diseased appearance, being twisted, broken, of a whitish color, and readily falling out; so that bald patches begin to appear, over which are scattered small bundles of the altered hair, which has been described, not inaptly, as resembling tow. This condition of the hair has induced some writers to describe the affection as a disease not of the scalp, but of the hair itself.

The eruption does not always present the exact characters now described. In the early stage—when, however, it is rarely witnessed by the medical practitioner—its appearance always agrees with the description given, except that in some cases there is more inflammation than in others; but in the advanced stages it varies much, both as regards the amount of desquamation and the appearance of the elevated patches: it is this fact which has led to so much confusion in the diagnosis and nomenclature of the disease. Yet in the most chronic or complicated cases, the circular form of the eruption, and the peculiar condition of the hair, render its diagnosis easy to even the tolerably experienced eye.

Bateman included this disease—by him termed porrigo scutulata—among the pustulæ; it has also been considered tuberculous, vesicular—as in this chapter—and parasitic.

Mr. Wilson believes it to be a disease of nutritive debility, and he calls the morbid result "granular or phytiform degeneration." The advocates of the parasitic theory believe the "phytiform" tissue of Mr. Wilson to be a vegetable fungus, which in the present case is called regard it as rather an affection of the hair follicles than of the skin.—See Wilson, Fox, Hillier, &c.

Herpes capitis does not cause baldness; the altered hair falls off the diseased patches, which, when the scales disappear in the progress of cure, are thus left in a bald state; but the hair eventually grows on them again, thereby constituting an essential difference between this affection and alopecia. The disease, unless when seen and properly treated in its early stages, soon becomes chronic and obstinate, and loses its inflammatory character. No constitutional symptoms either precede or accompany herpes of the scalp.

In some very rare cases the eruption in herpes circinatus assumes a singular arrangement, which, in the opinion of some dermatologists, entitles it to be considered as a distinct variety, receiving the appellation of herpes *iris*, or *rainbow ringworm* (Plate IV, Fig. 4). A small, round, inflammatory patch appears on some part of the cutaneous surface, and around it, but separated by a narrow band of healthy integument of the natural color, is a red slightly elevated circle, which in its turn is again surrounded by two or three other similar rings of inflamed skin; on the centre a few minute herpetic vesicles are developed in about twenty-four hours after its appearance, as also on each of the rings, but they are more numerous and more closely aggregated on them. The rings, which are usually four in number, differ in color, the inner one being of a darker red than the central patch, that next to it of a slighter shade, the third darker even than the first, and the outer ring paler than the second, being of a yellowish-red hue, fading at its outer border into the color of the surrounding skin.

The vesicles run the same course as in the milder form of herpes phlyctenodes, the crusts, which are small and thin, falling off on the eighth or ninth day, to be followed by slight furfuraceous desquamation, which lasts for a few days longer. Herpes iris seldom occurs except in very young children and in females; it usually appears on the backs of the fingers or of the hands, on the temples, and on the prominent parts of the joints, being sometimes associated with other forms of the eruption. It may occur singly, or several patches may appear simultaneously on different parts of the body; the only local symptoms are some trifling heat and itching, and it has no tendency to become chronic.

Causes.—Herpes is a disease almost entirely confined to young persons and to those in the prime of life, very rarely appearing in the old; among adults it affects females more commonly than males, but in children sex seems to have no influence in the frequency of its occurrence, those of a sanguine and lymphatic temperament, and in whom the skin is fine and soft, being most liable to it. Of the exciting causes of herpes phlyctenodes but little is known; it seems to be occasionally developed under the influence of strong mental emotions, and it is often connected with deranged conditions of the digestive and biliary organs. The season of the year, too, appears to have some influence on its occurrence, for it is most frequently met with in the spring and autumn. The connection of herpes labialis with febrile states of the system is usually very evident, and especially with those which affect the respiratory organs: thus it is an almost invariable accompaniment of catarrh, influenza, bronchitis, and pneumonia, in all of which its occurrence is a favorable symptom, whence has arisen the popular expression that the cold goes off in this way. It is also occasioned very frequently in travelling, by the direct effect of a harsh cold wind on the lips, or of the sun's rays; the action of local irritants, too, may produce herpes here, as is often witnessed in its being caused on the upper lip by the acrid secretions from the nostrils in coryza; this discharge, however, more frequently produces an eruption of eczema.

Herpes *præputialis* occurs only in adults, and most frequently in those in whom the skin of the prepuce is very sensitive; it is often caused there by the friction of the clothes. and when it appears on the mucous membrane. or on the glans penis. where I have occasionally seen it, by the irritation of the natural sebaceous secretion of the part. allowed to accumulate from want of attention to cleanliness. The connection between the occurrence of herpes on the prepuce and stricture of the urethra is very generally admitted, but many observers believe it to be only an accidental coincidence; others, with whom I agree. consider the existence of stricture to be a cause of this eruption. and the manner in which it acts may, I think, be easily explained. In persons affected with stricture. the last drops of urine are retained for some time in the urethra. the shirt is thus constantly wet, and the prepuce is irritated by the acrid moisture to which it is thereby so constantly exposed; hence also, in these cases. the eruption is usually seated on the verge of this fold of integument. In females herpes of the pudendum may occur at any age: it is invariably caused by local irritation.

Herpes *zoster* appears in adults more frequently than any of the other varieties. occurring also occasionally in old persons, in whom it sometimes becomes chronic, and terminates in troublesome ulceration: it seems to be generally occasioned by cold. acting on individuals suffering from hepatic derangements. In the summer and autumn of some years it would appear to be epidemic among children, and in them it is very frequently produced by sudden suppression of the perspiration.

Herpes *circinatus* is a disease of youth, being very rare amongst adults. and occurs with equal frequency in both sexes; it is very common in schools, or wherever many children are congregated together, amongst whom it spreads rapidly. The popular idea that ringworm is contagious is opposed by most English dermatologists on the grounds that no other form of herpes is so, and that the disease cannot be produced by inoculation. Now, neither of these reasons is sufficient to counteract, in my mind, the amount of direct evidence which an experience of some years in the treatment of diseases of the skin has afforded me of the propagation of this form of herpes by contagion, no matter on what part of the body it may be situated. I have elsewhere[1] published cases illustrative of the development of the eruption on the hands of adults engaged in the application of local remedies to the scalp of children who were affected with it, and to these I could now add several others; and I have seen too many instances of its direct communication from child to child of *different* families, when the argument of similarity of constitution and of dietetic arrangements could not avail, to have any doubt on the matter; but it must be remembered that, like all other contagious diseases, some families and some children are more prone to its attacks than others. My own opinion, too, is confirmed by that of M. Cazenave, who, in his *Leçons sur les Maladies de la Peau*, and in his more recently published *Traité des Maladies du Cuir Chevelu*,[2] adduces several cases from his own practice which exhibit in a marked degree the contagious nature of herpes circinatus.

Diagnosis.—The characters of the eruption in herpes are so well defined that, unless when it occurs on the scalp, it can scarcely be confounded with any other cutaneous disease. It differs from eczema *in the vesicles being larger, more globular, and distributed in patches; its eruption is unattended with constitutional symptoms, and in its advanced stages it is not accompanied by the copious serous exudation of that disease.* When the vesicles are very confluent it may be mistaken for pemphigus, but in that affection the eruption consists of bullæ, which do not in any of their stages present the pearly aspect of herpes, and are succeeded by hard, dark-brown crusts; the bullæ of pemphigus, moreover, are usually solitary and scattered over the cutaneous surface, not distributed in groups. Herpes labialis is diagnosed by the characteristic vesicles, and by their local situation. As already remarked, the serious error may be committed of confounding herpes præputialis with chancre; if the eruption is seen on its first appearance it is readily diagnosed by its vesicular character, but when the scab is formed, or

[1] *Dublin Quarterly Journal of Medical Science*, New Series, Vol. viii, p. 164, Note.
[2] Paris, 1850, p. 197. See also *Annales des Maladies de la Peau et de la Syphilis*, Tom. i, p. 37, *et seq.*

ulceration caused by irritation, the diagnosis is often not
unattended with difficulty. The ulceration in herpes, however. is always superficial, never deep, and presents a
smooth surface without raised edges and not coated with
a white, filmy membrane, appearances peculiar to chancre;
in very doubtful cases the question may with certainty
be decided by inoculating the integuments of the thigh
of the patient with some of the matter from the diseased
surface.   The same remarks, as regards diagnosis, apply
equally to herpes of the pudendum in females.   Erythema circinatum, or lichen circumscriptus, in their
advanced stages present some resemblance to herpes
circinatus, but neither of these are vesicular during any
period of their presence on the skin, nor do they spread
from their circumference in the manner that disease
does; they are, too, attended, with more thickening and
elevation of the integuments on which they are situated.
Herpes capitis, which corresponds with the herpes tonsurans of Cazenave, is, as I have already remarked,
described by many English writers as a variety of
porrigo, the yellow, cup-shaped, favus crusts so characteristic of which it, however, never presents.   It is diagnosed from the other eruptive diseases of the scalp by
its occurring in distinct circular patches, the slight serous
discharge from which dries into fine soft scales, that are
readily detached by the slightest touch, but are again
very quickly renewed, and especially by the peculiar
change, before described, which it produces on the hair.

The *prognosis* in any form of herpes is favorable, as
the eruption may be said almost never to endanger life,
and is but very rarely productive of any injury to the
general health; it is also not so liable as many other
eruptions to become chronic, unless when it occurs on
the scalp.   The local neuralgic pain, which not unfrequently is consequent on herpes phlyctenodes and herpes
zoster, is at times both severe and obstinate, often lasting
for many months.

Treatment.—The phlyctenoid form of the disease very
rarely requires any active constitutional remedies; in a
few cases, when it occurs in young persons of a full
habit of body, bleeding from the arm, or the application

of leeches in the neighborhood of the eruption, is attended with benefit, but neither should be had recourse to until the eruption is fully developed:[1] saline purgatives—preceded, if there is any biliary derangement, by a mild mercurial, five grains of blue pill, or two of calomel combined with a grain of extract of hyoscyamus—will, however, in nearly all cases, sufficiently meet the constitutional symptoms. In weakly individuals, tonics with antacids—as bark with the carbonate of ammonia—are indicated. With reference to local treatment, all that is requisite during the first two or three days after the formation of the vesicles is to protect them from being irritated by rubbing or scratching; unless there is much tingling and pain of the part, which will be relieved by smearing them over with a cerate consisting of two grains of acetate of zinc, an ounce of cold cream, and four minims of chloroform. Should there be any tendency to a copious discharge, finely powdered lapis calaminaris or starch will be dusted over the surface with benefit. As soon as the brown scabs form, a spirituous lotion, such as the following, should be substituted for the ointment:—

R. Olei Limonum, ... minima sex.
   Olei Corticis Aurantii, ... semi drachmam.
   Spiritus Vini rectificati, ... uncias quatuor.
   Aquæ Camphoræ, ... uncias octo. Misce.

The local pain consequent on this form of herpes or on herpes zoster is, as far as my experience enables me to come to a conclusion, but little relieved by external applications; those usually ordered for it are narcotics and sedatives; such as preparations of opium, of aconite, of belladonna, of arnica, &c. Regarding it as being chiefly neuralgic, I have prescribed with much benefit a combination of bark with hemlock, as thus:—

R. Tincturæ Cinchonæ compositæ, . . drachmas duas.
   Succi Conii, ... drachmas sex.
   Infusi Cinchonæ Flavæ, ... uncias septem. Misce.
     Sumat cochleare magnum quadrate indies.

---

[1] The Editor cannot concur in the propriety of bleeding from the

In herpes *labialis*, if a strong spirituous lotion—I
found none answer so well as *Eau de Cologne*—b
stantly applied to the part on which it is about to a
as indicated by dryness, heat, swelling, and tinglin
fore the vesicles are formed, the further progress
eruption may in most cases be arrested.

The only local application requisite, where the d
is fully developed, is some mild oleaginous oint
such as the cucumber cerate; should it, however, b
chronic, an ointment composed of ten grains of ca
to an ounce of simple cerate will be found useful.
sons who have once had an attack of herpes præpi
are fully aware of the premonitory local symptom
which it is ushered in; the development of the eru
may then be stayed by the continued employment o
water, the colder the better, which can be applie
plunging the penis several times in the day into ic
water, and retaining it there for a minute or two;
the vesicles are formed, no caustics or irritants shou
employed, as their use is apt to be followed by tr
some ulceration; the best local application is the
wash, or Turner's cerate if there is much discharge
the vesicles have burst.

The same treatment is adapted for herpes zoster
the phlyctenoid form of the disease. M. Cazenave, wi
view of preventing the premature rupture of the ve
recommends that the surface should be smeared wit
and then dusted with starch. The *ectrotic* plan of
ment, that is to say, opening each of the vesicles
needle, and introducing into them a finely pointed
of nitrate of silver, has been recommended in both
varieties of the eruption. If they are situated on a
exposed part of the body, and not in any way conr
with visceral derangements, it may be had recour
but it should be remembered *that an indelible mark*
times follows the application of caustic to herpes.

Most cases of ringworm require no treatment i
commencement except the use of mild mercurial p
tives, and protection of the eruption from local irrit
if, however, there is much heat or tingling in the
poultices prepared with bread and the weak lead

(see page 116) are productive of much benefit; when the scales have formed, the ointment of cold cream and acetate of zinc (see page 55) will be found an excellent application. If the disease become chronic, constitutional treatment is generally required for its removal, and preparations of iodine, with or without tonics, according to individual circumstances, are usually the most efficacious; as regards local applications, astringent ointments and alkaline lotions prove in most cases successful; thus an ointment consisting of four grains of the dried sulphate of iron, an ounce of white wax ointment, and a drachm of glycerine, should be smeared over the eruption three times a day, it having been previously sponged well each time with a lotion containing ten grains of the carbonate of potash in twelve fluidounces of rose-water; or, in very chronic cases, a dilute citrine ointment, containing from one to two drachms of *brown* citrine ointment (unguentum hydrargyri nitratis) to the ounce of prepared lead, may be substituted for that of the sulphate of iron. When herpes circinatus is inclined to spread rapidly, the progress of the eruption may be sometimes stayed by the application of strips of blistering plaster around the outer border of the rings, at a short distance from the inflamed surface; their effect seems to depend on a new action being excited in the part. The application of vesicating collodion will in like manner prove useful. In herpes of the scalp the same local applications will be requisite as when it occurs on other parts of the body, but the hair should be kept cut close with a pair of scissors during the entire progress of the treatment, and for at least three or four weeks afterwards; nor is it sufficient to cut the hair on the diseased parts solely, but it must be removed from the entire scalp, as otherwise the eruption is apt to appear in other patches on it. In herpes capitis in children, the green iodide of mercury, prescribed as recommended for eczema of the scalp, has proved in my experience the best alterative remedy. M. Bazin recommends an ointment of equal parts of lime and carbonate of soda to 30 of such parts of lard; and if the hairs are removed, an application to the hair follicles of one of the following forms:—

symptoms are succeeded on the second
the appearance of few or many bright sp
generally over the thighs and lower par
which are attended with heat and itcl
rapidly enlarge, and a minute, transpar
veloped in their centre, which in a few
as nearly to cover the previously inflam
ument, a border being left which forms
The bullæ thus constituted are round or
flattened at the summit, of a shining
being irregularly distributed, resemble
would be produced if boiling water wi
skin; on the day after their appearance tl
assumes a yellowish opaque aspect, and i
hours the bullæ usually break, giving ex
discharge, which continues to be secrete
longer, the surface thus exposed being
ated; the discharge then accretes into a t
lowish color, and a foliaceous aspect, wh
the sixth or seventh day from the first a
eruption, is succeeded by a slight epid
tion and yellowish stain of the surface;
from the tenth to the fourteenth day, bi
lasts for an indefinite period. In the a
phigus the eruption may occur in a sing
are more usually two or three in succes
of from twenty-four to forty-eight hours
them; and as each set of bullæ runs a si
duration of the disease is then prolonge
weeks. Two or more bullæ being oc
oped close to each other become confi
very large vesification is often formed.
inflammatory patches, on the other hand
urs, when, however, th
l a serous exudation

ntoms always abat
and the local hea
the appearance of
ed by their return
the bullæ is absorl

not break, and the disease terminates with epidermic desquamation, while in others superficial ulceration occurs, and then its duration is more prolonged, and indelible marks are often left on the skin.

Willan termed the disease *Pompholyx benignus*, when the premonitory fever was very mild, and the local inflammation trifling. He also described a very rare form of the eruption under the name, *Pompholyx solitarius;* in it "large vesifications arise on some part of the body, one after another, at nearly equal intervals of time; a disagreeable tingling is felt for several hours before the vesication arises, which is usually in the night. It enlarges rapidly, so as sometimes to contain on the following day a teacupful of lymph. Within forty-eight hours the cuticle breaks, the lymph is discharged, and a superficial ulceration remains. Near this another vesication arises in a day or two, and goes through the same process as the first. A third, fourth, fifth, and sixth vesication will sometimes appear, and proceed in like manner." This singular variety of pemphigus seems to affect women solely; it is extremely rare, yet Willan mentions that he witnessed three cases of it; Cazenave states that he saw one remarkable instance; and Copland records its occurrence under his observation in a man.

The most usual site of acute pemphigus has been already indicated, namely, on the thighs and lower part of the abdomen, but it may affect the arms, the backs of the hands, the legs, and the thorax; it has been also witnessed on the mucous membrane of the mouth and tongue.[1] It most usually occurs in adult life; but infants and children are not unfrequently attacked; and a variety has been specially described by some dermatologists under the denomination of pemphigus *infantilis*.

This corresponds with the form so admirably depicted by the late Dr. Whitley Stokes,[2] as being not uncommon in Ireland, and which he termed Pemphigus *gangrænosus*

---

[1] See Chausit, *Traité Elémentaire des Maladies de la Peau* (p. 95). Paris, 1853.

[2] *Dublin Medical and Physical Essays*, Vol. i, p. 146 : Dublin, 1808.

appended what Dr. Neligan termed a "graphic illustration" of the case which he afterwards transferred to his *Atlas of Cutaneous Diseases* (Plate V, Fig. 3).

Authorities are about equally divided as to the alleged syphilitic nature of this disease. On the affirmative side are found Paul Dubois, Devergie, Cazenave, Ricord, Dugés, Diday, Wichman, and Jörg: on the negative Krauss, Barnes, Cazeaux, Bazin, and Hardy. Fox believes that when it occurs on the general surface it is non-syphilitic; but on the hands and feet, when accompanied by ulceration, marasmus, and syphilitic history of the parents, "it is probably specific." See his *résumé* of the adverse statement at p. 118 of his work, from which the above is condensed.

Pemphigus *chronicus* (Plate V, Fig. 2) is of more frequent occurrence than the acute form of the eruption, and sometimes appears as an epidemic; of this a remarkable example is recorded by Dr. McBride, who witnessed it in the county of Wicklow in 1766. The disease, which corresponds with the *Pompholyx diutinus* of Willan, is not attended with any febrile symptoms, yet the outbreak of the eruption is preceded for some days by sickness, debility, and muscular pains. Red spots, as in the acute form, appear scattered over the skin, but the redness is of a livid color, and is not accompanied by heat or itching; on these spots the bullæ are rapidly developed, each bulla covering completely the reddened surface, so that to the naked eye they appear to have no areola, but when examined with a lens, a narrow red line will be seen to surround each. The vesications, which generally attain their maximum size in a single night, are much larger than in the acute form, and rarely become confluent; they come out almost invariably in successive eruptions, a second crop sometimes not appearing until the one which preceded it has completely disappeared from the surface, and thus the disease may be indefinitely prolonged.

The bullæ are irregularly globular, somewhat flattened at the summit, and contain a citrine-yellow, semi-transparent, serous fluid—in old persons or in broken-down constitutions the fluid is generally sanguinolent in some

13

cutaneous diseases, especially with prurigo or scabies, in either of which cases the sufferings it occasions almost baffle description.

The *causes* of pemphigus are more or less connected with constitutional derangements; the chronic form in particular rarely occurring except in persons who have been debilitated by distress, and by insufficient or bad diet, or in those who suffer from some chronic visceral disease, of which it seems at times to be symptomatic. Acute pemphigus is most frequent in children and young persons, infants even not being exempt from it, appearing rarely in adults or in the old; while chronic pemphigus is a disease of advanced life. The eruption is occasionally developed in children after a continued exposure to the heat of the sun; but it much more frequently seems to depend on the effects of moisture, most of those at any age who are attacked with it being persons who had lived in damp situations; this fact is well established in the country districts of Ireland, where it is most prevalent among the peasantry who dwell in mountainous districts, much rain falling there, and the hills being constantly enveloped in mists. The occurrence of the disease as an epidemic has been already adverted to; some of the ancient medical writers regarded it as being contagious; and Willan, by describing a variety of it under the name Pemphigus *contagiosus*, tended to perpetuate this erroneous view, one, too, which was contrary to his own opinion.

The *diagnosis* of pemphigus, whether acute or chronic, is, in most cases, unattended with difficulty. Although the bullæ resemble somewhat the vesications which occasionally accompany erysipelas, they are never situated on a diffusely inflamed portion of the skin, as occurs in that disease, nor are they attended with the constitutional fever. The diagnostic marks between pemphigus and herpes have been given in the description of that eruption. Rupia differs from pemphigus in there being in it a broad inflammatory areola to each bulla when it is first developed, and in the peculiar appearance of the resulting scab or crust. The foliaceous form of chronic pemphigus might be mistaken for psoriasis, but the scales in the latter desquamate more freely, are smaller, of a silvery whiteness, and are never preceded by an eruption of bullæ, nor attended with a serous discharge.

Prognosis.—Pemphigus in any of its forms is not unattended with danger, notwithstanding Willan termed one variety of it *Pompholyx benignus.* The chief apprehensions in the acute form are, the liability to relapse when it appears in children, or about the age of puberty; and, at an earlier age, that it may assume the characters of the pemphigus gangrænosus of Stokes. The chronic form is always a most dangerous disease, few old persons recovering from an attack of it. The more acute the symptoms, and the more inflammatory the constitutional disturbance, the more favorable the prognosis.

As regards the *pathology* of pemphigus, it is manifestly an atonic inflammation of the superficial layers of the derma, which terminates in serous effusion; the fluid contained in the bullæ is highly albuminous, becoming nearly solid when exposed to heat.

Dr. Fox states the fluid to be alkaline; adding, that Scherer (*vide Simon's Animal Chemistry*) declares it to be acid; that Professor Malmsten detected uric acid in it, while Bamberger thought the disease was due to an "ammoniacal dyscrasia." From the statements of several authorities, he concludes "that the urine is deficient in amount, of high specific gravity, very acid, and contains a large amount of urea, but is deficient in the earthy salts."—*Op. cit.*, p. 120.

Treatment.—The acute forms of this eruption demand but little medical interference—the accompanying fever being rarely such as to require any active antiphlogistics; should it, however, continue after the bullæ are fully developed, or inflammatory symptoms then appear, a small abstraction of blood from the arm may be requisite [? ED.]: but in the majority of cases, rest in bed, diluent drinks, reduced diet, and mild saline purgatives will suffice. The vesications should be as much as possible protected from local irritation, and, above all, from being prematurely ruptured; with this view they may be dusted over with flour or starch; as soon as they have burst they may be dressed with some simple ointment, such as the cucumber or acetate of zinc cerate, or collodion may be applied over them. When acute pemphigus presents the characters described by Dr. Whitley Stokes, all debilitating plans of treatment must be carefully avoided, good nourishing diet should be given in abundant quantity, the air be at once changed, and powdered bark, with minute doses of the pulvis cretæ aromaticus cum opio and of the hydrargyrum cum cretâ, administered internally. On the suggestion of Dr. Stokes, an ointment prepared with lard and the leaves of the common figwort, *Scrophularia nodosa*, was used as a local application in this form of pemphigus; he states that he derived his knowledge of its beneficial action from an inquiry into the applications which were popularly employed with success in the country districts of Ireland, in all of which he found that the leaves of this indigenous plant formed a principal ingredient; at his recommendation it was originally introduced into the *Dublin Pharmacopœia*, from the last edition of which, however, it was omitted. It was, in fact, but a mild astringent ointment, and its chief efficacy probably depended on the protection from the action of the air which it afforded; a weak cerate of tannic acid—two grains to the ounce of white wax ointment—melted, and applied to the surface with a camel-hair pencil, just as it is again about to become concrete, will be beneficially substituted for it.

In chronic pemphigus the chief indications are to allay both the local and constitutional irritation, and to support the strength; attention must also be directed to any visceral disease of which it may be symptomatic, or with which it may be complicated. I have experienced very great benefit in its treatment from the free use of opiates, which may be given, combined with bark, as in the following form :—

R. Liquoris Opii Sedativi, . . . minima decem.
Tincturæ Cinchonæ Compositæ, . minima quindecem.
Aquæ Camphoræ . . . . . unciam. Misce
Fiat haustus statim sumendus: repatur idem sextis-horis.

To allay the local irritation, the parts may be covered with raw cotton or dusted with starch; or, if the itching

and pain are very severe, they may be dr███████
on which has been spread the compound ███████
to every ounce of which a fluidrachm of glyc████
been added. By some it has been proposed to ████
bullæ as soon as they appear, and to apply to the ███
thus exposed a solution of nitrate of silver, conta███
scruple of the salt to an ounce of distilled water; inst█
of the solution, Dr. Graves proposed to employ the so
nitrate for this purpose, and mentioned a case in wh
its use was attended with complete success;[1] the practi
however, is only admissible when the eruption is of sm
extent, and not connected with constitutional deran
ment. In very obstinate cases arsenical preparations a
iodide of potassium are occasionally employed with b
efit. Wine and generous diet should be allowed in
cases of chronic pemphigus, and change of air (to a di
locality) enforced, if possible. When diarrhœa or dr
sical symptoms occur in the course of the disease, th
are to be treated on the ordinary principles. See ca
of Pemphigus Gangrænosus and Pompholyx Diutin
in Dr. William Moore's paper "On Some of the Mo
Aggravated Forms of Diseases of the Skin" (*Dub. Ho
Gaz.*, 1850, p. 35); also papers by Dr. James Russell,
Birmingham, in *The Medical Times and Gazette*, Oct.
1864, and Oct. 21, 1865.

RUPIA.

RUPIA (from Ρυπος, sordes, see Plate V) is characteriz
by the eruption of distinctly-separated and dispersed fl
tened bullæ, of the size of a small nut, on an inflamed ba
terminating in elevated dark-brown crusts, which, falli
off, are succeeded by atonic ulcers. The bullæ, whi
in most cases are not preceded by either local or cons
tutional inflammation, contain from the first a ser
opaque or ichorous fluid, which appears not to diste
them completely; this fluid rapidly becomes sero-pu
lent and more consistent, and the epidermic covering

---

[1] *Clinical Medicine*, Second Edition, Vol. ii, p. 354; and Repr
from Second Edition (1864), p. 709.

the bullæ, giving way usually on the second or third day, accretes into a wrinkled scab, more prominent in the centre than at the circumference. These varieties of rupia are in general described by dermatologists, but the third of these, rupia *escharotica*, as has been already mentioned when describing pemphigus, is a form of that eruption, being the pemphigus gangrænosus of Dr. Whitley Stokes—two forms, therefore, only remain to be considered here:—

Rupia simplex.
" prominens.

In *Rupia simplex* (Plate V, Fig. 4) the bullæ are but few in number, often not more than two or three, and situated remotely from each other; the inflammatory areola is narrow, and scarcely raised above the level of the surrounding integument, and the crusts, which are of a dark-brown color, only slightly elevated in the centre. The resulting ulceration is superficial, and scabs cover it in a few days; these scabs, which are wrinkled and raised at the edges, fall off and are renewed several times for from one to two or three weeks, when the surface heals, a livid stain, which does not disappear for some time, remaining on the part. The duration of the disease until the falling off of the scabs is, as above remarked, from two to three weeks, unless, as occasionally occurs, it is prolonged by the formation of new bullæ at the time those first developed are about to disappear. In some rare cases a slight degree of fever precedes the appearance of the eruption, and superficial redness, as in pemphigus, marks the spot on which each bulla is about to form

Rupia prominens (Plate V, Fig. 5) is so named from the characteristic appearance of the crusts or scabs which are formed in it. The bullæ are of larger size than in rupia simplex, the patches of the cutaneous surface on which they occur are previously swollen and of a dark red color, and the contained fluid, which is often ichorous or sanguinolent, sometimes as dark as chocolate, rapidly thickens and dries into a hard, wrinkled, blackish crust, surrounded by a swollen, inflamed border. From the

inner edge of this inflamed areola, unhealthy pus is secreted, which, concreting, forms additional crusts; these,
pressing on the original scabs, already somewhat raised
in the centre and corrugated, force them still more forward until they eventually attain such a prominence that
they bear an extraordinary resemblance to the shell of a
limpet, or in some cases—spreading from their circumference until they cover the entire of the inflamed border
by which they were surrounded—to the shell of an oyster.
These crusts, which are firmly adherent and slow in falling off, in a few days become somewhat raised at their
outer border, and permit the discharge of unhealthy pus
from the excoriated surface beneath; in the course of a
week or ten days they may be readily detached, or they
fall off spontaneously, when an excavated atonic ulcer,
the depth of which is usually proportioned to the thickness of the scab, is seen to occupy the site of the original
bulla. These ulcers are extremely indolent, pale, and
bleeding on the slightest touch, and either become covered
anew with the characteristic crust, which, however, does
not attain the same degree of prominence as in the first
instance, or, discharging an unhealthy ichorous pus, heal
slowly, leaving dark livid stains on the skin. Rupia pro-
mineus is always a chronic disease, lasting generally for
months, and its duration is often prolonged by successive
eruptions of bullæ.

The usual site of either form of rupia is on the lower
extremities, sometimes on the abdomen, the loins, or
the thorax; but, unless when occurring as a syphilitic
eruption, it is very rarely witnessed on the upper extremities or the face. The disease ma occur at any age,
but it most usually affects children and old persons, being
uncommon in adults.

The *causes* by which it is produced are sufficiently
obscure, but it appears to be connected with a debilitated
state of the constitution, and especially in children with
the scrofulous diathesis. It is also one of the sequelæ of
the eruptive fevers in young persons, and in the old it
not uncommonly occurs at the termination of some prolonged illness, such as fever or dysentery. Rupia is
sometimes complicated with other cutaneous diseases,

more particularly scabies, ecthy
last case the bullæ usually conta

Mr. Erasmus Wilson consider
mineua to be essentially syphiliti
in group XIV of his "Clinical (
head of "Syphilitic Affections."
variety, recognized by him, as
he considers to be the same as
already described.

Diagnosis.—Rupia may be
pemphigus or ecthyma. From
guished, even in its vesicular st
solitary, never confluent, and by
border which surrounds them;
its characteristic prominence se
nosis easy. Ecthyma is an infla
tion, and the resulting scabs a
rupia is distinctly vesicular at i
are large and prominent. The m
be made of mistaking idiopath
which is a much more severe di
different treatment; the latter
areola surrounding the bullæ b
hue; by the bullæ being mucl
covering nearly the entire body,
quently on the face; by there be
the same time, syphilitic sure t
cedent history of the case.

The *prognosis* in rupia is alwa
an obstinate but never a dange
injures the general health, unless
very numerous, and attended wit
a degree of low, irritative feve
presence.

Treatment.—Constitutional rer
relied on in the treatment of rup
adapted to the indications in in
especially preparations of bark
aud nourishing diet, are most us
the disease becomes chronic, hyd
given with benefit in equal parts

bark, of dulcamara, and of mezereon; a
scrofulous children, cod-liver oil shoul
As regards local treatment, it is general
to open bullæ at the earliest opportunity,
if possible, the formation of the crusts;
be covered with pledgets of lint, and sligl
on them, or they may be dusted with st
still preferable, as the chief object is to
collodion may be applied. When the cru
they should be removed as quickly as
been previously softened by the applicat
water, or of linseed-meal poultices; the
first few days, should be treated with wat
which oiled silk is placed; but if they d
position to heal, stimulating ointments o
requisite; of the former, the brown citr
one composed of equal parts of oil of ti
white wax ointment, may be used; or c
be found, as is often the case, that gre
disagree, solutions of the sulphate of copp
of iron, from six to twelve grains of eit
of distilled water, may be employed, lint
being laid on the ulcerated surface. Sor
dermatologists report that they have d
results from ointments of the iodides
drachm of the green or twelve grains of t
to the ounce of lard. By some practitio
mended to touch the ulcer every seeo
with the solid nitrate of silver, but the n
allowed to deliquesce, and then applied
camel-hair brush, will, in very obstinate
more beneficial. It must not be omit
that Rayer states he found the simple pr
the ulcers with finely-powdered cream
successful.

SCABIES.

Scabies, from *scabo;* supposed to l
Greeks; Gale of the French; Kratze o
Anglicè, the Itch; *Scotticè*, the Yuck

Ireland, the Scotch fiddle; Nethek in Leviticus xiii. 30 (Heb.); and θραυσμα by the LXX in the same passage.— See Plate VI.

SCABIES (*Itch*).—No little difficulty has been at all times experienced in classifying scabies; by some it is regarded as being papular, by others pustular, and by many modern dermatologists it has been made to constitute a division of cutaneous diseases of which it is the type—the presence of parasitic animalcules beneath the epidermis being considered by them as a necessary characteristic of the eruption. There can be no doubt but that during the course of the disease pimples and pustules constantly occur on the skin, mingled with the vesicles, and the vesicles themselves assume a purulent aspect in a few days after they are developed, yet on careful observation it will be found that the eruption is at first always distinctly vesicular, and that this character is never completely lost in any stage of the affection. The occurrence of the peculiar itch animalcule is very constant in scabies, and its existence easily demonstrable; but as cases do occur in which even the most experienced observers are unable to detect it, I cannot admit that its presence is necessary to and pathognomonic of the disease.[1] For these reasons, then, and also because the peculiar vesicle of the scabies is highly characteristic, I shall retain it amongst the vesiculæ. It has always been an eruption of much interest to the physician in consequence of its great prevalence, the rapidity with which it spreads by contagion, and the severity of the local symptoms with which it is attended.

The eruption in scabies, the development of which is unaccompanied by constitutional symptoms, is preceded by itching and tingling of the parts on which it is about to appear, usually the backs of the hands, the angles between the fingers, and the flexures of their joints; in about twelve hours afterwards there may be seen developed on them one or more conical vesicles, which rapidly enlarge until they not unfrequently attain the

[1] Wilson, Fox, and most of our modern writers, consider the disease to be dependent upon the presence of the acarus, but most surely it cannot always be found by careful observers.—[EDITOR.]

This insect—the *Acarus scabiei*, or, as it has been also termed, *Sarcoptes hominis*, being constituted into a new genus by Latreille—was discovered and described as existing in scabies in the twelfth century by Avenzoar; but although its presence was evidently known to the Greek and Roman physicians, little notice of it occurs afterwards in medical writings until the middle of the seventeenth century, when an Englishman, Mouffet, left in a posthumous work a singularly full and accurate description of the animalcule, especially as regards its anatomical characters, and in which many of the so called discoveries of modern days are anticipated. In our own times the natural history of the itch animalcule has been especially investigated by the French and German dermatologists, particularly by Renucci, Raspail, Albin-Gras, Hebra, and Bourguignon; amongst English writers Mr. Erasmus Wilson gives a very full account of its habits and structure, and from his observations the following description is condensed.

Examined with the naked eye the acarus scabiei looks white, shining, and globular in form. "There is no difficulty in extracting the little animal; the cuniculus is seen without difficulty; the end of the cuniculus is perceived to be a little raised, while a grayish speck is seen beneath it, as soon as this little eminence of epiderma is lifted, if the end of the needle or pin with which the operation is performed be examined, the minute, white, and shining globe will probably be observed attached to the instrument. If there be no such object, the point of the needle, placed again beneath the raised capsule of epiderma, will pretty certainly draw it forth. This facility of extracting the little creature is due to its great power of clinging to any object with which it comes in contact. When the aearus is seen running upon the surface of a plate of glass it may be perceived that its anterior margin presents a dusky tint of color, and the examination of this part of the creature with the microscope brings into view a head not unlike that of a tortoise, and a pair of large and strong legs on each side of the head. These organs are encased in a moderately thick layer of chytine, and have consequently the reddish-brown tint of the cases of certain insects, or of the bright part of a thin layer of tortoise-shell."[1] The general outline is sub-rotund, it being a very little longer than broad; the ventral surface is flat, and upon it may be seen the head and eight legs; the dorsal aspect is arched and uneven, and covered by numerous spines; and twelve hair-like filaments, some long and others short, project backwards from the posterior segment of the animalcule. Mr. Wilson, from a comparison of the measurements in ten specimens, found them to vary between $\frac{1}{147}$th and $\frac{1}{77}$th of an inch in length, and $\frac{1}{303}$d and $\frac{1}{214}$th in breadth.

This account refers to the female acarus, and with it are generally found some of the ova; the male insect seems to have eluded the research of many investigators; M. Bourguignon, writing in 1847, says, "that he has never found male sexual organs in the acarus, but in every specimen he examined has seen ovaries with the ova, it appearing that connection with a male is not requisite for the reproduction of the animalcule."[2] Gustav Simon, Physician to the Charity Hospital at Berlin, describes the male aearus, in the first edition of

[1] Erasmus Wilson on Diseases of the Skin. Third Edition, p. 499. See also p. 275 of the Fifth Edition of that work (1863); and the very full and recent account in his *Student's Book*, p. 118 (1864).
[2] *Recherches Entomologiques et Pathologiques sur la Gale de l' Homme.* Paris, 1847, p. 8.

14

his *Anatomical Description of Diseases of the Skin*, published in 1848; and in 1851, it was also discovered and described by M. Lanquetin, a pupil of M. Cazenave. It is much more minute than the female, and being always situated on the free surface of the skin, not taking up its abode in a cuniculus, accounts for its existence being overlooked by so many careful investigators.

A full and recent account of the male acarus will be found in Fox (*op. cit.*, p. 247), taken, for the most part, from the researches of Hebra and Hardy; and in Plate XVI of Dr. Neligan's Atlas will be found illustrations of both the male and female insect.

The eruption in scabies is invariably attended with severe itching—whence the name by which the disease is commonly known—this, causing the sufferer from it to scratch and tear the skin with the nails, increases the local inflammation, which already is considerable; fresh vesicles appear, often thickly set on the surface, and mixed with them large papulæ and pustules; a bloody serous and sero-purulent discharge flows from the torn integuments, in which deep fissures are also formed, and the eruption spreads rapidly, in severe cases attacking the lower extremities, the abdomen, and the trunk, as well as the hands and arms, but being very rarely, if ever, witnessed on the face. The sufferings occasioned by the disease are then extreme; sleepless nights are passed often for weeks together, the itching being always much augmented by the warmth of the bed; the constitution, consequently, sympathizes more or less, and in the old or the debilitated, prurigo, ecthyma, or pemphigus complicates the original eruption, rendering it more intractable, and in very aged persons even fatal.

Reference has been made to the "suffering" of the patient; but Mr. Wilson remarks that the pruritus is a kind of tickling itching which is said to be *pleasurable;* and so King James I. seems to have thought from delicious experience—for he is said to have declared "that none but kings and princes should have the itch, for the sensation of scratching was so delightful."—*Student's Book of Cutaneous Medicine*, p. 121. This sensation was not, however, deemed so pleasant by others, for Lorry (*De*

Morbis Cutaneis, p. 225) very graphically describes it as a
" pruritus enormis et scalpendi desiderium immane."

In some cases of scabies the eruption is apparently
altogether papular, but on examination with a lens it
will be found that a minute vesicle surmounts each
papule; from mistaking its true character, Willan and
Bateman termed this form of scabies *papuliformis;* when
the vesicles are perfectly transparent, and with little or
no inflamed base, they denominated the disease scabies
lymphatica; and when the pustular character predomi-
nated, they constituted it a distinct variety, under the
name scabies *purulenta.* The occurrence of the eruption
in broken-down constitutions is not unfreqnent, and its
aspect being then influenced by the physical condition of
the individuals attacked, the same dermatologists arranged
it in a distinct species, which they called scabies *cachectica.*

Causes.—Scabies occurs at all ages, in individuals of
every rank of life, and in all climates, being even more
prevalent in hot countries than in cold, and there it is
also a more severe disease; it is of much more common
occurrence among the poor than among the higher
orders, in consequence evidently of the less frequent
ablutions to which their bodies are subjected, and the
longer period during which their clothes are worn
without being changed, for the eruption is especially a
concomitant of filthy habits. That the spread of the
disease from individual to individual takes place by contagion is undoubted, but that this is the only cause some
have questioned, believing that it may be self-generated
in the system; however, such a doctrine is now nearly
obsolete, and the sole difference of opinion existing on the
matter at present may be said to be as to which is the contagious principle in scabies, the acarus, or the matter of
the eruption. Mr. Erasmus Wilson asserts his belief that
" the vesicle is a provision of nature to protect the derma
from the nearer approach of the *arator,* and the vesicle is
formed with the judgment which usually marks nature's
operations—namely, before a defensive operation would
be too late." Now, how the approach of the insect is to
be prevented by the formation of the vesicle, I must con-

fess I cannot understand; the *sillon*, or track ▉
cuniculus, always terminates in a vesicle, and obse
shows that the development of the vesicle prece
appearance of the animalcule: I therefore think 1
connection between them may be more simply ex
by regarding the *sillon* as being the track of the
in making its way from the vesicle—which he
caused by the irritative inflammation occasioned
deposition from the skin of another person, no
how conveyed, or in the fluid of which it he
hatched—to the cuniculus or burrow, for the pur
depositing its ova. The belief of those, then, who
with that dermatologist is, that scabies, being in a
dependent on and caused by the acarus, can al
propagated by the deposition of this insect, or of l
on the epidermis, and that the secretion from the v
will not of itself reproduce the disease. Direct
ment, however, proves that it may thus be propa
but to this they answer, that when it is so, the
lating matter employed must contain some of the ov
a similar argument is equally applicable to thei
namely, that when the disease has been produced i
viduals by the acarus being placed on the skin, it
be denied that the animalcule conveyed with it so
the characteristic secretion.

Dr. Frazer (*Treatment of Diseases of the Skin*,
doubts that the acarus, which so generally accom
this disease, is the cause of it. He states that it al
in cheese, flour, raw sugar, and other vegetable a
mal substances; and is convinced that it resorts
scabby skin to obtain nitrogenous food. Remarkin
all persons are not equally susceptible, he argues
the acarus be the exciting cause the itch would l
more general than it is. He also observes that the
are not always the same; *e. g.*, in Norway, where a
ent insect is associated with the itch; and states tha
who have once had the disease, obtain an almos

the treatment of this disease, is prepared to concur in what Dr. Neligan has advanced from the positive fact that the acarus cannot *always* be discovered in cases of scabies by *all* careful observers, and because the argument from a particular to an universal, which is that adopted by those who are convinced that *they* invariably discern the insect, is invalid.

For my own part, I am of opinion that scabies will be developed in a person whose skin has been previously free from the disease by the contact of either the itch-insect or the secretion from the eruption, but I believe the latter to be the most frequent cause of the contagion, and in this way only can we account for the many cases that occur in which the disease has been produced by contact with clothes, with gloves, &c., which have lain by for some time; in one instance which I saw, a lady was attacked with scabies on the palms of her hands, and as far as observation, which I freely admit is not indisputable evidence here, enabled me to judge, the contagion was conveyed to her from her servant-man, who was affected with the disease, by means of the handles of the knives which he was in the habit of cleaning.

From experiments which have been made it appears that scabies is more quickly developed in the young and in individuals of a full and robust habit of body than in the old, or those who are of a weak constitution; the period of incubation in the former being about four days, while in the latter it may extend to ten days or a fortnight, or even longer.

The *diagnosis* is, in some cases of scabies, extremely difficult, and in no other cutaneous eruption is it more important that a mistake should not be made, especially as a plan of treatment adapted for it is not at all suited for those diseases with which it is likely to be confounded; moreover, an opinion given with regard to contagion, if it prove to be incorrect, may seriously injure a physician's character. When eczema appears on the fingers or hands it is very often mistaken for scabies; in its early stages the minuteness and number of the vesicles generally suffice to render the diagnosis facile, but when it becomes chronic, the itching with which it is attended

14*

not unfrequently may lead to error. Eczema, however, never presents the conical-shaped vesicles of scabies, the discharge from the parts affected with it is more watery —being rarely sero-purulent except in eczema impetiginodes—is accompanied by a mealy epidermic desquamation, and it is rather a sensation of smarting and stinging than of true itching that attends it. The papular form of scabies may be mistaken for lichen, more particularly when the latter affects the backs of the hands; but the complete absence of vesicles and of a sero-purulent discharge in the latter, generally suffices to prevent the mistake from being made; the eruption, too, does not spread to the flexures between the fingers, the most usual seat of itch. Prurigo, which, like lichen, is a papular eruption, is liable to be confounded with scabies, chiefly in consequence of the severe itching with which it is attended; but it rarely affects the hands unless when it appears as a complication of that disease, its usual seat being the trunk of the body, the shoulders, and the thighs; and the small black crusts on the summits of the papulæ produced by scratching are highly characteristic; it is, moreover, very rarely accompanied by any discharge. When scabies assumes the pustular character, and the individual pustules attain a large size, it might be mistaken for ecthyma, but the latter is characterized by not being attended with itching, by its mode of development, and by the pustules being usually isolated. In fine, from all the cutaneous diseases now enumerated, scabies is especially distinguished by its contagious nature, and by the presence of the acarus; but it should be remembered that it may be complicated with any of them.

Prognosis.—As this eruption can scarcely be said to prove dangerous to life, except in the rare instances already referred to, the prognosis refers only to its probable duration, and this, when effective treatment is adopted, is always very short; but if scabies be left to itself, and not interfered with by the application of remedies, it may be indefinitely prolonged, as it never seems to exhibit a tendency to wear out, or to undergo a spontaneous cure.

Treatment.—If there be any well-established example of a *specific* in the whole Materia Medica it is that of the action of sulphur in the treatment of scabies; and as this medicine never fails to cure the disease, it is the universally admitted remedy for it; none other indeed would require to be alluded to, were it not that the unpleasant odor of sulphur renders its employment in some instances inadmissible. The general method of using this substance for the treatment of scabies is by the local inunction of ointments containing it, either alone or combined with alkalies; in the latter form it is generally employed in the present day in France, and found to be more efficacious than when used alone; the combination was first introduced by M. Helmerich, and the ointment, which is called after him, *Pommade d'Helmerich*, is composed of two parts of sulphur, one of carbonate of potash, and eight of lard. The surface of the entire body, but more particularly of the affected parts, should be first washed well with a strong solution of soft soap, the patient then placed for a quarter of an hour in an alkaline bath, containing a pound of the carbonate of potash to twenty gallons of water, at the temperature of 92°, the skin well dried, and this sulphuro-alkaline ointment afterwards thoroughly rubbed in; the disease may thus be effectually cured in two or three days, a single friction, preceded by the alkaline saponaceous bath, being used daily. Out of upwards of 700 persons treated on a plan nearly similar to this at the Hôpital St. Louis in Paris, M. Bazin only met with six unsuccessful cases, all the rest being cured on the third day.[1] M. Hardy, who succeeded M. Bazin in the charge of the itch wards in this hospital, has introduced a plan of using the sulphuro-alkaline ointment there, by which the period required for a complete cure is reduced to *two hours*. His method is as follows: "On the admission of the patient the entire surface of the body is rubbed, for half an hour, with soft soap—*savon noir;* he is then placed in a bath for an hour, and the body well rubbed while in it, and at the end of that time general friction made and continued, for half an hour, with Helmerich's ointment. The acarus," adds M. Hardy,

---

[1] *Journal de Médicine et de Chirurgie Pratiques,* Decembre, 1851, p. 529.

"is thus killed, and the patient consequently cure
400 patients thus treated, it is said that 4 only g
to return for further advice, and of these 2 §
tracted the disease.

A question arises as to whether it is advisable
thus suddenly a vesicular eruption, which in som
is attended with a rather copious discharge; M. D
a celebrated dermatologist, and one of the senio
sicians to this hospital, thinks it may be dangerou
so, but I cannot agree with him; for as scabies
attended with any constitutional disturbance, and i
symptomatic of an internal disease, the same can
not operate against the sudden cure of it as again
of cutaneous diseases the discharge in which is evi
dependent on some deranged condition of the
generally. M. Devergie, however, asserts that all
the contagious nature of scabies is destroyed by th
of treatment, a troublesome cutaneous eruption
mains—one, too, attended with much annoyance
patient, and often difficult of cure.

When any insuperable objection exists to the e
ment of sulphur for the cure of scabies, other appli
may be had recourse to which, although more tedi
their action, are equally efficacious; the use of
them will invariably be beneficially preceded by t
ployment of frictions with soft soap, and of the al
bath. Oil of turpentine made into an ointmen
eight times its weight of prepared lard, is a .very
application, but its odor is to many persons more
tionable even than that of sulphur; this may to
extent be removed, and its efficacy rather increas
the addition of eight minims of oil of bitter almo
each ounce of the lard, combined with it. The oi
of sulphuric acid, of the former *Dublin Pharma*
(1829), which is free from any unpleasant odor, rare
to cure the disease: stavesacre and white hellebor
ments, also, have been used with success; the for
prepared by mixing, with prolonged trituration, on
of the powdered seeds of the *Delphinium staphi*
with four times its weight of white wax ointmer
one part of glycerine, and the latter by combinin

ounces of the powdered root with half a pound of prepared lard, and adding twenty minims of oil of lemons.
Inunction with simple fatty matters even, such as olive
oil or lard, has been found sufficient to cure scabies, but
the duration of the disease is more prolonged than when
any of the above-mentioned remedies has been had recourse to.

In Lieutenant-Colonel Jebb's *Report on the Discipline
and Management of Military Prisons* (Blue Book, 1852)
it is stated that a cure can be made in two hours by
rubbing the skin with brick-dust, *to expose the acari ;*
next rubbing in sulphur-ointment for half an hour, .and
finally, washing with soap and 'water.—See *Braithwaite's
Retrospect,* Vol. XXIX, p. 260.

Dr. Decaisne, physician to the garrison at Antwerp,
affirms that oil of petroleum instantly kills the acarus,
and acts as a disinfectant against the larvæ in the
clothes.—*Glasgow Med. Journ.,* Jan., 1865, p. 428.

A strong objection often existing with some persons to
the use of greasy applications, lotions of the sulphuret of
potassium, or of chlorinated lime or soda, may be substituted for them ; of the former twenty grains, and of either
of the latter sixty grains to the ounce of distilled water,
should be employed.

With reference to internal treatment nothing more is
usually requisite than the administration of saline or sulphurous cathartics, and the use of the former should never
be omitted ; in very obstinate cases the combined employment of sulphur as an internal remedy and an external
application is not alone attended with benefit, but often
absolutely demanded.

Should the local inflammation run high in young
persons of robust constitution, bleeding from the arm
even may be indicated, but this is very rarely requisite.
[In the Editor's opinion it-is wholly unnecessary.]

In all cases of scabies constant ablutions with soap and
water constitute an essential part of the treatment, and
the clothes which had been worn previously should be
laid aside, as, from their retaining the contagious matter,
the disease may be reproduced after a cure has been
effected.

Since the publication of the first edition of this work in 1852, the mode of curing scabies has been so settled as to leave room for little or no further improvement. The Editor refers to the treatment with a preparation composed of a penta-sulphide of calcium, and a hypo-sulphite of lime ($3CaO + 12S = 2CaS_5 + CaOS_2O_2$). This is now in universal use in our military hospitals, where it has superseded every other method, and is prepared by boiling one part of quicklime, with two of sublimed sulphur, in ten of water, until the two former are perfectly united; stirring meanwhile with a piece of wood, and decanting the mixture into a well stopped bottle. The patient takes a hot bath, and then has some of this fluid rubbed diligently into his skin for half an hour, after which he takes a second bath, and comes out, cured, to dress in fresh clothing.

In the thirty-third volume of the *Dublin Quarterly Journal of Medical Science* (p. 474) the Editor called attention to the importance of this mode of treatment, and detailed several cases in point. Since then he has had it very often tried with unfailing success; and when he adds that he has had the experience of the senior medical officer of a militia regiment for more than ten years, it will be admitted that he is specially qualified to express an opinion in this matter.—See also *Braithwaite's Retrospect*, Vol. XXXIV, p. 266; and Dr. Frazer (*Treatment of Diseases of the Skin*, p. 68); also a paper on Scabies in the *Brit. and For. Med. Chir. Rev.*, Aug. 1865.

CHAPTER IV.

PUSTULÆ.

THE Order PUSTULÆ includes those cutaneous diseases that are characterized by the eruption of circumscribed rounded elevations of the epidermis, which contain pus, and are situated on an inflamed base—*pustules;* the pustules, which may be either psydracious or phlyzacious (see page 42), burst and form scabs or thick crusts, on the falling off of which a slight, not permanent depression or stain is left. Pustular eruptions are non-contagions, attended with more or less inflammation, usually of a subacute or chronic character, and their duration may be either very short or much prolonged. The local inflammatory action by which a pustule is produced affects the deeper structures of the derma as well as the epidermis, in consequence of which the sub-epidermic effusion is purulent, while in vesicular eruptions the superficial layer of the derma only being inflamed, the effusion is serous. In its early stage a pustule can scarcely be distinguished from a papule, inasmuch as the pus on which its specific character depends does not usually appear at the apex until the second or third day; the purulent secretion then gradually increases, distending the epidermie covering more and more, until, finally, it gives way, when the matter is effused on the cutaneous surface, and a scab is formed; of this process an excellent example is afforded in the case of the pustular eruption artificially produced by the local application of tartar emetic in the form of ointment or solution. While undergoing these changes, the pustule is said, in popular age, to be *ripening.* Some of the diseases included an and Bateman in this order were so classed by m an incorrect idea of their true characters;

thus scabies, for the reasons given in the last chapter, is
more properly placed among the vesiculæ; variola is one
of the eruptive fevers; and porrigo is not pustular in
any of its stages. Acne, included by them in the division which they termed Tubercula, presents the aspects of
a true pustule, according to the foregoing definition. The
group then comprehends four forms of cutaneous eruptions: Acne, Impetigo, Ecthyma, and Furunculi.

ACNE.

Acne (Willan and Bateman), Ἴονθος of the Greeks;
Varus of the Latins; Couperose of the French; Finnen
of the Germans. Acne is derived from ἀκμή, from its
appearance at the full growth and evolution (acme) of
the system. It is used by Ætius (*Tetrab.* II, serm. iv,
cap. 13) as a synonym for Ἴονθος, which not only means
a pustular eruption occurring during the growth of the
" prima lanugo," or first beard, but also means the lanugo
itself.—See plate IV.

Acne consists in the eruption of psydracious pustules,
with a hardened base, distinct from each other, but
usually aggregated in small patches on a circumscribed
inflamed portion of the skin; when they maturate,
bursting and giving exit to purulent matter, which dries
into thin, brownish crusts. The pus first appears as a
minute dot at the apex of each pimple, which is somewhat acuminate, then, gradually increasing in quantity,
the pustule becomes globular, and of a straw-yellow
color, its base still remaining hard, red, and painful, and
surrounded with an inflamed areola. At times, some of
the pustules, taking on an indolent action, little or no
matter forms in them, when they present the appearance
of hard, inflamed, minute tumors, about the size of a
small pea, and exquisitely painful to the touch, and are
slow in disappearing. The seat of the inflammatory
action in acne is chiefly in the sebaceous glands, and the
disease is not unfrequently produced by obstruction at
their orifices causing an accumulation of the natural
secretion and consequent irritation. By some modern
dermatologists it has, therefore, been made to constitute

a distinct class of cutaneous eruptions, *e. g.*, it is defined by Cazenave as consisting in "a diseased condition of the follicular secretion." Erasmus Wilson includes it in Group XX of his "Clinical Classification"—Affections of the Sebiparous System; M. Hardy includes it in his Second Order—Inflammatory Affections; and Hebra places it in his Fourth Order—Exudative. Acne is a disease chiefly of youth and of adult life, occurring with greatest frequency about the age of puberty, whence, as before observed, its name, derived from the Greek word ἀκμή, vigor. The several varieties of the eruption which have been described may, I think, be reduced to two forms :—

Acne simplex.
" rosacea.

Biett was the first to describe a rather rare cutaneous eruption as a variety of acne, terming it acne *sebacea*, in which the sebaceous follicles become hypertrophied and their secretion diseased; and nearly every dermatologist since his time has adopted his views, and retained the name proposed by him; as, however, it does not in any respect resemble acne, except in being an affection of the sebaceous follicles, it will be more correctly classed in the group of cutaneous eruptions which I propose to term Hypertrophiæ.

Acne simplex (Plate VI, Fig. 3) is a very frequent disease in young persons, especially in those in whom the cutaneous capillary circulation is active, appearing generally in the spring and autumn, and disappearing partially in summer and completely in winter; it may consist in the eruption of only a few scattered pustules on the face, or may occur in small patches, or pretty thickly disseminated over a large portion of the cutaneous surface, especially affecting those regions where the sebaceous follicles are most numerous. The pustules, whether few or many, are developed individually, and do not coalesce; each of them appears first as a small, red, acuminated elevation, hard, and somewhat painful, particularly so if the skin where it occurs is thick; within twenty-four or thirty-six hours the pustule, which has

15

continued to enlarge, presents at its apex a yello‌
point, which increases for a day or two, when the
dermis gives way or is ruptured, and pus, mixed ‌
the curdy sebaceous secretion of the follicle which
have been involved in the local inflammation, is
charged; although each pustule has an inflamed
there is no diffuse surrounding redness of the s
Many of these pustules do not maturate, but, remain
indolent for a few days, terminate by resolution,
lymphy effusion contained in them being reabsor
some slight hardness and redness, however, are
which gradually disappear.

In some persons, who are characterized for the
part by having a coarse, greasy skin, the sebaceous
hair follicles are peculiarly developed, and secrete
piously the thick curd-like matter which naturally ex
is them; individual follicles often become obstructed
the orifice, somewhat distended, and present a black p‌
at their apex; they then exhibit the appearance descri
by some dermatologists as a distinct variety of a
under the name acne *punctata.*—Plate VI, Fig. 4.
curd-like matter, when pressed out by the fingers, fo‌
a round cast of the follicle in which it existed, and, ow
to its size and shape, and the black point at its extrem
where it had been exposed to the action of the at
phere, bears much resemblance to a small maggot,
which it is commonly believed to be. Although
popular notion is, it need scarcely be said, erroneous,
Gustav Simon has discovered in the natural sebace
secretion a minute animalcule, from the 0.085th to
0.125th of a line (German measurement) in length,
about the 0.020th of a line in breadth; it was named
him *Acarus folliculorum,* but has more recently b
shown by Einsicht not to be an acarus, and is there‌
termed by the latter *Steatozoön folliculorum.*

The eruption in acne simplex is thus usually compo
of maturating and non-maturating pustules, and of
larged obstructed follicles characterized by black point
the latter are constantly present on the cutaneous sur

appear in successive crops, being consequently then of more prolonged duration. No constitutional fever or other disturbance attends the disease, even when it attacks many regions of the skin simultaneously; nor, although some pustules may be attended with pain, are the local symptoms troublesome, being chiefly annoying in consequence of their being situated on the face, and therefore causing a temporary disfigurement. The duration of individual pustules, when they run an acute course, is from five to eight or ten days; but when they are indolent, or appear in successive crops, the disease may be prolonged for as many weeks; in the latter case the marks left on the skin are slow in fading away. Appearing and disappearing with the seasons, being developed in spring and autumn, and receding in summer and winter, acne simplex becomes less frequent as youth changes into puberty, and with adult life either ceases altogether, or, becoming nearly permanent, is converted into the next variety to be described.

The usual seat of the simple form of acne is on the face, the neck, the shoulders, and the chest; it occasionally occurs on the scalp, where it is exquisitely painful, although the pustules are few in number, and very scattered; but it is very rare on the extremities.

Acne rosacea—Gutta rosacea; Rosy-drop; Carbuncled face; Brandy face—(Plate VI, Fig. 5) is a disease of more mature life than the preceding variety; it has especially attracted the attention of the French dermatologists, by many of whom it is described as a special disease under the name of *Couperose.* The eruption, which is invariably seated on the face, usually becomes chronic, but in all its stages is attended with more local inflammation than acne simplex; it generally commences in the form of a red patch on the skin, on which is rapidly developed a cluster of minute pustules, or rather pimples, hard, and but little elevated; these enlarge gradually, but are slow to maturate, and their base becomes harder, often painful, and much inflamed. Eventually giving way at their apex, a serous exudation, mixed with blood, oozes forth, which concretes into a hard, dry scab, and from beneath it a small quantity of a curdy pus escapes in a few days

after. The hardness at the base of each pustule,
ever, still remains, and the rosy or crimson-violet
of the skin, on which a varicose condition of the
ficial veins is sooner or later developed, is often pers
on the face for months, or even years, spreading grad
over the nose, cheeks, forehead, and chin, fresh crc
similar pustules constantly appearing on it.

When this form of acne is chronic, it assumes
aggravated character, and from its unsightly appea
causes great mental annoyance; the skin of the
of the face on which it is situated becomes thick
elevated, from effusion into the subcutaneous ai
tissue, caused by the repeated fresh attacks of infla
tion consequent on the development on each suea
crop of pustules; it presents a permanent rosente
which is deepened on every exciting cause—expos
the face to heat, indulgence in the pleasures of the
or mental emotions; and the surface is hypertrop
rugose, and seamed with the cicatrices from pustu
previous eruptions.

In its most chronic form it constitutes what has
termed acne *indurata* (Plate VI, Fig. 6), but I have
this variety of the disease not unfrequently succeed
simplex, and even sometimes appear as an indurated
tuberculated eruption from the first; it might, there
probably be made to constitute a distinct form of
eruption, but it has so many features similar to thos
acne rosacea, and so commonly occurs apparently a
advanced stage of it, that I have thought it bette
describe it as such. Acne indurata is characterized
the eruption being much elevated over the surface of
skin which is of a violaceous-crimson hue, and con
in conoidal pustules, about the size of a pea, extrei
hard and tuberculated, and presenting minute point
suppuration at their apex. These pustules are not
painful to the touch; they do not scab over; but w
ever they maturate and burst they leave a bluish cica
or pit, resembling that of smallpox. Those that ma
set closely together usually coalesce, and present thei
appearance of boils, but the contained matter is sma
quantity, the aggregated bases extremely hard and

nute, and superficial ulcers, covered with a yellowish soft scab, form on their apex. Acne indurata, when it is an advanced stage of acne rosacea, or when it occurs as an independent disease, is invariably situated on the face, affecting especially the alæ of the nostrils, and the most prominent portions of the cheeks; when it is consequent on acne simplex it may appear on any of the regions of the body mentioned as being liable to be affected by that form of the eruption.

Causes.—Acne simplex being, as already remarked, a cutaneous eruption of the period of puberty and of the prime of life, appears to be connected with the full development of the capillary circulation of the surface of the body, which at these ages usually prevails; it is also probably for the same reasons most frequently witnessed in individuals of the sanguine temperament; and when it occurs in others it is seemingly dependent on a naturally enlarged condition of the sebaceous follicles, the skin being then usually coarse, sallow, greasy, and shining. It is manifestly hereditary; and local heat, or anything which may determine to the surface, is a frequent exciting cause of the eruption in those constitutionally predisposed to it. Acne rosacea is frequently connected with the state of the uterine function in the female, in many cases appearing for the first time at the turn of life; it also occasionally, but much more rarely, attacks the face of young girls about the period of first menstruation; and when it does so, they are very liable to frequent returns of the eruption on the least exciting cause. It is also a constant accompaniment of a deranged condition of the digestive organs, especially when attended with constipation; and in many persons is evidently caused by indulgence in the pleasures of the table, particularly a too free use of rich wines or of spirituous liquors. Prolonged or extreme mental excitement is also a frequent exciting cause of acne rosacea. An attack of either form may be suddenly produced by the suppression of any accustomed evacuation, such as that arising from bleeding hemorrhoids; and they are very common attendants on pregnancy. Mr. Erasmus Wilson believes it to be essentially a disease of debility, and

If it be impossible to obtain the natural mineral waters for the baths, they may be artificially prepared by dissolving four ounces of sulphuret of potassium in thirty gallons of water.

No remedial measures can possibly prove of service in the treatment of acne rosacea until the habits by which the disease may have been occasioned are corrected, and in every case especial attention must be paid to the avoidance of all stimulating articles, both of food and drink, which occasion determination of blood to the face, such as rich meats, spices, spirituous and vinous drinks, shell-fish, pork, raw vegetables, etc., from the use of which the eruption is invariably augmented, if it had not been originally produced thereby; heated rooms, exposure of the face to the fire, continued stooping of the head, and mental excitement or anxiety, must be equally guarded against. When acne rosacea is seen in its early stages, or where there is much inflammatory action present, the application of from four to six leeches behind the ears twice or three times a week at bedtime will be found of much service, and at the same time saline cathartics should be used daily, preceded by mild mercurials, if there is any biliary derangement. The saline cathartic mineral waters are here, as in acne simplex, of especial service; and of them all I have found the Pullna water—which is now very generally imported—the most beneficial; it may be given in the dose of from one to two wineglassfuls, mixed with an equal quantity of tepid water, every morning. When they cannot be procured, one drachm of the compound saline powder, prepared as I have directed in my work on Medicines,[1] dissolved in half a pint of tepid water, may be substituted. The tendency to local inflammation being thus subdued, slightly stimulating applications may then be used, such as ointments of the ammonio-chloride or of the nitrate of mercury, of dried sulphate of iron, of the acetate of copper, etc.; the employment of the first of these will be found especially beneficial; it may be prepared as follows:—

[1] Sixth (Macnamara's) Edition, p. 157.

℞. Hydrargyri Ammoniati, . . grana duodecim ad grana triginta.
Unguenti Simplicis, . . . unciam.
Glycerini, ... drachmam.
Olei Amygdalæ Amaræ, . . minima tria. Misce.

The ointment should be smeared thickly over the affected part at night, and washed off in the morning with a weak spirituous alkaline wash, containing not more than twelve grains of the carbonate of soda to the pint of liquid, to which from half an ounce to an ounce of glycerine should be added if the skin be hard and dry and inclined to bleed. In every stage of acne rosacea the use of soaps should be carefully eschewed, as they are all more or less irritating; the bicarbonate of soda may be substituted for them, and in the case of men who are compelled to shave, a saturated solution of it mixed with an equal part of olive oil may be used. In chronic cases of the disease, preparations of iodine must be given internally; two grains of the iodide of potassium, dissolved in two ounces of the decoction of fresh elm-bark, with the addition of a quarter of a grain of iodine when the disease is very obstinate, taken at bedtime, will be found perhaps the most efficacious form of administering this remedy.

Should acne rosacea prove rebellious to these plans of treatment, the more active local medication proposed by some dermatologists may be tried; such as the application daily to each inflamed follicle of a small pledget of lint dipped in a concentrated solution of sulphuret of potassium, as proposed by M. Duchesne-Duparc,[1] the contact being continued for from fifteen to twenty seconds; of a concentrated solution of acetate of lead in *white-wine* vinegar, as recommended by M. Bretonneau;[2] or of a solution of two grains of the bicyanide of mercury in an ounce of distilled water, washed off in a few moments after with cold water; an application highly spoken of by Dr. Burgess.[3]

When acne assumes the indurated character which has acquired for it that special denomination, it requires

---

[1] *Nouvelle Prosopalgie.* Paris, 1847, p. 69.
[2] *Bulletin de Thérapeutique*, Tome xxxi. p. 285.
[3] *Eruptions of the Face, Head, and Hands.* London: 1849, p. 55.

active treatment, both constitutionally and locally;
may be removed by cupping from the nape of th
to the extent of from two to four ounces, once or twice a
week, according to the youth and constitution
patient, and daily purgation by active saline ca
had recourse to; unless, which rarely occurs, the disease
appears in an individual of a weak constitution, when
preparations of iodine with iron will be found more beneficial. Hebra recommends the application of soft soap to
the face, and then of a paste of sulphur in alcohol. He
also uses corrosive sublimate (five grains to one ounce of
spirit) with a compress for two hours; or a preparation
consisting of one drachm of tincture of benzoin, and one
grain of corrosive sublimate to six ounces of water. Mr.
Startin applies to the top of indolent tubercles with a
pointed glass-brush, one drop of this solution, mercury
one ounce, nitric acid (s. g. 1.50) one ounce.—*Braithwaite's
Retrospect*, Vol. XXXI, p. 343. The best local application is the iodide of sulphur in the form of ointment,
the strength of which may be gradually increased from
fifteen grains to half a drachm to the ounce of lard. Alkaline washes should also be used as in acne rosacea, and
change of air, with the internal use of the sulphurous
mineral waters, will be found of especial benefit. Blistering the face with glacial acetic acid or vesicating collodion
has been sometimes had recourse to, and it is said with
success, in cases of acne indurata which has resisted all
other methods of treatment.

Most of the lotions which are empirically employed in
acne of the face consist of corrosive sublimate dissolved
in bitter almond emulsion, in the proportion of from one
to two grains to the ounce; their use for a short time is
not unfrequently attended with benefit, but if continued
long they cause the skin to become harsh and scaly.

IMPETIGO.

Impetigo, derived, according to Pliny, *ab impetu, impetu agens;* Ψώρα ιλχώδης, ulcerated psora, of the Greeks;
Lepra squamosa, and Lichen vitiligo, of various Latin
authors (save Celsus, who uses the term impetigo); Kouba

(Arabic) of Avicenna; Dartre crustacée, Lépre humide, of the French; Zittermal, der kleienaussatz, of the Germans; crusted tetter.—See Plate VII.

IMPETIGO (*Crusted tetter*).—This term, like so many others applied to designate diseases of the skin, had no determinate signification previously to the time of Willan. It is now understood to indicate a cutaneous affection, characterized by the eruption of numerous psydracious pustules, occurring singly and distinct from each other, or in groups and confluent, with but little surrounding inflammation; they maturate rapidly, and discharge a thick purulent matter, which dries into a semi-transparent, greenish-yellow, irregularly-shaped, persistent, solid crust.[1] From beneath this crust, when formed, purulent matter continues to be secreted, often in considerable quantity, and the duration of the disease is thus usually prolonged for some time; the crusts are slow in separating; and when they at length fall off, a red mark or stain is left on the integuments, which, however, gradually wears away. Fresh pustules are developed in successive crops around the region of the skin originally affected, and the disease thus spreads, until it not unfrequently involves an extended surface of the body, which becomes covered with the characteristic, pellucid, soft, greenish crust, and from beneath which purulent matter oozes; when the eruption has existed for some time, cracks and fissures form, as in eczema, but they do not present the red color of that disease, nor are they accompanied by the serous exudation so characteristic of it. Impetigo is a highly inflammatory eruption, and may run either an acute or chronic course. Dr. Neligan was of opinion that it is not contagious; but Dr. Fox, in the *British Medical Journal* for May and June, 1864, has fully described a form of impetigo which was epidemic amongst the patients at the Farringdon General Dispensary, and which he believes

---

[1] "The pustule of impetigo is of the kind termed *psydracium*, and in the plural *psydracia*, ψυχρά ἰδρωτία, *frigidæ guttulæ*, that is, a pustule or pustules produced with little heat or inflammation, commonly aggregated or confluent, and, after pouring out 'a thin watery humor, which frequently forms an irregular incrustation.' "—E. Wilson, *Student's Book, &c.*, p. 115.

to be contagious. Wilson, Hardy, and Hebra all believe impetigo to be an eczematous affection.

M. Gendrin has carefully described the anatomical characters of impetigo and its seat, having had an opportunity of examining it after death—an opportunity which occurs with extreme rarity, as the disease does not prove fatal, and as inflammatory cutaneous eruptions generally disappear in the course of mortal diseases. The following is the account which he gives of the result of his observations: "At the parts corresponding to the eruption, the skin was more adherent to the areolar tissue than elsewhere, nevertheless, there existed on the external surface of the derma but a slight degree of capillary injection. The cutaneous tissue was more dense than natural, and was of a reddish-yellow hue, but this morbid color only extended for a short way into the chorion. On the edges of a section made through the diseased skin it could be observed that the small reddish, closely aggregated, but only slightly prominent granulations, which were situated beneath the crusts, were made up of minute grains about the size of the head of a pin, of a liquid and greenish-yellow cheesy-like substance; the surrounding cutaneous tissue was red, and matter similar to that which was secreted by the pustules of the eruption, and which, by drying, formed the crusts of the disease, oozed out of it when pressed between the fingers.[1]

The various forms of impetigo, which have been described by dermatologists, may, I think, be conveniently considered in two groups, named from the mode of development of the eruption. But as it presents certain peculiarities, when it occurs on the scalp, which require to be specially noticed, I shall describe it under three heads:—

Impetigo figurata.
"   sparsa.
"   capitis.

Impetigo figurata (Plate VII, Fig. 1) is so named from the disease appearing in patches of a circular or ovoid

_____
[1] *Traité des Inflammations*, Tome i.

shape. It usually sets in with feverish symptoms, which both precede and accompany the eruption, never severe but generally well marked, consisting in *malaise*, headache, loss of appetite, and occasionally slight shivering; in children the symptoms amount only to some heat of the surface, and general uneasiness; but at times there are no premonitory signs noticeable, when the disease usually assumes rather a chronic character from the first. Small, rounded, slightly-elevated, red patches appear on the skin of the face—where the disease is of most frequent occurrence—of the trunk, the shoulders, the arms, the hands, or the thighs; and on them psydracious pustules, closely set together, and more or less confluent, are rapidly developed, their appearance being preceded by much local heat and itching. The pustules attain their full magnitude, which rarely exceeds that of the head of a pin, in about forty-eight hours, when they burst and give exit to the contained purulent matter; this, which is very liquid, dries quickly into a pale greenish-yellow, or citrine-colored, soft crust, of a pellucid aspect, and bearing much resemblance to candied honey, so much so that Alibert, from this characteristic, named the disease *melitagra*. The crust generally covers completely the original red patch; it is very friable, and through cracks, which form from the motion of the part on which it may be seated, an ichorous pus oozes; this drying rapidly, adds to the volume of the first crust, until it often acquires a considerable thickness, still, however, retaining its semi-transparency, and kept constantly moist by the discharge from beneath. Should the crusts be removed, or fall off, the surface on which they were seated is seen to be raw, inflamed, and secreting pus, by which they are rapidly renewed.

The original patches of the eruption, should there be more than one, may remain distinct from each other, separated by healthy integument during the whole progress of the disease; but more usually those which are near become confluent, the eruption spreading by the development of isolated pustules or of successive crops on the intervening sound skin. The crusts in the more acute cases remain attached to the surface for three or

16

four week's, during which time the discharge contin....
they then gradually become drier, the secretion dim...
ishes in quantity, and, unless successive crops of p....
appear, the disease terminates by their becoming d....
in separate pieces as it were, a reddish-brown stain b...
left, which is slow in disappearing, and from which ...
some time an epidermic desquamation, accompanied o....
sionally by a slight serous oozing, takes place, ca....
the eruption, as well remarked by Cazenave, to rese....
somewhat, eczema. Until the crusts commence to d...
up and fall off, a constant heat and painful tingling ...
the affected parts attend the disease; these cause ch...
dren, and sometimes even adults, to tear the surface wi...
their nails, and thereby aggravate the malady.

In some cases of impetigo figurata the symptoms, b....
local and constitutional, are of a much more severe character than those now described. High fever marks the
outbreak of the eruption, which is characterized by active
inflammation that extends to the subcutaneous areolar
tissue, and affects a considerable surface of the integument, which is red and much tumefied. In its commencement it can scarcely be distinguished from an
attack of erysipelas, and was therefore named by Willan
and Bateman impetigo *erysipelatodes* (Plate VII, Fig. 3);
but on the second day the characteristic psydracious
pustules appear on the inflamed surface, when the disease
runs the course above described, except that the local
symptoms are throughout of much greater severity, the
discharge especially being much more copious, and so
acrid as to irritate and cause the development of pustules
on those parts of the unaffected skin over which it may
flow; there is also more or less fever present to the end,
and its duration is very prolonged.

Impetigo sparsa (Plate VII, Fig. 2) differs, as its name
indicates, from the preceding form in the arrangement of
the pustules, which are developed individually, and scattered or dispersed over the cutaneous surface, sometimes
pretty thickly on the legs, where it is of most frequent
occurrence; but it may affect any part of the body, in
children being often seen on the ears, the face, and the
neck. When the pustules in impetigo sparsa are nume-

rous and closely set together, as usually happens on the folds of integument in the neighborhood of the joints, although they may not coalesce, which they very rarely do, the intervening skin is inflamed, red, and slightly tumid, hot, painful, and tingling. The crusts which form present the same appearance as in impetigo figurata, but they are distinct on each pustule, or cover the site of two or three, rarely more, and are much thinner, softer, and more easily detached. The development of the eruption is attended generally with some fever, and always with an extreme degree of burning heat, sometimes almost insupportable, which remains, but in a less degree, until the crusts are about to fall off; then it returns, if possible, even with greater intensity, and a second crop of pustules is developed in the neighborhood of, and in the intervening spaces between, the first. This is in like manner followed by a third or fourth crop; and thus the disease becomes very often chronic, when the skin is hypertrophied, fissured with red cracks caused by tearing with the nails, of a crimson tint, and discharging a thin, unhealthy, bloody pus, which dries into dark greenish-brown crusts, that at times envelop an entire limb like the bark of a tree; when impetigo sparsa assumes this aggravated character it corresponds with the form described by Willan as impetigo *scabida* (Plate VII, Fig. 4). The duration of this variety of the eruption is always much prolonged, acrid, ichorous matter, of a heavy disagreeable odor, being secreted from the surface beneath the crusts, which are very permanent, and scattered pustules continuing to be developed in the neighborhood, often without any apparent fresh attack of local inflammation; superficial ulcerations also form, and if the limbs are the parts affected they become more or less œdematous.

Impetigo of either of the forms now described is very frequent on the face of infants and young children, and becoming chronic there presents these characteristics in their most aggravated form; the features are completely and the eruption covering them, as it were, with the disease has been termed impetigo *larvalis*.

capitis (Plate VII, Fig. 6) is the only pustular

time, being kept up by an eruption of fresh pust
other parts of the scalp. It not unfrequently pas
the second form, which is characterized by the e
occurring in groups of pustules. Their appear
attended with more decided symptoms of inflam
both general and local, and the heat and itching
many cases so severe that children tear the scalp a
vent the disease from presenting the truly pustular
ter of the first stage. The eruption usually com
on the forehead, involving at the same time some
hairy scalp; the inflamed patches vary in size a
in different cases; in some extending in their
measurement not more than from half an inch to
two inches, while in others the greater part of th
is involved from the very commencement; in
every instance the skin bordering on the scalp is
less engaged in the disease, and it often appears
same time on the ears or on some part of the fac
pustules are not so large as when they occur singl
coats are apparently thinner, and the pus whic
contain is not so consistent, and is of a richer
color. They usually become confluent before the
and the resulting greenish-yellow—if chronic, gr

brown — scab is consequently much more extensive. When the eruption has continued for any length of time, large quantities of bright yellow pus are secreted beneath the greenish crusts, which separate in cracks to give exit to the matter, exhibiting beneath the highly inflamed raw surface of the scalp from which the pus is secreted.

Mr. Balmanno Squire says that it is chiefly confined *either* to the anterior or to the posterior part of the scalp, and that where it occurs at the occiput it is associated with the presence of pediculi.—*Medical Times and Gazette,* Aug. 20th, 1864.

In either form of impetigo the hair is unaltered; it is usually matted together by the purulent secretion and the scabs, but it does not fall off or become changed in appearance, even in the most chronic cases.

Impetigo capitis is not contagious; it is met with at all ages, but most generally in early infancy, lasting for several years if not properly treated; it very rarely appears for the first time after the age of nine or ten, but I have seen some instances in which the eruption occurred in advanced life; in them the disease was of the form first described.

In the chronic stage of the eruption small abscesses very frequently form at the nape of the neck, close to the roots of the hair; and some of the chain of lymphatic glands, which lie behind the sterno-mastoid muscle, become enlarged, swollen, and tender, but they very rarely suppurate.

Bateman described a form of cutaneous eruption as a species of impetigo, terming it impetigo *rodens,* and in this he has been followed by Biett and Rayer; Wilson considers it to be syphilitic, and Hardy calls it " scrofulide pustuleuse;" but the disease is evidently a lupoid ulceration of the scalp, and as such will consequently be considered in the group Cancroïdes. Two other forms of the disease have been characterized by M. Devergie as impetigo *purifluens* and impetigo *pilaris;* the former is attended with profuse purulent secretion, and the latter affects those parts of the skin on which the hair grows, the pustules being frequently developed around individual hairs, which thus seem to penetrate them; these, however,

are merely accidental circumstances, and neither ~~can be~~
admitted as sufficient to constitute a special variety ~~of the~~
eruption. The impetigo *sycosiformis* and impetigo ~~lupi-~~
formis of the same dermatologist are identical, the ~~former~~
with sycosis and the latter with impetigo rodens.

Causes.—Impetigo is of most frequent occurrence ~~in~~
infants and children; when it affects adults, appearing
only on those who have a fine transparent skin, being
therefore more common in women than in men. In ~~all~~
persons it is usually seated on the lower extremities,
especially the thighs; in them it is developed in the form
of impetigo sparsa, and assumes a very obstinate character. The constitutional causes of the disease are more or
less connected with the scrofulous diathesis, and in children of this temperament it commonly appears about the
periods of first and second dentition, its eruption being
excited then by the general perturbation of the system
thereby occasioned. Anything which produces cutaneous
capillary determination of blood acts as a cause of impetigo in those predisposed to it; thus its origin may be
determined by irritants applied to the surface, such as
washing in very hot water—a frequent cause in infants
and children—the use of hard brushes or of fine-tooth
combs to the hair, stimulating soaps and cosmetics, and
solar heat, or that from a fire; the former accounts for
the frequently-witnessed recurrence of the disease in
summer and autumn, and the latter for its appearance
on the lower extremities of old persons. Prolonged constipation and menstrual irregularities are both frequent
exciting causes of impetigo in females.

Diagnosis.—Impetigo is well characterized in all its
forms by its truly pustular character, and by the peculiar
semi-transparent, soft, greenish-yellow, honey-like appearance of its crusts. From *eczema impetiginodes* it is
often with difficulty diagnosed, and both diseases seem
frequently in their advanced stages to be precisely similar; yet the copious ichorous exudation—so well described
by the French term, *suintement*—and the epidermic desquamation are present usually in all forms of eczema,
and in impetigo fresh psydracious pustules are in general
being constantly developed in the neighborhood of the

eruption. From *ecthyma* the disease is diagnosed by the small size of the pustules, those of ecthyma being phlyzacious, and for the most part scattered singly, or in twos or threes, over the cutaneous surface, and the scab resulting from them is of a dull brownish color; the parts usually affected are also different in the two eruptions. When pustules occur in *scabies* they are of a large size, and a conoidal shape, but that disease is especially distinguished from impetigo by the itching which accompanies it; burning heat, tingling, and smarting, not itching, being present in the latter; the detection of the acarus scabiei, of course, renders the diagnosis more precise, but it should be remembered that in some cases both diseases exist together on the same person. *Sycosis*, from its occurrence on the face, has been at times confounded with impetigo; but it invariably affects that part on which the beard grows, and its immediate neighborhood, is not truly pustular, and the crusts which form in it are hard, dry, and of a brown color, and, if examined under a microscope, exhibit the characters of a vegetable parasite.

As impetigo is the only pustular eruption which specially affects the scalp, it can scarcely be mistaken for any other eruptive disease that appears on this part of the cutaneous surface; the chronic form of *eczema* is that with which it is most likely to be confounded; in it the discharge, which is either serous or sero-purulent, dries into brownish-yellow scabs, through which the ichorous liquid forces its way, or into furfuraceous scales, while in impetigo the purulent discharge accretes into large, greenish-yellow crusts, by which the whole head, and even sometimes the forehead and part of the face, is in many cases covered as with a mask.

Prognosis.—The only question here to be considered is the probable duration of the disease, as its existence, when uncomplicated, does not either injure the health or endanger life. In children, although apt to become chronic and obstinate if neglected, it usually yields quickly to judicious treatment; and when situated on the scalp is, in my experience, more readily cured than any of the other eruptions peculiar to that region, if their relative duration previously to the employment of remedies be taken into account. It is in general more rebellious in adults; and when it affects the lower extremities in old persons is a most troublesome and obstinate disease, the form termed scabida by Willan not unfrequently lasting for years, notwithstanding the most careful treatment, at one time showing signs of amendment, but to break out with increased severity again and again. In young persons even the eruption is very apt to return in the summer and autumn months after it has been apparently cured. At all ages the obstinacy of impetigo is in proportion to its previous duration.

Treatment.—The acute stages of impetigo occurring in young persons of robust constitution require rather active antiphlogistic treatment—the daily use of saline cathartics, and local, or even in some cases general bleeding;[1] the local abstraction of blood should be by leeches applied in the neighborhood of the eruption, or behind the ears when it is situated on the face or scalp. When the disease, however, attacks the old or debilitated, bleeding is very rarely admissible; but should it be requisite in consequence of the inflammatory symptoms running high, with much heat and tumefaction of the part affected, a few leeches only should be applied, and the after-bleeding from the bites not allowed to continue; tonics are here more generally indicated, and the use of preparations of iron, combined with vegetable tonics and saline purgatives, as somewhat in the following form, will be found highly beneficial:—

R. Tincturæ Ferri Sesquichloridi,[2] . semi-unciam.
   Infusi Quassiæ, ... uncias octodecim.
   Tincturæ Calumbæ, ... unciam cum semisse.
   Maguesiæ Sulphatis, ... uncias duas. Misce.
     Sumat uncias duas fluidas omni mane.

In children or adults of the scrofulous diathesis, cod-liver oil is the best tonic; and if the eruption is attended

[1] The Editor thinks that the antiphlogistic plan is open to grave question; and he considers the proposal of general bleeding unnecessary.

[2] This—the Tincture of the *Pharmacop.*, *Dub.*, 1850—corresponds to the Tinctura Ferri Perchloridi of the *Ph. Brit.*; save that the latter is only one-*fourth* of the strength of the former.

with scrofulous enlargement of the glands of the neck, from a sixteenth to a fourth of a grain of iodine may be dissolved in each dose of the oil, which should not exceed a dessert-spoonful three times a day for children, or a table spoonful for adults; as when given in large doses the local disease is apt to be aggravated apparently from its over-stimulating action on the system.

In the chronic stages of the eruption, the administration of more decidedly alterative medicines is requisite, and a mild mercurial course is often singularly effieacious, especially when the mercury is combined with iodine and alkalies. With this view the green iodide of mercury may be given in the following form for adults, a proportionately smaller dose being prescribed for children :—

℞. Hydrargyri Iodidi Viridis, ... grana quatuor.
Hydrargyri cum Creta, ... rana duodecim.
Carbonatis Sodæ Exsiccatæ, . . . grana duodecim.
Pulvis Myrrhæ, ... grana sex.
Mucilaginis, quantum sufficit ut fiant pilulæ duodecim.
Sumat unam ter indies.

In the more obstinate cases, some practitioners recommend the employment of sulphurous preparations—especially in the form of sulphur-mineral waters; and others have recourse to the use of arsenic; of the latter the preparations most suited for this disease are the arseniates of ammonia and of soda: the dose of either is from the twentieth to the tenth of a grain; they may be given in infusion of dulcamara.

In the impetigo of infants and of very young children but little constitutional treatment is necessary: for infants at the breast, should the eruption exhibit a tendency to assume a chronic character, it will be advisable to change the nurse; and when the disease appears at the periods of dentition, the gums should be freely lanced. The state of the digestive organs must in all cases be strictly attended to, and mild purgatives, combined with alkalies, administered according to circumstances. The alkaline treatment is at this age of especial service; for children of a full habit of body the bicarbonate of soda may be prescribed in doses of from three to five grains, three times daily, in half a drachm of syrup of orange-peel and two drachms of orange-flower water, and for those of a weak or debilitated constitution, from one to three grains of the bicarbonate of ammonia in the same menstruum. Should diarrhœa or symptoms of any derangement of the brain accompany the eruption of impetigo, we should be most careful not to check the disease too suddenly, more especially if it is attended with discharge.

The local treatment of impetigo is of even more importance than the constitutional, for upon its judicious application, in the first instance, most frequently depends the duration of the disease. It is especially necessary to keep constantly in view that the eruption is of an inflammatory nature, and that even in its most chronic stages a fresh outbreak of inflammation, attended with the development of a new crop of pustules, may be readily excited. The very production of the disease in so many cases by the direct influence of irritants sufficiently proves this, and should warn against the use of irritating applications, which have been often too indiscriminately recommended. In the acute stages, no matter on what part of the cutaneous surface the eruption may occur, alkaline ointments are of especial service; and should there be much local tingling and irritation, chloroform will be beneficially combined with them, as in the following form :—

℞. Sodæ Bicarbonatis, ... grana viginti.
  Adipis præparati, ... unciam.
  Chloroformi, ... minima quatuor. **Misce.**

This ointment should be smeared pretty thickly over the pustules night and morning, the surface having been previously washed with equal parts of new milk and tepid water. To allay the irritation, unguents and washes, containing various preparations of lead, of oxide of zinc, and of hydrocyanic acid, are recommended by different dermatologists, but I have found none of them as useful as the above. Owing to the moisture from the purulent discharge which is so constantly present in impetigo, the addition of glycerine to the local applications, so far from being attended with benefit, usually proves injurious.

In the chronic forms of the eruption, the crusts or scabs should be always removed carefully before the use of medicated applications; this is done most effectually by the employment of linseed-meal poultices —wet with the weak lead wash (see page 116) when any tendency to local inflammation is present—changed twice in the twenty-four hours, .the parts being sponged with a warmed solution of half a drachm of carbonate of soda in a pint of distilled water each time the poultice is changed. The alkaline ointment above described may then be used ; or, should the disease be very chronic, an ointment of the dried sulphate of iron, in the proportion of from two to five grains to the ounce of cerate, employed ; this preparation even occasionally proves too stimulating, when the acetate of zinc cerate should be employed instead of it. In some cases of impetigo greasy applications are found to aggravate the local symptoms, and then lotions should be substituted for them, such as twelve grains of the acetate of zinc, or six grains of the acetate of lead, or four grains of either the sulphate of copper or the sulphate of iron, dissolved in eight fluid-ounces of elder-flower or of rose-water.

To the use of more active local stimulants, as ointments, baths, or washes of the sulphuret of potassium, of tar, of anthrakokali, of fuligokali, of the *huile de cade*, or of caustics, as the nitrate of silver, my experience is decidedly opposed ; as I have generally seen their application excite an outbreak of inflammation, and the consequent spread of the disease by the development of additional pustules.

When impetigo affects the scalp, the hair should always be carefully *cut* close, and the crusts removed by the application of poultices and the use of alkaline washes, as above directed ; afterwards the ointment of the bicarbonate of soda, and a lotion of milk and tepid water, will be employed with benefit: the green iodide of mercury, with the hydrargyrum cum cretâ, and the dried carbonate of soda should be given internally. This plan of treatment seldom fails to cure the disease, even in the most chronic forms, in from six weeks to three months, provided there is a careful attendant to carry out strictly

the employment of the local remedies. In any case the
salt should not be permitted to grow for some time after
the traces of the eruption have disappeared.

Dietetic and hygienic regulations are of much importance in the treatment of impetigo, particularly of its
chronic forms: all heating and stimulating articles of
food ought to be strictly prohibited, and everything
which could cause determination of blood to the surface
of the body carefully avoided. In children, the use of *a
poor, mild and farinaceous diet* will be found to expedite
the cure much.

ECTHYMA.

Ecthyma, ἔκθυμα of the Greeks (from ἐκθύω), literally *an
eruption*, used by them in a general sense, and synono-
mously with ἐξάνθημα, an eruption: Terminthus of various
Greek authors: Bouten of the French; Erbsenblattern of
the Germans.—See Plate VIII.

ECTHYMA (*Papulous scall*) consists in the eruption of
large pustules, on a hardened, more or less inflamed base, usually isolated, but occasionally in small
clusters, terminating in yellowish-brown scabs or crusts,
in many serious cases, of a livid hue—which, as they fall
off, leave small ulcers that heal with superficial cicatrices.
This cutaneous disease attacks the young and the
old, and is of an inflammatory character, but in the old
and debilitated it assumes from the first an asthenic
character. It is non contagious. In children it is rarely
seen, and more rarely in infants, occurring most frequently in old persons and in adults. The pustules may
appear on any part of the cutaneous surface, but they
chiefly affect the extremities, especially the thighs: they
appear with the next degree of frequency on the skin of
the trunk of the body or on the neck, being but seldom
witnessed on the face or the hairy scalp.

The division of ecthyma into varieties, as made by
Willan and those dermatologists who have adopted his
views, depended either upon the age of the patient or
upon accidental phenomena, having their origin in the
constitution of the individual attacked. This being so,

ifestly a bad foundation for a classification, though one not uncommonly followed as regards cutaneous eruptions, is now almost universally abandoned, and but two forms of the disease are described by most modern writers: these I shall adopt:—

Ecthyma acutum.
" chronicum.

The eruption of *Acute ecthyma* (Plate VIII, Fig. 1) is preceded by some degree of fever, usually very slight, amounting merely to heat of the surface, thirst, and head-ache; in about thirty-six hours afterwards, small, rounded, slightly elevated red spots appear on the skin, generally of one or both of the lower extremities, their appearance being preceded and accompanied by heat and sharp tin-gling of the parts about to be affected, the constitutional symptoms at the same time subsiding. These spots, which are nearly the size of a large pea, and few in num-ber, are scattered over the cutaneous surface distinct from each other, the intervening skin being healthy; on the second day of their development the centres are raised by purulent effusion, which, increasing rapidly, covers, within twelve hours, the entire of each inflamed spot, thus forming the characteristic *phlyzacious* pustule of the disease, surrounded by a narrow, inflamed areola, and situated on a hardened base; occasionally two or three of the pustules, from being developed close to each other, become confluent, and not unfrequently a few psydracious pustules form in the neighborhood, being evidently pro-duced by an intensity of the local inflammation. This stage of the eruption is attended almost invariably with severe lancinating pain and a burning sensation, both of which are much diminished, sometimes cease completely, on the maturation of the pustules. The maturation takes place from the fourth to the sixth day, the epidermic covering giving way and the contained pus being effused; a brownish-yellow crust or scab, occupying the site of the pustule, then forms rapidly, and if it be removed, a cup-shaped ulcer with hard edges will be brought into view. The scabs, if not interfered with, fall off sometimes in a few days, but they often do not separate for two or three

17

of the pustules, until at length the integuments of almost the entire body are involved in the eruption; the cutaneous surface then presents a most unhealthy aspect, large portions of it being covered with phlyzacious pustules in their various stages of development, hard dark-brown scabs, superficial ulcers, discharging unhealthy matter, and livid stains, the marks of spots that had healed. The constitution now, in most cases, sym· pathizes; in old persons extreme debility occurs, and dropsical effusions take place; and the disease in this, its most aggravated form, well deserves the name applied to it by Willan—ecthyma *cichecticum.*

Ecthyma chronicum lasts generally for four, five, or six months, or even longer, being often complicated in its advanced stages with prurigo, scabies, or chronic lichen, and being a frequent attendant on chronic organic diseases in old persons; although it spreads to all parts of the cutaneous surface, it is most thickly disseminated over the limbs, and least so on the face or scalp.

Either form may appear at any age, but the acute is most common in adults, the chronic affecting chiefly the very young and the aged; it attacks both sexes, but after the age of puberty males are more liable to the disease than females.

The *causes* of ecthyma are both constitutional and topical. The former are usually what may be termed hygienic and dietetic; thus residence in damp, ill-ventilated habitations, insufficient clothing, want of due attention to cleanliness, unwholesome food, habits of dissipation, &c., produce a state of the system in which the disease is often developed; and the direct action of substances which irritate the skin constitute the latter. Its association with chronic visceral diseases has been noticed above; it is also not an uncommon sequela of acute febrile diseases, more particularly typhus fever and dysentery.

Mr. Milton believes in the existence of a variety which he calls "vesicular ecthyma" (*Modern Treatment of Some Diseases of the Skin,* p. 87); and M. Hardy gives the name of ecthyma gangrænosum to an acute form which

Mr. Wilson thinks very probab
pemphigus gangraenosus of Dr. '

Diagnosis.—Ectbyma is in gen
by the *phlyzacious* character of
isolated manner in which they a
be confounded with either acn
characters by which it is disting
tions have been already describec
The smaller-sized pustules bear s
of modified smallpox, but the n
disease, its appearance first on f
of the body, and the accompanyi
diagnostic marks. The pustule
are, in many cases, very similar '
are with much difficulty diagnos
of the disease; the latter, howev
in very old persons, and the pr
comitant affections of the thro;
secondary syphilis, together with
of the case, marks the cutaneous
the venereal poison.

Prognosis.—When uncomplic;
disease dangerous to life; the
eruption is always of prolongec
continuance the general health is
injured.

Treatment.—In the acute stag
inflammatory symptoms that m;
dued by the use of diluents an
doses of tartar emetic dissolved in
of half a grain to the pint, will
and the solution may be made to
drink of the patient; or the '
ammonia may be given in decoct
with sugar, and flavored with ler
the bowels requires careful atten
if unhealthy, should be regulatec
of mild mercurial purgatives, cor
of taraxacum and of colchicum,
contraindicated. The only topi
the tepid bath, and from half ;

gelatine should be dissolved in each bath, if there is much local irritation; occasionally, in persons of a full habit of body, a few leeches will be applied with benefit in the neighborhood of the eruption.

The first requisite in the treatment of chronic ecthyma is to remove those causes by which the state of the system with which it is so frequently connected has been produced. In infants, the nurse should if possible be changed, or, if this cannot be done, the child ought to be weaned, and fed chiefly on ass's or goat's milk, mild alteratives, as the hydrargyrum cum cretâ, combined with myrrh and dried carbonate of soda, given, and the body warmly clad, but woollen clothing, as being apt to irritate, should not be worn next the skin. The best local application is calamine ointment, or the affected parts may be dusted with finely-powdered lapis calaminaris; emollient cataplasms or lotions generally aggravate the disease. When the eruption appears in old persons, the first and most important point is to change the air, or at least the locality in which the patient may have been residing: good and nourishing food should be given, and if there is much debility, wine or porter allowed. Should there exist any visceral organic disease, the line of treatment must be directed principally to its alleviation, if possible, and topical applications employed with caution, as the sudden repulsion of the eruption would be likely not alone to aggravate it, but might be dangerous to life. Tonics, combined with alkalies and sedatives, as in the following form, will in general be found useful:—

℞. Infusi Cinchonæ Flavæ, . . . uncias sex.
Liquoris Calcis, ... uncias novendecim.
Tincturæ Lupuli, ... drachmas duas.
Succi Conii, ... drachmas duas.   Misce.
Sumat uncias duas fluidas ter indies.

When, however, there is much debility present, alkalies should not be given, but the mineral acids, either the nitric or hydrochloric, will then be advantageously prescribed in combination with vegetable tonics; in the lurid form of the eruption, preparations of iron, more particularly the compound or aromatic iron mixture, generally prove most efficacious. For local applications many astringent and mildly stimulating ointments may be employed; a form that I have seen productive of excellent effect consists in the addition of half a drachm of oil of turpentine to the compound lead-cerate. This should be warmed and applied in the semi-fluid state, being gently smeared over the. surface with a feather. The ulcers which form may be touched daily with the solution of nitrate of silver—a scruple to the ounce, or dressed with lotions of sulphate of copper or sulphate of iron—from two to five grains to the ounce of distilled water.

The juniper tar soap has been also recommended; and the Editor has used with advantage Hebra's tinctura saponis viridis cum pice, already described.

In all forms of ecthyma the patient should be kept in the open air as much as possible, if extreme debility or accompanying organic disease does not prevent it. During convalescence, exposure to the sea air and the use of the chalybeate mineral waters for adults, will be found of especial service in promoting the restoration of health, and preventing a relapse; and for scrofulous children, the employment of cod-liver oil should not be omitted.

FURUNCULI.

Furunculi may be looked on as a sub-order, and may be briefly treated under three heads: FURUNCULUS, or boil; ANTHRAX, or carbuncle; and PUSTULA MALIGNA, malignant pustule, the Charbon of the French.

FURUNCULUS, furuncle, or boil, is, according to Dr. Macleod, "a circumscribed inflammation of the deeper portions of the true skin and the cellular tissue beneath, ending in suppuration and the sloughing of a portion of cellular tissue at its centre." It is generally multiple, occurs at any age, in the feeble and in the plethoric, is sometimes epidemical, occasionally critical, and attends convalescence from low fevers and the exanthemata. It is chiefly found in the loose cellular tissue of the shoulders, neck, back, and nates; as well as in the face, axillæ, thighs, and on the abdomen. It is said to be due to changes in diet, to the use of oatmeal food, and to derangement of

the biliary and digestive functions. It makes its appearance as a small, red, acuminated pimple, attended with
burning or throbbing pain, tension, and heat, and usually
ends in suppuration. It frequently causes irritation and
swelling of the neighboring glands, and may be attended
with febrile symptoms. Blind boils are furuncles which
do not result in suppuration.

Dr. Fox, following Mr. Wilson, observes that the treatment consists "in elimination, in the administration of
tonics, and the alleviation of local distress."

ANTHRAX, according to the excellent description of
Dr. Macleod, is "an inflammatory swelling, or carbuncle,
which consists of a circumscribed inflammation of the
subcutaneous cellular tissue, leading to its death and
expulsion." It may arise simply, or in connection with
glanders, plague, diabetes, Bright's disease, gout, and
various constitutional disturbances. It occurs chiefly in
persons of mature or advanced age, of plethoric or feeble
habit, and in those addicted to over-eating or drinking.
It is met with mostly on the posterior part of the trunk,
but sometimes occurs on the scalp. It is ushered in by
severe constitutional symptoms, accompanied or followed
by heat, itching, redness, swelling, livid discoloration, and
intense pain. The part gets brawny from the meshes of
the diseased tissue filling with plastic lymph. The tumor
remains flat, but slightly elevated. Openings soon occur
at several points, giving issue to unhealthy pus; sometimes these openings form one large opening, and gangrene
ensues. This affection is frequently fatal, especially when
it occurs on the head; and it is said to be originated by
various predisposing causes, such as old age, debility,
cachexia, and the like.

The treatment belongs more specially to the domain of
surgery; and the reader will find more full information
than is consistent with the scope of this work in treatises
on that subject. The supporting and stimulating plan
is that now usually followed in this country, with the
local application of yeast poultices and anodyne fomentations. The crucial incision has been long practised,
but latterly treatment by pressure, with the view of supporting the capillaries has been extensively advocated.

This plan was originated by Mr. O'Ferrall, of St. Vin cent's Hospital, and has been subsequently brought be fore the public by Mr. Collis, of the Meath Hospital. See *Dub. Hosp. Gaz.*, Vol. V, and *Dub. Quart. Jour.*, for 1864.

PUSTULA MALIGNA is a disease which man contracts from contact with the inferior animals affected with the *charbon* of the Continent, called in this country "joint murrain," black quarter, the quarter evil; and in German, "Milsbrand." "From one to three days after infection (observes Dr. Hillier) there appears on the part affected a small red spot, like a flea-bite, which is sometimes pre- ceded by, and always attended with considerable itching. After about twelve hours a small vesicle, about the size of a pin's head, appears; this contains a little brownish- red or yellow serum, and on its rupture the itching usually ceases, and the skin beneath is seen to be dry and of a dark color. This portion of skin is in reality dead. In less than twenty-four hours a fresh crop of vesicles ap- pears, distended with brownish-yellow serum, situated on an irregular circle round the dead skin. After twenty- four or forty-eight hours the parts beneath the eschar sometimes swell, harden, and form a solid lump, which is tolerably well defined ('bouton'). The mortification now extends to the circle of vesicles, or beyond it, and fresh ones form around, and the surrounding skin, which was pale, becomes of a livid color. Œdema now comes on in the surrounding integument, which gradually sub- sides into the healthy tissue. There is little pain, and but little elevation of temperature. The central slough enlarges, bullæ form over the central part, which is hard, and the surrounding œdema is very great." This disease runs its course in about eight or nine days, and is attended with constitutional symptoms, sometimes from the out- set; they are occasionally followed by the prominent symptoms of cholera, and the disease is frequently fatal, always serious, though only a local disorder. The head and neck are its most dangerous seats; and it is treated by the actual cautery, or caustic potash—with internal stimulants and nutritious food.

Further information may be had in a pamphlet published by M. Bourgeois, in Paris, in 1861, entitled, *La Pustule Maligne;* in Dr. Wm. Budd's paper in the *British Medical Journal* for August, 1862; in a paper by Dr. Burrows, in the *Medical Times and Gazette,* June, 1856; also in the *Medical Times and Gazette* for 1863 and 1864; and in Dr. Macleod's valuable work on *Surgical Diagnosis,* in which he points out (page 96) the diagnostic signs of anthrax from furuncle and pustula maligna.

CHAPTER V.

PAPULÆ.

THIS group of cutaneous diseases is characterize(
the eruption of minute solid elevations of the sk
papulæ, or *pimples*—generally reddish, but sometim(
the natural color of the part, or even paler, which co(
neither serum nor pus, terminate in the desquam(
of fine scales, and are almost invariably attended
intolerable itching.   The latter symptom is so mark
a characteristic of papular eruptions that it has ind(
Cazenave to place them in a subdivision of his (
group, the definition of which he gives as "gener(
local hyperæsthesia."   Mr. Erasmus Wilson distrib
the three varieties—strophulus, lichen, and pruri(
which were included in Willan and Bateman's (
Papulæ, into two of his groups—eczematous affec(
and nervous affections; Hebra includes them in his (
exudata; and Hardy places them in his order Inflam
tory Affections.

Papular eruptions are non-contagious, occur at all (
and in both sexes, and affect males more frequently (
females.   The papulæ, which are either dissemin(
and distinct from each other, or aggregated in patch(
as to form groups, may appear on a single region of
body, or may be diffused generally over the skin; (
vary in size from that of the head of a small pin to
of a pea, and are usually developed rapidly, gene(
coming out in successive crops.   They terminate in (
lution, with desquamation of the epidermis in fine mi
scales, which continues for some time; but occasion
superficial ulceration of the integuments occurs.

By most dermatologists three forms of cutaneous
eases, characterized by papular eruptions, are deser(

as originally arranged by Willan, namely, Lichen, Strophulus, and Prurigo; but the first two are manifestly merely varieties of the same affection, their characteristic phenomena are precisely similar, and the only difference between them is that the former occurs in infancy and childhood, and the latter at a more advanced age; I shall, therefore, follow the example of Rayer, Gilbert, Cazenave, Wilson, and others, and, speaking of strophulus as a species of lichen, reduce the number of papular diseases to two, namely, Lichen and Prurigo.

LICHEN.

Lichen; Λειχήν of the Greeks; Papulæ of the Latins; Dartre Farineuse, Poussée of the French; der Zitterich, Schwindfluken of the Germans.—See Plate VIII.

LICHEN (literally the moss of a tree)—including strophulus—may be defined to consist in the development of numerous minute papulæ of the color of the skin, or of a reddish hue, aggregated in patches or disseminated over the cutaneous surface, attended with heat, tingling, or even severe itching, and terminating in superficial ulceration or in epidermic desquamation. A great number of forms, both of lichen and of strophulus, have been described by Willan and other writers on diseases of the skin, and named by them either from the shape, as regards distribution, which the eruption assumes, from the color of the papulæ, from some of the attendant symptoms, from the particular structure of the portion of the integument, anatomically considered, that may be affected, and from the mildness or severity of the disease. Thus there have been constituted no less than nine varieties of lichen, and five of strophulus; they may, however, I consider, be all conveniently considered in three divisions:—

Lichen simplex.
" strophulus.
" agrius.

Lichen simplex (Plate VIII, Fig. 3) is at its outbreak very rarely attended with any constitutional disturbance; in some cases slight febrile symptoms, for a few days, precede the eruption, especially in females, but they seldom

of their phenomena resembling urticaria, and the er
tion, too, appears, as in that disease, in small patches.
is, however, distinctly papular, and has been well deno
inated lichen *urticatus*. It usually occurs on the neck a
side of the face, spreading in a few cases to the chest a
abdomen; is of an acute character, seldom lasting lon
than a few weeks, and is in general witnessed only
spring and summer.

Lichen strophulus (*Gum*).—This is a papular erupti
peculiar to the early periods of life, being rarely se
except in infants at the breast, and occurring most f
quently a few days after birth. The papulæ are of t
natural color of the skin, of a reddish or crimson hue,
white; they appear most frequently on the face and upp
extremities, but they also in some cases affect the bo
and the lower extremities. In one form, which has be
termed strophulus *intertinctus* (Plate IX, Fig. 1) popular
known as *red gum*, an eruption of very minute red papu
appears, generally a few days after birth, on the face a
the backs of the hands and arms; they are scattered ov
the surface, and intermingled with them are small er
thematous patches; for two or three days their col
becomes more vivid, they then gradually fade away, a
disappear in from a week to ten days, with some slig
epidermic desquamation. Smart itching would seem
accompany the eruption from the uneasiness the infa
exhibits.

When lichen strophulus appears on the skin at t
time the child is commencing to suffer from the irritati
attendant on teething, the papulæ, being still of a r
color, are much smaller and of a duller hue than in t
last described variety, but more numerous, and aggi
gated together in semi-confluent patches on the face, t
chest, the upper extremities, and often also on the abd
men and legs. The eruption is then denominated str
phulus *confertus*, and popularly known as *tooth-rash*; it ru
a somewhat similar course, though a little more prolong
than strophulus intertinctus, and not unfrequently, mo
especially if the child suffers much from teething, a fre
outbreak of the rash takes place as the first is fadin
away. In some cases the local and constitutional inflam

matory symptoms are tolerably intense, when the patches of papulæ are of a bright red color, and less disseminated, occurring in clusters, of not more than from five to ten or twelve, developed successively on various regions of the body, as they fade from one, appearing on another. This variety of the disease, which is rather uncommon, has been termed strophulus *volaticus—wildfire rash ;* it is often of tolerably long duration.

The papulæ in lichen strophulus are, as has been before mentioned, occasionally of the color of the skin, or even whiter, and under such circumstances have been regarded as characterizing a distinct variety of the disease—*white gum ;* of it two forms have been noticed: one—strophulus *candidus* (Plate IX, Fig. 2)—in which the papulæ are of tolerable magnitude, not surrounded by a red areola, and generally disseminated over the cutaneous surface, but at a distance from each other ; and the other—strophulus *albidus*—in which they are of small size, and occur in a few patches, each patch having a red border: in the former case they are usually distributed on the neck, the shoulders, the arms, and the lumbar region ; in the latter, on the face, the neck, and the chest. Both are attended, apparently, with much itching but no constitutional disturbance, and seldom last longer than for a few weeks.

Lichen agrius (Plate IX, Fig. 3) is occasionally a sequence of lichen simplex, but more frequently presents its peculiar phenomena from the first. In the latter case its occurrence is preceded for two or three days by smart febrile symptoms, and a remarkable burning heat and redness of the skin, so much so as at times to lead to the apprehension that scarlatina is about to set in ; the fever abates considerably, or altogether subsides on the appearance of the rash, which is developed in the form of numerous bright red, minute, acuminated, shining papules, clustered together on an uncircumscribed inflamed patch of the skin, often of considerable extent. The papules do not enlarge in size, but become more elevated from lymph being effused at their base into the subcutaneous areolar tissue, which is in consequence swollen and hard. An extreme degree of painful pruritis

attends the development of the eruption, and con
stantly present during the entire of its course, compell
the patient to rub and tear the skin; the itching wh
is incessant, is much augmented by anything a
increases the heat of the surface, especially the warm
of the bed, and thus renders rest or sleep in bed alm
impossible.   As the disease advances, the papulæ ulc
ate at their apex, and give exit to a sanious ichor, whi
concretes into thin, friable, yellowish scabs; the sk
becomes more and more inflamed, *thicker*, dry, and rugor
and eczematous vesicles and pustules of acne or impeti
appear, mingled with the lichenous eruption, or, owii
to the intense degree of local inflammation, are develop
on the surrounding integument. In this extreme for
of the eruption, the skin presents an hypertrophi
aspect, is of a dark livid color, uneven on the surfa
rugose, and fissured, and discharges a copious serosity.

In the comparatively milder cases of lichen agrius t
eruption commences to fade about the tenth or twelf
day, the subcutaneous effusion is absorbed, the local ir
tation diminishes, and the disease terminates in from
fortnight to three weeks with epidermic desquamatio
More usually, however, its duration is prolonged for s
weeks or three months, even in cases not at all aggi
vated; and it not unfrequently lasts for years, wi
occasional remissions during cold weather.

This form of lichen especially affects certain regio
of the body, more particularly the face—where its m
usual seat is on the forehead—and the backs of the han
and fingers; when it occurs on the face, the swelling
the integuments is usually much greater than when
attacks other regions of the body; the features, presenti
a tuberculated aspect, are completely altered in expre
sion, and the eyes are sometimes almost entirely clos
from the thickening of the upper eyelid. On the bac
of the hands and fingers (Lichen agrius, dorsi manû
see plate IX, Fig. 4) the eruption is in general attend
with much discharge, and in some cases complica
scabies, when it causes an extreme degree of suffering.

Heat seems to have a peculiar influence both in pr
ducing and aggravating lichen agrius; it is thus n

unfrequently developed in hot summer weather, in this
country, in persons predisposed to skin diseases; but it
is in warm climates that this influence is especially witnessed, and the eruption is consequently so frequent
there that it has been regarded as constituting a distinct
variety, termed lichen *tropicus*—the *prickly heat* of the
East Indies. The following graphic description of the
eruption, which is especially interesting as embodying
his personal experience of it, is from the pen of the late
Dr. James Johnson. "Among the primary effects of a
hot climate may be noticed the prickly heat, a very
troublesome visitor, which few Europeans escape. It is
one of the miseries of a tropical life, and a most unman-
ageable one it is. From mosquitoes, cockroaches, ants,
and the numerous other tribes of depredators on our
personal property, we have some defence by night, and
in general a respite by day, but this unwelcome guest
assails us at all, and particularly the most unseasonable,
hours. Many a time have I been forced to spring from
table, and abandon the repast which I had scarcely
touched, to writhe about in the open air for a quarter of
an hour: and often have I returned to the charge with
no better success against my ignoble opponent! The
night affords no asylum. For some weeks after arriving
in India I seldom could obtain more than an hour's sleep
at one time before I was compelled to quit my couch
with no small precipitation, and if there were any water
at hand to sluice it over me, for the purpose of allaying
the inexpressible irritation! But this was productive of
temporary relief only, and what was worse, a more violent
paroxysm frequently succeeded. The sensations arising
from prickly heat are perfectly indescribable, being
compounded of pricking, itching, tingling, and many
other feelings for which I have no appropriate appellation. It is usually, but not invariably, accompanied by
an eruption of vivid red pimples, not larger in general
than a pin's head, which spread over the breast, arms,
thighs, neck, and occasionally along the forehead close to
the hair. This eruption often disappears in a great measure when we are sitting quiet, and the skin is cool; but
no sooner do we use any exercise that brings out a per-

very chronic, desquamate, and disappear. On the healthy skin of other parts tubercular spots, resembling acne, appear, pustulate, and subside. L. ruber is characterized by the exhibition of small red papules, distinct, and on parts only of the body, chiefly on the extremities. It afterwards simulates psoriasis; and there are never any excoriations from it. Hebra has seen but fourteen cases of L. ruber.

Causes.—Lichen occurs at any age, but its different forms seem to prevail at different periods of life: thus, as has been already remarked, lichen strophulus is a disease of early infancy, very seldom appearing after the process of first dentition is completed, and being most frequent for a month after birth—in fact, few infants then escape it; lichen agrius is most usually an eruption of adult life and of old age; and lichen simplex affects young persons and those in the prime of life. The predisposing, and often also the exciting causes of this eruption are very obscure: it is certainly witnessed most frequently in persons of a nervous temperament, with a fine, easily irritated skin, and in whom the cutaneous capillary circulation is very active, but with deficient perspiration. Mr. Wilson believes it to be essentially a disease of debility. The occurrence of lichen strophulus in infants immediately after birth may be accounted for by the numerous local irritants to which their fine, delicate skin is then necessarily exposed, such as the effect of sudden changes of temperature, of the water and soap used in washing, of the friction employed in drying the surface afterwards, of the clothing, &c. The action of local irritants has a decided effect in the production of lichen at all ages and in most cases: thus it is caused on the forehead in men by the pressure of a tight hat, on the face and hands by harsh dry winds, and by solar heat or that arising from a very hot fire—the latter is a not unfrequent cause of the eruption in some trades, such as blacksmiths, furnace-men, &c.—and on the legs by the friction of worsted stockings, particularly when the veins are in a varicose condition. In certain occupations lichen is developed on the backs of the hands and on the fingers—in the same manner as other eruptions are—from the irritation of certain substances; thus it is witnessed in grocers, bakers, washerwomen, &c., when it is described as constituting one of the forms of the so-called grocers', bakers', or washerwomen's itch. In many cases lichen seems to be connected with derangement of the digestive organs, and its appearance on the skin in persons who had long suffered from painful affections of the stomach or head was noticed by Bateman and Biett as a favorable circumstance. The use of stimulating drinks, or of heating articles of food, or of spices, will, in some individuals, be followed by a lichenous eruption.

Diagnosis.—Lichen simplex is in general easy of recognition, in consequence of its distinctly papular character; the disease with which it is most likely to be confounded is prurigo, the elementary character of the eruption in both being the same; but in the latter the papulæ are larger and more globular—their apex being rather flattened than acuminate, and they are generally of the same color as the part of the skin on which they appear; the itching, also, which accompanies lichen simplex is not of the same acrid, burning nature as that which is so characteristic of prurigo. When the papulæ begin to fade and to desquamate at their apex, the eruption might be mistaken for psoriasis guttata, from which it is distinguished by the scales being much thinner, more minute and bran-like, and by the papular elevation of the surface from which they separate, as may be recognized with the aid of a lens, or felt by passing the finger over the part. From scabies and eczema, lichen **simplex** is diagnosed by the vesicular character of both **these eruptions** and the copious discharge with which they are attended. Lichen circumscriptus is liable to be confounded with herpes circinatus, or erythema circinatum; from both it is distinguished by the character of **the eruption**, *papulæ being never witnessed in any stage of either of these diseases.* From urticaria lichen urticatus **is often** with much difficulty diagnosed; the chief **distinguishing** characters are *the wheal-like elevations with the paler centres,* and the more decidedly evanescent nature of the former.

The only eruption with which lichen strophulus **could** be confounded is prurigo, but the age at which it **occurs** is sufficient to distinguish it from that disease; moreover, in those forms of strophulus in which the papulæ are red they are darker colored than in prurigo, and in the white varieties they are much paler.

The more aggravated cases of lichen agrius, in their advanced stages, bear much resemblance to chronic eczema rubrum, and are often with difficulty diagnosed from it; but careful examination will scarcely ever fail to detect *the popular character of the former;* in it, too, the integuments are much swollen, thickened, and tubercular, the serous discharge and the epidermic desquamation considerably less, while the itching is more intense; the peculiar red cracks and fissures from which the bloody ichor oozes are, moreover, not seen in eczema. On the face, lichen agrius may be mistaken for acne rosacea, from which it is distinguished by the *pustular nature and deep crimson or violaceous hue of the latter;* they also affect different regions of the face, lichen being generally situated on the forehead and the sides of the cheeks in front of the ears and lips, while acne rosacea occurs almost invariably on the nose and the most prominent portions of the cheeks. Impetigo occurring on the face in adults has been confounded with lichen agrius, but *the pustular character and greenish honey-like scabs of that eruption* sufficiently characterize it. This form of lichen is not so liable to be mistaken for psoriasis as lichen simplex, the attendant serous discharge and the characteristic itching marking especially the difference between them.

Lichen is a very frequent form of syphilitic eruption; it is then characterized by the peculiar dull coppery hue it presents, by its being always of a chronic character, unattended with any inflammatory symptoms, either local or constitutional, by the absence generally of itching, and by the presence of the other secondary symptoms of the venereal disease, together with the history of the individual case. In infants, hereditary syphilis must be carefully distinguished from lichen strophulus; the former rarely presents a papular form, and it occurs in patches or coppery stains, generally attended with a serous or sero-purulent discharge, on various parts of the body, but especially about the pudendal region, and on those parts of the skin on which the hair grows.

Prognosis.—In infants and young children the occurrence of lichen strophulus is quite unimportant, as it generally runs its course in a few days, not being attended with the least danger or injury to health, requiring notice merely in consequence of the accompanying itching, rendering the little patients fretful. In adults and old persons an eruption of lichen, though never attended with danger, is extremely troublesome, in consequence of the local annoyance and suffering by which it is accompanied, and the tendency, more especially of lichen agrius, to become chronic; like most other cutaneous eruptions, the longer its duration has been the more rebellious is it to treatment. The disease is also more obstinate on the face or hands than when it is situated on those parts of the body that are ordinarily covered; and the complication of other cutaneous eruptions with it invariably renders the treatment more difficult. In giving a prognosis in any of the severe forms of lichen it should be remembered that relapses are very liable to occur—the least exciting cause, such as even the heat of the sun in summer, being sufficient to reproduce the disease.

Treatment.—In all papular eruptions a manifest indication of treatment is derived from the hyperæsthesia of the cutaneous structure which accompanies them in their acute as well as in their chronic stages, and this should always influence our choice of remedies, whether tonics or antiphlogistics, according to individual circumstances,

may be required. In their early stages, local applications
will in general be found sufficient to check the progress
of the eruption, unless when symptoms of inflammatory
action are present, but these are usually of a trifling
nature and of short duration ; when, however, they have
become chronic, the most active constitutional alterative
treatment is required; and even under its most judicious
employment they not uncommonly baffle the physician's
art for a length of time.

In lichen simplex occurring in young persons of a
robust constitution, restricted diet should be enforced
at its commencement, together with rest in bed if the
eruption is at all extensive, and the administration of
diaphoretics, the bowels having been previously opened
by a mercurial purge, provided the papulæ are well
developed on the skin: the antimonial diaphoretics,
combined with guaiacum and Dover's powder, as in somewhat the following form, are usually productive of more
benefit than saline diaphoretics:— .

R. Antimonii Sulphurati, ... grana viginti.
    Guaiaci Resinæ, in pulvere, . . grana viginti et quatuor.
    Pulveris Ipecacuanhæ cum Opio, grana duodecim.
    Ope mucilaginis misce et in pilulas duodecim divide.
        Sumat unam sextis horis.

To allay the itching and local irritation, tepid baths of
fresh water may be employed daily, and the skin, having
been well dried, smeared afterwards with olive oil, to
every ounce of which twenty minims of chloroform have
been added. When the general inflammatory symptoms
are subdued by this treatment, if the disease exhibits
any tendency to become chronic, the compound lead-
cerate with glycerine may be applied to the surface, and
the ar s sponged twice daily with an alkaline spirituous
wash. t

In any of the forms of lichen strophulus medical
interference is scarcely required, and especial care should
be taken that no treatment, whether local or constitutional, be employed by which the eruption might be
repelled. If any derangements of the digestive organs
exist they may require the use of mild alteratives or

gentle mercurial purgatives; and when the eruption occurs at the period of dentition the gums ought to be lanced freely. The annoying pruritus, which so constantly seems to accompany strophulus, is best allayed by the use of the tepid fresh-water bath with gelatine, and the application of olive oil to the spots of eruption ; cold cream is also useful for this purpose, or the acetate of zinc cream, to every ounce of which two drops of oil of bitter almonds have been added, may be employed in more aggravated cases.

In the early stages of lichen agrius, while the inflammatory symptoms are present, the treatment should be decidedly antiphlogistic; but unless in strong, healthy, young persons residing in the country, general bleeding is not admissible, the local abstraction of blood, by means of leeches applied in the neighborhood of the eruption, being in most cases sufficient.[1] Even in the chronic stages of the disease this form of local bleeding is in general attended with the best results, as it relieves the congested state of the capillary circulation which is present, but the leeches should never be applied on any part of the skin which is affected, as their bites might give rise there to troublesome ulceration. At first the irritation caused by the eruption is best alleviated by gelatine baths and soothing ointments or lotions; of the former, the carbonate or acetate of lead cerate with chloroform, the compound lead cerate with glycerine, the oxide or carbonate of zinc ointment, with which oil of bitter almonds or hydrocyanic acid has been combined, or the hemlock ointment, will be used with benefit; of the latter, the weak lead wash, to which glycerine has been added in the proportion of a drachm to the ounce, equal parts of camphor mixture and distilled vinegar, a lotion containing a drachm of succus conii, half a drachm of glycerine, and a grain of carbonate of soda to the ounce of elder-flower water, or alkaline washes with hydrocyanic acid, as in the following form, may be employed :—

---

[1] The Editor cannot concur in this implied recommendation of general bleeding.

R. Boracis, ... grana triginta.
   Aquæ Rosæ, ... uncias octo.
   Acidi Hydrocyanici diluti, ... drachmas duas.
                          Misce.

If any connection can be traced between the appearance
on the cutaneous surface of the eruption and disease of
some internal organ, or deranged function, the remedial
measures employed must be especially directed towards
the alleviation of the former, and the correction of the
latter. With this view saline and mercurial purgatives
are generally required in most cases; and when debility
exists, their employment may be conjoined advantageously with chalybeates or vegetable bitters, and the
dilute mineral acids. Lichen is not unfrequently associated, in old persons, with the gouty or rheumatic
diathesis, and in such cases preparations of colchicum,
combined with the liquor potassæ or the carbonate of
ammonia, should be prescribed.

In the chronic stages of lichen agrius more active
constitutional treatment is usually required, while at
the same time attention is paid to any complication that
may exist. Iodine and arsenic, either separately or in
combination, in some of the forms described in former
chapters, will be found necessary, and they may be
given with tonics or diaphoretics, according to individual
circumstances. When there is general debility present,
more especially an anæmic condition of the system,
iodine combined with iron in the form of the syrup or
pills of the iodide of iron, is most useful. Tincture of
aconite is also an excellent remedy, more especially if
the hyperæsthesia of the cutaneous surface is well
marked, but its administration must, as in all other
diseases, be carefully watched; there is nothing to
contraindicate its employment at the same time with
the powerful alteratives above mentioned. Sulphur
and its preparations are highly recommended by many
practitioners, in chronic lichen, but I must confess that
they have not proved so successful in my hands as they
are stated to have done with others. It was at one time
too much the custom to administer sulphur in nearly
every form of cutaneous eruption, chiefly, I believe, in

consequence of its being evolved so manifestly by means of the insensible perspiration ; but for this very reason its use often proves highly injurious, owing to the direct stimulant action it thereby exercises in diseases which are of an inflammatory nature, or which are liable to be aggravated by determination of blood to the cutaneous capillaries.

Mr. Milton gives nitric acid with advantage, and speaks highly of arsenicals in refractory cases. In common with Wilson and Hardy, he prefers the omission of the spirit of lavender in Fowler's solution, and thinks the best mode of administering the latter is in plain water. In this the Editor fully coincides; and in the Dispensary for Skin Diseases, in Bishop-street, liquor arsenicalis is usually given in that way. Mr. Wilson thinks the following is the best form for an anti-pruriginous lotion : Pyroligneous oil of juniper and rectified spirit, of each an ounce; water six ounces. Mix.

Most of the local applications already spoken of will be found beneficial in chronic lichen agrius, but even in the same case they must be constantly varied, according to the severity of the local symptoms; when all inflammatory tendency has subsided, an ointment containing twenty grains of the iodide of sulphur to an ounce of white wax ointment, to which six minims of chloroform are added, will be found productive of excellent effect, an alkaline spirituous wash being at the same time used.

PRURIGO.

Prurigo (Lat. and Eng.); Κνησμός, of the Greeks; Prurit, of the French ; Das juckten, of the Germans.— See Plate IX.

PRURIGO.—It is very doubtful whether this disease should be termed an *eruption* of the skin or not, so frequently does it occur without any visible phenomena to indicate its existence, the only symptoms present being obstinate, intense itching, without heat, pain, or sensible elevation of the surface. But as in many cases it is attended with the development of papulæ, it must, in an artificial arrangement of skin diseases, be classed with

19

lichen. The papulæ, when they do occur, are of a some
what larger size, rounder, and less acuminate than thos
of lichen; and of the color of the skin, or of a yellow
ish hue. The disease is essentially of a chronic natur
is not contagious, and is neither preceded nor accon
panied by constitutional symptoms; nevertheless, whe
it has existed for some time, the health becomes more c
less deranged in consequence of the extreme suffe
ing caused by the itching and local irritation attendar
on it.

Three forms of prurigo have in general been describe
by dermatologists—Prurigo *mitis*, Prurigo *formican*
and Prurigo *senilis;* the first two are distinguished froi
each other merely by the degree of severity of the sym
toms, and may therefore be considered together; th
third, although denominated simply from its occurrenc
in old age only, yet requires to be noticed separately, i
consequence of some of its phenomena being peculis
and characteristic. I shall therefore describe the diseas
as consisting of two species, terming them—

Prurigo vulgaris.
" senilis.

Prurigo vulgaris (Plate IX, Fig. 5), then, may be eithe
mild or severe, the latter being the more frequent. Th
mild variety is developed by the eruption on the cut
neous surface of scattered papulæ, about the size of
millet-seed, without the least redness, inflammation, c
sense of heat; they are of the color of that part of th
integument on which they may be seated, but little el
vated, and scarcely to be distinguished unless with th
aid of a lens, or by passing the finger over the surfac
The attendant pruritus is not very severe, although suf
ciently sharp and stinging to cause the patient to scratc
the affected parts with the nails; the papulæ are th
torn, and a minute, blackish crust thereby formed o
their apices, which gives a remarkably characteristi
appearance to the affection.

In the severe variety of prurigo vulgaris the diseas
may commence with or without the eruption of papuls
but in all cases they are usually developed in some of it

stages; when they do occur they are more numerous
than in the mild form, of the same color, shape, and size,
or sometimes even larger. It is, however, the remarkable cutaneous hyperæsthesia and consequent intense
pruritus which especially mark the aggravated character
of the affection, and from whence it has derived its appellation—*formicans*, the sensations accompanying it being
often compared to those produced by the sting of an ant.
This comparison, however, very faintly expresses the sufferings attendant on the disease: not a single spot of the
skin in its entire extent but is more or less the seat of an
extreme degree of itching, which compels the individual
affected to tear with his nails and rub the surface all but
unceasingly; at times comparative cessation of the pruritus occurs, occasionally lasting for two or three hours,
more usually of shorter duration; but it is again exacerbated by the most trifling exciting cause—the friction of
the clothes, changes of temperature—especially the heat
of the fire or the warmth of the bed—mental emotions,
etc. In consequence of heat increasing much the local
symptoms, the itching is always remarkably aggravated
at night, rest is thus completely destroyed, sleep being
rendered impossible, hour after hour is passed tearing
the skin, and the sufferer is often compelled to seek relief
by lying on the floor without any covering. In one case
of extreme severity which I attended, the exacerbations
and remissions assumed a well-marked, intermittent,
semi-quotidian type; the itching commenced every after-
noon at about two o'clock, and continued until six
o'clock, when it generally abated, and there was comparative ease until the same hour on the following morning; it then returned, and lasted again for the same length
of time; but the night sufferings were tenfold more
severe than those of the day; this intermittent character
of the pruritus had lasted, at the time I saw the patient,
a young man of twenty-three years of age, for more than
two years, and his health, both mental and bodily, was
sensibly affected from the constant suffering and loss of
sleep.

When the disease has lasted for any time, the cutaneous surface is torn and fissured from the constant

scratching; if papulæ existed, their site is marked
minute, blackish crusts or small excoriations, and
skin is thickened, uneven and coarse, being found,
close examination, as remarked by Wilson, "raised i
small flat elevations, caused by the swelling of the li
angular compartments between the linear markin
The natural color of the skin is also much altered,
aspect being of a dirty brownish-yellow hue.

The milder form of prurigo vulgaris seldom lasts
a longer period than two or three weeks, but the durat
of the severe variety is in some cases almost indefinit
prolonged, recovery rarely taking place in a shorter ti
than from four to six months. The papulæ in both
developed, in the first instance, on the chest, the ne
the lumbar region, the shoulder, and the outside of
thighs, from whence, when the disease lasts for more tl
a month or two, they spread to the arms and legs, but
not appear on the face, the scalp, or the hands, althot
these parts, in aggravated cases, are rarely free from m
or less pruritus. Such of the papulæ as escape be
torn by the nails terminate in slight furfuraceous
quamation. The disease is not unfrequently complica
by the simultaneous occurrence of scabies and eczei
and in some cases, of ecthyma.

Prurigo senilis (Plate IX, Fig. 6) occurs, as its spec
name indicates, only in advanced life; the pruritus, wh
is usually of remarkable intensity, is attended alwi
with an eruption of papulæ; these are of larger size tl
in either of the forms of prurigo vulgaris, but thev
fewer in number, more dispersed over the surface of
body, and of a dull dingy-yellow color; soon torn w
the nails, small blackish crusts appear on their api
which also constantly bleed slightly when irritated.
chief peculiarity, however, in prurigo senilis is, that i
almost invariably attended with the appearance of in
merable pediculi on the integuments of every part of
body—a complication never absent in the poor, and
persons of filthy habits. Their presence aggrava
much the other symptoms of the disease: the skin l
comes of a livid color, thickened, rough, with a leathe
aspect, and covered with superficial excoriations, a

small pustules and indolent boils form in different regions of the body; the pediculi are renewed nearly as quickly as they can be removed from the surface, which has caused a controversy as to whether they are developed from the integuments or not. By some dermatologists the occurrence of the pediculi is considered, as only an accidental circumstance, and not constituting a symptom of the disease; by others it is regarded, more correctly I think, as an essential feature of the eruption, and they have, therefore, following Alibert, denominated the form thus characterized, prurigo *pedicularis.*

Many of the French schools describe, as a distinct disease of the skin, this development of pediculi on the cutaneous surface of the body, generally terming it *Phthiriasis,* and dividing it into three species, as it may be general or partial—Phthiriasis *corporis,* Phthiriasis *capitis,* and Phthiriasis *pubis*—considering the simultaneous appearance of the papulæ of prurigo as only a complication; but as I have almost invariably seen them occur together in old persons, I think it more correct to describe this singular affection as a variety of prurigo senilis. The pediculus in these cases has been called *Phthirius,* or *Pediculus pubis.*

Prurigo vulgaris very frequently affects some special region of the skin from which it does not spread, but becoming chronic there causes extreme suffering, and is very obstinate. It thus attacks the scrotum in males, and the pudendal region in females: the former, termed prurigo *scroti,* is a very troublesome affection, being attended with a constant itching, which, instead of being relieved, is much aggravated by scratching with the nails, yet the sufferer from it cannot resist the almost unceasing inclination which exists to attempt thus to alleviate the tormenting pruritus; the habit thence acquired can scarcely be got rid of, and even long after all apparent symptoms of the disease have disappeared, the integuments are continually fretted and torn. In females, prurigo *pudendi* is situated chiefly on the mucous membrane of the labia, but often extends to the entire surface, both cutaneous and mucous, of this disease; it is a most distressing and obstinate disease, and not uncommonly

19*

produces symptoms analogous to those of nymphomania. Another frequent form of local prurigo is prurigo *podicis;* in it a constant itching of the verge of the anus exists; and papulæ, which are often not present in the other local forms of the disease, are here almost invariably developed, and sometimes attain a considerable magnitude; occasional intermissions of the pruritus occur; but the least irritation, augmented heat of the surface, or derangement of the digestive organs, causes an exacerbated return of this tormenting sensation. Other regions of the skin are at times the seat of severe itching, and have been described, but without sufficient reason, as being then affected with prurigo; thus dermatologists have spoken of prur go *urethralis,* prurigo *præputialis,* prurigo *pubis,* and prurigo *palmaris;* the latter has been specially mentioned by Alibert as affecting the soles of the feet, of which he states that he witnessed many examples.

Causes.—Prurigo may occur at any age, but is most frequently seen in old persons, and more commonly in males than females: young persons are more liable to its attacks than adults, and it has been witnessed even in early infancy. That state of the constitution in which cutaneous irritability exists, as exhibited by the occurrence of troublesome ulcers from slight causes, and an inaptitude, so to say, of even the most trifling abrasion to heal, peculiarly predisposes to its development; there is usually in such a condition an impoverished blood circulating in the vessels, and a highly irritable nervous system. Bad or insufficient diet, want of care as to cleanliness, unhealthy habitations, sedentary occupations, or confinement to the house caused by ill-health, defective clothing, dissipated habits, &c., are both predisposing and exciting causes of prurigo. I have often thought that in gaols and workhouses, amongst the aged inhabitants of which the disease is so common, and also amongst the poor, it may be caused by the *sameness* of food, which, too often, is defective in nutritive qualities. Other cutaneous eruptions which are attended with local irritation, more especially scabies and lichen, not uncommonly are exciting causes of this affection; and it is in old persons a frequent accompaniment of convalescence from debilitating diseases, particularly fever, dysentery, and chronic diarrhœa.

Diagnosis.—The most characteristic symptoms of prurigo are the intense pruritus, the blackish crusts which are produced on the papulæ, and the alteration that takes place in the appearance of the integuments. The diseases with which it is most likely to be confounded are lichen and scabies, and the mode of diagnosing it from them has been already noticed when describing these eruptions, but, as has been before remarked, they often coexist.

Prognosis.—Prurigo, when it becomes chronic, is one of the most obstinate diseases of the skin ; in old persons seldom yielding to any treatment. Although prurigo vulgaris cannot be said to be attended with danger to life, yet it renders life miserable, sometimes for years, and from being a constant cause of irritation, may, to a certain extent, affect the mind, as is witnessed in some cases. The senile form of prurigo, although it is not in itself a mortal affection, nevertheless seldom disappears unless with life, and when it occurs as a complication of some organic or chronic disease, unquestionably hastens the fatal termination.

As regards the *pathology* of prurigo, it is evidently chiefly a hyperæsthesia of the cutaneous structure; the changes in the state of skin which attend it being usually produced by the local irritation thereby occasioned.

Romberg is of a like opinion; Bärensprung thinks it is primarily an affection of the papillæ, and looks on the pruritus as secondary. Fox considers it to result from an unhealthy state of skin, not a pure neurose ; and that the papules are determined in their formation by the local irritation ; " the effusion of blood upon their apices being a sufficient evidence of the badly nourished derma." Hillier believes P. senilis to be caused by the pediculus. Gout, rheumatism, and albuminuria are said, by various writers, to cause prurigo; and, in common with some physicians, the Editor has observed a modified form of it to be generally associated with jaundice, presumptively from the circulation of bile in the blood.

Treatment.—If Dr. Neligan's view of the pathology

be found useless. With this view mild mercurial and saline purgatives may be prescribed to correct the secretions from the digestive organs; and when there is a deficiency of bile in the discharges, as is not unfrequently the case in adults and old persons, dried carbonate of soda and extract of taraxacum should be combined with the mercurials. In females the association of the disease with derangement of the menstrual function is often witnessed; and when such exists there is generally an anemic state of the system requiring the use of preparations of iron, but they should never be prescribed except in combination with sedatives, as otherwise the stimulant action is apt to augment the pruritus; the same observation applies to the employment of chalybeates in the old and debilitated, for whom they are also generally indicated in prurigo. They may be advantageously combined, as in the following form :—

R. Misturæ Ferri compositæ, . . uncias octo.
Iufusi Lupuli, ... uncias tres cum semisse.
Succi Conii, ... semi-unciam. Misce.
Sumat semi-unciam fluidam sextis horis.

Or Dover's powder may be given in rather larger doses at night, preparations of iron being administered during the day. In very young persons antiphlogistics are sometimes needed as preludes to other remedies, but in no case should the strength be much weakened, as then the disease is more apt to become chronic. When prurigo has lasted for any time, or has resisted other plans of treatment, more active medicines of the class which especially influences the nervous system should be prescribed: nux vomica, or its alkaloid, and tincture of aconite, thus often prove useful; the former has succeeded in my hands when all other remedies seemed to fail; it may be given in the following form, a combination which will be found to promote a healthy condition of the digestive organs, and to correct the loss of tone which they exhibit usually in this disease:—

℞. Extracti Nucis Vomicæ, . . grana tres.
Fellis Bovini Purificati, . . grana sex.
Extracti Taraxaci, ... grana viginti et quatuor.
Pulveris Myrrhæ, ... grana octodecim.
Misce et divide in pilulas viginti quatuor.
Sumat unam ter indies.

The tincture of aconite should be given in the ordinary doses, from five to eight minims of the Dublin preparation,[1] or half that quantity of Fleming's tincture, and its effects carefully watched. I have also administered the *succus conii*, in doses of a drachm three times a day, in an ounce of the camphor mixture with magnesia, with excellent effect in some obstinate cases of senile prurigo. Preparations of sulphur are recommended by many in the treatment of this disease, and in the very chronic forms the sulphurous mineral waters, as those of Lucan, of Harrogate, of the Pyrenees, &c., prove of unquestionable benefit. Indeed, in all cases change of air, if possible, to the original sources of mineral waters—the saline in the early stages, the chalybeate in the more advanced, and the sulphurous when the disease is very chronic and obstinate—so that they may be drunk there, is highly advisable.

Mr. Milton recommends the administration of from $\frac{1}{80}$th to $\frac{1}{84}$th of a grain of strychnia every three hours until a decided effect is produced, or until nervous symptoms show themselves; he then follows up the treatment just mentioned with the administration of arsenic.

The local treatment is now to be spoken of: and at first nothing is requisite further than the daily use of the *hot* fresh-water bath, to which, if the itching is extreme,

---

[1] The tincture of aconite of the *British Pharmacopœia* is only *half* the strength of the above; so that a proportionately larger dose of *it* should be given. Professor Macnamara, however, gives the dose of the *Br. Ph.* tincture as 5 minims "cautiously increased" to 10.—*Neligan's Medicines*, Sixth Edition, by Macnamara.

Chapter on Urticaria, I have derived most excellent results; in fact, latterly I have seldom had occasion to employ any other application; but the substances mentioned above, as being used in lotions or washes, may also be applied as unguents, and the addition of glycerine will generally be found of advantage. In very obstinate cases the chloroform may be combined with iodide of lead, as follows:—

℞. Iodidi Plumbi, . . . grana duodecim.
Unguenti Simplicis, . unciam.
Chloroformi, ... minima octo, ad minima duodecim.
Glycerini, ... drachmam. Misce.

Mr. Milton recommends the Turkish or Roman bath; and so does Mr. Wilson, who advises the use of juniper tar soap. Dr. Frazer recommends a preparation composed of finely powdered camphor, with six or eight parts of rice or potato starch, and a small quantity of acetate or carbonate of lead, to be dusted on the surface three or four times daily, at the same time using calomel ointment. Hebra uses cod-liver oil externally and internally; Malmsten also advises the internal use of this oil. Bärensprung advises cold baths, ablutions, and applications, with a corrosive sublimate bath at 95° Fahr. every second day. —*Dub. Quar. Jour.*, May, 1860, p. 492. In cases of prurigo senilis the Editor generally finds a soft-soap hot-water bath, with the subsequent application of a diluted citrine ointment (one part to three of lard) to be very useful. These baths should be taken at night, thrice a week, and the ointment washed off in the morning. When greasy applications are used alkaline tepid baths should be employed daily to cleanse the skin, the patient remaining in the water for at least twenty minutes.

Strict attention to diet and regimen is requisite in all cases; stimulant food or drink being especially avoided.

CHAPTER VI.

SQUAMÆ.—(See Plate X.)

THERE is no class of diseases of the skin so well characterized by the apparent phenomena as that in which
the formation of a scale (*Squama*) constitutes the essential
feature; epidermic desquamation, as has been in the previous pages so frequently noticed, is present in many
cutaneous eruptions, but that differs in many respects from
the secretion and subsequent shedding of true scales,
which consist, according to the admirable definition of
Willan, of "a lamina of morbid cuticle, hard, thickened,
whitish, and opaque." Although in some of the forms
more or less change from the primitive characters of the
eruption takes place in the progress of the disease, it is
never such as to mask their scaly nature, and the diagnosis is consequently attended with less difficulty than
that of most other cutaneous affections. Squamous eruptions may be defined to consist in the secretion of dry,
laminated, whitish scales on the cutaneous surface, usually
occurring in patches, often of a circular form, but sometimes generally diffused, and covering an extended portion of the integuments. The scales, which are somewhat
elevated above the level of the surrounding skin, readily
fall off, to be again rapidly renewed, and the portions of
the cutaneous surface on which they are formed are of a
smooth, glistening aspect, reddish and dry.

Scaly diseases are essentially of a chronic, non-inflam-
matory nature, are slowly developed, and are not propagated by contagion. They may appear on any part of
the body, but they chiefly affect, at least in the first instance, the extremities, whence they usually spread to
other regions, being rarely confined to a single locality,
with the exception of pityriasis, which occasionally occurs

on some special portion of the skin. They are developed also at all seasons of the year, and are not apt, like other cutaneous diseases influenced by the atmospheric temperature, to disappear and again reappear at certain times.

The eruptions included in the order Squamæ are divided by Willan into four groups—Lepra, Psoriasis, Pityriasis, and Ichthyosis—and this arrangement has been followed by many modern dermatologists; recently, however, it has been very generally admitted that Ichthyosis was incorrectly classed by him amongst scaly diseases, and doubt has been thrown on the propriety of describing psoriasis and lepra as different forms, they being, moreover, evidently regarded by the ancient medical writers as constituting merely varieties of the same eruption. Of foreign authorities it may be observed that Hardy, Bazin, and Duchesne, among the French, and Fuchs, Riecke, Hebra, and Simon, among the German writers, look on them as identical. Mr. Wilson, in the last edition of his work, has applied the term psoriasis to the chronic stages of eczema; and he uses the term Lepra, or *Alphos*, which he prefers, to designate what is called psoriasis by most other writers. Fox, along with Wilson, looks on the Lepra and Psoriasis of Willan as identical in nature. Ichthyosis cannot, with any regard to accuracy in classification, be grouped in this class, for it is not attended with a separation—throwing off of scales, or desquamation, one of the most characteristic signs of this order of cutaneous eruptions; the epidermis is in it truly hypertrophied, and I shall therefore describe it as constituting one of that group of skin diseases which I have termed Hypertrophiæ. To even a superficial observer it must be evident that psoriasis and lepra have no essential differences, and they require a precisely similar plan of treatment; regarding them, therefore, as distinct affections could only tend to complicate their study. The number of scaly diseases of the skin is thus reduced to two— Psoriasis, Pityriasis.

20

PSORIASIS.

Psoriasis, or Lepra; from ψώρα (which is from the Hebrew, Tsorat); or more correctly, according to Liddell and Scott's Lexicon, from ψάω or ψωω to touch; λέπρα, of the Greeks; Vitiligo, of Celsus; Lepre, of the French, Der Aussatz, of the Germans; Sahaſati, of the Arabian writers; Sappachath of the Levitical Code (Lev. xiii, 2).—See Plate X.

PSORIASIS (*Dry tetter; Dry scale*)—under which term it will be understood I include Lepra—is characterized by consisting in the formation on the cutaneous surface, and subsequent desquamation, of true scales, the scales being of tolerable consistence, dry and friable, of a silvery or grayish whiteness, and separating in laminæ of about the size and consistence of particles of bran. The eruption appears in small, round, or irregularly-shaped spots, distinct from each other, scattered over the cutaneous surface in large, circular patches, depressed in the centre, or in masses so closely aggregated and confluent as to envelop an extended portion of the skin in one vast coating of scales in consistent layers. The surface of the integument on which they are situated is raised, reddish, and apparently inflamed, but unattended with any discharge; nevertheless, when the eruption has been of long duration, fissures and cracks through the deeper-seated tissues form, from which an ichorous, bloody secretion exudes. Psoriasis has been considered by many writers on diseases of the skin to be a special chronic inflammation of the cutaneous structures, the speciality consisting in the development of scales; it cannot, however, I think, be regarded as an inflammatory disease, for it is not attended with heat or other local sign or symptom of inflammation, except a slight degree of itching, unless when the affected surface is irritated by some cause.

With regard to the nature of the disease, Dr. Fox observes, on the authority of Hebra, Simon, and Rokitanski, that it is "the presence of an hyperæmic state of derma, connected specially with an excessive formation of epidermic scales; a morbid hypertrophy. The true derma appears not to be affected, except in long-standing cases, and then only as a secondary result of the long-continued congestion. The patches are made up of epidermic cells, imperfectly, because quickly formed—collected together; the papillary layer of the skin seems, however, to play the part most active in this change."—*Op. cit.*, p. 157. Dr. Wertheim, of Vienna, thinks it is due to the circulation of vegetable parasitic elements in the blood current; and he ascribes its greater frequency in *men* (?) to their habit of drinking more alcohol than women. Dr. Wertheim's observations, which appeared in the *Gaz. Heb. de Méd. et Chir.*, 1864, and are noted in the *Med. Times and Gaz.*, 24th July, 1864, are discussed at length by Dr. Fox, who thinks "such a theory cannot be maintained for a moment."—*Op. cit.*, p. 159.

The eruption appears in the form of minute, slightly-elevated papulæ, with a small scale apparent at the apex of each on careful examination; and, no matter what phenomena it may afterwards present, this is its primary aspect; coming on slowly, it runs generally a most tedious course, often lasting for many years, and sometimes even for a long life. The several varieties of both psoriasis and lepra which have been described may be conveniently reduced to three :—

Psoriasis guttata.
    "   aggregata.
    "   lepræformis.

Psoriasis guttata (Plate X, Fig. 1).—This, which is the mildest form of the disease, is unattended in any of its stages with constitutional symptoms; a slight degree of itching of the skin occasionally precedes its appearance, but even this is not a constant sign. Numerous minute, papular elevations of the epidermis, at first not exceeding in size the point of a pin, are developed on the cutaneous surface, scattered irregularly, but distinct from each other, except in the neighborhood of the joints, on the prominences of which they are usually more or less aggregated. On the apex of each little elevation a minute scale forms, which, at first slightly adherent, desquamates shortly after its appearance, to be succeeded by another somewhat larger and more consistent; this scale is shining, of a silvery whiteness, and about the thickness of thin writing paper. The raised spots on which the scales are situated enlarge slowly, not attaining the size of the head of a pin for several days, and very gradually acquiring a magnitude of from two to three lines in diameter, when they are of a somewhat circular shape, but irregularly circumscribed. In some parts two or more spots coalesce, and thus form small patches; rarely, however, in this form of the eruption, exceeding the size of a sixpence, except, as above remarked, near the joints, where they occasionally occupy a portion of the integument an inch or two in diameter. With the progress of the disease the scales continue to be continuously developed, and shed as rapidly as they are secreted; the affected spots are irregularly elevated, of a reddish color in young persons, but of a dull brownish hue in the old, contrasting well with the shining, grayish-white scales, and present an irritated aspect. The only annoyance accompanying the presence of the eruption on the body, the disfigurement it occasions excepted, is a slight degree of tingling scarcely amounting to itching, caused by the separation and shedding of the scales. The variety here designated as Psoriasis guttata is the Psoriasis punctata of Devergie and Hebra.

This form of psoriasis rarely becomes chronic; in three or four weeks after its first appearance the scaly desquamation begins to diminish in quantity, new spots, which continued to be developed on the sound skin amongst those which had previously existed, cease to form, the elevated patches gradually sink to the level of the surrounding integument, and the disease usually terminates in from six weeks to two months, faint reddish stains, which after a short time fade away, marking the site of the eruption. It may occur on any part of the body, but is most usually situated on the chest, the back, the arms, the face, and the scalp.

In some rare cases, as originally noticed by Willan, the eruption is developed in the form of narrow patches or stripes, consisting of the minute scaly elevations set closer to each other   ual. These stripes which generally appear on the trunk of the body, assume a singular shape: "some of them are nearly longitudinal, some circular or semi-circular, with vermiform appendages: some are tortuous or serpentine, others are shaped like earth-worms or leeches; the furrows of the cuticle, being deeper than usual, make the resemblance more striking by giving to them an annulated appearance."[1] This, which is manifestly only an accidental variety of psoriasis guttata, has, from its peculiar aspect, been named psoriasis *gyrata*.

Psoriasis aggregata (Plate X, Fig. 2).—I have ventured to change the specific appellation of this form of the eruption, which by Willan and his followers has been denominated *diffusa*, by Rayer *confluens*, and by many other dermatologists *vulgaris*. The latter term indicates correctly enough that it is the most common form of the disease, but does not afford any information as to its characteristics, while the first is not sufficiently specific, psoriasis guttata and psoriasis lepræformis being often as generally diffused with regard to locality over the cutaneous surface; the name applied by Rayer is objectionable, solely because, in the English language, the word "confluent" conveys the idea of the presence of fluid. Reluctant, then, as I am to alter the nomenclature of skin diseases, although anxious to reduce in number the terms used, I have thought it well in this instance to do so by employing a specific denomination, which, while being frequently employed to designate other diseases of the cutaneous structure, and thus, not being an innovation, would be both more correct and more expressive.

This form of psoriasis, developed like that last described, without constitutional disturbance, appears as numerous minute rounded elevations of the epidermis, closely aggregated together in irregularly circumscribed patches, varying in size from that of a silver fourpence to that of the palm of the hand, but very irregular, both as regards shape and extent; on these the scales are om the first, minute and tolerably adherent at

Cutaneous Diseases. London: 1808, 4to., p. 161.

20*

commencement of the disease, but gradually acquiring a greater magnitude, when they are shed and again secreted with astonishing rapidity. The scales are of the same color and consistence as in psoriasis guttata, but desquamate in rather larger pieces; their reproduction, too, takes place much more quickly, so that they are consequently desquamated in greater quantity. With the progress of the eruption, new patches form on the intervening sound skin, which, sometimes, coalescing with those that first appeared, increase their size often considerably; the diseased surface is now distinctly raised above the level of the surrounding integument, rather more so at the outer border than in the centre, of a dull, reddish color, and covered with shining grayish-white scales. There is no discharge, either serous or purulent, but fissures or cracks are generally found through the affected parts, which present an irritated aspect, and through which the blood occasionally exudes.

This form of the disease often does not attain its full development for many months, although several of the patches acquire their utmost magnitude in three or four weeks, after which time they do not increase in size, but continue to secrete the characteristic scales incessantly. Its duration is essentially chronic, lasting usually for years if not submitted to the employment of remedial measures. The disappearance of the eruption is in all cases slow and gradual, the first sign of amendment being the cessation of the development of new patches, a diminution of the scaly desquamation, and a sinking of the elevated surface to the level of the healthy integument; reddish stains remain for a considerable time on the surface, even after the disease is apparently cured, and from these a fine epidermic desquamation, though small in quantity, continues for some weeks.

Either of the forms of psoriasis now described, when they become very chronic, may assume an extremely aggravated character, and present local phenomena justly entitling them to the appellation which dermatologists then usually apply to designate their severity and obstinacy to treatment—psoriasis *inveterata.*—See Plate X,

Fig. 3. In it the various patches of the eruption coalesce, so as to cover completely the limb on which they may be situated, or even the trunk of the body; the entire of the cutaneous surface is one mass of dry, hardened, thick scales, or rather is enveloped in a case of them, which covers the integuments like a coat of mail. Through this deep fissures are formed, generally in straight lines, but sometimes following the course of the polygonal and lozenge-shaped linear furrows of the epidermis, so as to give the diseased surface a striking resemblance to a piece of tessellated pavement. From the fissures an ichorous and bloody pus exudes, the parts are constantly torn with the nails—itching, which is much aggravated by heat, being a constant accompaniment of this inveterate form—and the entire of the affected region is a mass of leprous irritation, attended with a foul discharge, and a shower of desquamating scales flies off on the least motion, the bed of the patient presenting an appearance as if bran had been thickly strewn in it.[1]

The most usual site of psoriasis aggregatâ is the extremities; but it at times affects the entire body, being least frequent on the face, where it is always less general than on other parts of the cutaneous surface. In some cases it appears on special regions of the skin, and under such circumstances has been particularly described, but the guttated form of the eruption is almost invariably present on the rest of the body at the same time. The local forms have been named, from the parts affected, psoriasis *labialis*, psoriasis *palpebrarum*, psoriasis *capitis* (Plate X, Fig. 6), psoriasis *scrotalis*, psoriasis *præputialis*, psoriasis *pudendalis*, psoriasis *palmaris*, and psoriasis *unguium;* of these the two last only require to be specially noticed.

Psoriasis *palmaris* has, in common with certain forms of lichen and eczema, been regarded as one of the varieties of the so-called bakers' and grocers' itch; it may appear on the palmar aspect of the hands, extending also to the wrists and the under-surface of the fingers. In its de-

[1] In Dr. Neligan's Atlas (Plate X, Fig. 4) is a very good illustration of Psoriasis inveterata presenting the *tessellated pavement* appearance, from a case under the care of Dr. Banks, in the Whitworth Hospital.

any other variety of the disease, inflammatory redness, accompanied by heat and itching, marking its advent; the skin on the palm of the hand then becomes swollen, irregularly elevated, and of a reddish hue, and the itching generally increases much, being at times as intense as in scabies or prurigo. Large, dry, whitish scales of tolerable thickness and consistency, are rapidly secreted on the affected surface; these soon desquamate, and are reformed again and again, as in the other varieties of the eruption. When it becomes chronic, the itching and heat diminish, but the integuments of the palm of the hand and of the palmar surface of the fingers become hardened, thick like leather, of a whitish-yellow color, corrugated, scaly, and fissured; the motions are then limited and painful, the fingers cannot be completely flexed or extended, and any sudden movement tears the fissured parts, and causes them to bleed. In a rare form described by Rayer, and termed by him psoriasis *palmaris centrifuga*, the eruption begins by the formation of a small, rounded, squamous elevation in the centre of the palm, around it a series of eccentric, raised, red circles are developed, from each of which epidermic desquamation takes place; the eruption spreads in this manner until it covers the entire palmar aspect of the hands, which is then deeply fissured and painful, and bleeds from the slightest cause. Psoriasis attacks the backs of the hands also in some instances, and occasionally the soles of the feet.

The eruption extends to the nails in most cases of chronic psoriasis of the hands; but what has been described as psoriasis *unguium* is a change from their healthy condition, with or without the existence of the disease, on remote parts of the body; one or more of the nails presents a brownish-yellow, scaly elevation near its root, which gradually extends so as to occupy the entire surface; its texture becomes brittle, breaking and sealing off constantly; it acquires a dirty-yellowish hue, and not uncommonly the entire nail is shed, to be succeeded by the growth of another equally diseased.

Psoriasis lepræformis (Plate X, Fig. 5), which, as al-

ready remarked, is the form of scaly eruption described
by most dermatologists as a distinct disease, and termed
by them "Lepra," is chiefly characterized by the development of the patches in usually a perfectly circular, but
sometimes in an ovoid shape. It commences without
either constitutional or local disturbance, in the form of
numerous small, round, reddish stains, perfectly distinct
from each other, and scarcely elevated above the surrounding skin, on which shining silvery-white scales
soon appear. Gradually, but slowly, the circles enlarge
from their circumference, which is somewhat more raised
than the centre, attaining a size varying from a few lines
to one or two inches in diameter; some of the patches
coalescing, they occasionally cover an extended surface
of the integument, and acquire an irregularly rounded
shape—this is almost invariably the case on the convex
aspect of the joints and in their neighborhood, on which
parts the eruption presents an appearance scarcely to be
distinguished from psoriasis aggregata; but the circumference of the patches, no matter how large they may be,
is always more elevated than the centre, which, after
some time, assumes a comparatively healthy condition,
its color becoming more natural, and but slight desquamation of fine epidermic scales taking place from it.
From the borders, however, the constant secretion and
shedding of true scales continues; they become thicker
and more solid, retaining their whitish aspect, and are
sometimes imbricated on each other at the outer border
of each patch; the integument on which the eruption is
situated also becomes somewhat hypertrophied.

Psoriasis lepraeformis always runs a very chronic
course, not exhibiting any tendency of itself to disappear,
the disease being kept up more by the desquamation of
scales from the patches of eruption originally formed
than by the development of new spots; at length, when
under treatment it begins to mend, the central healthy
surface extends towards the circumference, upon which
fewer and thinner scales are secreted; the eruption at the
same time ceases altogether to spread, and, finally, only
slight strains with furfuraceous epidermic desquamation
remain, as an indication of the parts which were affected:

rarely occurs on the scalp, unless when the eruption is present at the same time on some other part of the body; and this serves, to a certain extent, to distinguish it from other scalp affections; the scales, too, when they are secreted on this region, are thicker and more solid than when situated elsewhere on the cutaneous surface, and consequently much more so than those of any other eruption that may occur there, than which they are also more persistent, often constituting a firm, imbricated, adherent, dry crust, the outer layer of which only desquamates. Secondary syphilitic eruptions not unfrequently assume a scaly character, and are with difficulty diagnosed from the ordinary forms of psoriasis: the history of the case and the concomitant symptoms are the differential points to be chiefly depended on ; the color of the parts of the cutaneous surface which are affected is, moreover, of a dull coppery or livid hue.

From pityriasis the eruption is distinguished by the absence in that affection of elevation of the diseased parts, which are of a yellowish or reddish-yellow color, by the scales being fine and thin, and by their being generally diffused over the cutaneous surface, not in distinct patches or spots. The chief diagnostic marks between it and ichthyosis are the thick, hardened, and rugose condition of the skin in the latter, and the non-existence of any scaly desquamation. The aggregated form of psoriasis is distinguished from the guttated variety without any difficulty, but in some cases a distinction can scarcely be made between it and psoriasis lepræformis, a matter of but little import, as the treatment for both is in all respects similar.

Prognosis.—Squamous eruptions are essentially of a chronic nature; but even when of years' duration, scarcely ever affect in any respect the general health. Developed under the influence of a peculiar constitutional state of the skin, essentially of an obstinate character, and most apt to reappear even in months or years after they seem to have been completely cured, length of time is as important to their perfect removal as the most judiciously planned course of treatment. The physician should, therefore, in every case, be most careful not to promise a speedy cure, and always, before prescribing, explain to his patient the chronic character of the disease, and that it requires a steady perseverance in the use of remedial measures for at least two or three months before even an apparent amendment will be perceptible. The anxiety of mind which an individual laboring under a cutaneous eruption suffers is very great, and this, too, adds to the difficulty of treatment. The promise of an eventual cure, though after a lengthened period, tends to alleviate this anxiety, and prevents the repeated disappointment, changes of medical advisers, and trials of new plans of treatment, which the hope deferred, when a speedy cure has been promised, causes.

Pathology.—" It is an admitted fact," writes Cazenave, " that the therapeutics of these diseases rests upon purely empirical grounds, and that, unhappily, there exists no sure guide to direct to a rational mode of cure." This statement, sufficiently true of most eruptions of the skin, is equally so of many other diseases of the body, and it should teach us not to despise the light thrown on pathology by the experience derived from therapeutics. When it is found that a certain class of remedies acts beneficially on deranged conditions of the animal economy, concerning the true nature of which doubt exists, it cannot be termed a *petitio principii* to infer that such derangements have a similarity in a greater or less degree to affections the nature of which is known, and which are benefited by the same class of remedies. In the treatment of scaly diseases of the skin, iodine, in some of its various combinations, and cod-liver oil are especially useful; and I would, even from this therapeutic fact alone, be inclined to look upon the peculiarity of constitution in which they occur as nearly allied to the scrofulous; in fact, that their appearance is but one of the Protean forms in which scrofula may be developed. And, independently of the beneficial effects of iodine, if we look to the remedies ordinarily proposed as specifics for their cure—of course I speak only of those administered internally, or, so to say, constitutionally—what are they but tonics, alteratives, or diaphoretics, generally employed in the treatment of scrofulous affections?

Again, if we lay aside the analogy derived from the peuties, in how many points do not scrofula and sca eruptions of the skin agree?—their hereditary natu their slow development, the period of life at which th appear, their production by innutrition or mal-innervati of the system, their obstinacy, their liability to recur to be again reproduced, the diathesis of the individu in whom they appear, &c.

Treatment.—In consequence of its extreme obstina and usually chronic character, there is probably no eru tion of the skin for the treatment of which so ma varied remedies have been and still are proposed, as psoriasis. Some trust altogether to topical medicati for its cure, while others rely exclusively on the empl ment of constitutional remedies—both are needed, neither should be neglected; the former must be us when the eruption has lasted for any length of time where it affects an extended surface of the skin, to p duce a new local action, and to remove the diseas condition of the integuments; while the latter is requir to correct any deviation from a healthy state, whetl functional or organic, of the internal organs which m be present, and to alter the constitutional derangeme to the existence of which the eruption is due. Befc commencing any plan of treatment, therefore, it is neo sary to take into account the age, constitution, a diathesis of the patient, the extent of surface affect and the previous duration of the disease.

In strong, healthy, plethoric young persons of eith sex, when the eruption is of the guttated form, or affe only a small portion of the skin, Dr. Neligan was opinion that its progress will generally be stopped, an cure effected by the use of tolerably active saline cath tics every second or third day, preceded by a gene blood-letting, and the daily use of a *fresh*-water bath, the temperature of 98°. He also was of opinion that persons of a sanguine temperament, or of very plethor habit of body, the bleeding may be repeated, but that all cases only a moderate quantity of blood should drawn; for when much has been removed at a time, the operation frequently repeated, the eruption is apt take on an aggravated character, and to become chronic. Notwithstanding this opinion of Dr. Neligan, the Editor cannot look upon the system of general bleeding as any other than useless, if not positively injurious. The best cathartics that can be used are the saline purging mineral waters, such as those of Pullna, of Seidlitz, of Cheltenham, of Leamington, of Droitwich, of Kreuznach, etc.; or, in their absence, the compound saline powder may be given in the dose of two drachms, dissolved in half a pint of lukewarm water, to which from twenty to thirty minims of the liquor potassæ, or, preferably, Brandish's alkaline solution, and the same quantity of some aromatic tincture, as of orange-peel, should be added; in either case, the purgative should be taken in the morning early before breakfast. By these simple means, continued for five or six weeks, many of the milder cases of psoriasis may be cured; but more generally, and invariably when the eruption has existed for some time before it is submitted to treatment, it is only alleviated thereby.

When the disease affects old persons or individuals of a weak constitution, all debilitating remedies must be carefully eschewed; in its early stages, then, stimulating diaphoretics combined with tonics should be employed, and the tepid bath, or tepid douche if the eruption be local, used once or twice a week when the patient's strength admits, or the hot vapor bath may in some cases be substituted with benefit for the water bath. Guaiacum and mezereon often prove the best diaphoretics in these cases of psoriasis, and they may be given in combination, as in the following form:—

R. Tincturæ Guaiaci Ammoniatæ, . drachmam.
Tincturæ Serpentariæ, ... semi-drachmam.
Mucilaginis Acaciæ, ... minima viginti.
Decocti Mezerei, ... drachmas sex cum semisse.
Infusi Dulcamaræ, ... unciam.
Misce. Fiat huastus.
Sumat talem unum ter indies.

In scrofulous children, the progress of the disease may in its early stages be stopped, and a cure effected by the administration of cod-liver oil; and this medicine proves also very successful in many cases of the local forms of

the eruption in adults; but with children or young persons the employment of the tepid bath at the same time
should not be neglected.

In the more aggravated forms of psoriasis, however, or
when the disease has become chronic, recourse must be
had to the more active alteratives, some of which have
acquired a sort of *specific* reputation for the treatment of
scaly diseases; and of all that have been used none effects
a cure so frequently as arsenic, whether it be given alone
or its administration conjoined with the application of
various local agents. Dr. Neligan was of opinion that
in every case the beneficial action of this medicine is
more decided and more speedily manifested when iodine
or the iodide of potassium is employed at the same time,
or alternated with it, and that in those cases—not few in
number—in which arsenic, no matter how prescribed,
disagrees, the preparations of iodine suffice usually to
cure the disease. Arsenic may be prescribed either in
the fluid form or in that of a pill, but, however given,
the dose should be small, increased very slowly, and continued for a lengthened time, at least for several months.
Of the liquid preparations, the liquor arsenicalis of the
British Pharmacopœia, Fowler's solution—a convenient
name for prescribing when it is requisite to conceal from
patients or their friends that arsenical preparations are
being administered—is probably the best; or the liquor
arsenici chloridi, De Valangin's mineral solution—introduced into the last edition of the *London Pharmacopœia*—
may be used; they should not be given at first in a larger
dose than four minims, three times a day, in an ounce of
infusion of dulcamara, to which, except in persons of a
full habit of body, two drachms of syrup of mezereon
may be added. The arseniates of ammonia or of soda
may also be given in solution in water, with a little
syrup, or in some vegetable infusion or decoction, in the
dose of a twentieth of a grain, very gradually increased
to the fifteenth of a grain, three times daily. The arseniate of soda may also be given in the officinal form of
the *British Pharmacopœia*—liquor sodæ arseniatis—in
doses of from three to ten minims thrice daily, in some
vegetable infusion or decoction; or, better still, in plain

water. The following form, for the administration of the arseniate of ammonia, was first proposed by Biett:—

R. Ammoniæ Arseniatis, . . . granum cum semisse.
Aquæ destillatæ, . . . uncias tres.
Spiritus Angelicæ, . . . drachmas sex. Misce.

Signetur—"One teaspoonful, gradually increased to three, to be taken for a dose in some aromatic water."—See Sixth Edition (Macnamara's) of Dr. Neligan's *Medicines, &c.*, p. 521.

Notwithstanding the strongly expressed views of Mr. Hunt and others, Donovan's solution of the hydriodate of arsenic and mercury, which was officinal in the last edition of the *Dublin Pharmacopœia*, but which is no longer a Pharmacopœial preparation, is another liquid form that has been often employed successfully in the treatment of psoriasis; in consequence of its containing mercury it is especially applicable for those cases in which the eruption is either a secondary symptom, or is connected with a syphilitic taint in the system; but, from my own experience, I do not think that mercurial preparations in any form are generally applicable for scaly diseases, except in the local forms appearing in children, and I have not unfrequently seen their use followed by an aggravation of the symptoms. I have consequently, for some years back, substituted for Donovan's solution a compound in which mercury is replaced by the iodide of potassium; this mixture may then be termed an *Ioduretted solution of the Iodide of Potassium and Arsenic;* it is prescribed in the following form:—

R. Liquoris Arsenicalis, ... minima octoginta.
Iodidi Potassii, ... grana sexdecim.
Iodi puri, ... grana quatuor.
Syrupi Florum Aurantii, . . . uncias duas. Solve.

This solution,[1] which is of a rich wine-yellow color, and keeps unchanged for years, contains in each fluidrachm five minims of arsenical solution, a grain of iodide of potassium, and a fourth of a grain of iodine. Forty minims of it at first may be given three times a day in simple water, or in any tonic or diaphoretic vegetable

[1] See Sixth Edition (Macnamara's) of Dr. Neligan's *Medicines, &c.*, p. 598.

infusion or decoction, as individual circumstances may indicate, and the dose gradually increased to eighty minims; it is, of course, scarcely necessary to observe that this compound, as are all which contain iodine, is incompatible with vegetable preparations in which starch is present, or with the stronger acids. In cases in which from any reason it may be advisable not to prescribe arsenic, the Fowler's solution can be omitted from the above mixture; and, unless in the inveterate forms of the eruption, or when it has been of very long standing, the iodine preparations should in the first instance be tried alone. In some cases, in which neither iodine nor arsenic agreed either separately or conjointly, the Editor found a combination of arsenic and quina most useful; it may be prescribed in the form of arseniate of quina; or, better still, by adding Fowler's solution to an ordinary quinine mixture.

Where it is wished to prescribe arsenic in the solid form, the best preparation of it is the iodide, which may be given in pill, made with conserve of roses or with hard manna and mucilage, in doses of from the twelfth to the tenth of a grain, three times daily, very gradually increased[1] until the fourth of a grain is taken at each time; the arseniates of ammonia or of soda may be given in the same form. In the more rebellious cases of the disease, and especially when it occurs in persons of a debilitated constitution, an excellent and favorite formula for the administration of this powerful agent is what has been termed the *Asiatic pills*, in consequence of their being first beneficially employed in the East Indies, whence we derive our knowledge of their efficacy; they are prepared by rubbing together a drachm of arsenic and nine drachms of powdered black pepper, with sufficient liquorice powder and mucilage to make 800 pills. Each of these contains about a thirteenth of a grain of arsenic, and one or two may be given daily. No matter what preparation of arsenic is employed, it should be administered after meals, as it is then less apt to derange the stomach, and the effects should be

[1] As already observed, the Editor does not coincide in this proposal *to give gradually increasing doses of an arsenical preparation.*

carefully watched; the continuance of headache, of
sickness and pain in the stomach, of dryness of the
fauces, or of tenderness, with heat and redness of the
eyes for a few days, requiring its omission for a short
time, and the administration of an active cathartic, when
it may be again resumed. It generally occurs *that in
the treatment of scaly diseases by arsenic or by iodine, the
eruption at first presents an aggravated appearance, the
affected parts exhibiting an irritated aspect, and the scaly
desquamation being much augmented, but these symptoms
soon pass away, and signs of amendment begin to show
themselves.* In all cases the use of the remedies which
have proved successful should be persisted in for some
weeks after the disease is apparently cured, so as to
prevent a relapse. Mr. Hunt and Mr. Milton rely
almost exclusively on arsenic. Hebra uses it internally
in various ways, at the same time using local remedies.
Hardy believes in the use of copaiba, which Bazin
considers inferior to arsenic.

Chronic cases of psoriasis are very frequently complicated with derangement of the digestive organs, evidenced
by various dyspeptic symptoms; the most prominent of
these are nausea and vomiting immediately after meals.
This condition must be remedied by appropriate alterative and tonic treatment, previously to the employment
of medicines, with the view of acting directly on the
eruption; for if arsenic or iodine, in any form, be given
while this condition is present, they will tend to increase
the existing irritation, and their expected beneficial
action be thereby prevented. The tepid fresh-water,
the douche, or the vapor bath, should be employed at
least once or twice a-week, in addition to the use of the
internal remedies now recommended.

Hebra has found the hydropathic system of benefit in
severe cases. The patient is treated much after the
fashionable custom called "packing." At the end of
three or four hours perspiration he takes a cold bath,
then a cold douche, is rubbed dry, and takes walking
exercise. This he goes through twice in the twenty-
four hours, and lives on simple, nutritious diet, without
alcohol, but with plenty of cold water-drinking instead.

The so called Turkish bath is lauded to a great degree
by others.

But cases of psoriasis occur which resist with obstinacy
the administration, even though much prolonged, of either
or both of these powerful medicines, and then recourse
must be had to some of the many other remedies, both
constitutional and topical, which have at times proved
useful, and have consequently found warm advocates.
Sulphur and its preparations have been highly praised
by many practitioners for their efficacy; and, in the very
inveterate forms of the eruption occurring in languid
constitutions, or when there is no determination of blood
to the affected parts, nor local irritation, the sulphurous
mineral waters, both taken internally and employed in
the form of tepid bath, cure the disease when other
remedies have failed; but to derive the full benefit from
them their use should be continued for several months,
otherwise the eruption is sure to reappear. When the
mineral waters cannot be procured, or the patient is
unable to go to their sources, which is always most
advisable, sulphur may be given internally, and baths
or lotions of the sulphuret of potassium used. In the
local forms of the disease the iodide of sulphur ointment
is a most valuable topical application, but it should be
used only of moderate strength, from eight to twelve
grains to the ounce of white wax ointment, and its
efficacy is much increased by the addition of a drachm
of glycerine to each ounce.

M. Cazenave has administered the carbonate of ammonia, in the treatment of psoriasis, with marked success;
he prescribes it in the dose of about two grains and
a half, from one to three times a day, in a tablespoonful
of syrup of sarsaparilla. "In general, the symptoms it
causes are scarcely to be noticed; some slight disturbance
of the digestive organs, and occasionally slight heat and
tingling of the skin. Yet, after an interval of time,
varying usually from three to eight days, when good
results follow, the scales begin to be detached, those
which succeed them are more and more fine and of a
duller aspect, and the patches on which they are situated
lose their red tint and gradually fade away; after a

longer or shorter period a complete cure, and one which is often permanent, takes place."[1] When carbonate of ammonia was thus administered, M. Cazenave found it to occasion diarrhœa, preceded by colic, lassitude, sometimes headache, slight acceleration with diminished fulness of the pulse, alterations of heat and cold of the surface, &c.; these symptoms disappeared on omitting the use of the medicine for· a few days, and this fact, together with their similarity to those caused by arsenic, led him to draw an analogy between the mode of operation of the two medicines.

Among other constitutional plans of treatment proposed for psoriasis, bringing the system under the influence of mercury has proved successful in the hands of some practitioners; it is chiefly applicable, as already remarked, to those cases in which a venereal taint exists; but it may also be used in the milder forms of the eruption, when they do not yield to the more simple treatment recommended above. The preparations of mercury which are preferred are those that act slowly, and rarely produce salivation, such as the red iodide or corrosive sublimate; the latter is very frequently prescribed in decoction of cinchona bark, a good combination, although not strictly chemical.

Copland relies chiefly on the employment of emetics and purgatives at the same time, and their use is certainly attended with much benefit in most cases, previously to commencing the administration of the more active alteratives. The alkalies, especially the liquor potassæ, have also been highly recommended, particularly in the local forms of the eruption; but in any cases in which I tried them the result was not satisfactory. From its original use by Biett, and the favorable notice taken of its action by Rayer, tincture of cantharides has been rather extensively administered, especially on the Continent, in the treatment of psoriasis; it certainly succeeds in some cases in which other remedies have failed, but its employment, even in small quantity, must be carefully watched, in consequence of the dangerous effects it is apt to produce

[1] *Annales des Maladies de la Peau et de la Syphilis.* Tom. iii. p. 315.

on the urinary organs. It may be given in doses of five minims, gradually increased to fifteen or twenty, three times a day, in at least an ounce of some emulsion, or of decoction of linseed or barley. Numerous other medicines, especially diaphoretics, diuretics, tonics, and stimulants, have been employed in this disease, but none require mention here, with, perhaps, the exception of tar or pitch, which, when given internally, and at the same time applied to the affected surface, is regarded by some physicians as quite a specific; I consider it, however, much inferior in its medicinal efficacy to most of the other therapeutic agents which have been now noticed.

Local applications, ointments, lotions, baths, &c., have been at all times favorite methods of treating psoriasis, and many have attempted to cure the disease by their use alone; with this view, also, it has been proposed to destroy the eruption by the free application of nitrate of silver to the affected parts; but such a proceeding tends only to aggravate the morbid state of the cutaneous surface, and is not altogether unattended with danger. The simple *fresh*-water tepid bath has proved, in my experience, the best topical remedy—I might almost say the only one needed, and it should be employed at least once a week in all forms of psoriasis; its use tends to restore the natural secretion of the skin, and to prevent the accumulation of scales. When the eruption is local, and attended with symptoms of irritation or inflammation, soothing unguents, as those containing chloroform, preparations of lead, zinc, &c., or poultices prepared with the lead wash, often prove highly serviceable; and in the more chronic cases, when neither inflammation nor inflammatory irritation is present, stimulating applications are occasionally required; of these, probably the best is the iodide of sulphur ointment spoken of before, or the following, which was highly recommended by the late Dr. Anthony Todd Thomson :—

℞. Calomelanos, ... grana sexaginta.
Unguenti Picis liquidæ, . . . semi-unciam.
Adipis præparati, ... unciam. Misce.

Of other local applications it will be sufficient to enumerate blisters, creasote, turpentine, tincture of iodine, corrosive sublimate in lotion, black and yellow wash, citrine ointment, &c. The alkalies, when applied topically, generally, I think, prove injurious.

Dr. Moore applies sapo laricis, his preparation for which will be found in Chapter XIV; and reference may be made to his paper "On the Pathology and Therapeutics of Diseases of the Skin" (*Dub. Hosp. Gaz.*, 1860, p. 22) for details of cases exhibiting a useful combination of dietectics, constitutional and local remedies.

Strict attention to diet and regimen is especially requisite in the treatment of psoriasis; a milk diet should be, if possible, enforced, except in cachectic or broken-down constitutions, and when from this or any other cause it cannot be altogether adopted, farinaceous articles and milk should be made as much as possible a portion of the general food, and, in addition, fresh meat, plainly dressed, or poultry, should alone be allowed. From its being so much easier to carry out dietetic rules in hospital patients than with those in private or in dispensary practice, more satisfactory results are usually obtained in treating the former, and, consequently, perfectly accurate conclusions as to the effects of remedies in the treatment of any disease, whether of the skin or not, can only be drawn from hospital experience, except under unusually favorable circumstances in special cases.

PITYRIASIS.

Pityriasis, from πίτυρον, bran; Dartre tarmineuse of the French; Schuppen of the Germans.—See Plate XI.

PITYRIASIS is a scaly cutaneous disease, characterized by an abundant secretion and desquamation of minute, furfuraceous, white, and shining scales, from slightly elevated, irregular patches of the skin, of a yellowish, reddish-yellow, or dark-brown color, varying in extent, or from the surface of the body generally. It is attended usually with smart itching of the parts affected, sometimes with painful inflammatory tingling, and both are much augmented by any cause that may produce increased capillary circulation of the integuments. It is non-contagious, unaccompanied by constitutional symptoms; and

22

affected the body generally, into three varieties, according to the color which the diseased patches of integument presented, namely, Pityriasis *rubra*, Pityriasis *nigra*, and Pityriasis *versicolor*. Both Rayer and Erasmus Wilson consider the first of these only as being a scaly disease, and regard the others as simply alterations in the color of the skin, accompanied by a foliaceous or mealy desquamation, and not by the separation of true scales. As, however, in both forms there is a squamous secretion differing only in degree from the first, I prefer to regard them as sub-varieties of general pityriasis. Adopting, then, strictly the division of the disease into two forms—general and local—they may be termed :—

Pityriasis diffusa.
"   localis.

The early stage of *pityriasis diffusa* (Plate XI, Fig. 2) is marked by a sensation of heat and tingling on various parts of the cutaneous surface, usually on the neck, the chest, the abdomen, the back, and sometimes on the face and hands: uncircumscribed patches of a yellowish or reddish-yellow color, scarcely elevated above the surrounding integument, appear on the places which had been the seat of the itching, and on them minute, branny, micaceous scales soon form, at first in small quantity, but afterwards in very great abundance, desquamating freely when the spots are rubbed, or, should the eruption be general, on the least movement of the body. The affected patches vary much in shape and size, being often of an irregularly rounded form, separated at first by healthy skin, over which, in most cases, however, the scales gradually extend, and becoming confluent, cover the body almost universally; the furfuraceous desquamation is then extreme, and is attended with much itching, especially when the surface of the body is heated, and the disease assumes a very obstinate character. The skin from which the desquamation takes place—which in the commencement presents various shades of red and yellow intermixed, whence the specific appellation of pityriasis *versicolor* has been applied to this form—gradually becomes of a lighter shade of yellow, and in many instances the secretion of scales then ceases, yellowish stains remaining on the surface for some time; but in others the desquamation, attended with more or less itching, lasts with extraordinary obstinacy for months, or even years, after the skin has resumed its natural color.

In some cases the eruption is more partial, being confined almost exclusively to the integuments of the thorax, usually appearing on the chest; the spots or patches assume from the first a bright color, so marked that in the commencement they can scarcely be distinguished from erythema, they are also attended with much heat and itching, indicating the inflammatory nature of the disease; the characteristic scaly secretion and desquamation soon appear, however, and determine its nature. This form, which is also very obstinate, has been termed pityriasis *rubra;* it is of much less frequent occurrence than pityriasis versicolor, but oftener witnessed than the next sub-variety.

Pityriasis *nigra* is a very rare form of the eruption; it does not seem to differ in any respect from pityriasis rubra, except in the color of the diseased patches, which are dark-brown or nearly black, and usually appear on one or both of the lower extremities; according to Cazenave's observations, the black tint is in some cases so superficial that, on removing the epidermis, the derma is seen beneath, of a red, shining aspect; in others, however, the color affects the sub-epidermic layer of the derma. In both pityriasis versicolor and pityriasis nigra, the chromatogenous functions of the derma must be more or less disordered to account for the peculiar discoloration of the skin which accompanies them. As before remarked, Rayer considers the changed color as their essential characteristic, and he consequently terms the form Chloasma, and the latter Melasma; this view has been adopted by Wilson also.

Several local forms of pityriasis have been described chiefly by Rayer; thus he notices it specially as it affects the eyelids, pityriasis *palpebrarum;* the mouth and lips, pityriasis *oris* et *labiorum;* the prepuce and pudendum, pityriasis *præputialis* et *pudendalis;* the feet and hands, pityriasis *palmaris* et *plantaris;* and the scalp, pityriasis *capitis.* None of these, except the last, differ essentially from the eruption as it affects the body generally, and do not, therefore, require to be specially described; many dermatologists, indeed, and I think with much correctness, admit the existence of but one local variety of pityriasis—that of the scalp.

The development of pityriasis *capitis* (Plate XI, Fig 3) is not accompanied by any sign of constitutional or local disturbance, but soon after its eruption it gives rise to much itching, without heat or redness of the surface The disease consists in the secretion of numerous minute papyraceous, dry, and shining scales, in most cases scattered over the entire of the head, without any sensible elevation of the surface, and perfectly free from moisture. I cannot describe the precise manner in which the eruption originates, as I have never seen it until the squamous secretion was fully developed, there being no symptoms to direct the patient's attention to it until then. The presence of the scales produces much itching, compelling the individual affected to scratch the head, by which they are very readily detached in large quantity, in the state of a fine powder or *dandriff;* their removal is rapidly succeeded by a further secretion. If the condition of the scalp in pityriasis capitis be examined, the surface is found to be closely covered with the imbricated scales with small intervals here and there; the skin of the unaffected parts presenting a smoother or more polished appearance than natural. On removing one of the scales we find that the spot on which it is seated is raised, and that another finer scale may be removed from it; and it is not until after the removal of several scales, each finer than the preceding, that we arrive at the reddened and inflamed surface of the scalp which is somewhat depressed. The chief annoyance which it causes is itching; the patient, in scratching himself to allay this troublesome symptom, removes large quantities of dandriff; and in the child the irritation is often so great that the scalp is torn, becomes inflamed, eczematous vesicles appear, and the original affection is thus complicated.

Although the hair in this eruption is not apparently diseased, it grows weak and thin, and falls out on the slightest cause, so that, when of long duration, baldness may result, which, except in very old persons, is, however, only temporary.

Pityriasis diffusa may occur at any age, but it is most common in adults; it seems to affect both sexes with an equal degree of frequency. Pityriasis capitis is most usually met with in infants at the breast, the frequency of its appearance decreasing with the advance of years towards puberty, at which age it is of very rare occurrence, but it again appears at the approach of old age. It thus seems to be most frequent when the head is least covered with hair, and it is also most generally seen in individuals whose hair is naturally thin.

The *causes* of pityriasis are very obscure; in most cases it is manifestly a constitutional affection, but in some instances it is evidently produced by the action of local irritants. Thus its occurrence on the scalp may be often accounted for by the use of hard brushes or a fine-tooth comb, or from not drying the head sufficiently after it has been washed; appearing, too, most frequently at those ages in which the scalp is least covered with hair, it may be then caused by the sudden changes of temperature to which the surface is consequently exposed. The eruption, when general, appears to be more or less connected with some deranged state of the nervous system, especially when this state is accompanied by increased cutaneous susceptibility, and is also not unfrequently attendant on a disordered condition of the digestive organs. I can confirm the observation of Cazenave that in some cases, especially in nervous females, pityriasis capitis succeeds repeated attacks of nervous headache. The use of stimulating cosmetics,

22*

whether in the form of lotion or of pomade, bu
unusual exciting cause of the eruption. Dr. Fox
that it seems to be dependent on some peculiar st
the blood; M. Hardy believes it to be allied to ec
and that it results from the *dartrous* diathesis;
Hebra believes P. capitis to be due to an excessive
tion from the sebaceous glands. Fox, Hillier, and
believe P. diffusa—*i. e.*, P. versicolor, or Chloas
Wilson, to be a parasitic disease, and the merit
covering the fungus is claimed by Eichstedt (*Fr
Notizen*, 89 Band, July–Sept., 1846), according to
the plant is the *microsporon furfur*. Dr. Fox has n
the disease to be produced by implantation of the ol
and Hutchinson stated it to be produced from the f
of tinea tonsurans. Wilson does not believe the
sitic theory, but upholds his own—that termed *gr
degeneration.*

Diagnosis.—Pityriasis is distinguished from pa
by the fineness and thinness of the scales, which a
thicker than the healthy scarf-skin, even when tl
case is very chronic; by their being desquama
excessive quantity; by the parts affected being so
elevated above the surrounding integument; b
peculiar color of the surface of the skin on whi
eruption is situated; and by the attendant prurit
might be confounded with chronic lichen or ecze
consequence of the furfuraceous desquamation
attends the advanced stages of both these dis
pityriasis, however, is not preceded by any erupt
never accompanied by any discharge, and in it the
is never chapped nor fissured. From ichthyos
diagnosis is made without difficulty, the peculia
hard, rugose, and, so to say, horny condition of t
teguments being sufficiently characteristic of that
tion. Pityriasis capitis is distinguished from the
eruptions which occur on this region of the body
true scaly nature, the scales being minute, dry,
rugous, and imbricated, though scarcely, if at all, el
above the surface of the scalp, and readily separa
the form of a fine powder or dandriff; by there
no attendant inflammation unless it be produced by

irritating cause; by the absence of discharge; by the hair being unaltered, but falling out more easily than is natural; and by its not being contagious: it occurs, too, most generally in advanced periods of life, being rare in childhood, adolescence, and manhood.

Prognosis.—Trifling an eruption as pityriasis seems to be, it is one of extreme obstinacy, and not unfrequently, when it has continued long, causes more or less derangement of the general health, chiefly from the mental annoyance which its persistence occasions; this is especially witnessed when it affects the scalp of females at or about the age of puberty, to whom the falling out of the hair and the continued desquamation of dandriff are a source of constant distress; I have seen more than one instance in which extreme nervous and general debility was produced by this cause alone. The longer pityriasis has lasted the more difficult it is to cure, and relapses after apparent perfect recovery are very likely to occur. That the continued existence of the eruption generally over the surface of the body may not be altogether unattended with danger is proved by Rayer's narrative of a case in which he saw it prove fatal.

Treatment.—In the treatment of pityriasis, as of many other cutaneous diseases, it is too much the habit to resort to the indiscriminate use of active stimulants both internally and as topical applications; I do not mean to undervalue the benefit derived from their employment in many chronic eruptions, but I must protest against the custom which for some years back has become so general, of having recourse to them in all cases without regard to the fact that a majority of the affections of the skin are inflammatory in their origin, and that even in their advanced stages, when all tendency to inflammatory action has apparently disappeared, local irritation or capillary excitement often causes a fresh outbreak of the eruption, or an aggravation of the symptoms. These remarks, while they are true of many cutaneous diseases, are especially applicable to that now under consideration, which, though much less inflammatory than many others, is extremely liable to be reproduced by the action of stimulants—whether constitutional or local—a fact that every one, who has had any experience in the treatment of this class of affections, must, I feel certain, have observed.

When pityriasis is of the diffuse form, if it occurs in strong, healthy, young persons, a small general bleeding proves often of service in its early stages [? Editor], but the withdrawal of blood is not admissible otherwise; tepid gelatine baths should be used for at least half an hour daily, or every second day from the first, and purgatives be freely administered: of the latter class of medicines none prove so useful as the alkaline cathartic mineral waters, either thermal or cold, according to the age and constitution of the patient; for example, those of Carlsbad or Marienbad; but a combination of mild mercurials with alkalies, as in somewhat the following form, should be prescribed at the same time:—

> ℞. Pilulæ Hydrargyri, ... grana novem.
>   Sodæ Carbonatis exsiccatæ, ... grana sex.
>   Extracti Taraxaci, ... grana duodecim.
>   Extracti Hyoscyami, ... grana tres.
>   Misce. Fiant pilulæ sex.
> Sumat unam omni alternâ die semi-horâ ante prandium.

When the mineral waters cannot be procured, a drachm of the sulphate of soda—previously deprived of its water of crystallization, by exposing it to a red heat—and twenty grains of the bicarbonate of soda, dissolved in half a pint of tepid water, may be given in the morning after the pill.

Should the eruption resist this plan of treatment, and exhibit a tendency to become chronic, alkaline baths— four ounces of the carbonate of soda, or two ounces of purified carbonate of potash, in sufficient fresh water for an ordinary bath, at the temperature of from 80° to 92° Fahr., according to the season of the year—may be substituted for those of gelatine; and the surface of the body, previously well dried after leaving the bath, should be anointed with a pomade, composed of four ounces of prepared lard, well beaten up with an equal quantity of elderflower water, then squeezed as dry as possible, and half an ounce of glycerine added. The mercurials and alkaline saline cathartics must still be continued; but should the

eruption become essentially chronic, the more active constitutional alteratives, iodine and arsenic separately or
combined, as recommended for the treatment of psoriasis,
must be prescribed. In cases in which the pruritus is
extreme, chloroform, added to the pomade above recommended, in the proportion of from eight to twelve minims
to the ounce, will be found the most effectual application
for allaying it; lotions and ointments containing hydrocyanic acid or the preparations of lead have been employed usefully for the same purpose.

In some of the local forms of pityriasis, the vapor
douche bath is of especial service, and the constitutional
treatment applicable to the general disease is also indicated. When the scalp is the part affected, the hair
should be cut close—not *shaved* off—and so kept during
the progress of the treatment: this is not requisite in old
persons when the hair is thin on the head. In the early
stages, weak alkaline ointments and lotions, with the
addition of glycerine to either, will be found the most
beneficial applications; but when the eruption is of long
standing, or occurs in persons of debilitated constitution,
the tannic acid or dilute citrine ointment, should be substituted for the former, the lotion being still used each
time before the ointment is applied. When the eruption
appears on the scalp of scrofulous children, cod-liver oil
will be beneficially administered, but for those who are
not scrofulous the alterative powders of the iodide of
mercury and hydrargyrum cum cretâ, as I have recommended for other diseases of the scalp, are better adapted.
In very obstinate cases of any of the local forms of this
eruption more stimulating applications may be tried, such
as ointments containing calomel or white precipitate, in
the proportion of a drachm of either to the ounce of prepared lard or of white wax ointment, with the addition
of glycerine, or lotions containing the cyanide of mercury
or corrosive sublimate, but their effects must be carefully
watched, as they often cause a sudden aggravation of the
symptoms. For the same reason the sulphurous mineral
waters and sulphurous baths should be used with caution,
yet they unquestionably prove at times of much benefit

in chronic cases of the disease in persons of a languid circulation.

In general or diffused pityriasis Mr. Startin gives corrosive sublimate in infusion of elm bark. Hardy treats pityriasis capitis with soap and water and a solution of carbonate of potash, afterwards using an ointment of one part of sulphur to thirty of lard, or one *gramme* of nitric acid to thirty of lard. With old persons Dr. Frazer uses a weak solution of tannin in glycerine. Dr. Jenner uses a solution of corrosive sublimate, four grains to the ounce; and Mr. Hilton, commenting on all these, observes: "When these means fail, I believe there is just one remedy, and that is arsenic, which will, unless my experience has quite misled me, cure every case that is curable."

Dietetic rules are most important in the treatment of pityriasis, and when the digestive organs are deranged remedies calculated to restore their healthy tone should be employed. The food ought to be light but nourishing, as the strength must be supported, and therefore milk and farinaceous articles of diet are especially indicated; in the case of children, a strictly milk and vegetable diet should be enforced. Stimulating or heating drinks must be altogether prohibited, and the surface of the body kept as much as possible of a uniform temperature, extremes of heat and cold being avoided. In consequence of the liability to relapse, whatever treatment may be found to be successful should be continued for at least a month or six weeks after an apparent cure has been effected.

CHAPTER VII.

HYPERTROPHLÆ.

IN the Order HYPERTROPHIÆ I purpose to include all diseases of the skin which are specially characterized by an hypertrophied condition, attended with a morbid change from their normal state, of any or all of the anatomical elements which compose the tegumentary membrane. The affections to be described in this division are of a chronic nature both in their development and progress, rarely exhibiting in any of their stages signs of constitutional disturbance or inflammatory action, either local or general, yet some of them are unquestionably of constitutional origin, while others are manifestly produced by the direct action of irritant causes. I have already mentioned the objections which exist to the employment of the term "Tubercula," for the purpose of designating a group of diseases of the skin, or to its retention at all in cutaneous nosology; applied formerly to include several affections, nearly all modern dermatologists who still retain it have restricted its application to some forms of secondary syphilitic eruptions, to Lupus, and to Elephantiasis; now, of these it is evident that the first will be more correctly classed and more conveniently described with the other syphilitic diseases which affect the skin; the second is specially characterized by its malignant nature; and therefore the third only can, with any degree of accuracy, be designated as a tubercular affection, and yet although placed by Willan and Bateman in this class, it differs essentially from their own definition of a tubercle.

The appellation I propose ha bellairisch of not being an innovation in cutaneo   Schulz.   W a hype has a place in all modern natural systems of   cation of

affections of the skin, as constituting a special group, and I only seek to extend its signification as in any artificial arrangement may be correctly done—there being no necessity here for regarding the so-called natural affinities, similarly of elementary lesion or of external phenomena sufficing for the grouping of diseases. The order might certainly be made to constitute several groups were strict accuracy in arrangement the sole or even chief object in my inquiry; but regarding all systems of classification as altogether secondary, and useful more for the purposes of description than for affording any aid either in diagnosis or treatment, I think it better to make as few divisions as possible. The follo
the diseases I shall describe in this chapter: Ic
Molluscum, Stearrhœa, Elephantiasis, Verruca, Clavus, Callositates, Condylomata, Nævus.

ICHTYOSIS.

Ichthyosis (according to Mason Good more correctly *Ichthyiasis*), from Ἰχθύς, a fish; Ichthyose, of the French; Fischuppenkrankheit, of the Germans.—See Plate XI, Fig. 4.

ICHTHYOSIS (*Fish-skin disease*) is characterized by a morbid alteration and hypertrophied condition of the epidermis, by which it is converted into thick, dry, horny, adherent scales, the orifices of the hair follicles and of the sudiparous and sebiparous glands being thereby obstructed. This affection, classed by Willan and those who have adopted his views amongst the Squamæ, is, as I have stated in the last chapter, distinctly separated from the eruptions contained in that group by its not being attended with any desquamation of scales. Most modern writers on diseases of the skin differ as to what are the anatomical lesions by which it is constituted, and, consequently, as to the precise position which it should occupy in a nosological arrangement. Mr. Erasmus Wilson, in his earlier writings, regarded it as consisting in   r formation of the epidermis, but he has changed   pinion, and more recently announced his belief that the morbid condition of the integuments is composed of concretions of altered sebaceous substance; repeated observation, aided by microscopic examination, compels me, however, to differ from so eminent an authority, nor have I been able even to comprehend the grounds on which he has come to this conclusion. Dr. A. T. Thomson, who included it under *tubercula*, did not live to publish his opinions in the posthumous work which bears his name; but that he had not been able to satisfy his mind as to the nature of the disease is evident from the account of it given by his editor, Dr. Parkes. By Cazenave and the majority of the modern French dermatologists, ichthyosis is looked upon as a lesion of epidermic secretion, and is, therefore, made to constitute a distinct group, of which it is the type. Hebra includes it in his third class, scaly eruptions, "Die Schuppichten Hautaus Schläge"—Efflorescentiæ Squamosæ.[1] Gustav Simon, whose views I adopt, regarding ichthyosis as an hypertrophy or increased development of the epidermis,[2] places it, in his classification, among the Hypertrophiæ.

Willan and Bateman described two forms of the disease, terming the one ichthyosis *simplex*, and the other ichthyosis *cornea;* they differ, however, merely as to the degree in which the. epidermis is altered, and therefore cannot be correctly separated from each other for the purposes of description; other varieties have also been constituted by different writers according to the appearance which the altered integuments may present in certain cases: thus Wilson divides the disease into Ichthyosis *squamosa* and Ichthyosis *spinosa;* a form has been termed Ichthyosis *hysterix* by Fuchs; and another Ichthyosis *scutellata* by Schönlein. The Ichthyosis cornea of Willan (I. Squamosa of Wilson) appears to be the Seborrhœa sicca of Hebra, and the Acné sebacée cornée of Hardy. The literature of Ichthyosis is for the most part of an antiquarian, but highly interesting kind. The reader is referred to an excellent essay by Dr. Begbie, in the *Edinburgh Medical Journal* for July, 1861. In this essay

---

[1] *Diagnostic der Hautkrankheiten in tabellairischen Ordnung nach Dr. Hebra's Vorlesungen.* Von. Dr. Bendict Schulz. Wien: 1845, p. 36.
[2] *Die Hautkrankheiten durch anatomische Untersuchungen.* Berlin, Second Edition, 1851, p. 49.

will be found an enumeration of most of the old writers
on the subject, as well as a concise statement of the con-
flicting views of the moderns regarding its nature. Dr.
Begbie himself regards it as an "essentially scaly or
squamous disorder, and therefore correctly associated
with Lepra and Psoriasis." In the forty-sixth volume
of the *Medico-Chirurgical Transactions*, Dr. J. W. Ogle
details four cases of Wilson's Ichthyosis sebacea squamosa.

Ichthyosis may be congenital, but more usually, commencing a few months after birth, lasts for life, affecting
generally, after a short time, the entire of the cutaneous
surface, except the palms of the hands, the soles of the
feet, the eyelids, the lips, and the prepuce. It consists at
first of an hypertrophied condition of the epidermis,
which is dry, harsh, and corrugated, the natural linear
markings dividing it into distinctly separated, polygonal
and lozenge-shaped compartments. This change, except
in congenital cases, in which at birth it is very general
over the body, is first witnessed in certain regions only,
namely, the ankles, the knees, the backs of the hands,
the borders of the axillæ, and the neck; the morbid
alteration, becoming gradually more aggravated on these
parts, extends superficially also, affecting next the scalp,
the fronts of the legs, the backs of the arms, the folds of
the groins, the breasts, and the lower part of the abdomen; by degrees, however, if the disease be unchecked
by treatment, the epidermis of the entire body, with the
few exceptions noticed above, becomes engaged.

When ichthyosis is congenital, the skin of the infant at
birth is dry, rough, uneven, and of a grayish-brown
color, but the epidermis is little hypertrophied; this condition of it may continue for years, or even for life,
accompanied by a constant mealy exfoliation, without
being further aggravated, constituting the mildest cases
of the affection. More generally, however, the epidermis
soon becomes thickened, hypertrophied, and of a scaly
aspect, bearing at times much resemblance to the scales
of a fish—whence the name derived from the Greek
word, $ιχθύς$, a fish, was applied to the disease; the surface
is deeply furrowed, shining, and of a sallow or greenish
hue, free from hairs, and devoid of any secretion or

form, and in extreme cases the power of motion may be much limited. This form of ichthyosis is almost invariably congenital, not attaining its complete development, however, until it is about the age of puberty.

Since this disease of the skin was first noticed, it has at all times attracted much attention, owing to the singular condition of the integuments by which it is characterized; individuals affected with it in an aggravated form having been exhibited for money, in the case of males being termed *porcupine men*, and of females *mermaids*, the latter from the supposed resemblance of the skin to the scales of fishes; but it has been more aptly compared to the hide of an elephant or of a rhinoceros. Not being of frequent occurrence, moreover, in its full development some of these cases have been carefully described, the most celebrated probably being that of the family of the Lamberts, which occurred in the beginning of the last century. Of this family, John and Richard Lambert, two brothers, became notorious from their affliction with this disease. They travelled through various parts of Europe, exhibiting themselves as porcupine men. In their case the disease seemed to have been hereditary; for while their fathers for several generations had suffered from it, they had seven sisters who were entirely free from it, nor did it ever attack a female of their family. It is described as having attacked them about six weeks after birth, and at the time of their exhibition the only parts of their bodies not affected were the face, the palms of the hands, and soles of the feet; together with the interspaces and bulbs of the fingers.

Whether ichthyosis is general or partial the superficial layers of the hypertrophied epidermis are constantly being shed as a fine mealy desquamation; or, when softened by a warm bath, may be rubbed off with the hand, but are again rapidly renewed; the disease is always more marked on the regions of the body noticed above, as the parts where it first appears, and especially in the neighborhood of the joints; on the scalp the epidermis is not so much thickened as elsewhere, yet most of the hair is shed when it occurs there, and what remains is thin and weak. Although the general health seems to be unaffected in persons the subjects of ichthyosis, attacks of diarrhœa are of constant occurrence, probably owing to the nearly complete obstruction of the cutaneous transpiration, and for the same reason those parts of the integuments which are not engaged, especially the palms of the hands and the soles of the feet, are constantly bedewed with moisture; the urinary and pulmonary secretions are also said to be increased in quantity, but in four cases of the disease which I have had under treatment this was not so. The affected parts were constantly below the natural temperature, and persons afflicted with the disease usually suffer much from coldness of the surface of the body.

There is an excellent illustration of this disease in the Sydenham Society's edition of Hebra's plates.

The nature of the *anatomical changes* which constitute ichthyosis have been carefully investigated, both microscopically and otherwise. The following description of them is given by Franz Simon: "The scales were of a gray or black color; when placed in water they softened, and on then placing a section under the microscope, I found that the abnormal structure was formed of compressed epithelial scales. On incineration the scales left an ash containing carbonate and phosphate of lime and peroxide of iron; the latter was in such abundance as to communicate a yellow color to the ash. The ash yielded by the incineration of the ordinary thickened skin on the hands and feet is perfectly white, and contains a mere trace of peroxide of iron."[1] This account, directly opposed to the views propounded by Erasmus Wilson, which have been before referred to, is confirmed by Gluge, who states that on microscopic examination he found the scales to be composed of epidermic cells.

Causes.—Obscure as are the causes of skin diseases, generally speaking, there is probably not one of which so little is known as to how or under what circumstances it is produced, as ichthyosis. When congenital, it has been ascribed, like all the other deviations from a normal state which are observed occasionally in the fœtus, to the effect

[1] *Animal Chemistry;* Sydenham Society's Edition, Vol. ii. p. 483.

of the disease occur in children born of parents healthy in all respects, and in whose families, as far as could be ascertained, no trace of the disease ever existed. Dr. Sedgwick, in the thirty-seventh volume of the *British and Foreign Medico-Chirurgical Review* (1861, p. 478), relates a case of a man affected with this disease. It did not affect any of his five children, three males and two females; while it attacked four of his five grandsons, sparing his only two granddaughters. The seven grandchildren were the offspring of his daughters. It is seen at all ages, but is usually congenital, or developed within the first year of life, very rarely appearing for the first time after the age of puberty, yet it has been witnessed as a primary affection in old persons, but always in a modified form. All the examples of ichthyosis which I have seen have been in persons, whether children or adults, of a well-marked scrofulous diathesis.

In *St. Bartholomew's Hospital Reports*, Vol. I, 1865, p. 198, Mr. Church gives a curious "Report of a case of Ichthyosis, with a Congenital Malformation of the Aorta."

Diagnosis.—With no other disease of the skin can ichthyosis be confounded, so distinctly characterized is it by the abnormal condition of the epidermis : in the cicatrices of wounds and of burns a peculiar warty grow is occasionally developed, which, having been first w described by the celebrated French surgeon of the name, has been termed the *warty ulcer of Marjolin ;* this disease presents characters somewhat resembling those of ichthyosis, but it may be at once distinguished by its local nature, occurring only in those parts of the integuments which have been previously the seat of some severe injury.

Prognosis.—Ichthyosis has been in all ages regarded as being incurable; it is at all events a most grave affection, and one which usually lasts for years, if not for life. When it presents the aggravated characters of the severe form, as above described, it should be regarded as beyond the reach of medical skill, but if it be submitted to treatment in its early stages, and while it is yet of a comparatively mild form, affecting the surface only partially, the progress of the disease may be arrested, and its further development prevented, if it cannot be completely cured.

Treatment.—From the extreme obstinacy and general incurability of ichthyosis, many plans, as may be supposed, have been recommended for its treatment, both constitutionally and topically. The latter have consisted chiefly in means to soften and promote the desquamation of the altered and hardened epidermis, and the former in the administration of the most powerful remedies which experience has shown act specially upon the skin. Warm water and vapor baths, with the preceding or subsequent employment of oleaginous and greasy applications, constitute the chief part of any method which has proved at all successful in the treatment of ichthyosis; their action is evidently due to a direct effect in softening the hypertrophied integument, and thus promoting its separation; but experience has shown that unless the state of the constitution on which the abnormal secretion depends be at the same time changed, it is again rapidly reproduced in a similar diseased condition. "The easiest mode," says Willan, "of removing the scales is to pick them off carefully with the nails from any part of the body while it is immersed in hot water. The layer of cuticle which remains after this operation is harsh and dry, and the skin did not in the cases I have noted recover its usual texture and softness; but the formation of the scales was prevented by a frequent use of the warm bath, with moderate friction." More active local applications are recommended by some writers on the disease, such as sulphurous baths, stimulating lotions, containing corro- sive sublimate and other preparations of mercury, caustic potash, etc.

In an account, published by Professor Banks,[1] of two cases of the disease which he treated successfully, cod- liver oil was employed topically, and at the same time administered internally; at bedtime the patients were placed in a vapor bath, and the surface of the body well- rubbed afterwards with the oil, a flannel dress being always worn next the skin, with the view of keeping the surface constantly impregnated with it. The use of this remedy was, he says, suggested to him by the marked connection which he has seen to exist between the ichthyosis and the strumous diathesis.

In the first of these cases, which was *cured* under Professor Banks's treatment, the skin of the lower ex- tremities, save on the inside of the legs and thighs, was more like the skin on a fowl's leg than fish-skin. The second case was subsequently to the publication of Professor Banks's paper removed to Sir Patrick Dun's Hospital, where, during his attendance on Dr. Banks's clinique in 1853, the Editor had an excellent opportunity of watching its progress. It was decidedly benefited by the plan which proved successful in the former case; but of its subsequent history the Editor knows nothing.

The internal administration of pitch was highly recom- mended in this disease by Willan and Bateman, and their experience of its benefits has been confirmed, especially by Dr. Elliotson; they ordered it to be made into pills with flour, and increased the dose gradually, until from half an ounce to an ounce was taken daily and often con- tinued for months. But both Rayer and Biett state that although they gave this remedy a fair trial it failed com- pletely in their hands. The cold water treatment has also been tried in the treatment of ichthyosis; but in one case

---

[1] *Dublin Quarterly Journal of Medical Science*, New Series, vol. xii. p. 80.

which I saw it did not produce the least good effect; in this same case, enveloping the affected parts with wet lint, covered with oiled silk, also failed.

The following plan of treatment I have employed in four cases of ichthyosis, in three of which the disease was local, being confined to the lower extremities in two, and engaging the upper also in the third, and in these the recovery was complete and permanent; in the other the integuments of the body generally, except the face, the palms of the hands, the soles of the feet, and some patches of the trunk, were affected with the disease, which commenced five months after birth, and was of three years' duration when I first saw the child. Here, after a year and a half of treatment, the epidermis had regained a tolerably healthy condition, being only slightly hard and rough; but if the local applications were omitted for four or five weeks, it again began to present a somewhat thickened appearance; this case is, consequently, still (1852) under treatment. The remedies I used were the iodide of potassium and iodine, from one to two grains of the former, and from a sixteenth to an eighth of a grain of the latter, according to the age of the child, given once daily, in from one to two ounces of the decoction of elm bark, made with the recent inner bark, stripped from the growing tree; and an ointment, containing twenty grains, gradually increased to one drachm, of the iodide of potassium, a drachm of glycerine, and an ounce of prepared lard, with which the affected parts were well anointed morning and evening; an alkaline bath—one drachm of carbonate of soda to each gallon of fresh water at the temperature of 90° Fahr.—having been used for fifteen minutes previously to each inunction, the body being well rubbed by a flesh-brush while in the bath. An inner calico dress was worn constantly, and milk-diet was strictly enforced. I have had no opportunity, however, of trying the effects of this method of treating ichthyosis in adults, the four cases in which it proved so successful being children below the age of eight years.

MOLLUSCUM.

Molluscum ; Comedones, of some modern writ
Ecphyma mollusciforme, of Erasmus Wilson.—See F
XI.

MOLLUSCUM.—The origin of the employment of
term to designate a disease of the cutaneous struct
which is chiefly interesting in consequence of its extr
rarity, has been a matter of discussion. Used by Wi
and Bateman at a time when they themselves, not hav
seen the affection, obtained their knowledge of it from
account of a case—published in 1793 by Ludwig—
occurred in the practice of Professor Tillesius, of Leip
it is most natural to infer that its application was deri
from the description therein contained, in which si
tumors that constitute the disease are said to consis
" verrucis mollibus sive *molluscis ;*" yet nearly all
French dermatologists ascribe its employment to s
imaginary resemblance between them and the minute
crescences that form on the bark of the maple tree.]
characterized by the development on the skin of roi
slightly umbilicated, soft tumors, varying in size usu
from that of the head of a pin to that of a nut,
described as occasionally acquiring the magnitude i
pigeon's egg; they are of a yellow or pinkish-w
color, sessile, rarely pedunculated, scattered irreguli
over the surface, yet occurring not unfrequently in si
groups, of slow growth, and unattended with either li
pain or constitutional irritation. When pressed betw
the fingers, a small quantity of a thick, whitish fluid
udes from the minute aperture that forms the umbilic
apex of each tumor, the exudation being evidently alt
sebaceous secretion. They appear on all parts of
cutaneous surface, but are most frequently witnessed
the face, and most rarely on the extremities; their d
tion is uncertain, in some cases ulcerating and falling
spontaneously, their site being marked by a slight (
trix, in others lasting for life, without undergoing any
crease in size, but the skin covering them becomes da
colored or brownish, and the tumors themselves acq
a certain degree of hardness. The internal structui

the tumors of molluscum is cellular, a transverse section often exhibiting five or six divisions, each of which corresponds to a duct of the sebaceous follicle, and contains altered sebaceous matter.

Bateman, after witnessing some cases of the disease, described it as consisting of two varieties, which he named molluscum *contagiosum* and molluscum *non-contagiosum*, but inasmuch as it is doubtful that the latter, as described by him, was truly molluscum, and at all events as the distinction he drew cannot be regarded as sufficient to constitute a specific difference, his division must be abandoned. The eruption consisting admittedly in a hypertrophied state of the sebaceous follicles, and being therefore of the same nature, anatomically considered, as Acne, some recent French writers, especially MM. Caillault[1] and Bazin,[2] have regarded molluscum as a species of that disease, the former terming it Acne *molluscoides*, and the latter Acne *varioliformis;* the absence of local inflammation, however, clearly distinguishes it from that affection. The best division of the disease, I consider, is that proposed by Dr. Craigie, in an able essay published in the seventy-fifth volume of the *Edinburgh Medical and Surgical Journal,* namely, into

Molluscum acutum.
" chronicum.

Acute molluscum (Plate XI, Fig. 5) agrees, in all respects, with the form which is generally regarded as being contagious; it occurs usually on the face and neck of children, and from them is conveyed to adults, almost invariably, however, of the same family. It is developed at first in the form of minute papulæ, scarcely noticeable, and unattended with any local symptoms; these gradually increase, until, in from six weeks to two months, they attain the size of a small currant, which they resemble much in shape, being somewhat pellucid, and sessile on the portion of integument from which they grow. Their duration is seldom prolonged for more than six months,

[1] *Archives Générales de Médecine,* 1851, Vol. xxii. pp. 46 and 316.
[2] *Journal des Connaissances Médicales,* 1851, p. 277.

but their progress is often more speedy, terminating either
by ulceration, which first commences at the apex, an opening being there formed through which the altered sebaceous matter contained in them is discharged, when
the small tumors collapse and shrink away, or by an
attack of local inflammation, when they slough off, leaving
a pit like that resulting from smallpox.　In most cases
the molluscous growths are developed in successive crops.

In *chronic molluscum* (Plate XI, Fig. 6)—the molluscum *pendulum* of Willan—the tumors, which are more
generally distributed over the surface of the body, attain
a much larger size, and are more frequently pedunculated; they are sometimes very few in number, may even
be solitary, but occasionally several of them are developed
on different parts of the integument at the same time.
This form is most frequently witnessed in adults, and
runs an essentially chronic course, lasting often for life if
uninterfered with, yet with but little increase in size.
Occasionally, as in the acute variety, inflammation attacks
some of the tumors, and they slough off.

The chronic and acute forms of molluscum differ especially, to use the words of Dr. Craigie, "in the circumstance of the latter being propagated by a specific matter,
while the former is, so far as is hitherto known, entirely
incapable of such communication."　This contagious
property, though its existence is denied by many modern writers on the disease, is, I think, too well established by the numerous cases which have been recorded
by Bateman, Craigie, Thompson, Carswell, Henderson,
Willis, &c., to admit of doubt.　M. Caillault, in the essay
on disease published by him, to which I have referred
above, states that he himself did not believe in its contagious nature until it was proved to him in April, 1851,
in one of the wards of the Hôpital St. Louis, at Paris,
fourteen children out of thirty having taken the disease
in the course of three months from a little girl who had
been admitted with numerous molluscous tumors on the
face.　Mr. Erasmus Wilson, while denying the commu-
nicability of molluscum by contagion, narrates a case in
which one child of a family having been brought to him
affected with the disease, it appeared in a few weeks after-

last for life without the least injury to health or impairment of the constitution, but occasionally troublesome
symptoms may arise from attempts made to destroy or
remove the tumors. In one instance, communicated to
me by Dr. Lees, the case of a female, aged 18, who was
under his care in the Meath Hospital, the application of
potassa fusa was followed by erysipelas, which terminated
fatally. Acute molluscum generally disappears spontaneously in from four to six months.

Treatment.—Internal remedies do not appear to have
any effect over molluscum, and are therefore not required
in its treatment, except such as ·may be calculated to
restore a healthy condition of the system generally, should
it be deranged.   Local applications are not advisable in
the chronic variety of the disease, but the tumors may be
snipped off with a sharp pair of scissors, and the surface
then touched with lunar caustic, provided the patient be
in a state of good health ; but when such is not the case
this should first be attended to. ·In the acute form, the
employment of a slightly stimulating lotion, as of sulphate of zinc or sulphate of iron, ten grains of either to
an ounce of distilled water and a drachm of rectified
spirit, hastens the throwing off of the small tumors.

STEARRHŒA.

Stearrhœa, from στέαρ, tallow or suet, and ῥέω, to flow.—
See Plate XII.

STEARRHŒA is a disease of the sebaceous follicles, characterized—as the words στέαρ and ῥέω indicate—by augmented secretion and discharge of their natural contents,
the follicles themselves, and their exeretory ducts being
at the same time somewhat hypertrophied. The increased
secretion may consist merely in an excessive amount of
the natural oily matter or smegma destined for the pre-
servation of the skin from external irritants, or in its discharge on the cutaneous surface in a vitiated condition,
where it concretes and forms a thick adherent layer,
varying in color from a rich yellow hue to nearly black.
The former is of very frequent occurrence, and can
scarcely be regarded as constituting a disease, while the

latter, a rather rare affection, is of extreme obstinacy, usually resisting treatment for years. Three varieties of the disease, thus constituted, require to be noticed:—

Stearrhœa simplex.
" flavescens.
" nigricans.

Stearrhœa simplex (*Sebaceous flux*) is marked chiefly by an oily or greasy state of those parts of the integument in which the sebaceous follicles are numerous, as the nose, the cheeks, the ears, the scalp, and other regions where hair grows; it is an accompaniment usually of a coarse, sallow condition of the skin, and is generally witnessed in a class of persons who are liable to be affected with acne, as noticed in the description of that disease. The orifices of most of the sebaceous follicles are usually much dilated, but others, becoming obstructed, present the appearance regarded as being characteristic of acne punctata. This state of the cutaneous surface is manifestly hereditary in most cases, and is a constant accompaniment, or rather may be regarded as a sign of the scrofulous diathesis; it lasts generally during life, appearing in youth, but being less marked in old age; and although indicative, cannot be considered as a cause, of an unhealthy constitution; when it exists, the natural perspiration is deficient in quantity, and congestive or inflammatory affections of some of the internal organs, assuming, however, a scrofulous character, are more apt to occur.

Stearrhœa flavescens (Plate XII, Figs. 1 and 2).—It is only of late years that this affection, which is of rather rare occurrence, has attracted the attention of dermatologists; Rayer was the first to describe it under the name of sebaceous flux, and after him it was specially noticed by Biett, who, regarding it correctly as dependent on a diseased condition of the sebaceous follicles, although admitting the difference which exists between it and the true pustular acne, made it a species of that eruption, under the name of acne *sebacea*. Erasmus Wilson gives an illustration of the disease in his beautiful Portraits of Diseases of the Skin, where he terms it

Inflammatio Folliculorum, while in his octavo work he describes it under the name I have adopted.

It is characterized by an exudation from the sebaceous follicles, of their natural secretion, more or less altered, on the surface of the skin, where it forms a yellowish or greenish-yellow crust or layer—in the former case resembling the cerumen of the ear, of variable thickness and consistency, at times so soft as to be readily wiped off, but more generally hard and firmly adherent. By exposure to the action of the atmosphere the effused matter gradually acquires a darker tint, presenting at length a brownish hue, and numerous cracks or fissures divide it into small packets, which often correspond with the linear markings of the skin. The portion of integument on which the diseased secretion had been seated, if examined after its removal, is found to be more or less injected, not unfrequently inflamed, and the sebaceous follicles hypertrophied, with their orifices enlarged and filled with the peculiar matter, the presence of which constitutes the disease. The crusts on the surface are rapidly renewed after their removal, and, if uninterfered with, soon form a layer three or four lines in thickness. The parts affected are the seat of sharp tingling, occasionally of stinging pains, accompanied by heat and itching. There is generally also a deranged state of the health, evidenced more especially by the condition of the digestive organs, in those persons on whose skin the disease appears; and from its occurrence most usually on the face, causing, in consequence, much disfigurement, great mental distress is occasioned.

Stearrhœa flavescens, as is evident from the description now given, is an affection of the sebaceous follicles, and is, therefore, witnessed only on those regions of the skin where these glands exist, being of most frequent occurrence in the parts in which they are most numerous; it therefore appears usually on the nose, the cheeks, the eyelids, the ears, and the scalp, but is also seen occasionally on other portions of the integument. Mr. Wilson states it to be most frequent on ladies' faces. It runs essentially a chronic course, spreading, in general, but slowly

from where it is first developed, and, if removed by artificial means, being again quickly reproduced.

Stearrhœa nigricans (Plate XII, Fig. 3[1]), although differing from the form now described apparently only in the
color of the effused diseased secretion, which is nearly jet
black, deserves a special notice in consequence of the .
singularity of the appearance which it presents, and its
extreme rarity. In it the matter discharged from the .
follicles is of a thinner consistence than in stearrhœa
flavescens, and is from the first of the same dark color,
which, moreover, stains linen, or any other substance
with which it may come in contact. From the few cases
of the disease which have been recorded it would appear
also to be attended with more local irritation, at times
amounting to severe pain and burning heat. In the
twenty-eighth volume of the *Med.-Chir. Transactions* a case
is reported in which the skin was so sensitive that the
patient, a young lady, had to give up the attempt to wash
away the secretion. Its occurrence is accompanied by
general constitutional disturbance, and in one case recorded by Mr. Teevan,[2] which had been first under the
care of Dr. Read, of Belfast, if the secretion of the diseased matter on the surface was arrested by local treatment, black vomiting, and the discharge of a black
substance from the bowels and kidneys, took place immediately. The black secretion in this patient, a young
lady, was analyzed by Dr. G. O. Rees, and found to consist of carbon, iron, lime, albuminous matter, fatty matter,
and alkaline chlorides and phosphates. It sometimes (as
in Dr. Neligan's illustration, Plate XII, Fig. 3) gives the
patient the singular appearance of having what are popularly called *black eyes;* and Mr. Wilson draws attention
to a case published by Mr. Yonge, in the *Philosophical
Transactions* more than a century since, in which the face
turned suddenly black, and this frequently during the
twenty-four hours. The case is detailed at length, and in

---

[1] This illustration is from a case detailed by Dr. Neligan in the
nineteenth volume of the *Dublin Quarterly Journal,* where will be found
a lengthened statement of his views as to the nature and pathology of
this disease.

[2] *Medico-Chirurgical Transactions,* Vol. xxviii. p. 611.

the words of Mr. Yonge, in the *Student's Book of Cutaneous Medicine*, page 464. The instances of this peculiar affection which have been published were seemingly more obstinate than the second form of the disease which I have described: it was in all of them situated on the same region of the skin.

The *causes* of any of the forms of stearrhœa are very obscure; the first is both congenital and hereditary, but the others have not been proved to be either; they appear only in persons who have attained the age of puberty, and are very rarely witnessed in advanced life, yet I have seen one example in which stearrhœa flavescens was developed on the nose after the age of seventy; they occur, too, with much greater frequency in females than in males, and in the former their connection with suppressed menstruation, or uterine derangement, has been in some instances noticed; but in the majority of cases their development is preceded and accompanied rather by derangements of the digestive organs.

Diagnosis.—Stearrhœa simplex cannot be confounded with any other affection of the skin; the other forms, however, in consequence chiefly of their rarity, are often not recognized when they occur, and therefore occasion much doubt as to their nature. Thus, an account of five cases of what, from the description and accompanying illustrations I conceive to be stearrhœa flavescens, has been published by Drs. Addison and Gull,[1] but denominated by them *Vitiligoidea plana* and *Vitiligoidea tuberosa*, from a supposed correspondence between the affection and the incorrect definition of vitiligo which was given by Willan; and the case of Mr. Teevan, before referred to, was originally communicated to the Medico-Chirurgical Society of London, as being an example of Pityriasis nigra.

Prognosis.—Stearrhœa flavescens and Stearrhœa nigricans are both most obstinate affections, and appear to be equally rebellious to all plans of treatment, but are chiefly important in consequence of the disfigurement which they occasion, being not in the least degree

---

[1] *Guy's Hospital Reports*, New Series, Vol. vii. p. 265.

attended with any danger to life. In the former, I have seen the sebaceous follicles take on an active inflammatory action when caustic applications were applied to the diseased surface, and indolent pustules form, which, on the continuance of the irritation, terminated in obstinate ulcers, with hardened elevated edges.

Treatment.—The first and most important point to be attended to is the restoration of a healthy condition of the system; this is best effected by the internal administration of alteratives, combined with alkalies, such as the hydrargyrum cum cretâ with dried carbonate of soda, or cod-liver oil with lime-water, according to the circumstances of each case; the latter combination is readily taken in milk, from one to four drachms of the oil being given three times daily, in one ounce each of lime-water and new milk, previously mixed. As soon as the state of the digestive organs is improved, or the menstrual function restored, preparations of iodine—especially the syrup of the iodide of iron, or the iodide of potassium, in some tonic vegetable decoction or infusion—will be prescribed with benefit. Of course the employment of purgatives, when requisite, should not be omitted. The local applications that are found most useful are gently stimulating and astringent lotions and ointments. The affected surface should be sponged three or four times a day with the spirituous lotion recommended for acne simplex (see page 177), an ointment containing ten grains of the iodide of potassium to the ounce of cold cream being applied at night, or a solution of the iodide of iron—two grains to the ounce of rose or elder-flower water, and dilute citrine ointment may be used. No matter what remedies, however, are employed, they must be continued *for a very long time*, and local means will be found unavailing until the general health is restored. The application of caustics *I have invariablg seen productive of injurious consequences.* When the crust of effused sebaceous matter is hard, dry, and adherent to the surface, it should be removed by the application of poultices or of water dressing, previously to the use of topical remedies.

ELEPHANTIASIS.

Elephantiasis, ἐλεφαντίασις; Leontiasis and Satyriásis of the Latins; Elephant skin disease.—See Plate XII.

The term ELEPHANTIASIS has been applied, both in ancient and modern days, to designate two perfectly distinct diseases of the integuments; the one, which has been specifically denominated elephantiasis *Græcorum*, is by some believed to be the true lepra or leprosy of antiquity, and is the leprosy of the middle ages; while the other, which, from having been first accurately described by the Arabian physicians, has been termed elephantiasis *Arabum*, does not bear the least analogy to it. Both have been but rarely seen in these countries in modern times; though the former still prevails in India, Africa, Greece, Spain, Norway, and Iceland.

ELEPHANTIASIS GRÆCORUM (Plate XII, Fig. 4) is characterized by the development on the integuments of numerous globular tumors, varying in size from that of a pea to that of an apple, soft and yielding to the touch, at first of a dusky or livid hue, but afterwards becoming brownish-yellow or of a bronzed tint. They occur most usually and in greatest number on the face, but may appear also on every region of the body; the skin of the part affected is much hypertrophied, raised into irregular elevations, and of an unhealthy, diseased appearance, causing the sufferers from the disease to present a hideous aspect, described by those who have witnessed it to be revolting in the extreme, whence they have in all ages been regarded with abhorrence, as individuals specially afflicted. Both mind and body share at length in the local disease, the senses become obtuse, fatuity creeps on, and all the bodily functions are deranged. Eventually the tumors ulcerate, exude an ichorous matter, and form unhealthy open sores; the bones soften, and become affected with caries; mortification not unfrequently attacks the smaller joints, and death soon terminates sufferings which are extreme.

It is probable that the persecuted wretches mentioned by classic authors as affected with *satyriasis* had this disease; and it was sometimes called *leontiasis*, from the frowning and formidable aspect of the subject of it being supposed to resemble the lion as well as the elephant. Thus Aretæus, describing it, says " it is disgusting to the sight, and in all respects terrible, like the elephant;" and Avicenna affirms " it renders the countenance terrible to look at, and somewhat of the form of the lion's visage." The learned Dr. Mead (see *Medica Sacra*) thinks it was the disease of Job, and so does Dr. Mason Good. The comparison of Job's disease, as described in the Sacred Text, with the above description will tend to confirm this view; and the phrase " lazar-house," synonymous with "leper-house," was, probably, derived from the inmates of such a place being presumed to have the disease of Lazarus. In some MSS. of the English leper-houses the inmates are described as " Elephantuosi;" and Lucretius, following the common opinion of his time, ascribed the origin of the disease to Egypt:—

" Est Elephas morbus, qui propter flumina Nili,
Gignitur Ægypto in mediâ, neque præterea usquam."
De Rer. Nat. VI. 1112.

Dr. Simpson, of Edinburgh, published, in *The Edinburgh Medical and Surgical Journal*, Vols. LVI and LVII, a series of learned papers, entitled " Antiquarian Notices of Leprosy and Leper Hospitals in Scotland and England." From information collected by him from English and Scottish MSS. and records—from Dugdale's *Monasticon Anglicanum*, Semler's *Historiæ Ecclesiasticæ Selecta Capita*, Schilling's *Commentio de Leprâ*, and other authorities—he shows that a disease, popularly known as leprosy, was everywhere endemic from the tenth to the sixteenth century ; that against it princes and courts enacted laws and popes issued bulls, particularly Alexander III, who issued a famous bull—" De Leprosis"—regarding the ecclesiastical separation and the rights of the infected. A particular order of knighthood, that of St. Lazarus, was instituted to care for the sick, particularly lepers, one of whom they had to elect as their master, until countermanded by Pope Innocent IV. They separated from the Knights Hospitallers about the twelfth century.

Wilde's able reports, which the Irish people can never sufficiently value.

Sir William is of opinion that the Irish disease was elephantiasis.

In Waterford there was a leper hospital, which, though now used as an infirmary, is still known by its ancient name. The last recorded case of an Irish leper was found in it in 1775. There was formerly a "Leper's Old Hospital of St. Stephen's" in Cork. It was governed by a prior; and later (temp. Ric. II, and Hen. IV) by a guardian appointed by the King. It gave place to the parish church of St. Stephen, to which was attached, as an endowment, the landed property of the leper hospital. This parish, with some others, was ultimately incorporated into the parochial union, now known as that of S. Nicolas, while Baron Worth's Blue Coat Hospital was built on the site of the church. It is still known as S. Stephen's Hospital.—Caulfield's *Sigilla Ecclesiæ Hibernicæ Illustrata*, pp. 28, 29.

Mr. Erasmus Wilson (*Diseases of the Skin*, Fifth Edition) says the earliest records of this disease in Great Britain are those of the Welsh King, Hoel Dha, A. D. 950. In 1547–1553 (Edw. VI) a commission for suppressing colleges, hospitals, &c., reported most of the leper-houses as empty.

Dr. Simpson remarks that the earliest house in Scotland dates at 1150; and so late as 1604 a leprous woman was ordered into a lazar house at Aberdeen, by the town council; whilst there was a leper patient in the Edinburgh Infirmary in 1798. Mr. Erasmus Wilson says it still exists among us as morphœa (1, tuberosa; 2, alba atrophica; 3, nigra; 4, alopœciata), and that it has always existed in the north of Europe. Dr. Edmonston, of Lerwick, quoted by Dr. Simpson, says that it "was in Zetland sixty years ago (before 1848), and still is in Iceland and the Faroe Islands." So great a plague has it been in Sweden and Norway that a government commission investigated it, and the result is the best book on the subject (*Traité de la Spedalskhed ou Elephantiasis des Græcs*), by Dr. Danielssen, of Bergen, and Dr. Boëck, of Christiana, published at Paris in 1848.

Dr. George Macleod, of Glasgow, author of the scholarly and delightfully written book, *Notes on the Surgery of the Crimean War*, was in Iceland in the summer of 1868. In answer to a letter from the Editor he thus writes: "I saw a few cases (four) of leprosy when in Iceland, and was told by the chief surgeon (a government official as they are all) that it was very common, and all of the tubercular variety. The gentleman I refer to, and whose name was Hjaltelin (a most intelligent, well-read man he is), attributes the disease to dirt, badly ventilated house, and an unvarying diet; and if such causes are capable of producing this disease, I can speak for their powerful activity in Iceland. You are, perhaps, not aware that some years ago I paid some attention to the disease you write about, and that in Spain, Africa, and Palestine I saw much of it. I have always intended to give form to the scattered notes I possess upon it. There are now no leper hospitals now *in use* in Iceland, though the buildings remain, but the disease is still very common. By improving the hygienic condition of young persons Hjaltelin has arrested the complaint."

Dr. Mason Good states that this disease has been noticed by various travellers as existing in India, Madeira, and the Isle of France.

Dr. T. More Madden, of this city, remarked to the Editor that he had seen much of it lately in Spain; and in Tangiers, where the tubercular disease exists side by side with the skin affection. The latter prevails among the Jew residents, and his description of the ulcerated leprosy, as he saw it, was *totidem verbis*, that of the Levitical canon. He also remarked that it altered the countenance very little, except destroying the eyebrows; and the women remedied this defect by the use of certain pigments. The valuable treatise of Drs. Danielssen and Boëck on the SPEDALSKHED, of Norway, has already been noted. They believe it to be identical with Elephantiasis Græcorum; and they affirm that it is not the *Radesyge*, a Norwegian disease, with which it has sometimes been confounded. Elephantiasis, or Spedalskhed, is by them divided into E. *tuberculosa*, and E. *anæsthetica*. The former answers to the description already given;

25

the latter is characterized by the appearance of la
bullæ seated on livid patches; these break, and le
ulcers on which crusts subsequently form. After a wl
though not uniformly, white patches, accompanied
itching, diminished sensibility, and slight desquamat
appear irregularly scattered over the body. Hype
thesia and periodic shiverings follow, to be succeede
turn by a gradual, but finally extreme, and someti
general anæsthesia. The affected parts only are dry;
conjunctivæ are injected; vesicles form over them;
lids become atrophied; the lashes fall away; the n
mucous membrane dries up; ulcers form and destroy
septum; partial paralysis ensues; and occasionally a
forms on the sole of the foot, becomes blue, ulcerates,
seldom heals. The bones and periosteum gener
escape. Death is preceded by diarrhœa and someti
by tetanic spasms. During the progress of the dis
there is extreme thirst, occasional vomiting and pyr
with a feeling of cold, torpor, and drowsiness. In
sarcous cases, which are sometimes met with, the urin
albuminous. The disease is frequently complicated
scabies, eczema, and other skin affectious; it is ende
and hereditary, but is *not* contagious.

As to *treatment*, mercurials and arsenicals are decl
mischievous,[1] while iodine, bromine, cod-liver oil, sti
lant baths and ointments have been found occasion
useful. Bleeding has been also recommended, but ei
form of the disease must be considered hopelessly in
able. Such of our readers as may not have access to
valuable work of Drs. Danielssen and Boëck, or
French translation of it, will find a critical analysis c
of considerable value in the *Brit. and For. Med.-(
Rev.*, Vol. V (1850), p. 171.

In Ranking's *Abstract*, Vol. XLI, p. 77, will be fo
an abstract of Dr. H. V. Carter's most valuable pape
"Leprosy as seen in India."—See also the *Trans. of L
bay Med. and Phys. Soc.*, Vol. VIII (N. S. 1862),
Brit. and For. Med.-Chir. Rev., Jan. 1863.

---

[1] *Per contra see Dubli* _ _ _ *ical Press*, April 20, 1864, for the
treatment by arsenic pr   *lation.*

Dr. Carter states that it prevails extensively in the Bombay Presidency, and he mentions three forms of it: 1. An eruption of the skin, allied to lepra, and accompanied by anæsthesia. This form he conceives to be the *Leuke*, of the Greeks: the *Baras*, of the Arabians; and the *Barat-lebana*, of the Hebrews; to it belongs the *Shvet-Kusta*, or white leprosy, of India. 2. The *Guleet Kusta*, or Sunbahiree, of the Hindoos; the E. Anæsthetica of Danielssen and Boëck. 3. *Ructa-Kusta*, *Ructa-pitia*, of h e Hindoos; the E. tuberculosa already described.

Dr. Carter considers E. anæsthetica the typical and most invariable form, but he looks on them all as varieties of one disease, because they seldom occur separately, are almost always combined at certain stages, and different members of the same family may be affected with each. Contrary to Danielssen and Boëck, and others, he states that there are no special or invariable premonitory symptoms; the duration of the disease is from five to fifteen years; and according to the Norwegian writers nine and a half years. It mostly attacks males, and is limited to the lower classes of society. He also believes the disease to be a cachexia essentially related to syphilis; not transmissible by sexual intercourse, but clearly hereditary.[1]

Mr. Erasmus Wilson believes it to be essentially a blood disease, and the researches of Carter, Danielssen, and Boëck, and others, would generally lead to a like conclusion.

The MORPHIE, of Brazil, has been considered a variety of Elephantiasis. Dr. Fox remarks of it, that "the tubercles do not form a prominent feature; the usual erythema is succeeded by bullæ; ulceration is rather the rule; indeed the disease presents rather the anæsthetic form."

FRAMBŒSIA (so called from its resemblance to a raspberry, *Framboise*), Sibbens, of the Scotch, and Radesyge, of the Norwegians, is an ally of Elephantiasis. It is scarcely ever seen in England; is met with occasionally

---

[1] In the *Medical Times and Gazette* for 1st April, 1865, Dr. Hillier details ⸳ ⸳⸳⸳ of Elephantiasis Tuberculosa treated by him in University Hospital.

in Scotland, rarely in Ireland, but frequ
and the West Indies. It commences wi
toms, followed by an eruption of small fla
sometimes attain the size of half an in
This eruption prevails on the face, arm
and pudenda; becomes pustular in abo
crust forms, and beneath it a sloughing
ulcers appear simultaneously on variou
sometimes accompanied by ulceration of t
eruption may last from one week to abou
Emaciation, and debility; and frequently
vene. The disease is believed to be co
contagion and inoculation, occurs once di
prefers to attack the young, and appears
by misery, deprivation, and filth, engen
deterioration, as in Elephantiasis.

It is *treated* by external stimulants, witl
and nutritious food.

Elephantiasis occurring in Astrachan is
TAURICUS, or lepra Astrachanica, "the
It is noted as a distinct variety of tube
tiasis by Dr. Fox, who observes that,
attacked by it live very badly, eat stinki
like."—*Op. cit.*, p. 180.

THE ALEPPO EVIL, Bouton d'Alep,
Biskra, has also been noted as a variety (
Dr. Fox states that it is endemic at Alep
on the banks of the Tigris and Euphrates
itself does not seem to differ materially fr
It attacks every inhabitant of these dist
contagious. When the tubercle is *singl*
called the *male;* when multiplied, the *fe*
to be caused by the use of bad drinking-

The New Zealanders are affected with
NGERENGERE, which is by some believe
of Elephantiasis. From published accou
appear to be either tubercular or anæsthel
fact, a severe form of Psoriasis. As its m
is beyond the scope of this work, referenc
to Dr. Thomson's description of it in the

Med.-Chir. Review for April, 1854. Dr. Thomson believes it to be of strumous, not of syphilitic, origin.

Dr. Fox remarks that a similar disease has been described as existing in Jamaica. It is there called CACUBAY, and is characterized by the presence of white spots near the ends of the extremities, which ulcerate. The bones are destroyed by a "*quasi*-necrosis," after which the sore heals up until the next attack.

A remarkable ally of Elephantiasis Græcorum is PELLAGRA, Mal de la Rosa, Mal de Sole, or Elephantiasis Italica. This disease prevails endemically in the south of France, and in parts of Spain, but chiefly in Lombardy, Piedmont, and Venetia. It attacks the poorer members of the community, and is believed to be a peculiar diathesis, with three groups of symptoms: 1, an erythematous change in the skin; 2, general failure of power and nutrition; and 3, cerebro-spinal symptoms. The eruption appears on those parts of the body which are more generally exposed to the rays of the sun. The skin, without swelling or roughness, becomes red, with slight desquamation, and subsequent dark discoloration. The eruption disappears during winter, but returns with the spring in an exaggerated form. Failing appetite, indigestion, and diarrhœa, accompany or precede the disease from the outset. The cerebro-spinal symptoms are headache, giddiness, defect in the special senses, cramps, gradually progressive paralysis, delirium and despondency. The mortality is said to be from three to fifty-two per cent.; and the intellect is permanently and gravely injured in those who do not die of the disease. It is not contagious, is often hereditary, is more frequent in women than in men, and it usually occurs between the ages of thirty and fifty. Exposure to the heat of the sun is believed to be one of its exciting causes, as is also exposure to strong artificial heat. The use of maize is also said to be favorable to its production, which, no doubt, mainly depends on the physical degeneration caused by poverty, as in the other diseases of this class. Some pathologists have found, after death, opacity and thickening of the arachnoid, with atrophy and induration of the spinal cord; while others have not found any such appearances.

25*

The *treatment* may be said to be sanitary, and hygienic, and preventive. It is a poor man's disease, and improvement in the habits and supports of life constitutes the only sure safeguard against it.

For more full details see Dr. Gintrac's work, *De la Pellagre dans le Département de la Gironde*, Bordeaux, 1863. Dr. Fox in his work gives the substance of Dr. Gintrac's researches.

ELEPHANTIASIS ARABUM.

Elephantiasis Arabum.—Dal-fil (literally Morbus Elephas) of the Arabian writer; Bucnemia Tropica of Mason Good.

ELEPHANTIASIS ARABUM (*Barbadoes leg*).—Plate XII, Fig. 6.—The popular name for this singular affection indicates its frequency of occurrence in the West India Islands, where it is endemic, but cases of it are also witnessed in Egypt, in America, in various countries of Europe, and, as was remarked originally by Dr. Graves,[1] are not very uncommon in Ireland; it is, however, less frequently seen now than at the time his account of it was published, thirty-nine years ago.

The disease consists in an extreme degree of hypertrophy, affecting one or both of the lower extremities, the scrotum, the hands or arms, and occasionally even the face, and the mamma and pudendum in females; the enlargement affects equally the skin and the subcutaneous and deep-seated areolar tissue, so as to produce an enormous swelling of the part attacked, one of the legs not unfrequently exceeding in magnitude the girth of the body. It commences usually with symptoms of local inflammation chiefly engaging the lymphatic system, and general constitutional derangement; these attacks are of frequent occurrence, and after each, the parts engaged become more and more swollen, chiefly from effusion into the areolar texture; but in some cases, especially in temperate climates, the enlargement comes on slowly, and gradually augments without any apparent disturbance of

[1] *Dublin Hospital Reports*, Vol. iv. p. 54.

function, local or general. When the affection is fully developed, the integuments, which are enormously thickened, are generally of a whitish cólor, rough and swollen, and present deep furrows, occasionally the seat of ulceration, a thin, ichorous discharge, which concretes into hard, scaly incrustations, then issuing from them. To the great hypertrophy of the integuments is due the name of this disease, but in order to distinguish it from that last described, the term *Pachydermia*, first proposed by Fuchs, has been adopted by many modern dermatologists.

When the scrotum is the part affected, as it very frequently is in the colored population of tropical climates, it attains at times and enormous magnitude; Horner, in his *Medical Topography of Brazil*, narrates two instances in which the tumor situated there measured four feet in circumference. The upper extremities, when attacked by the disease, do not acquire as large a size as the lower, manifestly in consequence of their containing less areolar tissue. The palms of the hands and soles of the feet are never affected.

The *causes* of elephantiasis Arabum are altogether unknown, if we except its apparent connection with inflammation of the lymphatics; it is not contagious; it affects both sexes equally, and occurs at all ages, but is more frequent in adults than in children. Its much greater prevalence in hot countries, and its being more frequent there in those districts which are characterized by the presence of moisture, indicate the effect of heat and damp conjoined as an exciting cause.

There is no difficulty in *diagnosing* this disease in its advanced stages; in its commencement it might be mistaken for angeioleucitis, from which it appears to differ simply in its symptoms being less acute, and in its never terminating in the formation of purulent abscesses. Its *duration* is essentially chronic; but although its presence renders life a burden, it in very rare cases seems to prove fatal.

An anatomical examination of the parts in this form of elephantiasis exhibits the derma and epidermis usually much hypertrophied, the former sometimes constituting a layer an inch in thickness, but the enlargement of the affected regions is due chiefly to the change in the areolar membrane, from the deposit sometimes of fat, but more usually of a substance almost as firm as fibrous tissue, and of a lardaceous appearance, which to the naked eye resembles the natural structure compressed. Lebert and Gustav Simon, who examined the new deposit with the microscope, found it to consist in fibrous bundles of pure areolar tissue, fully developed or in the process of formation, with numerous fat cells in the interstices.

Treatment.—In the early or inflammatory stages of elephantiasis Arabum, antiphlogistic treatment is clearly indicated, but this must be constitutional and not local; if a limb be the part affected it should be kept at rest and placed in the horizontal position above the level of the body. Active purging seems to have been the plan of treatment most successful in those cases which have been reported, and even in the chronic stages, when other remedies generally fail to prove beneficial, it has been useful. When the disease becomes chronic, iodine frictions and firm bandaging have also been recommended, but they usually fail to produce any manifest effect; amputation of the parts, if possible, has been then advised, and ablation of the hypertrophied scrotum has, in many instances, been resorted to with success; but as regards the limbs, the removal of one of them has been usually followed by the development of the disease in another; thus in a case reported by Cazenave, in which a leg, the seat of elephantiasis was removed, the arm became affected soon afterwards.

Professor Carnochan, of New York, originated the practice of ligaturing the main artery of the affected limb; and Mr. Butcher, of this city, believing Barbadoes leg to be a blood disease, performed the first operation of that kind in this country. In the thirty-fifth volume of the *Dub. Quar. Journ.*, and more recently in his large *Treatise on Surgery*, Dublin, 1865, p. 409, he details the successful ligaturing of the femoral artery in a case in Mercer's Hospital; and his example has been followed by others. See also a more recent case of "Elephantiasis of the Leg, Treated by Ligature of the Femoral

Artery," by Mr. Fayer, of Calcutta.—*Ed. Med. Journ.*, Nov. 1865.

THE LEPROSY OF THE HEBREWS (*Lepra Hebræorum*).

In the preceding remarks on Lepra or Psoriasis in Chap. VI, and on Elephantiasis in Chap. VII, no particular mention has been made of the Leprosy of the Hebrews. Modern writers, and particularly Mr. Erasmus Wilson, have revived the discussions of former times regarding this disease, and the general impetus given to the study of modern elephantiasis by the researches of Danielssen and Boëck, and of Carter, makes it desirable that a short dissertation should be here given on the vexed question, "What was the Leprosy of the Hebrews?" For a more full discussion of the subject the Editor must refer the reader to two papers of his in the *Dublin Quarterly Journal* for 1864 (May and Nov.), entitled respectively— "The Hebrew, Mediæval, and Modern Leprosies Compared," and "Remarks on the Hebrew Catalogue of Skin Diseases."

In the thirteenth chapter of the Book of Leviticus we find an exact description of three varieties of "leprosy;" and although the Arabic and Greek writers notice them all, yet it is difficult to identify their descriptions with those of the Levitical Canon. This proceeds, in a great measure, from the use of synonyms and inexact renderings of medical terms from one language to another, from the various terms applied in successive ages to the same diseases, and from variations and total changes in the meaning of some of them. The light which modern science has thrown on the origin and causes of leprous diseases, be they squamous or tubercular, will readily account for the generally received opinion, that the peculiar employments and hardships to which the Hebrews were subject during the last and most oppressive stage of their Egyptian bondage, rendered them peculiarly liable to contract the Egyptian endemic leprosy ; and also that this predisposition was retained by them in their own land where it was, probably, in no small degree fostered by hereditary descent, to which all their laws and customs indirectly tended. *Justin Trogus* (*Hist. Lib.* XXXVI,

C. 2) and Tacitus (*Hist.* Lib. V) join Strabo, who f
the Egyptian historian, Manetho, in asserting that
was communicated to the Egyptians by the H
who, in consequence of it, were driven out of the c
but Josephus (*Antiq.* Lib. III, Cap. XI, Sec. 4)
shows their statements to be incorrect, and so
result of narrow prejudice. Whatever may ha*
its origin, it is quite clear that, when a free nat
Hebrews had leprosy as an endemic; and respe
we find some of the most remarkable of the ena
of their great lawgiver, Moses.

Following the Hebrew original, we find that
speaks of three varieties of "leprosy," to all of w
applies the generic term *Bahereth*, or bright sp*
divides them into—*Bohak*, or dull white, and tw*
ties of *Tsorat*, or malignant disease, viz., *Bahere*
or dusky Babereth, and *Bahereth lebhana*, or brigl
Bahereth. *Bohak* was not seriously regarded
Jewish law: "If a man also or a woman have
skin of their flesh bright spots (Bahereth), *eve*
bright spots, then the priest shall look: and be
the bright spots (Bahereth) in the skin of their
darkish white; it *is* a freckled spot (Bohak) *that*
in the skin: *he* is clean." Lev. xiii. 38, 39. The
variety *Bahereth Kehe*, nigrescent or shadowed
similis, Celsus) leprosy, was more serious than
but the third variety *Bahereth lebhana*, or brigh
leprosy, was the most serious of all. The pathogr
characteristics of this disease were: "A glossy
and spreading scale upon an elevated base; the el
depressed into the middle, but without change of
the black hair on the patches, which is the natur
of the hair in Palestine, participating in the wl
and the patches themselves perpetually widenir
outline."—Mason Good.

When any one of these appeared on a person
brought before the priest; and if, in connection wi
a blemish, the specific marks of a *tsorat*, or m*
leprosy, were found, he was declared unclean; or,
of doubt, he was remanded for further examinatio
disease, particularly the bright white variety, ter*

either favorably or unfavorably. In the former case it spread over the body without ulcerating, and, having run through its course, exhausted itself. In such case, while the scales were yet dry on him, the leper was declared clean, and restored to society. If the case terminated unfavorably, the patches ulcerated, producing quick and fungous flesh, and the patient was pronounced unclean for life. He was clothed and otherwise treated as one dead, while the Hebrew theocracy compelled him to forsake the haunts of men, proclaiming to all passers-by the hopeless and irrevocable sentence—"Unclean, unclean."

According to Dr. Mason Good, the Arabians still know *Bohak* by the same name and with the Levitical meaning. *Bahereth lebhana* they termed *Beras Bejas;* and *Bahereth Kehe* they termed *Beras Asved.* The Greeks called *Bohak*, λίπρα ἄλφος; *Bahereth Kehe*, λίπρα μίλας; and *Bahereth lebhana*, λίπρα λευκή. In course of time the Arabians used *Bohak* and *Beras* indiscriminately, confounding their symptoms and qualities, and added a term of wider extent, *Kouba*, designating scaly eruptions of every kind.

The Greeks derived their ψώρα—whence our term *sore* —from the Hebrew Tsorat,[1] but it soon gave place to the older term λίπρα, which is a synonyme of the Hebrew generic term *Bahereth*. In its secondary sense ψώρα was used to express scaly eruptions in general, and particularly the scaly state of the skin which sometimes accompanies scabies. The LXX, or translators of the Septuagint, use the generic term *lepra* indiscriminately. For example, the Hebrew tells us that the priest shall examine the *Bahereth*, or general morbid appearance, and if it have the specific marks which are accurately defined, it is a *tsorat* or malignant disease—*i. e.*, either *Bahereth Kehe* or *Bahereth lebhana*. The Greek merely reads: "The priest shall examine the λίπρα, and if it have the specific marks it is a λίπρα." Not only was the Hebrew *Bahereth* translated into λίπρα by the LXX, but it also stands as *lepra* in the Vulgate; further, it is described by Celsus (Lib. V, cap. XXVIII, Sec. 19) under the name *Vitiligo*. It

---

[1] Or from τάω or τάω, to touch—See *Liddell and Scott's Lexicon.*

will be remembered that, in the time of Augustus (
Celsus collected the works of the principal Greek m
writers; and respecting this vitiligo, or lepra, h
writes: "There are three species of it. It is 1
ἄλφος when it is of a white color, with some deg
roughness, and is not continuous, but appears as i
little drops were dispersed here and there. Som
it spreads wider, but with certain intermissions
continuities. The μέλας differs from this in color, b
it is black, and like a shadow (umbræ similis), but in
circumstances they agree. The λευκή has some sim
to the ἄλφος, but it has more of the white and r
deeper, and in it the hairs are white and like down
these spread themselves, but in some persons
quickly, in others more slowly. The alphos and
come and go off some people at different times, b
leuce does not easily quit the patient whom it has
The cure of the two former is not very difficult; tl
scarcely ever heals."

Rhenferdius, an older medical writer, in his tr
"De Leprâ Cutis Hebræorum" (to be found in Meus
Nov. Test. ex Talm., illustr., pp. 1057, &c., classed D-
in library T. C. D.) plainly proves from ancient ai
Talmudists and others, that lepra Hebræorum was
disease denoted by every name implying cuticular
tion. He asserts that one pathognomonic sign—
præternaturalis—was common to all the species
and, quoting from Maimonides, he observes that
albus, diffusio, et vivacitas" were the distinguishing
observed by all Jews to mark the different varietie
remarks that λέπρα (of the Greeks), "præternatural
porum albedo non longe recredit ab illa Maimonid
data;" and that vitiligo of Celsus "proxime acced
lepram Hebræorum;" that it is the alphos and m
the Greeks, and the lepra in S. Matt. viii. Iu Schi
De Leprâ Commentationes (Leyden, 1778) the autl
prints the philologico-medical dissertation, "Ph
Ouseelii, M. D., de Leprâ Cutis Hebræorum." I
treatise the points prominently remarked on by
ferdius are duly noticed. Thus, at p. 77, he obs
"Generale Lepræ signum omnibus ejus speciebu

petens est; *Albedo prœternaturalis*, externæ superficiei partis affectæ." He pursues this part of the subject at some length, and shows from numerous authorities that the *whiteness* was pathognomonic, and that in the different varieties of the disease it varied as the whiteness of snow varies from that of gypsum, which varies from that of wool, which again varies from the whiteness of a sheep's fleece.

The learned Mead, in his *Medica Sacra*, identifies the vitiligo of Celsus with lepra; Lorry (*De Morbis Cutaneis*, p. 373) remarks that the addition of the symptoms described by Celsus to those defined by Moses makes the identity of the two complete; Galen and Hippocrates considered leprosy and λευκη[1] to be the same; and Dr. Mason Good, who has fully treated the subject, considers the description of Celsus to approach nearer to that of Moses than any other known to him. The word used by the LXX, λέπρα from λέπις *a scale*, also confirms the preceding remarks. Because of the *white* scales, it was likened to snow, and this where the disease was distinctly *penal* and therefore it may be presumed of the severest and most typical kind. Hence, it is recorded that the hand of Moses was leprous *as snow* (Exod. iv. 6); that Miriam became "leprous (white) *as snow*" (Numb. xii. 10); and Gehazi went out from Elisha's presence "a leper as (white as) *snow*" (II Kings, v. 27).

From what has been already stated it would appear that lepra Hebræorum was a white scaly disease, answering to Lepra or Psoriasis described in Chapter VI; and it may be asserted that *Bohak* was the *alphos* of Celsus, and the Lepra (or Psoriasis) guttata already described in Chapter VI; that *Bahereth Kehe* was the *melas* of Celsus and the Psoriasis Nigricans of Chapter VI; and that *Bahereth lebhana* was the *leuce* of Celsus, and a very intense kind of psoriasis lepræformis already described. It must be borne in mind that the varieties of lepra detailed in Chapter VI are those occurring in this country in the

---

[1] The λέπρα λευκή, or white leprosy of Celsus, and the (substantive) λεύκη, or white cutaneous eruption of Hippocrates (*Prædict.*, Lib. ii., Sec. 2) are synonymous terms.

26

present day; and therefore that the difference of th
Jewish disease in *degree*, but not in *kind*, is just what th
history of that historic and oriental nation would lead
to expect. It has, however, been alleged, and not witho
some show of reason, that elephantiasis Græcorum w
the leprosy of the Hebrews. As we have already see
elephantiasis was the leprosy of the middle ages, and
called leprosy by many of the moderns; and not only
but several of the ancient writers so confuse and jumb
names and terms as to perplex the reader exceedingl
How this came to be so may be shortly explained.

  The Arabian writers described elephantiasis Græcoru
by the term *Juzam*, literally disjunction, or erosion; at
they called elephantiasis Arabum *dal-fil,* literally *morb
elephas.* The Greek translators of the Arabian medic
writings finding two diseases described by one nar
(their own elephantiasis, and the Arabian elephas
which they knew nothing) rendered both into the wo
ἰλεφαντίασις and, in common with some of the Arabia
deeming elephantiasis to be an advanced stage of lep
they applied that term (λίπρα) to elephantiasis als
though the word λίπρα from λίπις a scale, is never me
tioned by them except as a scaly eruption. This, as
should now call it, pathological error of deeming the o
disease to be an advanced stage of the other, was readi
copied by the Latins, until ultimately both diseases ca
to be placed in the same nosological order. In the pi
sent day, however, while it is contended that they are n
in the same nosological order, it is at the same time urg
that λίπρα and ἰλεφαντίασις were identical; and to suppe
this view, a forced and unnatural construction is put o
only on the Sacred Text, but also on the descriptions
Celsus and others. From what has been already a
vanced, it has appeared that the pathognomonic sign
the Hebrew leprosy was *a white scaly eruption.* In t
Mosaic description we find nothing that at all likens it
the thick, rugose, tuberculate, or anæsthetic skin of e
phantiasis, to say nothing of the other prominent sym
toms of that disease, which find no counterpart whatev
in the Mosaic description. So different, indeed, are t
two affections that Mr. Erasmus Wilson, in his earne

endeavors to explain the Sacred Text according to his views, does not seem to have satisfied himself, for he remarks: "The Sacred Writings usually exact and accurate in their description of events, are so confused on the subject of elephantiasis as to require to be put out of the pale of reference when treating on this subject; and the pages of the Greek and Arabian authors are equally uncertain." Also Dr. Henderson (*Iceland, or a Journal of Residence in that Island*) while calling the Icelandic elephantiasis Jewish leprosy, apologizes for Moses that he " has not noticed the very striking anæsthesia or insensibility of the skin, which is an inseparable attendant of the genuine elephantiasis." Now it may be noted that it is not Moses who is "confused," or who omits to "notice" an important symptom of a disease known for thousands of years, but his modern critics, who very illogically assume the truth of their own position, and then try by that standard the great Hebrew lawgiver and the fathers of medicine, who wrote of another disease altogether. Celsus' description of vitiligo, and his division of it into alphos, melas, and leuce, has been already referred to. This description, which appears plain enough, Mr. Wilson endeavors to accommodate in a rather strange manner to elephantiasis. The Editor is the more surprised at this because any reader of Celsus will see that among his descriptions of some fifty skin diseases there is no mention of elephantiasis. On the other hand, a full and very accurate account of it will be found in Cap. XXV of his third book, in which, be it observed, is no mention of any of what he considered cutaneous diseases. It is placed between descriptions of "morbus arquatus," and ἀποπληξία, and it is obvious to the reader that so far from Celsus having considered it to be the *leuce* of the Greeks described by him in his fifth book, he had no idea of elephantiasis being a skin disease at all; and so little did it resemble the leuce, or *bright white* leprosy, that of its pathognomonic signs he writes: "Summa pars corporis crebras maculas crebrosque tumores habet; ruborearum paulatim *in atrum colorem convertitur.*"

In Spain, elephantiasis is called *mal rojo*, from the

dark-red color of the skin: and in other countries it is named *mal mor*, clearly following the description of Celsus. After this it may well be asked, how can *mal rojo* or *mal nir* be identified with the bright white Bahereth of Moses, with the white scaly (λιπίς) λίπρα of the LXX. or with the disease of Gehazi, who "went out from Elisha's presence a leper (white as) snow?"

From all this it is urged that the leprosy of the Hebrews and that of the middle ages (Elephantiasis) were as dissimilar as atrophy and hypertrophy, and as black and white can be.

The confusion of writers accounts for the contrary opinion in great part: and the fact of the tubercular disease, by Dr. Mead believed to be the disease of Job, being anciently supposed to follow the cuticular, and both being endemic in the East, would further tend to confusion in the minds of readers and writers.

How far the idea of Galen—that they were kindred diseases—may be found true it is not easy to say; but, like most remarks of the ancient keen observers, there is probably much truth in it; and Dr. Carter's recent researches point in that direction. Although Lepra Hebræorum and Elephantiasis Græcorum were different. in their appearances, symptoms, and effects, yet if both be constitutional maladies, or the results of exposure to conditions unfavorable to health, there is nothing impossible or improbable in the opinion that elephantiasis may have found an easier victim in the Hebrew leper than in any one of sound constitution; for then, as now in Tangiers, both diseases existed side by side.

It is not within the scope of the question here discussed, to inquire into the alleged contagiousness of the Hebrew leprosy, or into its property of infecting clothes and houses. This part of the subject, and the other skin diseases of the Levitical Canon, are fully treated in the two papers of the Editor, already referred to; and the reader may consult with advantage the following authorities beside those already quoted: Dean Alford (of Canterbury)—*Greek Testament*—Note on S. Matthew viii; v. 1, 2, &c.; Archbishop Trench (of Dublin), *Notes on the Miracles*, p. 210; Robinson's *Biblical Researches in*

Palestine; the articles LEPROSY and MEDICINE, in Smith's
Dictionary of the Bible (1863); Shapter's *Medica Sacra*
(1834); and Bartholini (Thom) *De Morbis Biblicis Miscellanea.* This last curious treatise is to be found in Ugolini's *Thesaurus Antiquitatum Sacrarum* (Vol. XXX, p.
1521), published in folio, at Venice, in 1765; and classed
Fag. W, 1-30, in the library of T.C.D.

VERRUCA.

VERRUCÆ (*Warts*), both in consequence of their
appearance being familiar to all from their extreme
frequency, and of their unimportance, scarcely require
description; they consist in a hypertrophied condition of
a small patch of the papillæ of the skin, by which a
round tumor, with a flattened top, varying in size from
that of the head of a pin to that of a large pea, is formed.
They are of most frequent occurrence on the hands,
next on the face, and are rarely witnessed on those parts
of the body which are ordinarily covered. They are
generally placed singly on the integuments, but occasionally two or three originate close to each other, and
these sometimes coalesce. Warts appear in the early
periods of life, being seldom developed for the first time
in adults; they often disappear spontaneously, and even
suddenly, at the approach of puberty, but sometimes,
becoming indolent, are permanent.

Some persons are peculiarly liable to warts, and the
tendency to them seems to be hereditary; their immediate cause has not been satisfactorily ascertained; but
that it is more or less connected with local irritation,
and the effects of the atmosphere on the skin, is evident
from their being almost altogether confined to those
parts which are ordinarily exposed to the action of the
air. Small growths, soft to the touch and slightly pediculated, are of frequent occurrence on the face and neck,
particularly of females, and are also regarded as a variety
of wart; they appear to me to consist in the hypertrophy
of a single papilla, but Mr. Erasmus Wilson believes
them to be "the emptied tegumentary sacs of small
sebaceous tumors."

26*

Corns occasionally become the seat of active inflammation when irritated by any cause, or when they have been cut too freely, and afterwards subjected too soon to compression and friction by the shoes in walking; purulent matter then often forms beneath them, and, from its being firmly bound down by the hardened superincumbent tissues, extreme suffering results, followed sometimes by inflammation of the lymphatics and the formation of buboes in the groins; they have thus ended even fatally, from the occurrence of erysipelas, and in some instances from the supervention of tetanus.

Although, as above remarked, corns are almost invariably confined to the feet, they may also be developed on other parts of the body, but then they partake more of the nature of callosities; I have in a few cases seen them on the knuckles of the fingers in persons, too, in whom the hands were not exposed to any manual labor that could exert pressure on the parts affected.

The *treatment* of these morbid growths consists in their ablation, by means of the knife patiently and gradually employed, until all traces of hardened tissues are removed, and afterwards protecting the parts for some time from pressure; this is the only effectual remedy, and is the one always adopted by the self-styled chiropodists. The application of caustics never succeeds in destroying them completely, but is of use in enabling the hardened surface to be pared off without causing hemorrhage. Corns, whether hard or soft, may generally be kept in abeyance, as regards troublesome symptoms, by removing the superficial layers with the knife from time to time, according to the rapidity of their growth, or by rasping them with a file, the surface having been previously softened by maceration in warm water. Most of the corn plasters which are ordinarily sold in the shops contain carbonate of potash, the alkali of which dissolves partially the horny substance which constitutes the outer layer of the growth, or, a round hole being cut in the centre of each piece, they act by removing pressure from the most prominent point of the corn, which is directed to be pared previously to their application.

CALLOSITATES.

CALLOSITATES.—Callositas consists simply in thickening of the epidermis, which becomes of more or less hard consistence, produced by friction or continued pressure. They are usually witnessed on the palms of the hands or on the soles of the feet, when their cause is in general sufficiently evident. Occasionally they are attended with some degree of inflammation of the derma upon which they are developed, which may result in the formation of pus or in the effusion of a serous fluid beneath the hardened integument. They are witnessed also when thinned and enlarged mucae mucosae, especially on the membrane joint of the great toe, where they are most likely produced by pressure from the boot or shoe, and their presence tends to aggravate and increase the original disease.

Their treatment in the chronic stage should be the same as that for corns; but when inflammation is present, emollients and warm applications should be employed, and in all cases the exciting causes should of course be removed.

CONDYLOMATA.

CONDYLOMATA.—Generally the result of the syphilitic poison, but at times developed in persons in whom no such taint exists, these soft fleshy tumors appear on those parts of the integument where the skin and mucous membrane meet, at the verge of the anus, on the prepuce, at the vulva, and occasionally, though very rarely, on the lips and nostrils. They are of a soft consistence, and a reddish white color, varying in size from that of a pea to that of a marble, and have usually a broad base, with a flattened or rounded apex. They consist of numerous papillæ in a highly vascular condition, though apparently not much hypertrophied, and the epidermic covering is unchanged, except in being more vascular than in its healthy state. Various opinions have been propounded as to the nature of condylomata; Simon and Rokitansky regard them as being a new formation,

consisting chiefly of areolar tissue, while Lebert believes
that they are epidermio or epithelial growths.

Treatment.—They may be destroyed by the application of caustic, or strangulated with a ligature, which,
by means of a needle, may be passed through the centre
of the tumor, and then tied firmly at either side around
the base.

NÆVUS.

NÆVUS (*Mother mark*)—Plate XIV, Fig. 1.—Of the
several varieties of this adventitious production which
have been described, but one only can be regarded as
a disease of the skin, namely, that which consists in a
hypertrophied condition of the capillaries of a portion
of the cutaneous structure; the others, in which the
vascular system of the areolar tissue, and sometimes
even of deeper-seated parts, is engaged, are truly surgical
diseases, requiring usually surgical interference for their
removal, and are consequently treated of in all works on
surgery. All the forms are usually congenital, and are
popularly believed to be occasioned by the effect of the
mother's imagination upon the foetus in utero, an opinion
shared in by the profession even until modern times, and
not yet altogether exploded.

The illustration of Nævus which Dr. Neligan supplied
in Plate XIV of his Atlas, subsequently to the publication of the first edition of this work, may be here
remarked on. The subject, a boy, aged seven years, was
covered along the neck and back with long silky hair,
that along the spinous processes of the vertebræ being
arranged somewhat like the mane of a horse. The boy's
mother was the wife of a coachman, and when about six
months pregnant of this child—as she stated—the stables
took fire during the night, and she went to the assistance
of her husband, who was endeavoring to get the horses
out. In the midst of the smoke she had to hold one of
the horses around the neck for some time, and try to
restrain his violence. This alarmed her very much at
the time, but she soon thought no more of the occurrence
until the child was born as marked in the illustration.

The variety of nævus to be described here is char
terized by a permanent discoloration and slight elevati
of the part affected, on which the minute veins of 1
cutis appear dilated and slightly tortuous, becomi
gorged with blood from any exciting cause, and thus 1
color varies at different times, being dark red, or purpl
when the circulation is hurried or impeded.   They vi
in size, sometimes consisting of a small central poi
from which several minute vesicles ramify, a form term
nævus *araneus*—in other cases covering a patch of
surface from the size of a shilling to that of the palm
the hand, when they are usually irregularly circu
scribed, but often roundish.   They seldom enlarge mu
after birth; but, occasionally affecting the deeper vas
lar structures, they become converted into one of
other forms of the disease, which consist of erectile tiss
when they acquire a greater magnitude, and are
unfrequently attended with troublesome or even dang
ous symptoms.

Treatment.—If the nævus which engages the cutanee
capillaries be wounded, copious hemorrhage, often di
cult to check, ensues, but otherwise .they are of no
portance, except from the disfigurement which th
presence occasions, the more especially as they are usua
situated on the face.   On this account attempts have be
at times made to remove them by caustics and ot
means, but a greater deformity is thereby often oc
sioned; unless, therefore, they exhibit a tendency
spread much, or to be converted into one of the ot
forms of the disease, they should not be interfered w
Mr. Startin has cured them by subcutaneous ela
strangulation.   Elastic bands are sewed with a nee
beneath the skin in a triangular form, including
nævus.—*Med. Times and Gaz.*, 3d July, 1852.

Where the nævus is large, Mr. Spencer Wells ties
knot of a ligature over a piece of bougie, or other s
stance which can be twisted daily until the thread c
through the base of the tumor.—*Med. Times and Gaz.*,
Nov. 1854.

Mr. Hunt considers the nævus araneus to be cor

nal, and treats it successfully with arsenic. Dr. end, of Berlin, applies strong acetic acid, and then es compresses soaked in vinegar. Mr. Milton remarks *vaccination* succeeds in some cases by producing a cicatrix.

CHAPTER VIII.

HÆMORRHAGIÆ.

THE single disease which constitutes the order
ORRHAGIÆ might perhaps be more correctly regar
an affection of the system generally, but as its chief
acteristic phenomena become apparent to the eye th
the medium of the skin, custom has sanctioned its
described as a lesion of that structure.   In cuta
hemorrhages the blood does not escape from the s
of the body, but, being bound down by the epider
effused beneath it in variously sized and differently s
spots or patches.   At times, in certain diseases, espe
in fevers characterized by low vital power, of whic
constitutes one of the most important signs, the h
rhagic effusion is in the form of perfectly distinct n
dots, termed *Petechiæ*, from their resemblance to
bites.   In the division of Continued Fevers, now
rally recognized, into Typhus, Typhoid, and Relapse
we have the mulberry rash, a macula in Typhus; th
spots, or rash, in Typhoid; while the Relapsing
does not present any specific eruption.—See Murc
On Continued Fevers.   In other cases, occurring alo
complicating the diseases above noted, it appears in
ularly circumscribed patches, often of large exten
blood escaping chiefly into the subcutaneous a
tissue; these are denominated *Vibices* or *Ecchymos*
latter term being especially applied to them when
succeed a blow or injury.   And in a third form, v
constitutes *Purpura*, the only one here to engage ,
tion, the hemorrhage is in perfectly circular spots;
mingled with them, however, are usually several patc
vibices or ecchymoses.
    The very minute points of extravasated blood are e

stigmata; those next in size, *petechiœ;* those larger again, *vibices;* and the largest are denominated *ecchymoses,* or blotches.

PURPURA.—(See Plate XIII.)

PURPURA (*The Purples*) is characterized by the appear-ance on the integuments, generally over the whole body, of small, perfectly circular spots of the color of the blood, attended with more or less derangement of the vital func-tions. The spots vary in size from that of the head of a pin to that of a small pea; on their first appearance the color is bright red, but augmenting slightly in extent, still preserving their circular form, they gradually acquire a deep purple hue, which, as they fade away, passes through the various shades of greenish-yellow discolora-tion ordinarily presented by blood effused beneath the skin from a bruise. They are generally very numerous on the cutaneous surface, and often aggregated in masses on certain regions, yet perfectly distinct from each other, except in some parts which may be exposed to pressure, where, becoming confluent, they constitute vibices or ecchymoses. Each individual spot of purpura runs its course from its first appearance until it fades away in from five or six to ten or twelve days, a slight stain remaining for some time to mark its site; but the disease may last for many weeks, or even months, its duration depending upon the development of successive crops of the eruption, an occurrence which takes place in the mildest cases. The spots or patches are not in the least degree elevated above the cutaneous surface, their pre-sence being caused by an extravasation of blood into the derma or beneath the epidermis, from the capillaries of the skin.

The appearance of purpura is most usually preceded by slight febrile symptoms and general depression—hot skin, quick yet comprehensible pulse, thirst, anorexia, *malaise,* and headache; but in some cases no premonitory symptoms are noticed. The circular spots are, in the majority of instances present on the several mucous membranes of the body, and sometimes also on the

27

serous, at the same time that they exist on th
the blood being in them effused beneath their ep
covering, through which structure, so much mo
cate and fine than the epidermis, it commonly m:
way, and hemorrhage, often to a great extent
place, complicating the disease, and rendering i
more dangerous.

Several varieties of purpura have been descri
dermatologists, all of which may, I think, be conve
arranged in two divisions:—

Purpura simplex.
"   hæmorrhagica.

Purpura simplex (Plate XIII, Fig. 1).—The s
this form of the disease, which may be regarded a
chiefly characterized by its mildness, appear for tl
part on the extremities, and are developed very su(
often in the course of a single night, and usually v
any preceding or accompanying constitutional d
ance. Vibices or ecchymoses are seldom intern
with them, and they are generally much disperse
the surface, not aggregated in masses; successive
rarely, however, more than two or three, appear i
cases with an interval of from twenty-four to fort;
hours between each, and some spots then occur s
various regions of the body, the shoulders, the
the face, &c., but they are always most numerous
extremities. The disease runs its course in from
or eight days to a fortnight or three weeks, at t.
of which time the stains it occasions have totally
peared.

In some cases the extravasation of blood into the
or beneath the epidermis, instead of occurring in d
circular spots, without any elevation of the surface
place in raised wheals, resembling exactly in fot
eruption of urticaria, and accompanied often by m
less of a stinging and tingling sensation, in conse(
of which it has been termed purpura *urticans* (Plate
Fig. 2); the patches, owing to their extent, are of a (
·rple color than in the ordinary form of purpur;
) and their duration is for the same reason prol

to five or six weeks, although they are almost invariably developed in a single crop. Purpura urticans usually occurs on the lower extremities, and most frequently in persons laboring under some organic disease, and in those who have taken much mercury; it also appears at times in females when the menstrual function is deranged.

· Purpura simplex occurring in old persons, especially of the female sex, when it appears very much intermingled with large vibices and some ecchymoses, was described by Bateman as a distinct variety, under the name of purpura *senilis;* it is usually confined to the arms and legs, is developed in a single crop, unattended with any constitutional or local symptoms, and is an affection of but little disturbance, not impeding the usual avocations of life, and running its course in from a week to ten days or a fortnight.

When any of the varieties of simple purpura now described is accompanied by hemorrhage from the mucous membranes it then constitutes a form of the second division of the disease. Occasionally purpura simplex is attended with some trifling febrile symptoms, rarely exceeding slight heat of skin, thirst, and anorexia, yet by some writers it has then been described under the name purpura *febrilis simplex.* The duration of the simple form of the disease, as has been above remarked, seldom exceeds a few weeks, but cases occur in which successive crops are developed for from eighteen months to two years or upwards.

Purpura hæmorrhagica (Plate XIII, Fig. 3) is especially characterized by the escape of blood from some of the passages of the body which are lined with mucous membrane; occasionally it takes place from the serous membranes also, when hemorrhage into the shut sacs occurs. The spots on the integuments are usually much more numerous, and generally acquire a larger size than in the former variety, and vibices and ecchymoses are more frequent; they appear on every region of the body, being most generally witnessed first on the neck and shoulders, the face, and the upper extremities; they also occur on the conjunctiva, on the gums, the tongue, and the inside of the cheeks, and are found after death to be

as thickly dispersed over the mucous membrane of the
entire digestive track as on the external integument.

The disease is ushered in usually by much consti-
tional perturbation, the chief symptoms being that
general oppression; in from twenty-four to forty
hours the spots begin to appear on the cutaneous sur-
at first of a bright red color, but assuming a deep pu
hue in about twelve hours; they are very numerou
most cases, and are rapidly developed; whatever pa
of the body is exposed to pressure, there large hæmo
rhagic patches are developed beneath the epidermis;
if the surface is scratched or torn, copious bleeding t
place from them; in some cases the slightest pres
even that caused by feeling the pulse, will produce
ecchymosed spot.

Hemorrhage from the mucous membranes takes p
often from the very commencement of the disease; so
times it precedes the appearance of the spots of pur
on the integuments, but more frequently does not o
for several days after they are visible. Its most u
and most manageable form is that of epistaxis, but
bleeding is also very common from the lungs whe
constitutes hemoptysis, and from the stomach and bo
whence it is rejected by vomiting, or escapes by s
In some cases of purpura hæmorrhagica, the blood ex
from the gums in great quantity, apparently by a
of oozing, which it is almost impossible to check,
which not unfrequently proves fatal. The hemorrh
may take place also from the kidneys, the bladder,
urethra, the vagina, &c. The losses of blood are usu
very great, and recurring constantly produce extr
depression and prostration, with a marked pallor
anæmic condition of the entire surface of the body,
throws out into marked relief the purple spots and st
which are thickly scattered over it.

The duration of this form of purpura is very varia
the local hemorrhages may be checked in seven or n
days, but they are very apt to recur, and thus the dis
is often prolonged for several months, the cutaneous sp
and patches continuing to be developed in constant, s
cessive crops. When it has lasted for any time, the v

powers become extremely depressed, dropsical effusion takes place into the lower extremities, and uncontrollable bloody diarrhœa not unfrequently sets in.

When the constitutional symptoms attendant on purpura hæmorrhagica assume a more febrile character than has been above described—a general redness of the surface, with burning heat, preceding the appearance of the purple spots—the disease has been specially noticed under the denomination of purpura *febrilis hæmorrhagica*. This variety is chiefly remarkable from its not unfrequently appearing as an epidemic, especially where many persons are crowded together, as in gaols, poorhouses, &c.

In many cases of purpura the cutaneous phenomena are so trifling as to be scarcely noticeable, while the hemorrhages from the mucous surfaces are excessive; these constitute, in my experience, the most dangerous and uncontrollable cases, and death often occurs in them from extravasation of blood into some of the serous cavities. Dr. Graves describes a form of the disease resembling this, in which, however, there was an exanthematous rash on the skin, resembling the red efflorescence so often seen in maculated typhus fever; in consequence of its presence he proposed to term the affection *Exanthema hæmorrhagicum.*[1]

In the earlier editions of his large work, although not specially noticed in his latest production—*The Student's Book*—Mr. Erasmus Wilson describes as a form of purpura, under the designation purpura *cachectica*, the occurrence of petechiæ and ecchymoses on the skin, "as the consequence of a reduced and debilitated state of the system, from whatever cause the latter may arise." We frequently see instances of this kind during the latter stages of various diseases, as of dropsies, or whenever the venous circulation is obstructed. The purpura *contagiosa* of Bateman corresponds with the petechial-eruption of typhus fever.

Purpura may occur at any age, but is very rarely witnessed in infants or very young children; it affects both

[1] *Clinical Lectures on the Practice of Medicine,* Second Edition, Vol. ii. p. 362; and reprint from Second Edition (1864), p. 715.

pin. The *proximate cause* of purpura is manifestly
ly in the capillary system of bloodvessels, combined
h an abnormal fluidity of the blood.

Diagnosis.—This disease is so well marked by the visible phenomena that it can scarcely be confounded with
any other; but it is necessary to distinguish the occurrence
purpura in the course of fever, or as a complication of
any other affection, from its existence as an individual
disease. The diagnosis between it and *scurvy*, or scorbutus, is unattended with difficulty—the characteristic
condition of the gums, the extensive brown and purple
discoloration of the integuments, and the absence of the
round purpuric stains in the latter, are sufficiently distinctive marks. The spots of purpura are distinguished
from flea-bites, with which a careless observer might con-
found them, by the presence of a central punctum in the
latter, and their almost total disappearance on firm pressure being made with the finger, the marks of purpura
being thereby unaffected.

Prognosis.—Even cases of purpura that, in their commencement, do not present symptoms of severity, are not
altogether free from danger, for the simple form of the
disease not unfrequently becomes converted into the
hemorrhagic, and whenever bleeding from the mucous
surfaces takes place in this affection the prognosis must
be cautious. When death occurs it is either directly or
indirectly consequent on the loss of blood: in the former
case it may be sudden, as when apoplexy results from
hemorrhage into the substance of the brain, or from its
membranes, and in the latter it is generally less immediate, the patient dying with the symptoms usually
caused by repeated losses of blood. The hemorrhage
being profuse, or continuing unchecked by treatment, is
always an unfavorable sign; and until it ceases completely, and fresh spots no longer appear on the cutaneous or mucous surfaces, the patient cannot be regarded
as safe. Bleeding from the gums, particularly when at
all excessive, is, in my experience, one of the gravest
symptoms of the disease, even although there may be
but little eruption on the integuments; I have rarely

l extent, in the very commencement of the dis-
at once stop its progress;[1] these are cases of pur-
plex, affecting plethoric young persons of a
)us temperament; but the bleeding should
; used with caution, and is rarely, if ever, admis-
n hemorrhage occurs spontaneously, to any ex-
ι the mucous membranes. In that form of the
·hich has been described as appearing on the
:tremities of old persons, whatever tends to
n the constitution generally should not be
n the treatment; but if preparations of bark, or
ics, be administered too freely, and without the
:ous employment of remedies calculated to re-
hemorrhagic tendency, the symptoms are often
aggravated, purpuric spots are developed over
generally, and bleeding takes place from the
:avities, the simple form of the disease being
l into the hemorrhagic.

years since I published an essay[2] on the treat-
)urpura by *large* doses of oil of turpentine, and
l the efficacy of this remedy, when thus admin-
y a report of several cases in which it proved
7 successful. Since then I have continued to em-
)th in the simple and hemorrhagic forms of the
nd my additional experience is fully confirma-
ιe views then propounded. It must be given in
iciently large to act as a purgative—from one to
es, according to the age and strength of the pa-
adults, and a proportionate dose for children;
its purgative action I was at first in the habit
· it in combination with castor oil, but this, so
being necessary, interferes, I think, more or less
special effect of the turpentine, and therefore I
:ribe it combined simply with mucilage, as in
7ing form :—

t here entering on the *vexata quæstio* as to the change of
)ase, the Editor cannot concur in the above advice. He
lieve that bleeding can stop the progress of the disease.
Journal of Medical Science, First Series, vol. xxviii. p. 189.

℞. Olei Terebinthinæ, . . unciam.
Mucilaginis Acaciæ, . . unciam.
Aquæ Menthæ Piperitæ, . unciam cum semissé.
Misce. Fiat haustus.

This draught may be taken once or twice daily, accor
to the degree of its action on the bowels; and sh
there be much hemorrhage from the intestinal can
the stomach reject the draught, the same or a larger q
tity of the oil of turpentine, suspended by means of
of egg in decoction of barley, may be administered
enema. The beneficial action of the turpentine in
disease is twofold : first, it is a diffusible stimulan
styptic, which, when conveyed into the circulation thr
the digestive organs, is exhaled from the system by n
chiefly of the mucous surfaces, as is manifested b
odor of the breath, and of the various secretions an
cretions; it is thus consequently brought directly
contact with the capillary circulation, from which in
disease the hemorrhage takes place; and, second, the
employment of purgatives in the treatment of pu
having been long since proved to be attended with
successful results, the administration of oil of turpe
to fulfil this indication is especially serviceable in c
quence of its not being a debilitant.

In cases in which from any cause—excessive de
or tendency to diarrhœa, &c.—purgatives are co
indicated, the turpentine may be given in smaller
and repeated at shorter intervals; thus from twer
thirty minims to a drachm may be prescribed every
or fourth hour, or three times a day, according t
amount of hemorrhage which accompanies the di
Should there be extreme debility present, preparati
iron—those which are astringent being preferre
other tonics, may be administered conjointly wit
turpentine; but, on the other hand, when there is
vascular excitement or general plethora, bleedin
other evacuants should be had recourse to at the
time that it is prescribed.

The employment of numerous other astringent
styptics has been recommended for the treatment of
pura; in cases attended with much hemorrhage fro

stomach and intestines, or from the lungs, acetate of lead combined with opium often proves useful; the combination may be given in a pill—two grains of the former with a fourth of a grain of the latter every fourth or sixth hour. But of all this class of medicines which have been used not one has proved so beneficial as gallic acid; it is especially of service in cases attended with profuse bleeding from the mucous surfaces, and may then be given in alternate doses with the oil of turpentine. Thus, a pill containing five grains of gallic acid made with sufficient mucilage or conserve of roses, should be administered every fourth hour, the turpentine draughts being given two hours before and after each pill.

When excessive hemorrhage takes place from the mucous membrane of the gums and the inside of the mouth, it is, as before remarked, a most dangerous symptom, and the bleeding is extremely difficult to check—the most active styptics applied directly often failing to diminish it in the slightest degree. I have in such cases tried, unavailingly, nitrate of silver, saturated solutions of alum, of sulphate of iron, of gallic acid, &c., Ruspini's styptic, nitric acid, and even the actual cautery; pieces of lint dipped in oil of turpentine seem to have the most effect, but the general treatment above recommended can alone be then relied on.

Sponging the surface of the body repeatedly during the day with cooling lotions—such as equal parts of vinegar and water, with the addition of a sixth part of rectified spirit, should there be much febrile heat—is an adjunct, too often neglected, of much value in the treatment of purpura. Acidulated drinks—lemonade, raspberry vinegar and water—should be always freely allowed, and the diet, though rather small as regards quantity, ought to be nutritious and tonic, but easy of digestion, consisting chiefly of milk, farinaceous food, and strong beef-tea; all food and drink being taken rather cold than warm.

Scorbutus.—A passing reference has been already made to *scorbutus*, or sea scurvy; chiefly with the view of showing that it should not be confounded with purpura. Though popularly spoken of as a skin disease, it is not properly so, and therefore the reader must refer to works on general medicine for an account of it. It may, however, be here stated, that in one of the most elaborate and scholarly papers ever written on a hotly controverted question, the late Professor Osborne of this city (in the *Dub. Qu. Journ.* May, 1855) demonstrated the plague at Athens, as described by Thucydides, to have been none other than scorbutus or sea scurvy. Lucretius (*De Nat. Rer. VI., 1104*) described this plague by the name of "Sacer ignis," and Eusebius, the Ecclesiastical historian, gave the same name to the plague which raged in Syria A. D. 302.

CHAPTER IX.

MACULÆ.

THE group of cutaneous affections classed in the order MACULÆ (spots) is characterized by a morbid condition of the color of the skin, dependent on some deranged state of the secretion of the pigment cells of the derma. The change may consist in either an augmentation or a diminution of the natural color, or it may be altered in hue or totally absent; in some instances it affects the entire surface of the body, but more usually occurs in spots or patches that vary much in shape and in extent; in either case there is no sensible elevation or depression of the surface. The several affections belonging to the order may be congenital, or they may be developed at any period of life; in the former case they usually consist in the total absence of coloring matter, constituting what has been denominated *Albinoismus*—individuals being born so termed *Albinoes*—or there may be only a deficiency of coloring matter in large patches, a condition which is rare, but most frequently witnessed in children of negroes, who are thus piebald at birth. In certain diseases, as in jaundice, in chlorosis, in malignant and in most chronic affections, a peculiar alteration in color of the integumentary membrane takes place, which is regarded usually as one of the most important signs of the special diathesis or constitutional derangement which characterizes or accompanies the disease; but it is readily recognizable and cannot be confounded with the pigmentary alterations of the cutaneous structure here to be considered, which do not influence in any way the general health, and are therefore to be regarded solely in consequence of the disfigurement which they occasion, in many instances a cause of greater annoyance than a real disease.

28

... apparently described in
... Achroma: and
... literature of the

... — See Plate ... Fig. 4

... a deficiency or total
... matter in the skin, in
... with ... and sometimes
... this is adopted by Willan
... have been derived from the
... the arrangements thus affected bear
... being sanctioned by
... have been unwilling
... in importance more strictly
... with ... is employed by many modern
... it must be borne in mind, however, that
... vas not the disease here under
... As already remarked in Chapter VII, his
... with the Greek ..., and it will be
... that in the present work, the latter term is
... to be synonymous with Psoriasis.—See Chap.
... may be limited to certain regions
... of the body, occurring in patches, or may be general
... the absence of pigment is witnessed in the hair,
... &c. In the former case, the peculiar condition
... of the skin is often congenital, but it may be developed
at any period of life: it constitutes the *Achroma vitiligo*
of Alibert; the latter, the *Achroma congenitale* of the
same author is always congenital; it is denominated, as
before remarked, *Albinoïsmus.*—Plate XIII, Fig. 5. Albinoïsmus cannot be regarded as a disease, and therefore,
not coming within the scope of this Work, need not be
described here; it, moreover, is not within the sphere of
medical art, being altogether an unalterable, and consequently an incurable, affection.

What then may be termed *true* vitiligo, when not congenital, is developed in the form of rounded spots or
patches, few or many, on some special region of the body,

or on several parts at the same time; the spots are at first usually small, not more than a few lines in diameter, and nearly circular, but they gradually augment in size—often acquiring the magnitude of the palm of the hand, and become irregular in shape. It appears most frequently on the chest, the back, the scalp, and about the genital organs, but it may occur on any part of the integuments. The portions of skin affected present simply a white aspect, in some cases dull, in others bright and glistening, without any sensible elevation or depression of the surface; if hairs grow naturally on the part they also become perfectly white, no matter of what color they may have been previously, and not unfrequently fall out after a short time, leaving a bald, colorless patch. When the hairy scalp is thus affected attention is at first usually attracted to it by a single lock of the hair, generally on the back part of the head or temples, turning white; this gradually becomes larger, and at length the hairs, which have lost their color, fall out, and one of the forms of *alopecia*, or what has been termed a variety of *porrigo decalvans*, is thus constituted.

The *causes* of this singular affection of the skin are perfectly unknown: it occurs at all ages, and is most frequent in the prime of life, especially when it appears on the head, but it is developed on the genital region usually in old persons; it is witnessed, too, in individuals of all temperaments, yet I think it is more common on the scalp of those who have dark than of those who have light hair; it is also, in my experience, more usual on the head in females, and on other parts of the body in males. Congenital vitiligo is rare in the white races, occurring with a much greater degree of frequency in negroes, infants at birth sometimes presenting a completely pied appearance.

The *diagnosis* of vitiligo is unattended with difficulty; the longitudinal white furrows on the abdomen of females who have borne children or of those who have had ascites, and on the breasts of nurses, might, by a superficial observer, be confounded with it, but their site and the history of the individual case are in all cases sufficient to prevent such a mistake. A form of lupus, to be herein the proportion of a drachm to the ounce of white wax (simple) ointment, rubbed in twice daily. Sulphuret of potassium and other preparations of sulphur, in the form of lotion or ointment, employed locally, sometimes succeed when other remedies fail; but next to tannic acid I have found oil of turpentine prove most useful as a local application: a pomade may be prepared with it as follows:—

℞. Olei Terebinthinæ, ... drachmas duas.
  Sevi Præparati, ... uncias duas.
  Balsami Tolutani, ... drachmas duas.
Simul liquefac lento igne, dein adde,
  Olei Rosmarini, ... minima viginti.
  Olei Amygdalæ Amaræ, . . minima quinque.

A small portion of this pomade should be rubbed into the affected spots, twice or three times a day, with a piece of flannel, the part having been previously well washed with an alkaline wash—a drachm of carbonate of potash to eight ounces of distilled water.

EPHELIS (*Melasma* of Plenck).

EPHELIS.—This term, as its derivation (ἐπί, upon, and ἥλιος, the sun) indicates, was originally employed to designate all discolorations of the skin caused by the direct action of the solar rays, but latterly it has acquired a more extended signification, and may, I think, now be understood to include all those affections in which the natural pigment-hue of the skin is augmented or altered. Some of these changes being congenital and unalterable, need not be described here, while others are due and can often be traced to specific causes. Ephelis may be conveniently considered as consisting of three varieties:—

Ephelis lenticularis,
" hepatica,
" violacea;

to which, perhaps, should be added a fourth, known of late as *Morbus Addisonii*, or Melasma Supra-renale, or Ephelis Melaina.

Ephelis lenticularis (*Freckles*).—This discoloration of

28*

the skin is too well known to need description; in many persons the buff-colored or reddish-yellow spots which constitute it are congenital, when they are beyond the reach of medical art; but in others they are developed on those regions of the body which are uncovered, by exposure to the weather, but especially to the direct action of the sun's rays. They are seldom witnessed except in those who have a very fine and fair skin, and are of the sanguine temperament. Appearing usually for these reasons, on the skin of young persons of the female sex and on those parts of the surface which are most exposed to observation, freckles cause very serious annoyance and a host of applications have been employed for their removal, which is often a matter of some difficulty; persons who are liable to them should therefore protect themselves as much as possible from the causes by which they are produced. The various empirical lotions which are sold for the removal of these spots are composed chiefly of corrosive sublimate, or of the solution of the subacetate of lead in bitter almond emulsion, in the proportio of a fourth of a grain of the former, or six minims of the latter, to each ounce of either of them; they are often very useful. Mr. Erasmus Wilson recommends the application of a liniment "composed of equal parts of lime-water and olive oil," to which, if the heat of the surface is considerable, he adds "liquor plumbi in the proportion of twenty minims to the ounce." I have found the following lotion of much service:—

R. Liquoris Sodæ Chloratæ, . drachmas duas.
Aquæ Sambuci, ... uncias septem.
Aquæ Lauro-Cerasi, . . drachmas sex. Misce.

And the application at night of a pomade, consisting equal parts of cold cream and cucumber cerate, to every ounce of which half a drachm of the solution of chlorinated soda is added.

Ephelis hepatica (Melasma figuratum of Wilson) is characterized by the appearance of one or more patches, tolerable extent, on some portion of the cutaneous surface; they are of a dull yellow or buff color, occasiona of a bronze hue; at first distinct from each other, wh

more than one occurs, they grad... ...
escing often acquire a consi... ...
cases the neck, the face. the ... ...
the hands, being the part... ... ...
brown color. On the first... ...
are not unfrequently att... ...
tingling, and a fine mealy ... ...
scratching or rubbing ... ...
is no sensible elevati... ...
affected. The colorati... ...
through all the shades of ... ...
often evidently depend... ...
vidual: at times, when ... ...
is so remarkable that ... ...
appear as if they were ... ...
    Ephelis hepat... ...
cases lasting for many ... ...
is occasionally ... ...
disappearing ... ...
In the latter ... ...
rally appear ... ...
menstrual ... ...
It is a more ... ...
female than ... ...
attendant ... ...
menses ... ...
prime of life ... ...
In ch... ...
hepatic ... ...
... ...
... ...
... ...
... ...
... ...
... ...
... ...
Purp... ...
... ...
... ...
... ...
... ...

Diagnosis.—This affection is often confounded with a form of pityriasis, and, as already remarked, when describing that disease, Rayer and Wilson consider pityriasis versicolor, and pityriasis nigra, as being nothing more than discolorations of the skin, and therefore to be classed with ephelis: my reasons for differing with them have been there given.—See Chap. VI. The stains of ephelis hepatica may be confounded with those which are symptomatic of a syphilitic taint in the system, from which they are chiefly to be diagnosed by the history of each case, and the concomitant symptoms.

In the *treatment* of this affection it is requisite, in the first place, to direct attention to the general especially the state of the digestive organs, with a deranged condition of which their presence is often associated, and to use remedies calculated to restore to them, if requisite, a healthy tone; in females, moreover, should there exist any irregularity of the menstrual function, appropriate means to correct it must be employed; but when the patches are developed in the course of pregnancy, no treatment ought to be had recourse to, for they usually disappear after delivery. The local applications that prove most successful are those which have been recommended for the last described variety of ephelis; when, however, the discoloration of the surface is very extensive, hot baths containing the sulphuret of potassium, or of the natural sulphurous waters, will be found of service: these mineral waters also should be used internally, and if drunk at their sources so much the better. When a single large patch of ephelis hepatica becomes chronic, repeated blisters applied over it will sometimes remove the discoloration of the part.

Ephelis violacea.—When the internal administration of the nitrate of silver has been continued for a lengthened period, without prolonged intermissions, the derma becomes chemically stained with it, and the entire surface of the body then presents a slate-colored, bluish-gray or leaden hue, causing a frightful disfiguration, more especially as the face and those parts constantly exposed to the light are most deeply tinged. This discoloration is much less frequently witnessed now than it was some years since, when this medicine was so universally employed for the treatment of epilepsy and other nervous and convulsive diseases. The most certain way to prevent this result—one of so grave a character as almost to counterbalance any good effects which might be derived from the administration of nitrate of silver as a medicine—is not to continue its use for a longer period than six weeks or two months; and should it be thought proper to resume its employment again, to permit at least a month to elapse before doing so.

Treatment.—This discoloration when once produced is permanent, and becomes even deeper with time; nor have any means hitherto tried for its removal had the slightest effect on it. The iodide of potassium, when applied to the skin, even some days after it may have been stained by the direct application of the nitrate of silver, effectually removes the discoloration; its use in various ways has therefore been proposed for the general staining of the cutaneous surface above described. Professor Melsens, of Brussels, has given it in enormous doses, half a drachm, or even more, three times daily, exposing the patient at the same time to a hot vapor bath: the iodine is thus brought to the surface, when it may be readily detected in the perspiration by the ordinary tests. He continues this plan of treatment for months; but in one case that I am cognizant of, which was treated by himself, the discoloration was not in the slightest degree removed. This, I think, was to be anticipated, for it is as iodine, and not as iodide of potassium that the preparation is given off by the skin after its use has been continued for some time; I would, therefore, suggest that the patient, while under the influence of the remedy, should be placed, during half an hour or an hour, in a warm bath containing carbonate of potash in solution, instead of employing the hot vapor bath, as thus the iodide of potassium might be brought into direct contact with the derma.

Mr. Wilson, and others, have noticed a blue tint of the skin, and have called it *Cyanopathia:* That it exists at all as a special affection is doubted by many; the alleged cases of it are very rare, and Dr. Fox very graphically

"3. La coloration bronzée doît être considérée coi
un épiphénomene ; elle est indépendante de l'état
capsules surrénales.

"4. La maladie d'Addison peut-être considérée coi
une névrose ayant son siége dans la grand sympatheti
névrose soit primitive, soit symptomatique.

"5. L'altération des capsules surrénales dans (
maladie peut, á l'example de ce qui a été fait
l'abuminurie, le goître exophthalmique, être consid
comme secondaire.

"6. Les capsules surrénales ne me paraissent
nécessaires à la vie."

As it is obvious that the discussion of this intere;
malady belongs rather to general medicine than t
special subject of this work, the Editor can only
to some books and papers in which more com
information may be found. Besides those already n
the reader may consult Dr. Greenhow's remarks ir
Lancet for April 1, 15, and 22, 1865; Report of a
at the Radcliffe Infirmary, Oxford, in the Lance
'18th February, 1865; Dr. Wilkes, in Guy's Ho;
Reports, Third Series, Vol. VIII; Drs. Cotton
Harley, in Med. Times, 1857; Dr. Parkes, in Med. 7
1858; Dr. Barton, in Dub. Hosp. Gaz., 1859; Dr.
rison, in Brit. Med. Jour., 1861; Dr. Fricke, in Brit
For. Med.-Chir. Rev., 1857; Jaccoud's French editi(

29

CHAPTER X.

CANCROÏDES.

ᴛʜᴇ order CANCROÏDES (from καρκίνος cancer, and like) includes two diseases of the skin, which ₑₛₛ a certain degree of malignancy, inferior to that ᵤe cancerous affections, yet in many of their fea-ₜ bearing much resemblance to them, especially in ₷ usually characterized by a slow and insidious ₐtive process, often attended with severe stinging , and by a marked tendency to return in the same ᵢ some other part of the skin, after they have been rently cured, or even after the diseased portion of nteguₘent has been excised. These diseases are, by , dermatologists, classed among the Tubercula of ₐn, but for the reasons already stated in the intro-ₒry remarks to the seventh chapter, I have omitted order altogether; and even if it were to be retained, ₐffections now to be described could not, with any ₙsion to accuracy, be included in it. The term ₜroïdes, a more correct term than Cancrodes, which Neligan adopted from Copland's Classification of ₐses of the Skin,[1] expresses well their peculiar ₗres above referred to, and is at the same time ₚiently distinctive for all purposes of arrangement. two diseases to be described in the order are: Lupus, ₗis.

LUPUS.

ₗpus (the Wolf); Dartre Rougeante of the French; ₷ende Flechte of the Germans.—See Plate XIV. ₗPUS (*Eating letter*) appears on the skin usually of

[1] *Dictionary of Practical Medicine*, Vol. iii p. 799.

the face, but often on the scalp in various forms: it is generally developed as an inflammatory affection with more or less hypertrophy of the integuments attacked, and terminating in ulceration, which may be either superficial or deep-seated, but is always painful, slow, and insidious, and especially characterized by a destructive tendency, whence the name Lupus, "*a wolf*," was originally applied to the disease. The ulcerative process may be confined to the epidermis and the superficial layers of the derma, may extend quite through the cutaneous integument, or may even affect the deeper-seated parts, destroying areolar tissues, muscles, cartilages, and even osteum, laying bones bare, and thereby causing caries of them. The disease is thus naturally divided into three forms, but in general two only are described by writers on the subject as affections: the one, in which the ulcerative process attacks the deeper-seated tissues being termed lupus edens, and the other, which affects mere superficial structures only being for contrast denominated lupus *non-edens*. Here, however, a similar form of ulceration, differing in degree, occurs—and this division is, therefore, not strictly accurate. I shall describe the three forms, the leading features of which have been noticed under the following specific denominations:—

Lupus superficialis.
" serpiginosus.
" devorans.

Lupus superficialis (Plate XIV. Fig. 2) commences by the development of a slight thickening or elevation of the skin, not larger than a small pea, usually on the most prominent part of any direct: it presents a somewhat indurated appearance, is soft to the touch, rather painful if pressed hard, and is of a very indolent nature. A thin, hard, brown-red scab appears on its surface after some weeks, or even for months, but is seemingly not preceded by any ulceration, when the scab is picked off with the nails, as it almost invariably is by the individual himself, the part on which it rested is seen to be superficially ulcerated, with thickened and slightly elevated edges: it is soon reproduced, a little more consistent than before, but still of small extent, and increases very slowly in size, even when irritated by the use of stimulant applications or by other local causes. Generally, after several months, the dry crust or scab falls off that part of the integument on which it first appeared, while it is spreading slowly to the neighboring surface. The portion of the skin on which it had existed is white and seamed, resembling much the condition which results from destruction of the superficial layers of the cutaneous structure by a burn. With slow but steady progress the disease advances over the cheek, usually in one direction only, leaving its trace behind in the white seaming of the skin; at times it becomes the seat of active inflammation, generally from being rubbed or torn with the nails, when a small, painful ulcer results; but the local symptoms are never very severe, the chief annoyance it causes being due to the unsightly deformity which it occasions on the face. The progress of this form of lupus is so slow that the resulting superficial cicatrix above described, which is somewhat circular, does not attain a larger size than that of a shilling in from two to three years after the first appearance of the disease—at least such was the case in two persons affected with it whom I have had under my care.

Lupus superficialis, as here described, is a rare affection, and has escaped the notice of many writers on diseases of the skin; Dr. Copland gives the best account of it that I have met with, under the appellation of Lupus *superficialis non-tuberculosus*.[1] Its duration may be almost indefinitely prolonged; when it terminates in cure the scab falls off, and is not succeeded by another, but the mark on the cutaneous surface is indelible.

Lupus serpiginosus (Plate XIV, Fig. 3).—This variety of the disease—well named by Alibert, *Esthiomenos* (from ἐσθίω, " I eat") *ambulans vel serpiginosus*—is well marked by highly characteristic phenomena, which distinguish it from either of the other forms of lupus; but it must be noticed that the specific name "superficialis" has been applied to it by some dermatologists who do not appear

---

[1] *Dictionary of Practical Medicine*, vol. iii. p. 790.

...in the manner above described ... matrix or pit ... disease continues to ... —whence the ... irregular ... cases reattacks ... and they again may thus ... or even oftener, the seat ... as at the first, but each time the surface heals the resulting cicatrix is deeper and more uneven. It not uncommonly occurs that two or more patches of the lupoid ulceration coalesce in consequence of the disease spreading from the circum-

ference of each, and an extended portion of the integuments may thereby be affected.

Lupus serpiginosus occurs, as already remarked, with
greatest frequency on the face and scalp, often extending,
too, from one to the other, and being confined to them,
but it is also witnessed on both the upper and lower extremities, and occasionally on the trunk of the body; it
is usually attended with more or less local pain in all its
stages, which is much aggravated at times by attacks of
acute inflammation when it spreads more rapidly; but
the constitution very rarely participates, those affected
with the disease being often apparently in excellent health,
even although it may have lasted for years. It is always
of a chronic nature, and its duration is extremely prolonged. When it terminates in cure the intra-dermoid
ulceration ceases to spread; healthy granulations, at times
rather exuberant, form on the surface, and cicatrization
of the affected part takes place; the annular edges being
elevated over the healthy skin, and of course much more
over the cicatrized portion, and being of a bright-red
color, which they retain for a long time, contrast remarkably with the shining white aspect of the latter; much
disfigurement consequently results.

Lupus devorans (noli me tangere), Plate XIV, Fig. 4.—
This variety of the disease commences in various ways;
but no matter what appearance it may present at first, is
in its progress characterized by destructive ulceration of
the various structures situated beneath the skin—areolar
and adipose tissues, muscles, tendons, cartilages, and
periosteum being equally destroyed; the bones even do
not escape, for where they are laid bare caries attacks
them. It may be developed, like the last-described form,
by the appearance of one or more rounded, dusky-red
elevations of the integument—tubercles—on the alæ nasi,
on the cheeks, or on the roof of the mouth, which, however, run a somewhat more rapid course than in lupus
serpiginosus, are the seat of more active inflammation,
and are attended with a more destructive ulcerative process, which extends to the deeper-seated structures. In
other cases one of the alæ of the nostrils becomes slightly
swollen, painful to the touch, and of a violet-red color;

being attended with itching, it is soon scratched with the
nails, a brownish crust or hard scab results, which is
surrounded by an inflammatory œdematous base, and,
purulent matter forming beneath it, ulceration of the
destructive character peculiar to the disease commences.
In a third class of cases the tip of the nose swells, and
presents a dead-white color; gradually but slowly enlarging, a black crust forms at the very apex, the mucous
membrane of the nostrils becomes thickened, chiefly from
effusion into the areolar tissue beneath it, and at length
ulceration takes place. And, lastly, the thickening and
subsequent ulceration first appears in the soft palate or
posterior nares, and, proceeding from within outwards,
eventually attacks the septum naris and the other cartilages of the nose.

In whichever way the disease may commence, the
resulting ulceration presents much the same character,
its tendency is to spread from the surface inwards, not
unfrequently undermining in its progress the healthy
integuments before it attacks them, and being attended
with a foul, unhealthy, purulent, often ichorous, discharge.
The parts first affected usually cicatrize in the course of
the disease, when the cicatrices present a similar appearance to what is witnessed in lupus serpiginosus, but indicate a greater loss of substance beneath. This is especially remarkable on the nose, the most usual seat of this
variety of lupus, this feature assuming then a peculiar
pinched appearance, from a deficiency of some of its
natural proportions. The amount of destruction caused
by the ulcerative process varies much in different cases
—in some removing only a small portion of the cartilages
of the alæ nasi, while in others the entire soft part of the
nose, the alæ and septum naris, and the soft palate are
destroyed, frightful deformity being thereby occasioned.
As in the other forms of lupus, parts that have been cicatrized not unfrequently again become the seat of fresh
ulceration, which runs a similar course to what it did at
first, being then, however, more difficult to check.

Lupus devorans most generally runs a very chronic
course, its progress being slow, years often elapsing
before it causes much destruction of the part it appears

on; but cases occur, happily very rarely, in which it destroys with extreme rapidity those portions of the integuments and of the neighboring structure it attacks; thus, in from a month to six weeks the entire of the nose may be eaten away: this variety of the disease has been appropriately enough termed lupus *vorax*.

In some cases lupus devorans attacks the lower eyelid first, commencing by the development of a single rounded elevation of the skin, of a livid aspect; its progress is extremely slow, but in the course of years it eats away all the structures around the eyeball, laying the orbit almost completely bare, but sparing the eye itself, which appears just as if it had been dissected out by the ulceration. This variety of the disease was first accurately described by Professor Jacob, who, however, regarded it as a malignant ulcer, and not as a form of lupus, and it has been ever since known to the profession in this country by the name of "Jacob's ulcer."—Plate XIV, Fig. 5. Rayer, who also gives an accurate account of it, believed it to be lupus, and with him my experience, derived from the prolonged observation of several cases, compels me to agree. The following graphic account of this lupoid ulceration is given by Professor Jacob:[1]— "The edges are elevated, smooth, and glossy, with a serpentine outline, and are occasionally formed into a range of small tubercles or elevations; the skin in the vicinity is not thickened or discolored. The part within the edges is in some places a perfectly smooth, vascular, secreting surface, having veins of considerable size ramifying over it, which veins occasionally give way, causing slight hemorrhage; in other places the surface appears covered by florid, healthy-looking granulations, firm in texture, and remaining unchanged in size and form for a great length of time. The surface sometimes heals over in patches, which are hard, smooth, and marked with venous ramifications. . . . The discharge from the surface is not of the description called by surgeons unhealthy or sanious, but yellow and of proper consistence; neither is there more fetor than from the healthiest sore,

---

[1] *Dublin Hospital Reports*, Vol. iv. p. 232.

if the parts be kept clean, and be dressed frequ
It is surprising how little suffering, either local c
stitutional, attends this frightful affection, the du
of which may extend to an advanced old age.

Lupus in all'its forms is a disease of youth and
prime of life, being rare before the age of ten, ane
seldom developed for the first time in old age.
regards its *causes*, there is abundant evidence to sho
it is intimately connected with the scrofulous diat
especially when it is hereditary; and many cases
to prove that a constitutional syphilitic taint also
frequent predisposing cause of it. In the major
instances it appears at or soon after puberty, withor
manifest exciting cause, but sometimes it follows
jury or other local irritant. It is, on the whole, :
a rare disease, and is perhaps somewhat more fre
in females than in males.

Diagnosis.—The differential diagnosis of the v
forms of lupus now described is unattended with diffi
but some of them may be mistaken for other dise
the skin. Lupus superficialis is of such very rare
rence that it is not often recognized when met wit
its phenomena are highly characteristic, and it is
portance, with reference both to prognosis and treat
that it should be diagnosed; *the peculiar cicatrizat
seaming of the surface over which it has passed* is its es
mark; a similar result is not met with in any other
neous affection. Lupus serpiginosus may be confor
with impetigo, from which it is distinguished by tl
structive ulceration which attends it, by its spreadi
rings and undermining the integuments as it *cree
wards; pseudo-pustules are constantly developed on
parts of the skin which it attacks, but they differ
the pustules of impetigo in being flattened, more c
uncircumscribed, and presenting from the first a
paratively large quantity of purulent matter, with a
thin covering. This variety of lupus is in gener
scribed by dermatologists as being with difficulty
nosed from scrofulous ulceration of the integuments
this is a matter of little import, for it rarely occur
cept in persons of a well-marked scrofulous diathesi

by many it is termed *Esthiomanic scrofula.* A somewhat similar form of ulceration constitutes at times one of the phenomena of secondary syphilis, but it is not of the same indolent and destructive character, is attended with other symptoms which mark the presence of this poison in the system, and is always more or less amenable to specific treatment. Lupus devorans may, in its early stages, be mistaken for acne indurata, but the distinctive signs have been already pointed out in the description of that disease (see page 174). From the syphilitic affections which occur on the face it is distinguished by its malignancy, by its slow progress, and by its not directly implicating the bony structures; but in many cases the diagnosis is made with extreme difficulty, and then the results of treatment—more especially when the history of the individual case cannot be satisfactorily obtained—afford much aid in arriving at a conclusion.

The form of lupus described above under the name of "Jacob's ulcer" is regarded by many as being nearly allied to, if not a variety of, cutaneous cancer; by most surgical writers the latter view is taken, and Copland regards it as a connecting link between the two diseases. But its chief characteristic phenomena, especially its tedious but onward ulcerative progress, not implicating the bony tissues, the freedom from pain which marks its course, the non-contamination of the constitution generally, and the absence of the hypertrophied condition so characteristic of cutaneous cancer, sufficiently identify it, in my opinion, with the other lupoid affections.

Prognosis.—In every form of lupus, the prognosis, though favorable as regards the general health, must be more or less unfavorable with respect to the local disease, the latter being by many regarded as altogether incurable; yet, although most tedious and obstinate, in the majority of cases resisting even judiciously applied and appropriate treatment for.years, it not unfrequently eventually yields, the destructive process of ulceration is arrested, and the affected parts heal. The superficial variety of lupus is the least important in all respects; but even it is most rebellious, and the diseased surface rarely takes on a healthy action until after several months of treatment; and after apparent cure it is very apt to re-appear in the old cicatrix. Lupus serpiginosus, when of small extent, is in some cases very amenable to treatment, but when it affects an extended portion of the integu-ments it is rarely cured in a shorter period than from a year to a year and a half or two years; and, often after the disease is apparently perfectly removed, it breaks out afresh in one or two of the spots which had healed, when it lingers obstinately for months. Lupus devorans is both the most severe and the most obstinate of the several varieties of the disease, its destructive progress, unless when submitted to treatment at a very early period after it commences, is scarcely to be arrested, nor does it seem ever to tend to spontaueous cure; the form de-nominated "Jacob's ulcer" is, in my experience, perfectly incurable in all its stages. Like most other cutaneous diseases, the longer the duration of lupus the more diffi-cult is it to treat it successfully.

As regards the *pathology* of lupus, it is manifestly nearly allied to cancer, especially by its malignancy, and the appellation for the group of diseases of the skin in which it is here placed has, I think, been therefore happily chosen by Dr. Copland; yet they differ remarkably, in the latter being almost invariably marked by a general contamination of the system, which is never witnessed in the former; this is well evidenced by the glandular sys-tem in the neighborhood of the disease not becoming affected in the course of lupus, even when it has existed for years.

Treatment.—The administration of constitutional re-medies, in the treatment of lupus, is regarded by many as being useless, and the employment of local applica-tions is solely relied on, but I agree with those who con-sider both to be requisite, and it is only from a prolonged perseverance in remedial measures, judiciously selected, that good results can be expected to follow in this ob-stinate and malignant affection. The intimate connection that exists between the disease and scrofula being an admitted fact, the general treatment should consist in the use of those remedies which are calculated to correct that vitiated condition of the system, and the avoidance of all medicines which experience has proved to disagree with scrofulous individuals, or to aggravate any local derangement under which they may labor. The preparations of iodine and of iron, cod-liver oil, and the vegetable tonics are, therefore, especially indicated in the treatment of the different forms of lupus, and general hygienic measures, calculated to invigorate the constitution and to remove its vitiated condition, should never be neglected.

Iodine in some form, given in combination with tonics or alteratives, according to individual circumstances, is the remedy which, in my experience, is most to be relied on; for the majority of cases the iodide of potassium is the preparation best adapted, but, as I have already remarked in a previous part of this work, its beneficial results are more certainly obtained by being administered in rather small doses, continued for a long time, than if it be prescribed in large quantity at first—a practice which has been recently much followed in the treatment, especially of secondary syphilitic diseases. In persons in whom the constitution is unimpaired, and the muscular and adipose tissues are well developed, it may be prescribed in somewhat the following form :—

R. Iodidi Potassii, ... grana duodecim.
Infusi Cascarillæ, . . . uncias duodecim.
Succi Taraxaci, ... drachmas duas. Misce.
Sumat unciam fluidam ter indies.

The quantity of the iodide of potassium should be increased by the addition of a grain to the mixture each time it is renewed, until it contain twenty four grains, when it should be omitted for a few weeks, and again recommenced in a small dose. For weakly persons or those of a broken-down habit of body, the iodide of iron should be substituted for the iodide of potassium, and it may be given in decoction of fresh elm bark; when the scrofulous diathesis is very well marked, and the lupoid ulceration extensive, threatening to engage the deeper seated structures, iodide itself will be advantageously combined with the iodide of potassium or iodide of iron: if with the former, it may be prescribed according to the formula at page 247, the arsenical solution being omitted.

30

Cod-liver oil also proves an excellent remedy in the treatment of lupus, especially when the disease occurs at an early age; from my own experience of its effects I do not think it is attended with so much advantage when given in the enormous doses recommended by some; it when administered in smaller quantity, and its use persevered in for a very long time: a teaspoonful, three times a day, and increased so gradually that at the end of six months, two tablespoonfuls, as frequently given, will be the amount arrived at, a dose which need not be exceeded, is the manner of administering the medicine that I have seen prove eminently successful in lupus. By some of the French dermatologists, however, many of whom speak in rather extravagant terms of its efficacy in this disease, the dose is increased as rapidly as the stomach will admit, until from a pint and a half to two pints are taken in the twenty-four hours.

Arsenic alone, or combined with iodine, has been highly recommended by many practitioners for the treatment of lupus; the late Dr. Anthony Todd Thompson was in the habit of relying chiefly on it in the form of the iodide of arsenic. I have found this preparation very useful in the form described above as constituting lupus superficialis, but in the other varieties of the disease it has not proved so beneficial in my hands as iodine and the iodide of potassium. The liquor arsenici et hydrargyri hydriodatis, of the last *Dublin Pharmacopœia*, proves of especial service in those cases in which there may exist in the system an hereditary or acquired syphilitic taint.

So many other medicines have been at different times, and still are, proposed for the treatment of lupus that it would be almost impossible even to enumerate them; a few, however, require to be shortly noticed. The animal oil of Dippel—obtained in the dry distillation of harts-horn shavings in close vessels—has acquired some character on the Continent; it is given in doses of five or six drops at first, gradually increased to twenty or twenty-five. The chloride of barium and chloride of calcium have both been much used; that they possess some efficacy, due certainly to their anti-scrofulous powers, has been proved by the publication of several cases in which a cure resulted from their administration. Various preparations of mercury have also been tried for the treatment of lupus, and the red iodide is especially recommended by M. Rayer for those cases in which there is much hypertrophy of the integuments; but in consequence of the injurious effects so often occasioned by the administration of mercurials to persons of the scrofulous diathesis, I cannot agree with those who advocate their use in this disease.

The general hygienic measures to be adopted require merely to be alluded to; they consist, of course, in attention to every circumstance which can fortify the constitution, and remove the depraved condition on which the presence of the local disease depends: the chief of these are, breathing a dry, pure air, the use of nourishing, unstimulating diet, residence on the sea-shore, and when the strength admits, cold salt-water bathing.

The *local* treatment of lupus has at all times attracted more attention than the constitutional, and, as before remarked, many consider that the disease can by it alone be cured. It may be considered under two heads: first, the ablation of the affected portion of the integuments by the knife, or its destruction by caustics; and, second, the employment of astringents or other medicinal agents, calculated to promote cicatrization, or excite a new action in the parts. In the superficial variety of lupus, the chief object being to prevent disfiguration by arresting the progress of disease, the use of the knife is not admissible, for, were its employment even certain to effect a cure, the resulting eschar would occasion as much, if not greater deformity; for in the serpiginous form it is not applicable, nor has it been recommended, except by a few surgeons, to remove the hypertrophied edges; and, therefore, it is only in lupus devorans that excision holds out any prospect of being useful. An almost insurmountable difficulty, as regards its application, however, is experienced in all cases in which the disease has existed for

duration, and the deeper-seated structures are not
volved, the operation has occasionally proved
especially in "Jacob's ulcer," but the employment of
constitutional treatment above recommended should
be neglected at the same time, as thereby alone can i
expected that the return of the disease will be preven

The stronger caustics, from being more easy of ap
cation, and more certain than the knife in their effectu
the uneven, penetrating ulceration which characteri
this form of lupus, have been more generally emplo
Those chiefly used are the nitric and hydrochloric ac
the acid nitrate of mercury, caustic ammonia, chloride
zinc, chloride of gold, caustic potash, solution of
terchloride of antimony, and arsenical pastes or powd
The chloride of zinc has many advocates; and, where
edges of the ulcer are ragged and unhealthy, and
surface discharges a sanious pus, it in many cases pro
useful by exciting a new action; as much of the sur
as it is wished to destroy should be touched lightly v
the solid salt, and the application renewed every altern
day until the desired effect is produced: the stron
acids may also be applied in the same manner. I b
generally known the employment of caustic applicati
prove injurious in lupus serpiginosus, yet they are hig
praised by several writers, nitrate of silver being usu
preferred to any other; in many cases in which I b
seen them used the parts to which they were immedia
applied healed up temporarily, but the serpiginous u
ration from the circumference continued to spread
checked, undermining the surrounding integuments,
erally with increased rapidity. In lupus superfici
caustics, if effectually applied, cause a worse disfig
ment than the original disease, which, moreover, the
not check.

Under the second division of local applications
be noticed, first, those which, though not actually cau
are highly stimulant and resolvent, such as the di
acids, Donovan's solution, the animal oil of Dippel
tions or ointments containing the chloride of zinc, nit
of silver, caustic potash, &c. The oil of Dippel is
ployed very extensively on the Continent, and, it is

der the influence," he says, "of the applicat
biniodide of mercury, frequently repeated, 1
, after the disappearance of the sharp but fl
inflammation produced by it, and as a consec
ably of its general action, the hypertrophied
me resolved, the tubercles disappear, and soft,
, smooth cicatrices, on a level with the rest
form; in short, I have seen the most frightful
pus cured without leaving any other traces th
rently thinned skin, with white or red spots
there, according to the length of time whic
ed from the formation of the cicatrices."[1] M.
applies a thin layer of the powder, undilutec
on only of the diseased surface at a time; it
re pain and much inflammation, the former l
ix or eight hours, and the latter for three c
; a thick crust is left, which falls off at the c
ight, or ten days, when, should there be occ
pplication may be renewed.
e topical remedy which I have found most
e treatment of lupus serpiginosus is the acet
; the ulcerated surfaces should be touched wi
salt—care being taken to use a crystal whic
effloresced—twice a day, daily, or every secc
day, according to the degree of activity of th

nnales des Maladies de la Peau et de la Syphilis, Tom. ii

inflammation, and a lotion containing from three to ﬁ
grains to the ounce of distilled water should be used ﬁ
wet with it being applied, and the parts covered ﬁ
oiled silk when practicable. In this form, as well as
lupus devorans, the local inﬂammation, of which ﬁ
time to time rather smart attacks occur, should be check
by the application of leeches as near the affected parﬁ
possible, but sufﬁciently distant to prevent the bites ﬁ
becoming involved in the disease ; and emollient po
tices should be used occasionally with the same intentio
and to remove the hard crusts which form.

No matter what local treatment be employed in t
treatment of lupus, attention must be especially pa
when the nose or mouth is the seat of the disease, to p
vent the natural outlets from becoming obstructed duri
the progress of cicatrization. •

In conclusion, I may again repeat that, as the result
considerable experience in the treatment of this obstin
and serious disease, I regard the employment of topic
agents as altogether secondary ; they are unquestionab
useful in modifying the diseased process that is going
and in exciting a new action in the parts, but they m
be regarded as only auxiliary to the constitutional tre
ment, which should engage the chief attention of t
practitioner, the fact being always kept prominently
view, that it is alone by the *prolonged* use of remedi
and diligent attention to general hygienic measures, t
a favorable result can be expected. See Hutchins
Jonathan, " A Clinical Report on Rodent Ulcer."—
Times and Gaz., 18th Aug. 1860; and Paget, Ja
" Three Cases of Rodent Ulcer."—*Ibid.*

KELOÏS.

Keloïs, or Kelis, from χηλή a crab's claw, or from ﬂ
a scar, or from Κήλη a tumor.

KELOÏS (*Cheloïd tumor*) is an extremely rare dis
of the skin, which was first noticed, in the latter end
the last century, by Retz, and was soon afterwards f
described by Alibert, who applied this name to it f
a fancied resemblance which he thought it bore to

w of a crab (χηλή, "forfex cancrorum"): for a similar
son he first denominated it *Cancroïde*, and also because
a latter term expressed the analogy which he believed
exist between the disease and cancer; it is for the
ter reason that I have included it with lupus, in the
ler Cancroïdes. It consists in the development on the
aneous surface of an irregular-shaped, or somewhat
ll, hard, and prominent excrescence, slightly depressed
l uneven in the centre, the edges being raised and
kened; the surface has a polished and shining aspect,
a rose or reddish-white color, marked with bright-red
white lines, and corrugated so as to present nearly
appearance of an old much-hypertrophied cicatrix,
ten pressed with the finger it is somewhat resilient,
the part pressed upon becomes momentarily color-
. The morbid growth, which varies in size from a
lines to an inch or more in diameter, is extremely
erent to the integuments, roots projecting from it into
deeper layers of the skin. It first appears in the
n of one or more small, hard, wart-like tumors, accom-
ied by itching and some pain; as it increases in size
pain becomes much augmented, being of a severe
ging character, and in some cases has been described
being almost unbearable.

he cheloïd tumor is most generally solitary, being,
the majority of cases which have been reported, de-
pped on the anterior surface of the thorax, either
ow the clavicle on either side, or on the sternum, but
a few instances several of them have been witnessed
xist at the same time on different regions of the body;
growth is comparatively slow, it does not ulcerate,
is it painful to the touch, and may continue indolent
years; but in a few cases it has been reported to have
ome gradually smaller by interstitial absorption, until
inally disappeared altogether, its site being marked
a white cicatrix. Dr. Fox is inclined to confirm the
nion of Dr. Carter, that it is a form of Elephantiasis;
Mr. Balmanno Squire considers it to be allied to
ous.

he *causes* of this disease are very obscure; in one or
instances it has been stated to have followed local

injury, and some cases have been published in which the tumor was developed on the old cicatrix of a burn or wound, but many have with sufficient reason questioned the fact of these being examples of true keloïs. No proof exists of its being hereditary, or of its occurring in persons whose parents had been affected with cancer or scrofula, nor does it appear to be connected with any special temperament or diathesis. It would seem to affect both sexes nearly alike, but it has not been observed in early life, those who labor under it being individuals usually of mature age. Dr. Fox is of opinion that the cause of it is "a special diathesis similar to, if not a modified phase of, that of Elephantiasis."

The extreme rarity of the disease is very remarkable, and consequently its nature, history, and characteristics are not well understood, from the want of sufficient opportunity for their being studied: Mr. Wilson states that the total number of cases recorded amounts only to 24, of which he himself has seen 7; but it has been witnessed also in Ireland, casts and drawings of it existing in the Museum of the Richmond Hospital in this city, although the cases have not, as far as I am aware, been published.

Since the preceding remarks were written several other cases have been recorded, and observations written on this disease. Of these may be noted Dr. Addison, in *Med.-Chir. Trans.*, Vol. XXXVII. 1854; M. Gillette's monograph on "*Sclerema*," in the *Archives Générales de Médecine*, Dec. 1854; Dr. Robert M'Donnell, on "*Sclerem a*," in the *Dublin Hospital Gazette* for 1855 and 1856; Mr. Sedgwick, in *Path. Soc. Trans.*, Vol. XII, p. 234; Dr. Alderson, and Dr. Valentine Mott, in *Med.-Chir. Trans.*, Vol. XXXVII, 1854; Dr. Henderson, in *Med. Times & Gaz.*, 14th July, 1860; and several other papers, particularly in the foreign journals, noted by Dr. Fox.

Diagnosis.—The only affection with which keloïs is likely to be confounded is cancer; it is distinguished from it by its indolent nature, its indisposition to ulcerate, the absence of contamination of the glandular system, and its peculiar site.

Prognosis.—Were it not for the extremely painful sensations which usually attend this affection it would be little moment, there being no risk to life, nor local ﾟgerous symptoms likely to be occasioned by its pre-ﾟce. The duration of the disease is almost invariably ﾟlonged; years elapsing in those cases in which it has appeared spontaneously, before absorption had com-ﾟnced.

Treatment.—Excision of the cheloïd tumor has been ﾟposed and practised, but such a course seems to have ﾟn invariably unattended with successful results; the ﾟund made was difficult to heal, and the disease returned ﾟer some time either in the cicatrix or in the integu-ﾟnts of some other region of the body. The sponta-ﾟous cure of the affection by absorption having occurred comparatively speaking, many cases, should inculcate ﾟpropriety of abstaining from meddlesome interference, ﾟd teach that reliance ought to be placed chiefly on ﾟstitutional treatment by means of alteratives and cor-ﾟents where necessary, and the local use of mild stimu-ﾟts or sedatives to allay pain. With the latter view I ﾟuld suggest the employment of an ointment containing iodide of potassium and chloroform. Cazenave re-ﾟmends the sulphur douche; Wilson the application ﾟollodion and the tincture of iodine; and Rayer, that ﾟn and constant compression should be made on the ﾟor when its situation permits.

CHAPTER XI.

DERMATOPHYTÆ.

THE general application within the last few years of the use of the microscope in investigating diseased conditions of animal structures has afforded most important and valuable assistance to the morbid anatomist and pathologist, by throwing new light upon much that was before obscure; our knowledge of cutaneous affections has, along with other subjects in practical medicine, been advanced thereby, and chiefly by the discovery that in certain of them a vegetable production—a cryptogamic plant—is present on the surface of the skin. It is in consequence of this discovery that a necessity has arisen for constituting the present group or order of diseases of the skin, which is termed *Dermatophytæ*—from δέρμα, "the skin," and φυτόν, "a plant:" it includes, then, *those cutaneous affections which are dependent on, or are characterized by, the presence of parasitic plants on the diseased surface of the integuments.* By some the existence of these vegetable growths is altogether denied, while others, who admit their existence, regard them as being accidental productions, a consequence and not a cause of the disease which they accompany; the investigations, however, of Dr. Hughes Bennett, of Edinburgh, Dr. Tilbury Fox, of London, Dr. M'Call Anderson, of Glasgow, and of Robin, Gruby, Lebert, and others, on the Continent, in my opinion, place it beyond doubt not only that these parasites are developed in certain diseases of the skin, but that they constitute their essential nature. In addition to the two affections, Porrigo and Sycosis, which I shall include in this order, the presence of a cryptogamic plant has also been ascertained in Pityriasis versicolor (Chloasma); but I agree with Dr. Bennett in the opinion that

although this disease frequently presents epiphytes
among the scales, it owes none of its essential characters
this circumstance." It has been already noticed in
chapter VI.

Other writers have included, as Dermatophytæ, herpes
circinatus, plica polonica, and alopecia areata; but of
these the first has been already referred to in Chapter
II, and the last two will be found noticed in Chapter
III, where also will be found a notice of onychomy-
osis, a parasitic disease of the nails.

Several modern writers of note devote a special order
or group to "Parasitic diseases," which are by them believed to be caused by *animal* or *vegetable* parasites. As
the former, called dermatozoa or ectozoa, are not here
noticed in a special division, it may be well to observe
that the group is held to comprehend the acarus scabiei,
already noticed in Chapter III; the pediculus capitis,
asserted by Mr. Balmanno Squire to be a common cause
of impetigo; the pediculus corporis, asserted by the same
authority to be a common cause of prurigo and urticaria;
the phthirius, or pediculus pubis, noticed in Chapter V;
the pulex irritans, or common flea; the acanthia lectularia, or common bug; the leptus autumnalis, or harvest
bug; the steatozoön folliculorum, noticed in Chapter IV;
the pulex penetrans, chigoe, chigger, or jigger, common
in the West Indies and in South America; and the filaria
medinensis or dracunculus, the guinea worm of tropical
countries. Dr. Fox also notices the œstrus, bots, or gad-
. For a full account of the leptus autumnalis see *Amer.
Month. Jour. Med. Sci.,* N. S., Vol. XX, p. 91. Dr. Fox
gives, from the *Social Science Review,* an account of the
disease caused in the West Indies by the pulex irritans;
Hillier refers to the researches of Carter, Busk, and
others, respecting the guinea-worm disease, and most
writers refer for full information respecting it to Mr.
Bastian's paper in the twenty-fourth volume of the *Transactions of the Linnæan Society,* p. 101.

The *treatment* of the guinea-worm disease consists in
gently extracting the worm by winding it gradually on
a piece of card, during which process, if the worm be
broken, much inflammation and sloughing occurs.

Dr. Fox quotes several notices respectir
ment of the œstrus or gad-fly, e. g., Et
April, 1854 (Dr. Londre's paper), and Ran
Vol. XXIX, p. 91.[1]

A paper on "Animal Parasite Disease
has also been recently read before the I
Association, by Mr. Balmanno Squire; ;
of it see Med. Times and Gaz., 19th Aug.

The consideration of skin diseases of ;
has of late years been so zealously pursu
anything like a full discussion of the sub
in the limits of a practical work.   Dr. Fox
of Parasitic Origin, and Dr. M'Call Ande
The Parasitic Affections of the Skin ma
with advantage on the one side; and on
Wilson's paper "On the Phytopatholog
and Nosophytodermata, the so-called Para
of the Skin," Br. and For. Med.-Chir.
1864.   See also, Dr. W. Abbots Smith (
tozoa, Lond., 1863; Mr. T. Spencer Co
Lond., 1864; Küchenmeister's treatise or
Vegetable Parasites of the Human Bc
Soc. Trans., Lond. 1856–57; and Dr. Geo.
worm, Scall-Head, Baldness, and other Par
of the Head and Face.

PORRIGO.

PORRIGO (Favus; Tinea; in German, E
wabbengrind; Scall-Head—Plate XV, Fi
This peculiar affection, which, from its ;
frequently on the scalp, is generally desc
peculiar to that region of the body, is cl
phenomena so distinct from those of all
tive diseases which are apt to occur there
possibly be mistaken for any of·them.
in the form of small, elevated, dry spots
of a pin's head, of a bright yellow coloi

---

[1] On the Occurrence of Bots in the Human Subje
and J. Matthews Duncan.

rface of the skin, which is depressed slightly by them;
ch spot is distinct, hemispherical. slightly concave or
ıp-shaped on its free surface, and convex beneath, where
is adherent to the skin. On removing the small, dis-
sed mass, that portion of the scalp on which it was
ated is found to be somewhat depressed, smooth, and
ining. A single crust of the disease, or *favus*—as it
ıs been termed, from its resemblance both in color and
ntral depression to the superficial surface of a honey-
mb—is often traversed by one, and sometimes by two
iirs, which appear to grow, as it were, from the very
ntre or most depressed portion: this has given rise to
e notion that the disease is one of the bulbs of the hair;
ıt the fact of its appearance on other parts of the body
iich are quite free from hair affords a sufficient refuta-
ın of this opinion. The eruption spreads by additions
the outer edge or circumference of each crust, which
ıs retains its hemispherical character, until it acquires
diameter of two or three lines, or sometimes more;
ne of the favi on the trunk at times attain fully half
inch in diameter; on the head, however, they rarely
eed the size above mentioned. The adjacent favi, as
y increase, unite with each other, and form large,
'gular-shaped masses, in which the original circular
ʼn of the individual crust is in a great degree lost;
centre also of each is changed in appearance, and,
ead of the cup-shaped depression, the entire surface
overed with alternate elevations and depressions, or,
ʼo speak, ridges and furrows, concentrically arranged.
ɜ eruption thus increasing, the whole of the scalp,
n, too, the forehead, the neck, and parts of the trunk,
ome encased in one large yellow crust, at the edges
vhich some favi, of the peculiar characteristic appear-
e, are invariably to be seen.
ʼhe crusts of porrigo are of a pale sulphur-yellow
ɔr; they are hard and dry, and break with a short
ıture, exhibiting within a mealy powder, of a paler
low than the external surface. They may generally
remov   ʼacility from the scalp, but they bring
                 thin layer of epid   which is
                 r under surfac   ı which

small projections may be seen with a moderate lens;
sometimes with the naked eye. These projections, or
processes, pass into the dermis beneath, and when the
crusts are torn forcibly away blood issues from the actual
orifices into which they were inserted. From the very
commencement of the eruption the hair becomes altered;
much of it falls out, and the straggling hairs that remain
are thin, broken, weak, whitish, and readily removable
with the crusts of the disease, in which they are firmly
imbedded. When this affection has continued for any
length of time, bald patches are left after cure, on which
the hair does not again grow; and even where it has
been cured at an earlier stage the hair seldom regains its
proper character, being often weak, thin, of a diseased
appearance, and of a whitish-yellow color. Porrigo, in
its first stage, does not give rise to either heat of the
scalp or itching, and, consequently, is very rarely noticed
until it is fully developed. It usually commences on the
forehead, at the edge of the hairy scalp, but it spreads
rapidly over the head, soon involving nearly the entire
surface, the healthy patches which are left between the
diseased spots being but very few, and small in extent.
The eruption is also met with on various parts of the
body, the trunk, or extremities; but I have very
rarely seen it there except when it existed at the same
time on the scalp. As the disease advances much irritation of the surface is produced; small pustules form
here and there in spots as yet unaffected with the eruption: the tingling and heat are so unbearable as to compel
the patient to tear the surface with his nails, even to such
a degree as to cause ulceration; innumerable pediculi
are endangered; the favus crusts emit an abominable
odor, resembling that of mice; and a copious offensive
discharge is secreted by the pustules and ulcerated spots:
in short, an individual affected with this disease in its
aggravated form becomes a loathsome and disgusting
object.

I have already referred to the vegetable nature of this
eruption; it is in the spongy, friable contents of the favi
that its characters are best seen. "Reduced to powder,
and placed under the microscope, it presents," says Robin,

cture—1, of tortuous, branching tubes, without
)na, empty, or containing a few molecular granules
ium); 2, straight or crooked, but not tortuous tubes,
mes, but rarely, branched, containing granules or
ounded cellules, or elongated cellules, placed end
so as to represent partitioned tubes, with or with-
nted articulations (*receptacles or sporangia, in vari-
les of development?*); 3, finally *sporules*, free or
into bead-like strings. The mycelium is very
nt near the inner surface of the external layer,
ch it adheres. The spongy, friable mass of the
of each favus is principally formed of sporules
e different tubes containing mycelium already
ed (*sporangia or receptacles?*). We often find
with them *mycelium* tubes, but in small quantity.
se elements pass insensibly into each other: empty
mycelium); tubes containing small round corpus-
ubes with corpuscles as large as the smaller spo-
sporules placed end to end, so as to resemble a
partitioned cylinder, with a tendency to separate
joints; and free sporules." Bennett has given a
rawing of this arrangement. M. Robin[1] gives a
description of the various parts of which the
is composed, as well as faithful and well executed
tions of this vegetable parasite, the correctness of
I have had repeated opportunities of verifying,
nes with the assistance of Dr. Lyons, of this city,
as devoted so much time and talent to promote
copical medical investigations in Ireland. The
al characters of the plant are appended in a note.[2]
is a rather rare affection, appearing, however,
e observations of those who have written specially
;, to be more common on the Continent and in Ire-

Végétaux, qui croissent sur l'Homme et sur les Animaux Vivans,
Robin. Paris : 1847.
HORION SCHONLEINII. *Remak.* Orbiculare, flavum, coriaceum,
nanæ presertim capitis insidens ; rhizopodion molle, pellu-
.occosum, floccis tenuissimis, vix articulatis, ramosissimis,
oticis (?). Mycelium floccis crassioribus subramosis, distincte
is, articulis inæqualibus, irregularibus, in sporidia abeuntibus ;
rotunda, ovalia vel irregularia, in uno vel pluribus lateribus
atia."

land than in England. When I first wrote on this disease in 1848,[1] my experience was drawn from a limited number of cases; since then, however, I have had under my care a comparatively large number of examples—twenty-three.

It may appear at any time of life, but is very seldom met with except in childhood, from the age of 3 to 12; it may be developed on almost every part of the body, but, as already remarked, occurs with much the greatest frequency on the scalp, and next to it on the back of the trunk. When it appears on those portions of the integument which are not covered with hair the favus crusts acquire a larger size, and increase more rapidly than when it is seated on the scalp, but it presents precisely similar characters.

Great confusion long existed amongst dermatologists as to what special disease was understood by the term "Porrigo;" the many eruptions which have their seat on the scalp were at one time described as being merely varieties of a single genus, which was indiscriminately denominated Favus, Tinea, or Porrigo; this confusion has, however, been lately much removed, and the latter appellation—the others being synonymous with it—is now strictly confined to the cutaneous affection above described, which corresponds with the Porrigo *lupinosa* of Willan. Cazenave divides it into two species characterized by the form in which the crusts are developed, the one he terms *Favus disseminé*, and the other *Favus en cercles;* this is, I think, an unnecessary refinement, tending to complication, and presenting no advantage in practice. Wilson, who denies the vegetable nature of the morbid production on the scalp, describes favus, which is the name he adopts, as being a disease of the hair follicles.

The *causes* of porrigo have given rise to much difference of opinion, especially with reference to its contagious nature; the correctness of my adhesion to the views of those who hold that it is so, which I avowed some years ago in the little work already referred to, has

[1] *Eruptive Diseases of the Scalp.* Dublin, 1848. 12mo.

been confirmed by almost every day's experience since, for I have seen numerous instances of the propagation of the disease from individual to individual, by direct contact, in the majority of cases from children to children, but sometimes even from children to adults. The mode in which I believe the contagion to be conveyed is by the propagation of the vegetable parasite, by means of the *mycelia*. But its contagious character has been denied by many on the grounds of the rarity of the disease, and the failure to produce it by inoculation, as tried by Gruby and others; the former of whom produced the disease only once out of seventy-six trials on vegetables, and not at all on animals. But Remak succeeded in inoculating his own arm in August, 1842;[1] and Bennett, who had previously failed in his own person after repeated trials, succeeded completely in 1845, in producing the disease in one of his class by inoculation and close contact of the favus crusts, obtained from the head of a boy at that time in the Royal Infirmary. An account of his experiment, and also of Remak's, will be found in the *Northern Journal of Medicine* for September, 1845, p. 202, and the account of the former will also be found in Bennett's *Clinical Lectures on the Principles and Practice of Medicine*, second edition, p. 799. Hebra has also proved its contagious property in the same manner.

Now in all these trials to generate the plant, one important fact connected with the natural history of parasitical fungi has been overlooked by all, namely, *that they require for their growth a peculiar soil;* thus we find one genus is found only on snow, another on cheese, another in yeast, different varieties on different decaying vegetable matters, and individual genera and species on various living animals and plants; nay, even different sorts on different parts of the same animal. This holds true with the Achorion Schönleinii; it requires for its reproduction to be planted in a peculiar soil, that is on an individual whose system is in a peculiar cachectic condition; and until it is ascertained what this exact constitution is, a single instance of its propagation by con-

---

[1] *Medicinische Zeitung* for 1842.

integuments, but they are evidently due to the
inflammation caused by the morbid growth on
neous surface, on the application of acrid or st
unguents, lotions, &c. In its very early sta
seated on the scalp, porrigo might be mistakı
commencement of an attack of impetigo, but
development of the pustules in the latter soo
the diagnosis simple; and it does not present
tures in common with the other eruptive disea
scalp. Should a doubtful case, however, occur,
culty that may exist will be at once cleared
microscopic examination.

Prognosis.—A disease of great gravity, an
regarded with extreme abhorrence in consequne
disagreeable symptoms with which it is att
unsightly aspect, and its contagious nature
nevertheless in no respect tends to shorten lif
to injure the general health, unless in so fi
almost necessitates strict confinement to the b
isolation. The fatuity which is so commonly
to accompany its advanced stages is certainly
extent a consequence of its existence, for it is
in any remarkable degree in individuals in
affection has been of short duration. The effect
on the growth of the hair must also be t

account in forming a prognosis, as its loss is often regarded as one of the most grievous consequences of the disease; when the crusts cover the head completely, and their duration has been at all prolonged, the pressure produced by them causes absorption of the superficial layers of the derma, and consequent destruction of the hair follicles, permanent baldness then necessarily results; but when the morbid growth is removed at an early stage, although the hair is usually deteriorated and its subsequent growth injured, no ill consequences to it follow in some cases. As regards the eruptive diseases of the scalp, porrigo is the most obstinate and most rebellious to treatment of them all; by many dermatologists it has been regarded as being almost incurable, and, consequently, the most violent remedies have been proposed for its treatment, but I have never failed in curing it permanently by the simple method to be now described.

Treatment.—There is probably no disease of the skin which has been subjected to a greater variety of plans of treatment, some of them of the most painful character, than this, chiefly in consequence of its extreme obstinacy, and the opposing views which have been and are even still held as to its nature: before proceeding to speak of the remedies used by others, I shall first describe the method which has invariably succeeded in my hands, and the efficacy of which has been now for some years proved by the testimony of others. It consists in the simultaneous employment of constitutional remedies and local applications: the former, used with the intention of correcting or altering that vitiated condition of the system generally, to the existence of which is due the development of the morbid growth on a congenial soil: and the latter, to remove the diseased mass constituted by the peculiar vegetable parasite, and to prevent its reproduction.

A combination of the two alteratives which experience has proved to be the most powerful in the removal of cutaneous diseases—arsenic and iodine—has, in my experience, effectually fulfilled the requirements of the constitutional treatment. They may be given in the fluid form, as already recommended for the squamous erup-

intment is, at the expiration of this time, replaced
containing the iodide of lead, in the portion of
lrachm of the iodide to an ounce of prepared
iich is to be renewed morning and evening, the
iing well washed with the carbonate of potash
rery time before the ointment is reapplied. In
ses it will be found that the iodide of lead oint-
xcites a certain degree of inflammation of the
of the scalp after it has been used for some days;
ich occurs it should not be applied for a day or
; the lotion may be employed alone three or four
iily. After this first attack of inflammation dis-
iit rarely recurs, although the use of the ointment
ited in for months. The strength of the ointment
be increased after a fortnight; and if the disease
ipear, even to double that above indicated. The
cap should be kept on the head until a cure is
; the advantage derived from it is twofold: in
t stage of treatment, by keeping the hard and
ilanted crusts of the disease in a constant atmos-
if warm moisture, it softens, and thus renders
ore easily removable; and in the after-treatment
cedinous vegetable being retained by it in the
contact with the iodide of lead and the emana-
ising therefrom, is more certainly destroyed, and
iduction prevented.

continuing . this treatment for at least three
ir a month all external applications should be
and the hair allowed to grow, so as to ascertain
ingus will be reproduced; for it often lies dor-
id suddenly shoots forth, increasing rapidly when
er subject to the action of the iodide of lead.
it again return, the local applications must be
ourse to as before, immediately on its appearance.
ministration of the iodide of arsenic should be
ed until we are quite satisfied that the cure is
e.

ig the entire progress of treatment the patient
kept on a strictly milk and farinaceous diet, and
els regulated by the administration of mild mer-

curial alteratives and saline cathartics—especially
saline mineral waters—when necessary.

A most cruel, almost barbarous, method of trea
porrigo, when it occurs on the scalp, originally prop
in the ancient days of medicine, is still followed
great extent on the Continent. It consists in the a
cation to the hairy surface—the crusts of morbid gr
having been previously removed as much as possible
poulticing, &c.—of some adhesive plaster, such as
gundy or common pitch, or ammoniacum, spread
strips of stout calico, which, being caused to ad
firmly, and left on for several days, are torn off
direction opposite to that in which the hair grows, a
to remove as much of the latter as possible; and the
applied again and again until the entire of the sca
completely deprived of hair. The sufferings occasi
by this proceeding are, as may readily be imagined, s
thing horrible, and the Brothers Mahon, who stro
advocated its employment in a somewhat modified f
mention that even death has resulted from it. /
remedial measure, it originated in the false idea tha
disease was an affection of the hairs solely, and th
their total ablation it would of necessity be cured;
in modern days it has been continued chiefly fr
theory which found many supporters, that the produ
of perfect baldness would suspend the morbid a
sufficiently long to allow the diseased surface to retu
a normal state.

A host of powerful topical applications have been
in the treatment of porrigo:—the strongest cau
blisters; ointments containing quicklime, the sulp
of lime, tartar emetic, arsenic, pepper, &c.; lotio
corrosive sublimate, and of other irritants and stimul
but inasmuch as the method of treatment which I
recommended above has proved invariably success
my experience, this simple enumeration of them
suffice here.

In addition to the preceding remarks of Dr. Ne
it may be observed that epilation is frequently res
to, and is even considered necessary by some physi
Dr. Jenner uses sulphurous acid locally; Dr. Be

makes a similar use of cod-liver oil; Hebra applies alcohol; and in two cases treated by the Editor, during the present year, the tinctura saponis viridis cum pice of Hebra was found very useful. The tincture was smeared over the scalp, and the entire mass was easily removed by a poultice, leaving the surface quite clear. Thus it answered the purposes of the pitch-cap without the barbarity of that horrible application. The admirable remarks of Dr. Jenner in the *Med. Times and Gazette*, for 20th August, 1858, p. 181, and Dr. Corrigan's concise and comprehensive clinical lecture in *Dub. Hosp. Gazette* for August 15, 1845, may be consulted with great advantage; as also Dr. Moore's paper on Cutaneous Diseases, *Dub. Hosp. Gaz.*, 1859, p. 117.

No matter on what part of the cutaneous surface porrigo may be developed, the constitutional and topical remedies to be employed are the same.

SYCOSIS.

SYCOSIS (Plate XV, Fig. 1).—It is conjectured that this term, which is of very ancient origin in medicine, was applied to designate the cutaneous affection which is now understood by it, or one nearly allied thereto, from a fancied resemblance which the eruption bears to the rough exterior of a fig (σῦκον): from the special seat of the eruption it has, by many modern writers, been denominated *mentagra*, which must therefore be regarded as synonymous. By Bateman the disease was classed in Willan's order of the Tubercula, from which it has been removed, together with Acne, to the order Pustulæ, by those dermatologists of the French School who have adopted an artificial arrangement of diseases of the skin. Mr. Erasmus Wilson, who in his latest work (*Student's Book*, p. 457) describes it as "a dermophytic disease," formerly regarded it as being nearly allied to Acne, and consequently described it with that affection in the group of "Diseases of the Sebiparous Glands" in his earliest classification. As regards the appearance of the eruption, in one of its stages it certainly bears much resemblance to acne in being more or less pustular, but the pustules

... ... the result of irrita-
... ... the absence of a parasitic
... ... described by Gruby, and, since
... ... in 1842, by other
... ... the result of repeated microscopic
... ... M. Gruby and Dr.
... ... the absence of this parasitic cryp-
... ... I have therefore placed it with
... ... diseases to which the
... ... has been applied. In this view most
... ... agree.

... ... which is limited to that por-
... ... the beard grows—the chin, the
... ... lip—rarely extending to the integ-
... ... adjacent, is developed at first by the
appearance, around the roots of the hairs, of slightly inflamed, itching elevations, on which a dry, grayish scurf
soon appears: this increases pretty quickly, and its presence exciting inflammation, which is much augmented
by the use of the razor in shaving, conical pustules soon
form, and mask much the original character of the disease. The eruption escaping notice in most cases in its
early stage has caused it to be described as being pustular from the first, but careful observation has convinced
me that the pustules are secondary, and that they origi-
ate from the irritation caused by the vegetable parasite,
which must therefore be regarded as the essential characteristic of this affection. The crust or scurf increases
very slowly in extent, but, the attendant inflammation
attacking the subcutaneous structures, is accompanied
much heat, pain, swelling, and tension, which are furt
... ... by the formation of the pustules; these p
... ... slowly, and when they at length bu
... ... brown scab forms, which is very persiste
... ... be attempted, the surface to which
... ... is very painful.
... ... the disease a small porti
... ... which the attack is often
... ... and
... ... redi
... ... growi

but most usually the eruption returns after a short time, when it spreads more rapidly and engages a much larger extent of surface, the local symptoms also being more severe. After repeated outbreaks, thus characterized, the integuments of the chin become generally much hypertrophied, of a dusky-red color, hard, and covered, in patches of a greater or less extent, with a thick, grayish crust pierced by the hair of the beard, with hard, dry, brown scabs, from beneath which pus exudes here and there, and with conical, elevated pustules, many of which, in consequence of their being developed over the site of a hair-follicle, are perforated by hairs. The inflammatory action, when sycosis presents these aggravated symptoms, is usually very severe, small abscesses sometimes form in the subcutaneous areolar tissue, and engaging the hair-follicles, the beard falls out in patches, and permanent bald spots on the face result. Although the disease is in the majority of instances confined to that portion of the chin on which the beard grows, in very severe cases the upper lip and the surface covered by the whiskers are also engaged, and occasionally it is confined to these parts alone.

In 1842, M. Gruby first announced to the French Academy of Sciences his discovery of the existence of a cryptogamic plant[1] surrounding the roots of the hair of the beard in sycosis, and he believed that its presence constituted a previously undescribed variety of the disease, which he proposed to term *Mentagra contagiosa*. This parasitic vegetable does not appear above the surface of the integument, and thus differs altogether from that of Porrigo. "On examining the crusts or scabs under the microscope," writes M. Gruby, "they are seen to be composed of epidermic cells; but a microscopic examination of the hair demonstrates that the entire of that part of it which is inserted in the skin is surrounded by cryptogamic plants, which form a layer between the sheath of the hair and the hair itself, so that the hair is placed, as it were, in a cryptogamic sheath, just as a finger in a glove. But it is a remarkable fact that the parasitic growths never extend

---

[1] Microsporon mentagrophytes.

32

chin or the lips, are not unfrequently confounded with sycosis, especially when they become chronic, and, indeed, by some dermatologists, all pustular eruptions when seated on that part of the face on which the beard grows, are denominated sycosis; this term, however, should, I think, be restricted to designate the disease above described, as being characterized by gray and yellow crusts or scales and a thickened and indurated condition of the integuments, and attended with the development of conoidal pustules, terminating in dry, brown, adherent scabs; in doubtful cases a microscopic examination of the roots of the hairs will aid the diagnosis.

Prognosis.—Although seemingly not injurious to the general health, sycosis is a cutaneous disease of much gravity in consequence of its extreme obstinacy, the great suffering it occasions, and the repulsive appearance which it gives to the face of those who suffer from it. If submitted to treatment in its early stages, it is in most cases readily cured, but it is extremely apt to return, and almost invariably in a more severe form than at first; when once it has become chronic it usually resists every plan of treatment for years and sometimes lasts for life; or, if removed, leaves its disfiguring traces behind, in the form of hypertrophied livid-red patches, on the parts which had been affected, and often in the existence of irregularly-shaped, uneven, bald spots, on which the beard is not reproduced. Such being the character of sycosis, as regards its duration and ultimate results, it is of the utmost importance that the disease should be carefully diagnosed before a prognosis be formed.

Treatment.—The first point to be attended to in the treatment of sycosis is the state of the general health, which will be found more or less deranged in most persons affected with the disease; and the condition of the digestive organs especially demands attention. To regulate it, mild mercurials, purgatives, alteratives, or tonics should be prescribed, according to the indication in each case; and when the eruption has been of long standing, and engages an extended portion of the integument, preparations of iodine with the vegetable tonics and diaphoretics should be administered. As regards the local treatment, the first indication is to counteract, as far as possible, the irritation caused by the growth of the hair; with this view the use of the razor should, from the first, be altogether omitted, and the hair kept out as much as practicable with a sharp pair of scissors during the early progress of the treatment. The application of three or four leeches beneath the jaw or behind the ears, either twice a week, during the inflammatory stages of the disease, or whenever the affected parts present a swollen or irritated appearance, is productive of especial benefit; in the more chronic stages, or when it has been of long duration, they should be used with caution, and their application repeated not oftener than twice a month. Numerous topical remedies have been recommended for the treatment of sycosis: that which I have found most useful is a cerate containing calomel and chloroform, as in the following formula, applied three times daily :—

R. Calomelanos, ... grana triginta.
   Cerati Galeni,[1] . . . . unciam.
   Chloroformi, ... minima duodecim.
                                          Misce.

But in very obstinate cases, or those which resist the use of this combination, the iodide of lead ointment, as recommended for the treatment of porrigo, with the addition of the quantity of chloroform above prescribed, will be found of much service. Whichever be employed, the diseased surface should be well sponged previously to each application with equal parts of new milk and the weak alkaline or lead-wash. The ointment of the iodide of sulphur, also, has been highly recommended by many for the treatment of this disease, and in some very obstinate cases, I have found it of service. Attention to diet and regimen is particularly demanded in all cases, the use of spirituous liquors and of all rich or heating articles of food being carefully eschewed.

Madura Foot.—Most modern dermatologists notice an affection peculiar to India, called the *Madura foot, Fungus foot of India,* or *Mycetoma.* Dr. Fox believes it to depend on the presence of a parasite which makes its way beneath

[1] See Sixth (Macnamara's) Edition of Neligan's *Medicines,* p. 291.

the integuments of the foot to the bones, producing symptoms closely resembling caries. Numerous sinuses lead to the diseased bone, and give exit to fungous elements in the form of little black or white masses, together with their sero-purulent or viscid secretion. The structures of the foot are found studded with masses of various sizes, black, red, or white, and they may be picked out from apparent cavities lined by a speeial membrane. Dr. Fox, from whose description this account is condensed, remarks that the joints are healthy, and that no caries exists. The fungus is called *Chionyphe Carteri*. The disease is of no special interest to practitioners in this country.—See Carter, H. V., "On Mycetoma," *Br. and For. Med.-Chir. Rev.*, July, 1863.

Mention has been already made of the propagation of epiphytic disease by contagion; parasitic germs are also believed to be transmissible from men to animals, and *vice versâ.* In the *Dub. Qu. Journ.* for May, 1865, Dr. Frazer has given instances in point, in a paper of his entitled, "Remarks on a Common Herpetic Epizoötic Affection, and on its 'Alleged Frequent Transmission to the Human Subject;" and that it is not a rare condition we see on the authority of Von Bärensprung (*Brit. and For. Med.-Chir. Rev.*, July, 1857, p. 263), and Bazin (*Leçons sur les Affections Cutanées Parasitaires*, second edition, p. 126). In the course of a paper on Onychomycosis, by Mr. Purser, M.B., of this city (referred to in Chapter XIII), the writer remarks that "Dr. Lowe has found epiphytic disease with great frequency among brewers, and attributes it to contact with the growing yeast. I may mention, however, that with unusual opportunities for observing the diseases of brewery laborers, I have been unable to confirm the observations of Dr. Lowe."—*Dub. Quart. Journ.*, Nov. 1865, p. 359.

32*

CHAPTER XII.

THE SYPHILIDÆ.

... the time of the distribution of the syphilitic ... in the system during the existence of the primary ... constitutional symptoms of the venereal disease, several ... which are in most cases developed in a space ... the exact limits of which experience has not yet ... but a period that usually varies from six ... even in some to from six to twelve months; ... these cutaneous eruptions hold a prominent ... in consequence of their extreme frequency ... their lingering effects. The diseases of the skin ... might in this cause present the same ele- ... characters as those which are so produced, and ... different cases the form of nearly every ... eruption which has been described in the pre- ... pages ... they have certain specific features by ... they are really distinguished. and the treatment ... their removal is to be effected consists in the ... of remedies calculated to eradicate from the ... to counteract the effects of the constitutional taint ... their existence is due. It is for these reasons ... most modern dermatologists have thought it neces- sary to describe the syphilitic eruptions as constituting a distinct group of cutaneous diseases.

Secondary syphilitic symptoms, more especially those which affect the skin, may also be developed in individuals who have never had the primary disease, the venereal virus being transmissible from parent to child; thus, a cutaneous eruption is not uncommonly witnessed soon after birth, the origin of which may be traced to the previous occurrence of syphilis, whether primary or secondary in either parent, it may have been even many months previously. Secondary symptoms are also by many practitioners, chiefly those of the English school, believed to be directly communicable by contagion, as in the breast of a nurse being affected by suckling an infant who has a venereal eruption on the mouth, by the act of kissing, &c.; but the truth of this view, one so difficult to be proved, has been ably impunged by M. Ricord—an analysis of whose observations has been given in the twelfth and thirteenth volumes of the *Dublin Quarterly Journal of Medical Science*—and his arguments, fully cor- roborated by my own experience, incline me to agree with the opinion, that secondary symptoms are not con- tagious.

Syphilitic cutaneous eruptions have certain features in common by which they are specially characterized and distinguished from other diseases of the skin; these it will be well to consider shortly before speaking of the indi- vidual varieties.

Since they were first recognized as being dependent on a special cause, it has been noticed that although the syphilides may differ in the elementary form which they assume, they invariably present a peculiar dull tint of a brownish or coppery hue, which is more or less evident in all their stages, and also that they are rarely accompa- nied by the active, local inflammatory symptoms which often attend other cutaneous eruptions. The shade of color by which they are marked varies in different cases from a pale brown to a dull copper, the difference depend- ing both on the natural color of the complexion and on the degree to which it is effected by the syphilitic ca- chexia; thus, when the secondary eruptions appear in a short space of time after the occurrence of the primary symptoms, the hue of the diseased surface is of a less dull tint than when they are not developed for several months, the venereal virus affecting the system more, and conse- quently producing a more decided constitutional effect, the longer it has lain dormant in the system. For the same reason the more acute forms of syphilitic eruptions, or those which are occasionally attended with some degree of local inflammatory action, occur either when the primary symptoms are still present, or shortly after they have disappeared.

Another remarkable feature which the syphilides possess in common is a tendency of the eruption, no matter where situated or of what form, to assume a circular or annular shape as regards its distribution, and to spread over the surface of the body in rings or crescentric-shaped patches: this is especially remarkable when they are of the papular, the squamous, and the hypertrophic types, and least manifest in the syphilitic maculæ and pustulæ.

They are also characterized by their more general occurrence on the exposed regions of the skin, especially on the scalp, the forehead, the cheeks, and the alæ nasi, than on those parts which are ordinarily covered; the eruption, too, is more thickly disseminated there. They appear, however, more frequently on the trunk of the body than on the extremities, being especially developed on the back and the shoulders.

Lastly, syphilitic eruptions engage the more deeply seated cutaneous structures to a greater extent than the non-specific diseases of the skin, as is evident by the greater hypertrophy of the integuments that attends them, the firm, indurated feel by which they are characterized, and the greater elevation over the surface of those which are papular or pustular. They are, moreover, essentially chronic in their nature; the stains which remain on the skin after they have been cured are usually very permanent; and they are even more apt to return than the other cutaneous eruptions, which are complicated by no special constitutional taint. Ricord has noticed sternal tenderness as a symptom of acquired syphilitic taint; and Dr. Broderick has more recently called attention to this, which he believes to be a diagnostic sign.— See *Madras Quarterly Journal*, New Ser., Oct. 1862.

The development of the secondary symptoms of syphilis, in the form of a disease of the skin, is almost invariably preceded and accompanied by well-marked signs of derangement of the system generally. The individual about to be affected has have recovered in all effects from the immediate consequences of the primary

ack, and even a considerable period of time may have
pssed, during which he seems to be and feels in the
joyment of his ordinary health, when, without any
nifest exciting cause, a degree of cachexy is esta-
shed: the complexion becomes sallow and earthy-
king, unwillingness to take part in any active exertion,
ether of mind or body, is experienced, the appetite
a, thirst becomes constant, often extreme, pains in the
soles and bones, much exacerbated at night, are com-
ined of, and venereal periostitis and sore throat in
he cases precede and in others accompany the cuta-
us eruption which now appears; the outbreak being
general immediately preceded by a pretty smart fever-
attack. To a certain degree the syphilides resemble
eruptive fevers, and by many writers the analogy
ween them has been made a subject of special ob-
vation: the similarity consists in both having a stage
incubation following the contagion, a period of febrile
ression preceding the eruption, and a characteristic
er attending its development, which ceases to a greater
less extent when the eruption appears fully on the
face.

As the scope of this work does not admit of any ac-
nt being given of the other secondary symptoms of
venereal disease which usually accompany the syphi-
s cutaneous affections, and which in many cases aid
ch in arriving at a correct diagnosis between them
l the non-specific affections of the skin, I shall now
ceed to speak of the special characteristics of the
ividual eruptions, describing them in the order of
ssification which I have adopted, as they present the
nptoms of the groups therein contained.

Reference may here be made to Cazenave's *Traité des
philides*, in which the whole subject is discussed at con-
srable length, and to the beautiful plates accompanying
t well known work. With regard to the importance
a knowledge of the secondary symptoms of syphilis in
nection with the diagnosis of the subjects of this
pter, a most concise, brief, and intelligible definition
them and of the syphilides will be found in the valua-

gh it is less prominent, during the day. It is an
mon form of syphilitic eruption, but when it does
is extremely obstinate. By some dermatologists it
ed that syphilitic urticaria is not unfrequently de-
d on the skin as a symptom of the primary disease,
sequence of its appearing while a blennorrhagic
rge is present; but when an eruption of urticaria
essed in such cases, it most probably always de-
on the administration of copaiba, which has been
noticed as being the cause of the disease.

hilitic Roseola (see Cazenave's Plate I).—This is
st common of the secondary eruptions belonging
group; it generally appears in from four to six
after the apparent cure of the primary symptoms,
metimes even months elapse before the outbreak.
ave and Wilson both describe it as occurring on
in while chancres still exist on the genital organs,
so as a frequent concomitant of blennorrhagia; but
, with whose views my experience coincides, re-
its causation in such cases to be rather referable to
ious venereal attack; at all events all must admit
most total impossibility of arriving at a true his-
f the precedent occurrences in individuals laboring
any of the symptoms of syphilis. The eruption
loped usually on the forehead, and the upper part
face, but sometimes on the trunk and extremities
the form of small circular patches, scarcely ele-
above the surface of the skin; they are of a dull
d or bronze hue, and fade but slightly on pressure.
dividual rings do not at first exceed the size of a
g, but, gradually increasing, two or more coalesce,
form large circumscribed patches, the borders of
however, still retain an annular character. The
ak of the eruption is in general preceded by some
febrile symptoms; it comes out rather rapidly on
n, being often fully developed in twenty-four hours,
runs a more acute course than most of the other
itic cutaneous affections. Occasionally slight itch-
ends it, but this soon disappears with some super-
pidermic desquamation; in all cases copper-colored
for some time mark the site of the eruption after

roseola, a similar
present in the
usual secondary
roseola occurs
the symptoms of

appear in the form
by some
venereal eruption,
Herpes, also occurs,
descriptions of
more applicable

secondary symp-
from time to time
characteristic example
eruption appears
the trunk of the
rarely extend-
are developed some-
patches of skin,
these patches gradually en-
are developed on them:
they may attain by coalescing,
more or less of a circular
spreads in an annular form,
appearing at the edges. The
and are accompanied by com-
discharge: the stains attended
exudation remain on the surface
considerable period, and fresh crops of
time to time developed on them; the
however, do not become thickened and
as in non-specific eczema. In some cases, when
the eruption has existed for a long time, or is attended
with more active inflammation than usual, it presents
many of the characters of eczema impetiginodes, but the
crusts or scabs which form are dark brown or blackish,

hard, dry, and very persistent. Syphilitic eczema is generally late in being developed after the disappearance of the primary symptoms, several years not uncommonly elapsing, so that if we were to reckon, as some do, from time, and not according to order of occurrence, it might be classed in most cases as a tertiary and not a secondary affection.

Syphilitic Pemphigus is a very rare form of venereal eruption, which occurs more frequently, however, in new-born children than in adults. It is not preceded by any apparent constitutional disturbance; several moderately sized bullæ are simultaneously developed generally on the palms of the hands and the soles of the feet, but I have seen them on the buttocks also; each bulla is surrounded by an areola of a dull violet tint; the contained fluid is turbid from the first, does not completely distend the epidermis under which it is contained, and is rather slowly absorbed, the dark stain, remaining. After the absorption of the effused serum, the spot on which the bulla was situated most generally becomes the seat of an unhealthy ulcer, and then the disease almost invariably proves fatal.

That Syphilitic Pemphigus occurs at all in the adult is doubted by some; and others extend this doubt to its existence in children. M. Diday believes the first condition to be rare—" if it occur at all;" and MM. Gibert and Bazin deny its existence altogether. M. Ricord, however, does believe in its existence in the adult, and so does Dr. M'Call Anderson.[1]

Syphilitic Rupia (see Cazenave's Plate III) presents nearly the same characters as the prominent variety of the non-specific eruption. The vesicles, which are rather large and flattened, are developed in successive crops, especially affecting the face, but appearing also on nearly every region of the body, being most rare on the hands and feet. Each bulla is surrounded at first by a tolerably broad margin of a dull red or copper color, over which, as in ordinary rupia, the characteristic crust gradually

---

[1] Syphilitic Pemphigus in the adult. Is there such a disease ?— *Glasg. Med. Journ.*, July 1st, 1864.

itutional derangement immediately attends the out-
of syphilitic ecthyma, and the local symptoms which
de amount merely to slight itching, there being
er heat nor pain. It is one of the most frequent of
syphilitic eruptions in infants and young children,
s witnessed more commonly in old persons than in
in the prime of life.

SYPHILITIC PAPULÆ.

e SYPHILITIC PAPULÆ (see Cazenave's Plate VIII)
leveloped always in the form of the non-specific
en simplex or Lichen agrius; they constitute a very
non secondary cutaneous eruption, and occur usually
early period after the contamination of the system
the venereal poison, being often present on the skin
the primary symptoms still exist, or being devel-
in a few weeks after they have disappeared. In the
er case the affection runs a much more acute course
in the latter.

chen syphiliticus is usually preceded by some fever
general heat of the skin; the eruption comes on very
ly, the entire cutaneous surface of the body, includ-
the face and extremities, being sometimes covered
innumerable, minute papulæ, within twenty-four to
eight hours. They are placed so close together,
in patches or groups of a circular form, as to coal-
and present the appearance of large elevations, which
re the aid of a lens to prove that they are made up
e minute papulæ which are so characteristic of this
ion. At other times they are scattered over the sur-
perfectly distinct from each other, when, however,
h less numerous, they are individually of large size;
her case they present a bright copper color. The
læ generally disappear in a few weeks, with slight
rmic desquamation, as in the ordinary forms of the
se, but the surface remains spotted with dull coppery
, which fade away very slowly; and not uncom-
y a second outbreak of the eruption takes place
ly after the first has commenced to decline. In some
ns, especially those of a full habit of body, and in

33*

face, the scalp, and the entire trunk, especially affecting the chest and shoulders; the surface of the skin on which the squamous eruption is seated is of a dull violet or dark coppery-red color, and is elevated somewhat above the surrounding integuments. In the leproid form the edges of the circular patches are much raised, and the centres, which are always of a more dingy hue, depressed and free from scales, or with a few thin scattered scales on them. In the aggregated variety the outer border of the patches assumes more or less of an annular character, and, as Biett has remarked, it is separated in the majority of cases from the surrounding non-affected integument by a narrow white rim; the central portions are much more elevated than the edges, and the scales on them are thicker and of a dull gray color. Syphilitic psoriasis differs especially from the non-specific disease in not being more thickly developed around the joints than elsewhere on the extremities. In some cases, when the eruption has been of long persistence, it presents the tes-sellated pavement character described at page 235; but fissures do not form in the scales, nor is it attended with an ichorous discharge, or the symptoms of local irrita-tion which characterize the inveterate variety of the ordinary disease. Syphilitic scaly eruptions are of ex-treme obstinacy, and their duration is invariably much prolonged; when they begin to disappear the desquama-tion—which, however, is never in such quantity as in the non-specific squamæ—gradually diminishes, the ele-vated surface becomes flatter, until it at length sinks to the level of the surrounding integument, but still retains its peculiar copper color, which disappears very slowly, years often elapsing before it fades away completely.

Syphilitic psoriasis is in some cases confined to a single region of the body, especially the palms of the hands, when it presents most of the phenomena characteristic of ordinary psoriasis palmaris, but the scales are thicker, of a duller hue, more persistent, and the portion of integu-ment on which they are developed is more elevated, drier, and of a copper color; the general appearance of the palm of the hand when affected with the eruption is

such that Biett termed it *horny*, the affection
the *Syphilide squameuse cornée* of that dermat

The squamous syphilides are very rarely s
dren, and are still more rarely developed
time in old persons, being an affection of in
the prime of life, liable to accompany either t
secondary or tertiary venereal symptoms.

SYPHILITIC HYPERTROPHIÆ.

In the SYPHILITIC HYPERTROPHLÆ a fo
neous affection occurs which has no parallel
non-specific diseases of the skin; custom
pletely sanctioned the application of the ter
its different varieties that it is almost hope
think of changing this denomination, and for
notwithstanding the great objections, so freque
to in the preceding pages, which exist to re
word in the nomenclature of cutaneous nosolog
attempt to substitute another for it. Condylo
belong to this group of diseases of the s
already noticed, most frequently of syphilitic
as, when of this nature, they fall altogether
domain of general surgery, no further de
them than what has been given at page 308
here. For the same reason warts which re
venereal source will not be noticed. Th
tubercles will therefore alone engage attent
sidering this group of cutaneous diseases as s
of secondary syphilis.

Syphilitic tubercles (see Cazenave's Plates,
and XII) are among the most frequent of th
symptoms of the venereal poison which affe
they may be developed in a very short tin
disappearance of the primary disease, or thei
may be deferred for many months, or even
tubercles vary much in size and in their ap
nomena, and thus constitute different varie
they may occur in the form of large papul
from lichen chiefly as regards their size,
equal to that of a small pea; they are rounde

elevated above the level of the skin, appearing in small groups, most usually of a circular shape, with healthy skin intervening, and not unfrequently forming a centre to each patch. These groups are irregularly disseminated over the surface of the face, the neck, the trunk, and the extremities, especially the first; but are often symmetrical as regards the two sides of the body. The individual tubercles, which are of a violaceous or dull coppery hue, soon secrete a thin scale at their summit, beneath which, if rubbed off or torn with the nails, a slight watery exudation takes place; this dries into a thin, reddish-brown, persistent scab, which eventually falls off, leaving a characteristic syphilitic stain that for a long time marks the seat of the eruption.

Second, the tubercles are of greater magnitude, varying in size from that of a nut to that of an olive, of an ovoid shape—hard, distinctly elevated, and disseminated over the surface; they may occur on a single region of the body, especially affecting the face and neck, or may be generally distributed over the surface. In some parts, being more closely set together than in others, they sometimes coalesce and form a tolerably large tumor, uneven on the surface, but distinctly circular at the margin. The tubercles in this variety are of a deeper and duller shade of color than in that first described; neither desquamation nor serous exudation takes place from them; they remain stationary for a very long time, not unfrequently for years, and at length, being absorbed, often rather suddenly, the characteristic stain, slow to fade away, marks their site.

Third, a still larger tubercle than the last appears isolated, on some portion of the integument, most generally of the extremities, but sometimes of the body and face; it is rather soft to the touch, slightly painful, scarcely elevated above the surrounding skin, of a dull violaceous tint, with a bronze or copper-colored margin. It increases very slowly in size, exhibiting an appearance as if about to suppurate, and the margin assumes an uncircumscribed erythematous blush. At length the most prominent part ulcerates slightly, a thick, blackish, adherent crust forms on it, which is very gradually detached, usually not for

weeks, when the entire tubercle falls out, leaving an unhealthy, indolent ulcer, with excavated edges, painful and
slow to heal. At first rarely more than three or four
tubercles of this character are developed on the body, but
they come out in successive crops, so as at length to
amount to a considerable number. When the ulcer
which they leave heals, a permanent depressed cicatrix
results, which for a long time exhibits a rather bright
copper-red stain. This variety of tubercle rarely appears
for years after the primary symptoms, is generally met
with in old persons, or those of a broken-down habit of
body, and in individuals in whom there exists extreme
syphilitic cachexia.

Fourth and last, several tubercles, about the size of a
sixpence, but little elevated above the surface, and rather
soft to the touch, are developed, distinct from each other,
on some special region of the body, usually on the scrotum
in males, and the pudendal region in females, on the face,
particularly on the lips and nose, and around the arms;
they are perfectly circular, and of a dull reddish tint.
Small superficial ulcers soon form on them, appearing
first at the outer margin; these gradually extend so as to
cover the entire surface of the tubercle, retaining, however, their superficial character, and from them there
exudes an extremely fetid, sanious liquid, which irritates
and inflames the neighboring integument over which it
may flow. Eventually the discharge ceases, copper-colored crusts form, and the parts heal without any marked
cicatrix. By many modern writers, particularly of the
French school, this form of syphilitic tubercle is regarded
as constituting, in some cases, one of the varieties of primary symptoms.

SYPHILITIC MACULÆ.

Under the head of SYPHILITIC MACULÆ some of the
forms of secondary roseola are not unfrequently described;
but they should not be confounded with the peculiar pigmentary alterations of the cutaneous structure which in
many cases accompany other secondary eruptions, and in
some constitute the only affection of the skin present.

hey resemble most, in their apparent phenomena, ephe-
hepatica, but differ from it in being developed in the
jority of cases on the legs, or in the region of the gen-
organs, occurring only in a few instances on the face
the trunk of the body. They are also characterized
their color, which is distinctly of a copper shade, at
nes approaching to black, and in assuming from the
st a well-marked circular form, spreading from the cir-
mference in ring like patches. These morbid altera-
ns of color do not appear on the cutaneous surface
ally until several months or even years have elapsed
er the cure of the primary symptoms; they are inva-
bly attended with well-marked syphilitic cachexia, and
extremely obstinate to treatment, sometimes remain-
for life. Syphilitic maculæ occur at all ages, both in
sons in the prime of life and in old age, and are a not
frequent result of congenital syphilis.

Diagnosis of Syphilides.—Under this head little remains
be said after the observations which have been made
the commencement of the chapter on the general char-
ristics of the secondary eruptions. The history of
individual case, where it can be arrived at satisfac-
ily, which, however, in the majority of instances is
te impossible, is the aid chiefly to be relied on; in
btful cases assistance is often gained by an examina-
n of the glans in males, and the external organs of
eration in females, when the cicatrix or induration
ulting from a chancre, if it had previously existed, will
ord satisfactory evidence; inspection of the throat and
k of the pharynx also should never be omitted, the
racteristic venereal ulceration existing there usually
connection with the eruption on the skin.

Prognosis in Syphilides.—The prognosis in secondary
aneous affections must be guided much by the degree
syphilitic cachexia present, by the length of time
ich they may have previously existed—for in propor-
n to their duration is their obstinacy—by the severity
l extent of the concomitant circumstances in other
uctures of the body, and by the nature of the eruption
lf: the latter point has been noticed in the description
the individual forms.

Treatment of Syphilides.—As in all other affection which have their origin in the absorption of the syphiliti poison into the system, the secondary eruptions of th skin demand a specific mode of treatment, directed to the eradication of the constitutional taint on which the depend. Formerly it was believed that this could alone be effected by the action of mercurials, but the discove of iodine and of its medicinal properties has wrought complete revolution in the therapeutics of the consecu- tive symptoms of the venereal disease. This has in so me respects, however, been attended with an evil result, th a of inducing many practitioners to discard mercury al to gether as a remedial agent in the treatment of the sypl hi lides, and to trust to the employment of such sim pl measures as may be indicated by the local and gene ra symptoms, independently of their specific character; o to rely solely on the administration of preparations o iodine to correct the constitutional contamination. Bu as in nearly every other disease to which man is subj ect it should always be kept prominently in view that an exclusive system of treatment cannot be expected to be invariably successful, for the same affection often requi res the use of even the most opposite remedies in differ ent individuals, or in the same person under different circu m- stances.

The remedies to be employed in the treatment of *the* syphilides may be conveniently considered under th ree heads: the general, the specific, and the topical.

The *general* treatment consists in the employment of means, calculated to meet the indications dependent on the special symptoms which may arise or be present in individual cases. Thus, when the outbreak of an erup- tion is attended with distinctly febrile symptoms or well- marked local inflammatory action, the employment of antiphlogistics is demanded before the administration of specifics can be commenced. Under such circumstances, in young plethoric persons, Dr. Neligan was of opinion that general bleeding will be resorted to with advantage, and that topical abstraction of blood by means of leeches is almost invariably necessary. Active saline purgatives should be given also, and in no case should they be

omitted; with very few exceptions their effects are productive of the most beneficial results in the early stages
of every syphilitic eruption : the only instances in which
they occasionally prove injurious are, when the syphilitic
cachexia is extreme in very old persons or individuals of
a broken-down habit of body.   They seem to act chiefly
by determining to the intestinal mucous tract, and thereby
diminishing excessive cutaneous action, the quantity of
the eruption, and consequently the local inflammation,
being thus checked; but they also lessen the general
febrile symptoms.   The neutral purgative salts are best
adapted to fulfil these intentions, and their administration
will be advantageously preceded by a full dose of calomel
or blue pill.

On the other hand, should the vital powers be low, and
the depression of the system very manifest, as is very
frequently the case, the vegetable tonics must be given;
and if there are deep-seated pains present, especially the
nocturnal pains so characteristic of the disease, opiates
in full doses should be prescribed in combination, or if
the suffering is extreme their use may precede the employment of the tonics.   No preparation so well relieves
the deep-seated pains which so frequently accompany
secondary symptoms, whether of the skin or not, as crude
opium : it may be given in the dose of a grain made into
a pill, three or four times, or even oftener, in the twenty-
four hours, according to circumstances.   Of the vegetable tonics, those which determine to the skin, such as
the elm bark, are especially useful ; or cinchona bark or
quina may be combined with the tonic or stimulating
vegetable diaphoretics—dulcamara, mezereon, sarsaparilla, guaiacum, &c. : the mineral tonics, especially the
stronger acids, and iron and its preparations, are also
often highly serviceable in the Syphilides, when the employment of this class of remedies is indicated.   The
former were largely given by Biett in the syphilitic
exanthemoid and papular secondary eruptions, much
reliance being placed by him on the nitric and sulphuric
acids: the latter are especially indicated when much
anæmia is present, and they are often usefully prescribed
in combination with iodine, as in the chemical compound
34

of the iodide of iron, or of the iodide of iron and quina, When a specific eruption occurs in an individual of a scrofulous diathesis, or with a strumous tendency, cod-liver oil will be administered with decided benefit; and should the debility be extreme, preparations of iron are usefully given at the same time.

The *specific* treatment of the syphilides consists in the employment of the preparations of mercury, of gold, or of silver, and of iodine alone or in combination with any of them. Dr. Neligan was of opinion that mercurials are unquestionably the remedies on which most reliance is to be placed, but that the amount of benefit to be derived from their use depends much on the manner in which they are administered, and the preparation that is employed. They should not be given on the first appearance of the eruption, the more especially if its outbreak is connected with general febrile symptoms; these must be previously removed by the means already referred to: and in all cases the state of the digestive organs requires special attention before their employment is commenced. The several forms of the secondary eruptions serve as indications as to what preparation of mercury is best suited, but it may be laid down as a general rule *that those which have the property of pro-ducing salivation quickly or freely, such as blue-pill, calomel, and the allied compounds, are rarely adapted for these conse-quences of the venereal disease.*

For the scaly and tubercular syphilides, corrosive sublimate and the red iodide usually prove the best preparations of the metal; either may be given in pill with opium, in doses of from 1-12th to 1-8th of a grain three times daily, the quantity of opium being propor-tioned to the degree of the characteristic venereal pain which may attend; or the former may be preferably prescribed in some vegetable decoction, such as that of dulcamara, of elm-bark, of mezereon, of sarsaparilla, &c., as in the following formula:—

R. Corrosivi Sublimati, ... granum.
Infusi Dulcamaræ, ... uncias quatuor.
Decocti Mezerei, ... uncias duodecim.
Infusi Sassafras,[1] . . . . uncias octo. Misce.
Sumat uncias duas fluidas ter indies.

When these or any other of the syphilitic eruptions become chronic, or return frequently after they have been apparently removed, it will be necessary to have recourse to the administration of arsenic, in combination with the mercury and iodine, and under such circumstances Dr. Neligan was of opinion that Donovan's solution—the liquor arsenici et hydrargyri hydriodatis of the last *Dublin Pharmacopœia*—proves singularly beneficial. It is for the chronic forms of secondary diseases of the skin that this combination is especially adapted, and in these cases its therapeutical efficacy is undoubted; indeed (he adds), in my hands, it has very rarely failed to effect a permanent cure, but it must be given in moderate doses—from ten to twenty minims three times daily—the quantity increased very gradually, and its use continued for a long time. even after the disappearance of the eruption. It may be administered in some of the vegetable tonic or diaphoretic decoctions, according to individual circumstances.—[? Gradually increased doses.—ED.]

For the pustular and papular syphilides the green odide of mercury of the last *Dublin*—the iodide of the last *London—Pharmacopœia*, has proved, in my experience, the best preparation of the metal. It may be given in pill, combined with opium, should circumstances indicate the use of that drug, in the dose of from half a grain to three grains, three times daily, but its effects must be carefully watched, as it is in some persons apt to produce salivation, even in small doses; and in the treatment of any form of syphilitic eruption it is most important to administer as little mercury as possible, and to introduce it very gradually into the system; the precise quantity requisite can only be judged by watching the effect produced in each individual case, but the

[1] See Macnamara's (Sixth) Elition of Neligan's *Medicines, &c.*, p. 248.

mildest action on the mouth is always an indication that for the time enough has been given. An excellent way of prescribing this preparation for adults is to substitute it for the calomel in Plummer's pill, and the vegetable decoctions before referred to may be given at the same time.

The syphilitic exanthemata do not require the employment of specific remedies in their acute stages; but should they exhibit a tendency to become chronic, the green iodide of mercury is the preparation best adapted for them. The occurrence of maculæ as a secondary symptom indicates the necessity for a prolonged administration of a mercurial, and, therefore, either the chloride[1] or the red iodide should be used.

When any of the forms of syphilitic eruption appear on infants at the breast, it is desirable, when practicable, to introduce the specific medicine into the system of the child by means of the nurse's milk; but as in the majority of cases it is essential to change the nurse, and is, consequently, often requisite to wean the infant, the hydrargyrum cum magnesiâ, or hydrargyrum cum cretâ, may be given in doses of from one two grains daily, according to the age; and with each dose from a twelfth to an eighth of a grain of the green iodide of mercury may be combined, when the eruption is extensive.

The preparations of gold and of silver were at one time proposed by the French school as substitutes for those of mercury, but they were found not to possess at all the same efficacy, and they have, consequently, fallen into almost complete disuse for the treatment of secondary symptoms. The former were supposed to be especially adapted for persons of a scrofulous diathesis, with whom mercurials very generally disagree; and their effects are highly spoken of by Legrand and Chrestien, but they have not, that I am aware, been employed in this country.

Iodine or its preparations should not be trusted to alone with the intention of producing a specific action in

---

[1] Hg Cl, Hydrargyrum Corrosivum Sublimatum.—*Brit. Pharma-copœia.*

the treatment of the second[...]
been already said it is an [...]
with mercurials is of espec[...]
prescribed, they usually [...]
their administration sh[...]
mercurial must be given w[...]
the evidences of syph[...]
much the more must the [...]
rations predominate in the [...]
tion of iodide of potass[...]
results as soon as the prepar[...]
have been given evidence[...]
the mouth being affected an[...]
when given to nurses with [...]
real eruption in an infant a[...]
case, it often suffices to [...]
nurse is at the same time affected w[...]
symptoms or not.

The employment of [...]
of the syphilides is co[...]
non-specific eruptions [...]
majority of cases, that the [...]
second or third day, to al[...]
matory action which may a[...]
healthy functions of the sk[...]
in the progress of any of the [...]
black-wash is the best appl[...]
it takes place on the sa[...]
but on the face, an [...]
calomel to an ounce of [...]
applied and is more eff[...]
symptoms are usually more [...]
they are easily calmed by [...]
powder, containing twenty gr[...]

[1] Lorsque les syphilides [...]
utiles pour consolider la guéris[...]
monie des principales f[...]
Pour obtenir ce dernier résul[...]
avantageuse; elle est indiqué[...]
avec accidents nerveux con[...]—*X. [...]*
et les Scrofulides et sur [...]
P. 211.

lead, half a drachm of the oxide of zinc, and an ounce of starch, reduced together to a state of the minutest division; a tepid bath of fresh water, containing from two to four ounces of size, should be at the same time employed every night, or every second night, according to circumstances. The dispersion of the stains in syphilitic maculæ is much hastened by inunction with mercurial ointment while the constitutional treatment is being followed out.

Dr. Hillier notices " a very good way of administering mercury without disturbing the digestive organs." This is effected by means of a vapor bath, in which from ten to twenty grains of calomel are volatilized and brought in contact with the skin, together with steam. In Holmes's *Surgery*, Vol. I, p. 422, Mr. Henry Lee describes a simple form of apparatus. It consists of a tin case containing a spirit lamp; immediately over the wick of which is a small circular tin plate on which the calomel is placed; around this is a circular furrow, in which hot water is placed. This is placed on the ground; the patient, closely wrapped in a cloak from the neck down, sits over it in a cane-bottomed chair. Dr. Hillier very strongly recommends this; and in a case recently under the observation of the Editor its judicious use effected an apparent cure.

The practice of *Syphilization*, or inoculating with the syphilitic virus, has, of late years, been advocated by Professor Boëck, of Christiania, and others. As it is connected with the treatment of secondary syphilis, and so is beyond the scope of this work, the Editor can only refer to copious analytical reviews and papers on the subject in the *Dublin Quarterly Journal* for Feb. and Nov. 1857, and May, 1861; also, Professor Boëck's papers, in the *Lancet* for Aug. 1865.

In all cases of secondary syphilitic eruptions, as soon as the first inflammatory symptoms, if any occur, are subdued, the diet should be nutritious, and wine and other stimulants should be allowed; if the syphilitic cachexia be extreme, and much debility present, the chief points to be attended to are, to support the strength and at the same time to allay both general and local

ritability. Change of air, especially to a dry and
arm climate, is an aid to the treatment of the utmost
portance in chronic and obstinate cases.

It may not be out of place to mention here "the Zitt-
ann treatment," advocated by some Continental authors,
d by Mr. Wilson, who gives it "with the strongest
commendation in its favor." Mr. Wilson 'concisely
lls it "a triple compound of starving, purging, and
reating." The plan, as follows, is given in the words
' Dr. Fox, who, however, does *not* recommend it:—
First day, a purge (calomel and jalap), and three meals
' broth; up to the fifth or sixth day four pints of the
ittmann decoction are taken daily; of these four, two
nts are made of the strong and two of the weak decoc-
on (*vide* formulary following), with each day two ounces
' meat and two of bread; on the sixth day an active
urge, with broth as before; the seventh till tenth, repeat
e drinks, and meat and bread; this continues till the
urteenth day or so, and then the patient is kept on low
iet, allowed to get up, but still continues to take a small
uantity of the decoction. If convalescence is tardy
r insufficient, the same treatment must be recom-
ended."—Fox, *op. cit.*, p. 289. The formula Mr. Wilson
ives thus in his latest work—*Student's Book, &c.*, p.
74:—

DECOCTUM ZITTMANNI FORTIUS.

B. Radicis Sarsæ concisæ, . . ℥xij.
    Aquæ fontanæ, ... libris (libras) lxxij.

Digest for twenty-four hours; then add, tied up in a piece
f linen:—

Sacchari Albi,
Aluminis, ... aa ʒvj.
Calomelanos, ... ʒiv.
Hydrargyri bisulphureti rubri (Cinnabar) . ʒj.

Simmer down to twelve quarts; towards the close of the simmering
dd:—

Seminum Anisi, contus.,
Seminum Fœniculi, contus., ... aa ℥ss.
Foliorum Sennæ, ... ℥iij.
Radicis Glycyrrhizæ, concisæ, ... ℥ss.

Press and strain, and, after standing until cool, decant the clear
quid and bottle twelve quarts.

The bottle of the stronger injection is to be taken *warm* every twelve ...... in the day; and one bottle of the weak solution is ... between twelve o'clock and bedtime. The ... objects to this plan of treatment that it is inapplicable in a general way, because of the very great inconvenience to the patient, for such he literally is when undergoing all this physic. The system itself is nothing more than a perpetuation of the old plan, not yet disused elsewhere, of ...ring what is popularly termed "an apothecary's shop" down a patient's throat.

CHAPTER XIII.

DISEASES OF THE APPENDAGES OF THE SKIN.

In this chapter I shall describe affections of the hair and of the nails. They constitute a class of morbid changes, concerning which the regular medical practitioner is but rarely consulted, and therefore a short notice of them must here suffice; yet the former, especially, are not uncommonly a cause of as much anxiety to those who suffer from them as a really grave cutaneous disease.

In Plenck's Classification of 1776, Morbi unguium and Morbi pilorum were the last two orders. They were rejected by Willan, but there is no doubt that they might have been retained with advantage. Dr. Neligan's supplementary group, "Diseases of the Appendages of the Skin," it is obvious, is nothing more than a return to the principle, and almost to the letter, of Plenck's nosology.

DISEASES OF THE HAIR.

The DISEASES OF THE HAIR consist in alterations of its natural color or characters, and in its partial or total loss. Some few cases have been recorded in which the hair has undergone a sudden change of color from a light to a dark hue, or the reverse, without any apparent cause, or after some acute disease; and not unfrequently when it is reproduced after it has been removed for some febrile or other affection, it grows of a much darker color than it had been originally; this is usually the case when it has been kept cut close for any length of time in the treatment of any of the eruptions of the scalp.

Loss of color in the hair—*Canities* (grayness)—is one of the natural results of old age, but it often occurs at a

comparatively early period of life, either from con:
tional causes or from extreme mental anxiety.   The e
of the latter is often well marked, and some cases
been witnessed in which the hair has become perf:
white in the space of a few hours, while an indivi
was laboring under some violent emotion of the m
these, which have often furnished a theme for the~
and the popular writer, demand no other notice here
that of a mere reference.[1]   The most important of
constitutional causes of canities is hereditary predis
tion, and examples of premature grayness of the
descending through several generations in certain fam
are very numerous.   Blanching of the hair is somet
associated with debility of the vital powers, but that
very rarely so is evident from the fact of its bein
seldom witnessed in those who die young of consum;
or other lingering diseases.

While, as a general rule, canities is one of the ac
paniments of old age, yet the cases of very old per
are numerous in which no sign of it can be dete
The editor believes this will be found true occasion
with insane persons, who have lived for many yea
a state of mental aberration, and have died a
advanced age.   In a recent case which he had u
observation for several years, an old lady who had
more or less insane for nearly fifty years, died at the
of ninety-three with as beautiful tresses of brown ha
any young woman could have.   She had not a si
gray hair.   A full account of this remarkable case
read by the editor before the Medical Society of the
lege of Physicians, in 1863, and was subsequently
lished in the *Dublin Quarterly Journal* for February, 1
under the title of "A Short Biographical Sketch
Remarkable Case of Insanity."

Canities of the beard is in the present day chiefly no
in persons who have abolished the irrational and unm
use of the razor.   In such cases it very frequently

[1] The well-known case of Queen Marie Antoinette, of France, v
beautiful hair turned to a silvery gray color in one night, is a ca
point.

pens that that portion of the beard which had been pre-viously shaved at first appears gray when allowed to grow. This canities, however, in many cases disappears as soon as the newly-grown beard has lost its coarse appearance—a process which sometimes takes so long as two or three years. The reader will find more full information respecting the beard in a paper by the editor, entitled, "The Hygienic Aspects of Pogonotrophy," published in the *Dublin Quarterly Journal* for February, 1864.

Treatment, whether topical or general, has, in my opinion, no effect over any of the forms of canities except that last described, and in it the indications are manifestly to restore the system to a state of robust health, if practicable, by the use of such remedies as may be appropriated for the individual case. But numerous local applications and other means have been and still are recommended, with the view of preventing the hair from turning gray; should it be dry and crisp, and the surface of the scalp appears bloodless, any gently stimulating pomade may be used; cutting the hair short, or removing it altogether by shaving the scalp occasionally, proves useful. The preparations which are used for dyeing the hair are very numerous, and formulæ for them are given in all druggists' or perfumers' receipt books.

The occurrence of white hair in patches on the scalp has been already described—See Vitiligo.

The only alteration in the character of the hair which can be strictly regarded as a disease is that peculiar felting and matting of it together which constitutes the singular affection that has been named *Plica Polonica*. This disease, which is "der weischelzopf" of the Germans, is an affection of the hair endemic in Poland and the surrounding countries, where it is said to be produced by the bad living and unclean habits of the inhabitants. After inflammation of the scalp, which becomes swollen, red, and sore to the touch, a viscid exudation takes place from it, matting the hairs together, so that, as Dr. Fox observed—"Lice, pus, blood, and fungous elements are found mixed together in the plicose felting." This disease affects the scalp, pubes, nails, and sometimes the

chin and axillæ; and after some months the diseased mass
is said to be "pushed off." Dr. Fox, from whose description the above is for the most part condensed, considers
it to be of the same nature as the Pellagra, or modified
forms of elephantiasis, viz., a result of action of deteriorating influences upon the general nutrition at large.
He also observes that a.fungus—the trichophyton sporuloides of Günsburg—has been found, and is supposed to
be the real cause of the disease, the soil favoring the
development of a parasitic fungus. On the other hand,
Gustav Simon could not find any vegetation in the hairs
themselves, and he regards the disease as consisting
chiefly of an abnormal secretion from the surface of the
skin, not especially implicating the hair follicles. Fuchs
believed the sticky material to come from the hair follicles. Hillier thinks that the real nature of the disease
is not fully proved, and Hebra suggests that it is not a
distinct disease, but eczema or some other skin affection
much neglected. Dr. Neligan never saw a case of it, nor
has the Editor had that advantage.

Loss of hair or *baldness*, termed "Alopecia" by the
ancient writers on medicine,[1] would appear to have been
of much more frequent occurrence and to have attracted
more attention formerly than at present; it may be eithe
partial or general on the hairy scalp, or on the other
parts of the body which are naturally covered with hair.
In the former case, it was termed *Porrigo decalvans* by
Willan, but then it is manifestly due to the occurrence
of Vitiligo on these regions of the skin, as before described. General baldness is in many persons the accompaniment of old age, being usually associated with gray
hairs, nor can it be regarded as a disease except when it
occurs in comparatively early life; some few cases have
been recorded as being congenital, in which, however, it
was due to non-development of the hair follicles. Permanent baldness, as has been remarked in the preceding
pages, is also at times a result of the eruptive diseases of
the scalp, especially of Porrigo, and is then a consequence

---

[1] From ἀλώπηξ, a fox; because foxes suffering from the *mange* are
more or less bald.

of the inflammatory action which may exist extending to the bulbs; after most diseases of the scalp, however, although the hair falls out, it is reproduced. Loss of hair, partial or general, is also a not unfrequent sequence of fevers and acute inflammatory affections, and of syphilis; in the former case it generally grows again, but in the latter the baldness is usually permanent. Loss of hair from natural causes at an early age is, like the premature change of its color to gray, hereditary in the majority of instances, is also caused by violent emotions of the mind, or prolonged mental anxiety, and is connected pathologically, in some individuals, with general debility, or diminished vital action.

It has been frequently remarked in this country that Alopecia is common among young men of the middle and upper classes in England, while in Ireland it is comparatively rare. This has been sometimes attributed to the custom of wearing hats indoors, particularly in merchants' offices, in clubs, and places of public resort; but whatever may be the true cause, the fact of the general prevalence of Alopecia among young men in England is notorious.

Alopecia sometimes occurs as a consequence of mental anxiety. In another work[1] the Editor has noticed a curious case which happened in the South of Ireland about the middle of the seventeenth century, and is recorded by Dr. Stearne, founder of the College of Physicians, as having come under his own observation. A young man was successfully operated on for a stone in the bladder. The stone was in one piece, and weighed eleven ounces; yet after six days, during which the urine flowed through the wound, the natural function of the urethra was restored, and the parts healed without suture or plasters. The young man's father, who was aged sixty-three and in robust health, was present at the operation, and was so violently affected by fear of his son's death, that within twenty-four hours every hair on his head fell off. Afterwards he complained of extreme heat in his head, was

[1] *Memoir of John Stearne, M. & J. U. D., with a Review of his Writings.* Dublin: 1865.

deprived of vision for two hours, and lo! his hair began to bud forth anew.[1]

Congenital and senile baldness are incurable, as is also that form of it which is hereditary. In other cases, repeated shaving the head, or keeping any hair that may remain constantly cut close, and the application of stimulating spirituous washes, such as either of the following, sometimes prove useful :—

R. Spiritus Vini Rectificati, ... uncias sex.
Ammoniæ Hydrochloratis, . . . grana triginta.
Olei Rosmarini, ... semi-drachmam.
Infusi Armoraciæ compositi,[2] . . uncias sex.
Misce. Fiat lotio.

R. Tincturæ Cantharidis, ... drachmas duas.
Aquæ Sambuci, ... ; . . uncias undecim.
Spiritus Rosmarini, ... drachmas sex.
Misce. Fiat lotio.

The turpentine pomade, as ordered at page 329, not unfrequently proves of service also, and each time, previously to its application, the scalp should be washed with an alkaline lotion, containing a drachm of carbonate of potash to eleven ounces of water, and one ounce of rectified spirit or of rum. The following pomade, as recommended by Dr. Copland, I have frequently used with excellent effect :—

R. Adipis præparati, ... uncias duas.
Ceræ Albæ, ... semi-unciam.
Lento igne simul liquefac, tunc ab igne remove et ubi primum lentescant,
Balsami Peruviana, ... drachmas duas.
Olei Lavandulæ, ... minima duodecim.
Adyce, et assidue move donec refrixerint.

In cases of what he calls *Symptomatic* alopecia, M. Hardy recommends the application of the following preparation : Ox marrow, one ounce : castor oil, half an

[1] "Illius pater annum agens sexagesimum tertium, robustus tamen, huic periculosæ operationi interfuit : mox vehementiori mortis filii sui, capitis pili universæ intra horas viginti quatuor defluxere. Dein de aegerti capitis ardore conquestus est, et ad binas horas visu orbatus fuit, et crines jam regelascit."—*Sturæ Johannes, Animi Malica,* p. 43, Dubl. 1835.

[2] *Pharmacop. Lond.*

Ounce; gallic acid, twenty grains; tincture of rosemary, half a drachm.—See *Journ. de Méd. et Chir. Prat.*, Sept. 1864; and Ranking's *Abstract*, Vol. XL, page 123.

Mr. Wilson (*Student's Book of Cutaneous Medicine*, p. 432) notices a variety of alopecia which he terms *Area*, or *Alopecia areata*. This consists in total loss of hair in a circular patch, and sometimes in the form of an elongated band which, from its resemblance to the trail of a serpent (ὄφις), has been called *ophiasis*. The sudden discovery of one or more bald spots is the first intimation of this disease, which Mr. Wilson believes to be essentially a *neurosis*. It is not limited to the scalp, but also occurs in the beard, whiskers, and eyebrows, as well as on the body and limbs. The Editor has known it to be cured by repeated shaving, once weekly for months. There is a very good illustration of it in the Sydenham Society's edition of Hebra's Plates. Dr. Fox believes it to be parasitic, the fungus being the microsporon Andonini.

In all forms of alopecia the scalp should be kept warm, and consequently wearing a wig is often of service when the hair first begins to fall off.

See Dr. Ross *On Ringworm, Scall Head, Baldness, &c.*, quoted in Chap. XI.

DISEASES OF THE NAILS.

Most of the DISEASES OF THE NAILS are of such a nature as to demand surgical interference, and are consequently described in the works of surgical writers. Perhaps the most important of them all is that in which the nail of some of the toes grows into the surrounding fleshy integuments, and by the irritation thus occasioned gives rise to the formation of a foul, unhealthy ulcer. It would not be in accordance with the plan of this work to say anything here of the surgical treatment requisite to cure this most obstinate and painful affection; but I cannot avoid remarking on the importance of preventing the *ingrowing*, as it is termed, of the nails, by always cutting them straight across, parallel with the extremity of the toe, as when they are cut at the edges the pressure of the boot or shoe not uncommonly gives rise to this disease. The nails both of the hands and feet are also subject to inflammation attacking their matrix, to hypertrophy and to atrophy, and they occasionally fall off completely, and are not reproduced. This last affection, which has been termed by the French writers *Alopecia unguale,* is sometimes congenital, children being born without nails; but such cases are extremely rare. When the nails become hypertrophied, the application to them of caustic potash, and the daily use of a strong lotion of carbonate of potash is often useful; the nitrate of silver is the best application when the nails, being brittle, split and break readily; and it is also productive of much service should a foul discharge continue from beneath the nail, as a consequence of previous inflammation of the matrix. As has been remarked already, the nails at times become engaged in some of the eruptive diseases of the skin, more especially psoriasis and eczema, when, however, they require no further treatment than that applicable to the existing affection.

Onychomycosis.—From ὄνυξ and μύκωσις, and that from μύκης, a fungus.

This term is applied to cases in which a parasitic disease of the nails is believed to exist. As already remarked, the instances are not rare in which diseased nails accompanied cutaneous affections, but a few cases have been noted where what was believed to be parasitic disease of the nails existed alone. Some of these, as noted by Meissner and Virchow, will be found in Küchenmeister's *Manual of Parasites* (Vol. II, p. 228), already referred to; and, more recently, two cases ard detailed in an interesting paper in the November number of the *Dublin Quart. Journ.* for 1865, by Mr. John M. Purser, M. B., of this city.

In one of these cases the patient had, three years before, suffered from a skin affection of uncertain nature, which was confined to the dorsal surface of the left thumb, on which the skin reddened, and small blisters formed. The nail became thickened and discolored, and, after a considerable time, small collections of matter formed under and near the root of the nail, and discharged by its edge, or became absorbed. The nail now presented the following appearance: "It was of a dirty brownish-yellow color, streaked with lines of a darker brown, greatly thickened, and at its free extremity separated from its bed by a mass of soft nail substance which could be easily picked out. The entire nail was somewhat roof-shaped, a prominent ridge running along its centre, from which it sloped down on each side towards its attached edge. Its sides were concave from above downwards; its surface was very rough, and marked by deep transverse grooves; the longitudinal striæ also were strongly marked; it was very hard, more brittle than natural, and inclined to split longitudinally, and in flakes. Near the root was a small portion of nail of a pink color, but rough and thickened; there was no trace of lunula; a small abscess existed at the root, and the skin in the neighborhood was slightly red and swollen."—Purser, *Op. cit.*, p. 353.

Microscopic examination.—Mr. Purser removed a portion of the nail and some of the loose substance lying under it, and found that the superficial horny part presented nothing remarkable in its appearance, save its thickness. "Some of the cells, however, were opaque and granular, and others were of a brownish color; but in the deeper layers of the nail the elements of a fungous growth were found in abundance. These were: I. *Spores*, circular or oval, either scattered, collected in groups, or forming moniliform chains. In some of them a central nucleus-like spot was apparent. II. *Tabular filaments*, tortuous and branching; these were for the most part jointed at intervals, and many of them contained small shining bodies. III. *Larger, less branched filaments*, of a brownish color, and containing spores at regular and close intervals; the walls of these filaments were sometimes indistinct, the spores being apparently attached to each other, end to end, forming a moniliform chain, which was often seen to terminate in a dense cluster of minute spores, or in a mass of granular matter. IV. *Granular matter.* All these were mixed up with tolerably healthy nail plates, and were rendered very clear by caustic soda or potash." Space would not admit of a detailed account of Mr. Purser's second case, in which the microscopic appearances differed slightly from those seen in the first.— The microscopical appearances in both cases, and the appearances of the nail in Case I, are well figured in good woodcuts accompanying his excellent descriptions and commentary, which convey the impression that in both cases the fungous growth was secondary to disease of a non-specific kind.

Treatment.—In cases where the disease appears to be connected with cutaneous or specific disease—*e. g.,* syphilis—the treatment resolves itself mainly into attention to the primary affection; where it is non-specific, blisters have been tried, but with small success. If its parasitic nature be admitted in a given case, as it clearly must be in Mr. Purser's cases—of course the parasite should be destroyed as soon as possible, and the recurrence of its growth prevented by raising the tone of the system and improving the general health. In the first of Mr. Purser's cases he cut and scraped away some of the thickness of the nail, and then applied a weak solution of corrosive sublimate as a parasiticide.

CHAPTER XIV.

THERAPEUTICS OF DISEASES OF THE SKIN.

In describing the individual eruptions of the skin I have spoken of the treatment adapted for each, yet there are some general points in therapeutics especially applicable to this class of affections which require a separate notice, and to their consideration I propose to devote this chapter: it will, therefore, consist in a review of the remedies most generally used in cutaneous diseases, and the manner in which they should be employed; a few formulæ which may prove suggestive in prescribing will also be appended. The remedial measures ordinarily required may, for convenience of description, be considered in two divisions—the *topical* and the *constitutional;* it is true that some of them, baths for example, produce their effects by acting both locally and on the system generally, but as their mode of application is external they will be considered in the former division.

Several objects are in general expected to be fulfilled by the employment of *topical* medication in the treatment of cutaneous eruptions. It may be used with the view simply of cleansing the skin from the scales or crusts which form on the surface, so as to ermit the direct application of remedies to the diseased parts: for this purpose cataplasms, baths, alkaline washes, and soaps are usually had recourse to. It may be employed with the intention of protecting the affected portions of the integument, from the action of the air; or a directly therapeutical effect may be expected from its application. Some topical remedies fulfil only one of these indications, while the benefit derived from the use of others depends on their mode of operation combining the three.

The treatment of diseases of the skin *by the total exclu-*

sion of air has, of late years, more especially since the discovery of collodion, been much employed and highly recommended by some practitioners, while in the hands of others it has completely failed. The practice is chiefly applicable to local eruptions, and to those which are not attended with much discharge. Its employment in erysipelas and in smallpox has been referred to when speaking of the treatment of those diseases, but it has not as yet been sufficiently tested by experience to enable a satisfactory conclusion as to its therapeutical efficacy to be arrived at. So far as regards the application of collodion to form an impermeable covering, it has been productive rather of injury than of benefit in any cutaneou eruptions in which I have used it; this appeared to me to depend chiefly on the uneven compression and contraction of the integument which it occasioned, causing much local irritation, and sometimes even a degree of inflammation. Such effects being due principally to the rapidity of evaporation of the ether in which the guncotton is dissolved, these resulting injurious consequences will, to a considerable extent, be prevented by adopting the plan of the late Dr. Graves, who, in the *Dublin Quarterly Journal of Medical Science* for August, 1852, recommended the employment of a solution of gutta percha in chloroform for this purpose. Moreover, the gutta percha forms a less brittle, firmer, and thicker, though still transparent, covering to the skin, and exerts an even and more complete compression on the surface; the latter effect also being regarded by Dr. Graves as of importance with reference to its beneficial action. In his paper on the use of this substance, above referred to, Dr. Graves illustrates its therapeutical efficacy by the narration of some cases in which it proved remarkably successful; but the experience of other practitioners is more in favor of the use of a solution of India-rubber in chloroform.

The advantage to be derived from the application of *bandages* to either the upper or lower extremities, when they are the seat of cutaneous eruptions, is too often overlooked; they fulfil to a certain extent the indication of excluding the action of the air, but they also prove beneficial by exerting an equable amount of compression on the overloaded and congested vessels, as has been already noticed when speaking of erysipelas; and they afford, in addition, a useful means of applying medicated lotions, as referred to in describing the treatment of eczema.

The various remedies which are employed topically for the treatment of diseases of the skin may be applied to the surface in the form of baths, cataplasms, caustics, lotions, ointments, powders, and soaps. These will now be considered in succession.

Baths, both simple and medicated, have at all times been very extensively used as remedial agents in cutaneous eruptions, and have by many been supposed to be sufficient for their cure, without the administration of any internal remedies. To the reader of the foregoing pages it must be evident that I place comparatively little reliance on their efficacy, and that I recommend a resort to their employment with the intention of acting, so to say, medically on the disease in but few cases: yet it cannot be denied that abundant testimony exists to prove that persons affected for years with chronic eruptions, more particularly those of a scaly character, have been cured by the prolonged use of medicated vapor, steam, or water baths. But they are not at present employed to at all the same extent that they were formerly, and modern writers do not recommend baths in the same laudatory terms as those who preceded them—a proof that their efficacy was, to say the least, somewhat overrated. As a cleansing agent, and to promote the discharge of the healthy functions of the skin, and a return to its normal state, the fresh water tepid and warm baths are of especial service in many cutaneous eruptions, chiefly those in which the surface is dry and hard, as in the exanthemata, the scaly diseases, and ichthyosis; and when these affections are local, they are often advantageously employed in the form of douche; but they seldom agree with those cases which are attended with a discharge, whether it be serous or purulent. In addition to their cleansing effects they also often prove useful, as antiphlogistics, in allaying local irritation and inflammation.

Vapor baths, being slightly stimulant, are not indicated until the chronic stages of cutaneous diseases are fully established, when, in consequence of their possessing this property, they are frequently used with advantage. A *vapor bath* may be advantageously given on the plan described by Mr. Grantham in the *Brit. Med. Journ.*, 20th August, 1864. In this bath the patient sits on a cane-bottomed chair, with his feet in a foot-bath, while he is covered from the neck downwards with a blanket which envelops the chair also. He is, of course, quite nude, save this covering. A quantity of boiling water in an open vessel is placed under the seat of the chair, and in the pan is placed a red-hot brick. A *sulphur bath* may be given in this way by boiling six ounces of sulphur in the water; or an *ammonia bath* by introducing two ounces of the strong liquor ammoniæ before the introduction of the red-hot brick.

The portable Oriental vapor bath of Messrs. Benham and Froud, of Chandos street, London, is noticed by Dr. Fox, as a *modified* form of the above. It contains a complete set of apparatus for all kinds of fumigation, and it costs about thirty shillings.

Salt water bathing, in my experience, proves injurious in most diseases of the skin; for although it often appears at first to produce a beneficial action, the eruption usually returns afterwards with greater obstinacy, and is much more rebellious to treatment; but usually, and always when the affection is of an inflammatory tendency, it aggravates the disease: the only cases in which I have seen it almost invariably serviceable are when maculæ or stains of the integument become persistent after the removal of any of the syphilitic eruptions. The following are formulæ for some of the medicated baths usually employed:—

GELATINE BATH.

℞ · Gelatinii (*vulgo dicti "Size"*), . . . libras sex.
Aquæ (Caloris gradu, 75° ad 92° F.) . oongios triginta,
Solve.

This bath is employed with excellent effect to allay local irritation and itching, and is especially useful in the cutaneous diseases in children. The temperature must be proportioned to the indications in each case. The above are the quantities requisite for a bath for the entire body in the case of adults.

ALKALINE BATHS.

℞. Sodæ Carbonatis, ... uncias octo.
Aquæ Pluviæ (Caloris gradu, 84 ad 96°
F.), ... congios triginta.
Solve.

℞. Potassæ Carbonatis, ... uncias sex.
Aquæ Pluviæ (Caloris gradu, 84° ad 96°
F.), ... congios triginta.
Solve.

℞. Sodæ Carbonatis, ... uncias sex.
Boracis . . . . uncias duas.
Aquæ Pluviæ (Caloris gradu, 75° ad 98°
F.), ... congios triginta.
Solve.

These alkaline baths are often usefully employed as detergents of the surface when it becomes covered with thick crusts or adherent scales. They should be used with caution when any tendency to inflammatory action exists in the skin. They are also of service in chronic scaly eruptions, especially pityriasis, and in ichthyosis.

IODINE BATHS.

℞. Iodi, ... grana triginta.
Iodidi Potassii, ... semi-unciam.
Glycerini, ... uncias duas.
Aquæ (Caloris gradu, 86° ad 94° F.), . . congios triginta.
Solve.

℞. Iodi, ... grana sexaginta.
Liquoris Potassæ, ... unciam ad uncias
duas.
Aquæ Pulviæ (Caloris gradu, 86° ad 94°
F.), ... congios triginta.
Solve.

℞. Brominii, ... minima viginti.
Iodidi Potassii, ... uncias duas.
Glycerini, ... unciam.
Aquæ (Caloris gradu, 86° ad 94° F.), . . congios triginta.
Solve.

Iodine baths are used in very chronic cutaneous eruptions, when there is much hypertrophy of the integuments. They may also be employed in aggravated cases of prurigo.

which they may be seated; caustics have been thus used, especially in the treatment of the eruptive diseases of the scalp and in squamous affections; my experience of their effects, however, is not in accordance with the opinion of those who report favorably of their application. Besides nitrate of silver—which is the favorite caustic in skin diseases—chloride of zinc, and caustic potash, some practitioners use a strong solution of iodine, which may be prepared as follows:—

R. Iodi, ... grana triginta.
   Aquæ destillatæ, ... drachmas quinque.
   Iodidi Potassi, quantum sufficit ut fiat solutio.

The following formula for a compound caustic solution is contained in the Pharmacopœia of the London Hospital for Diseases of the Skin:—

R. Zinci Chloridi, ... semi-unciam.
   Antimonii Chloridi, ... grana centum et
      viginti.
   Pulveris Amyli, ... grana sexaginta.
   Glycerini, ... quantum sufficit.
      Misce.

Vienna paste is also frequently used. It consists of equal parts of caustic potash and unslaked lime; mixed *for use* with alcohol.

Dr. Burgess' bicyanide of mercury caustic consists of two grains of the salt to one ounce of water. He recommends it for acne rosacea; to be painted on the affected parts for a few minutes, followed by the application of cold water. Dr. Hillier uses a "biniodide of mercury caustic," composed of equal parts of red iodide of mercury and prepared lard; he also gives a form for preparing "chromic acid caustic"—100 grains to an ounce of prepared lard. Dr. Frazer uses "corrosive collodion," as may be expressed in this form:—

R. Collodii, ... drachmas duas.
   Hydrargyri Corrosivi Sublimati, . . . grana sexdecim.
      Misce.

He also gives a very useful preparation, "glycerine with iodine." It may be thus expressed:—

R. Iodi, ... grana triginta.
   Potassii Iodidi, ... grana viginti.
   Glycerini, ... semi-unciam.
      Misce.

Whether caustics be resorted
of diseases of the skin, they sl
exclusion of other remedial m

Lotions, were it not for the
effectually in many cases and
body, constitute the best form
tion in the treatment of a gr
eruptions. Their special appli
when treating of the individu
are to be used, and several for
have been given. They are
means of bandages kept const
as this method is applicable
when the eruption is situated
integument, they may be appli
linen or lint, covered with a t
which is preferable for this po
not keep the surface so hot,
mitting a certain degree of ev
spirituous or other cooling lot
course admissible, and then t
moistened with the wash as oft
addition of glycerine to lotion
in consequence of its non-evap
the part to which they are ap|
moisture; this is peculiarly t
lotions, which tend to render t
an evil that in many cases wou!
effects that might result from
pendently of their use with th
direct medical action, lotions
ficially employed to cleanse
viously to the renewed applica
this purpose they are applied
should the crusts or scales that
adherent, a roll of lint wet with
over the part. When the
lotions which are used for the
irritating or astringent they
diluted by adding to them ar
In addition to the formulæ fr

tained in the several preceding chapters, the following
may also be employed for the purposes indicated:—

STIMULATING ALKALINE LOTIONS.

R. Liquoris Ammoniæ, ... unciam.
Glycerini, ... drachmas sex.
Spiritûs Lavandulæ, ... drachmas duas.
Aquæ destillatæ, ... uncias sex.
                                          Misce.

R. Liquoris Ammoniæ Sesqui-Carbo-
natis,[1] . . . . uncias decem.
Glycerini, ... uncias duas.
                                          Misce.

R. Sodæ Carbonatis, ... grana viginti.
Spiritûs Rosmarini, ... unciam.
Aquæ Rosæ, ... uncias septem.
                                          Misce.

These lotions are adapted for all eruptive diseases in
which the external application of alkalies is indicated,
when their chronic stage is attended with atony of the
cutaneous surface.

SEDATIVE ALKALINE LOTIONS.

R. Boracis, ... grana centum et
                                          viginti.
Aquæ Sambuci, ... uncias undecim.
Aquæ Lauro-Cerasi, ... unciam. Misce.

R. Sodæ Bicarbonatis, ... grana triginta.
Aquæ Aurantii, ... uncias undecim.
Succi Conii, ... unciam. Misce.

Chiefly used in eruptive diseases of a dry nature, which
are attended with much itching.

Hardy's sedative lotion, for use in lichen, prurigo, and
pudendal irritation, is as follows:—

R. Potassi Cyanidi, ... grana quindecim.
Aquæ, ... uncias octo.
                                          Misce.

This should be kept in a dark place.

ANODYNE LOTIONS.

R. Acidi Hydrocyanici diluti, . . . drachmas duas.
Aquæ Lauro-Cerasi, ... semi-unciam.
Glycerini, ... uncias duas.
Aquæ Sambuci, ... uncias novem.
                                          Misce. [Frazer.]

[1] Of last London Pharmacopœia.

℞. Spiritûs Chloroformi, ... uncias du
    Glycerini, ... uncias du
                      Misce. [

GLYCERINE WASH.

℞. Glycerini, ... uncias du
    Misturæ Amygdalæ, ... uncias sex
    Aquæ Rosæ, ... uncias oct

ASTRINGENT LOTIONS.

℞. Tincturæ Acetatis Zinci (*Ph. Dub.*,
    1829), ... drachmas
    Aquæ Rosæ, ... uncias oc
                      semisse.

℞. Acidi Tannici, ... grana qua
    Aceti Gallici, ... semi-uncia
    Aquæ destillatæ, ... uncias sep
                      semisse.

℞. Creasoti, ... minima oc
    Tincturæ Krameriæ, ... drachmas
    Acidi Hydrocyanici, ... minima oc
    Aquæ destillatæ, ... uncias qu

In using this lotion the bottle in which it i
should be well shaken before it is applied to

CAZENAVE'S ALUM LOTION.

℞. Aluminis, ... grana cent
    Infusi Rosæ Acidi, ... uncias vig

DUPEY'S SULPHATE OF COPPER LOTIC

℞. Cupri sulphatis, ... grana sex
    Zinci Sulphatis, ... unciam cu
    Aquæ destillatæ, ... uncias vig
    Aquæ Lauro-Cerasi, ... semi-unci

For use in Sycosis.

SULPHUROUS LOTION.

℞. Sodæ Hypo-Sulphitis, ... semi-unci
    Potassæ Sulphuratæ, ... grana sex
    Aquæ destillatæ, ... uncias un
                      semisse.
    Aquæ Lauro-Cerasi, ... semi-unci

STIMULANT WASH.

℞. Tincturæ Nucis Vomicæ, . . . semi uncia
    Spiritûs Camphoræ, ... drachmas
    Essentiæ Carui (Ph. Dub.), . . drachmas
    Aquæ destillatæ, ... uncias sep

This last wash is sometimes a useful application in the chronic stages of lichen simplex, when the disease is very obstinate, of prurigo, and in inveterate psoriasis, provided there is no tendency to local inflammatory action.

Ointments, under which appellation I include cerates and pomades, are more generally employed than any other form for the application of topical remedies in the treatment of diseases of the skin; this is owing chiefly to the facility with which they can be used, and the readiness with which their strength may be increased or diminished—both matters of great practical convenience and utility; yet they have the disadvantages of being easily rubbed off, of affording but little protection to the diseased surface, and soiling the clothing with which they come in contact. In some cutaneous eruptions the application of any greasy matters disagrees remarkably, but this appears to depend, in the majority of cases, rather on some constitutional cause in the individual affected than in a specialty of the eruption which may be present; it also seems to be to a certain degree influenced by the region of the skin on which the disease is situated; thus, I have seen them prove injurious more frequently in the eruptions of the scalp than in those of any other part of the body. With affections which are accompanied by excessive serous discharge, as in most forms of eczema, they also, in my experience, generally disagree more than with any others. We can, however, seldom ascertain the existence of this peculiarity except by direct trial; but when it is once discovered to exist, the use of ointments should then be carefully avoided. Prepared axunge, in consequence of its greasy nature, does not, therefore, form a good basis for ointments to be used in the treatment of cutaneous diseases, except in cases attended with much hypertrophy of the integuments, as in ichthyosis, and in the chronic stages of some obstinate eruptions which are not accompanied by copious discharges; and the white wax ointment—which is employed for the preparation of nearly all the ointments contained in the last edition of the *Dublin Pharmacopœia*— is often not well adapted for this purpose in consequence

... I have therefore, latterly ... either cold cream or the ... of the French pharmaceutists, as the ... ointment I prescribe: the latter pre... already remarked when speaking of the ... in itself a ... local application, possessing ... and healing properties. As ... of either of them are contained in but very few English works on Materia Medica, it will be well, I think, ... —

... (Cold Cream).[1]

... ...	. . . .	uncias sexdecim.
... ...	. .	uncias quatuor.
... ...	. . .	uncias sexdecim.

'Let the wax ... the oil with a gentle heat, in an earthen vessel; ... the mixture into a marble mortar, previously heated, and stir it ... until it is nearly cold; then, by beating up the cerate ... incorporate with it the rose water, added in small quantities at a time.'

... wax may be substituted for the white wax in ...

... (Cucumber Pomade).[3]

...	. . . . .	libras duas.
... ...	. . .	semi-libram.
... ...		
... ...	. . . . .	uncias viginti et quatuor.

'Mix and bruise them well with the hand: set aside for twenty-four hours, then pour off the juice, and replace it by a similar quantity of fresh juice, and repeat this process ten times, adding fresh juice, each time. As soon as the pomade has acquired a well-marked odor of the cucumber, melt it in a water-bath, and add an ounce of finely-powdered starch, which will combine with the water and precipitate it. Allow the entire to settle, and then pour off the pomade into small vessels. To render it more white and smooth the French pharmacists usually prepare it for use by melting again in a water-bath, and beating it for two hours, or even longer, with a wooden spatula; but when submitted to this treatment it does not keep fresh for a longer period than a month: while in the former case it will keep for a year, or even longer, in a cool place.''

---

[1] The "unguentum simplex," of the *British Pharmacopœia*, is, to some extent, free from this objection to its predecessor—unguentum ceræ albæ.

[2] French Codex.

[3] Henry and Guibourt—*Pharmacopée Raisonnée.*

I shall now append some formulæ, in addition to those already mentioned, for ointments which are ordinarily employed in the treatment of diseases of the skin. And first, I may mention that an excellent calmative ointment, especially useful in the cutaneous eruptions of children which are attended with heat and itching, may be prepared by substituting cherry-laurel water for rose-water in the above formula for cold cream.

SEDATIVE OINTMENTS.

R. Chloroformi, ... minima sex.
Cerati Cucumis, ... unciam. Misce.

R. Carbonatis Plumbi, ... grana triginta.
Cerati Galeni, ... unciam.
Chloroformi, ... minima quatuor.
Misce.

R. Glycerini . . . . drachmam.
Unguenti simplicis, ... grana tercentum
et septuaginta.

Chloroformi, ... minima octo.
Cyanidi Potassii, ... grana quatuor.
Misce.

The great advantage derived from the employment of chloroform, alone or in combination with other sedatives, as an external-application in the treatment of cutaneous diseases, has been frequently referred to in the foregoing pages. In the preparation of ointments it should always be the last ingredient added, in consequence of its volatility, and for the same reason the ointment *should be dispensed in bottles* and not in boxes or pots.

ASTRINGENT OINTMENTS.

R. Carbonatis Calcis præcipitati, . . . grana centum et
viginti.
Cerati Galeni, ... uncias duas.
Extracti Belladonnæ, ... grana viginti.
Glycerini, ... drachmas duas.
Misce.

R. Oxydi Zinci, ... grana viginti.
Cerati Galein, ... unciam.
Tincturæ Myrrhæ, ... semi-drachmam.
Misce.

R. Creasoti, ... minima decem.
Adipis præparati, ... uncias duas.
Pulveris Opii, ... grana octo.
Misce.

... the preceding remarks must be held to qualify, ... as to the use of soaps. ... ... as to the beneficial results ... ... Emulsine Dispensary *Soap*, and the ... ... *Tar Soap*, before referred to in ... ... *Edinbl. Gazette*, for 1859, ... of this city, described the prepa- ... ... will be found very useful in ... ... affections—such as pityriasis, psoriasis, ... herpes. This soap is composed of ... ... of white curd soap, 3 oz. of ... ... extract of birch bark, and 12 oz. ... ... In the expressed liquor the glycerine is ... ... will be found elabo- ... ... Mr. ...'s paper above referred

... ... which are administered *internally* in ... ... of the skin, with the view of ... ... system require but little notice ... ... described, and several ... ... prescriptions in the preceding ... ... the individual diseases.' The ... ... constitutional treat- ... ... one which has been before ... ... in most cases, a prolonged ... ... which may be employed, ... should be given at first in ... ... steadily increased afterwards ... ... Dr. Neligan held that this ... ... in respect to those powerful alter- ... ... which are still valuable agents ... ... produce injurious conse- ... ... and a tendency to ... ... being given at first in ... ... such is true of cod-liver oil and ... ... which are of daily use in the ... ... of the skin.

... ... giving the above opinion of Dr. Neligan ... ... to the principal prescriptions in with regard to the administration of arsenic in gradually increasing doses, the Editor is convinced that it is better administered by not giving large doses at any time ; but by beginning with the largest dose intended to be given, and continuing the same, unless it should appear desirable either to diminish or discontinue it.—See also Hunt *On Diseases of the Skin, in loc.;* and Cummins *On the Use of Arsenic—Dub. Qu. Journ.,* Nov. 1864.

During the employment of any of these remedies their administration should be occasionally omitted for a day or two, whether they cause constitutional manifestations of their effects or not, and the bowels freely acted on by purgatives, those of a saline nature being preferred if the patient's strength admit of their use.

The following formulæ may, in addition to those already given in the preceding chapters, serve to aid the practitioner in prescribing the medicines which are ordinarily used in the treatment of this class of affection :—

DIAPHORETIC PILLS.

℞. Antimonii Oxidi, ... grana nonaginta.
Morphiæ Hydrochloratis, ... granum cum semisse.
Confectionis Rosæ, quantum sufficit ut fiant pilulæ, viginti et quatuor.

Sumat duas sextis horis.

℞. Antimonii Sulphurati, ... grana sexaginta.
Pulveris Ipecacuanhæ cum Opio, . grana sexaginta.
Guaiaci Resinæ, ... grana centum et viginti.
Theriacæ, quantum sufficit ut fiant pilulæ sexaginta.
Sumat unam sextis horis.

ALKALINE MIXTURE.

℞. Liquoris Potassæ, ... semi-unciam.
Infusi Dulcamaræ, ... uncias undecim.
Tincturæ Chiratæ, ... semi-unciam. Misce.
Sumat unciam fluidam ter indies.

ALKALINE CATHARTIC DRAUGHT.

℞. Solutionis Alkalinæ (Brandish), . drachmam.
Potassæ Sulphatis cum Sulphure,
(*Ed. Ph.*), ... grana nonaginta.
Aquæ destillatæ, ... uncias duas.
Tincturæ Aurantii, ... drachmam.
Misce. Fiat haustus, primo mane ante jentaculum sumendus.

DIAPHORETIC MIXTURES.

R. Tincturæ Guaiaci Ammoniatæ, . . . drachmas du
Mucilaginis Tragacanthæ, ... drachmas sec
Misturæ Amygdalæ, ... uncias tres.
Sumat unciam sextis horis.

R. Sarsæ, ... unciam eum
Aquæ destillatæ ferventis, ... octarium.
Per horas duodecim in vase clauso macera, subinde ag
cola, et

R. Hujus infusi, ... uncias decd
Infusi Sassafras,[1] . . . . unciam sem
Decocti Mezerei (Ph. Dub.), . . . unciam ound
Syrupii Hemidesmi, ... unciam. Mi
Sumat uncias duas fluidas ter quaterve indies.

ALTERATIVE MIXTURES.

R. Hydrargyri Bromidi,[2] . . . . . . semi-grammu
Infusi Dulcamaræ, ... uncias octo.
Sumat unciam fluidam ter indies.

This preparation may be administered in obstir
of secondary syphilitic eruptions; in its action if
allied to the red iodide of mercury.

R. Hydrargyri Iodidi Rubri, ... grana quinqi
Spiritûs Vini rectificati, ... drachmam.

Tere simul dein adde.

Aquæ destillatæ, ... unciam cum
Iodidi Potassii, ... grana centui
Syrupi Aurantii, ... semi-unciam
Sumat guttas viginti ter indies in cyatho vinoso infusi

This is a preferable form to that of a pill for th
istration of the red iodide of mercury in vene
tions.

R. Ferri Bromidi,[3] . . . . grana sexagi
Liquoris Arsenicalis, ... minima sexi
Syrupi Aurantii, ... semi-unciam
Aquæ Aurantii, ... unciam cum

Sumat drachmam fluidam ter indies in cyatho vinoso dec
Ulmi recentis.

---

[1] Vide Macnamara's (Sixth) Edition of Neligan's Medic
248.

[2] Vide Neligan's Medicines, &c. (op. cit.), p. 128.

[3] Vide op. supra cit., p. 640.

A useful form for the administration of arsenic in chronic cutaneous eruptions, attended with anæmia or much debility.

The publication of the *British Pharmacopœia*, since the appearance of the first edition of this work, has rendered necessary a very material alteration in the mode of expressing the numerous prescriptions scattered over these pages. These prescriptions have been translated into the existing language of officinal pharmacy, except where (chiefly owing to their being quotations) such was impracticable, retaining, of course, the essential identity in every case. With two or three exceptions, which sufficiently explain themselves, the directions for use have been put into Latin, as the Editor thinks they should be. The system of writing names and quantities in Latin and the directions in English he entirely disapproves of, on the grounds that, irrespective of its being unworthy of an educated man, it is a sop thrown to ignorance, and that by encouraging ignorance in a learned profession it directly tends to promote the evils which the writing of directions in English is intended to prevent.

Some men, whose scholarship is above reproach, deliberately adopt the plan here objected to for special reasons, as in the case of a friend of the Editor, who does so in order to impress the directions on the friends of the patients with whom the prescription is left. With many, however, it is the result of ignorance; a large number could not, if they would, express their directions in Latin, while a still larger number conceal the weakness of their Latinity under abbreviations and symbols, the use of the latter being altogether illegal in Ireland. The present confusion respecting the use of symbols should be set at rest by loyal obedience to the statute law, which provides thus: "And in order to prevent the uncertainties and dangers which may attend the setting down the quantities of medicines in chemical and numeral characters, in prescriptions, be it enacted by the authority aforesaid, That every physician, chirurgeon, or other person or persons, who now do, or hereafter shall, take upon him or them to prescribe internal or external remedies for the health of man's body in this kingdom, shall hereafter set down the

37

quantity or quantities of all and every medicine or ingredient, whether simple or compound, which he or the shall prescribe in any *recipe, formula,* or prescription, in words at length, and not in chemical or numeral characters, under the penalty of forty shillings for every such omission."—Stat. 1, Geo. III, cap. xiv, sec. 19 (Lucas' Act), made perpetual by 30 Geo. III, cap. xlv, sec. 11. For a more full discussion on this subject the Editor may refer to a paper of his in the *Dublin Quarterly Journal* for Aug. 1864, entitled "Brief Considerations respecting the Weights and Measures, and the Nomenclature of the Pharmacopœia."

Inasmuch as the pharmaceutical revolution caused by the appearance of the *British Pharmacopœia* renders a clear understanding of the doses of some important medicines imperative on the practitioner, the editor appends a posological table compiled from that in Professor Macnamara's valuable sixth edition of Dr. Neligan's well-known work *On Medicines:—*

POSOLOGICAL TABLE.

MEDICINE.	DOSE FOR AN ADULT.	FORM OF ADMINISTRATION.
Acidum Hydrocyanicum Dilutum,	1 to 2 minims,	In draught or mixture.
Ammoniæ Arsenias,	$\frac{1}{12}$ to $\frac{1}{6}$ of a grain,	In pill or solution.
Arsenici Iodidum,	$\frac{1}{16}$ to $\frac{1}{8}$ of a grain,	In pill.
Arsenicum Album,	$\frac{1}{16}$ to $\frac{1}{8}$ of a grain,	In pill.
Creasotum,	1 to 5 minims,	In draught or pill.
Ferri Arsenias,	$\frac{1}{12}$ to $\frac{1}{8}$ of a grain,	In pill or mixture.
Ferri Iodidum,	2 to 5 grains,	In pill.
Hydrargyri Iodidum rubrum,	$\frac{1}{16}$ to $\frac{1}{8}$ of a grain,	In pill.
Hydrargyri Iodidum viride,	1 to 3 grains,	In pill.
Hydrargyri Iodo Chloridum,	$\frac{1}{16}$ to $\frac{1}{12}$ of a grain,	In pill.
Hydrargyri Oxydum Rubrum,	$\frac{1}{16}$ to $\frac{1}{8}$ a grain,	In pill.
Liquor Arsenicalis,	2 to 8 minims,	In draught or mixture.
" Arsenici Chloridi,	3 to 10 minims,	In draught or mixture.
Liquor Arsenici et Hydrargyri Hydriodatis,	10 to 30 minims,	In draught or mixture.
Liquor Sodæ Arseniatis,	3 to 10 minims,	In draught.
Potassi Iodidum,	3 to 15 grains,	In draught or mixture.
Quiniæ Arsenias,	$\frac{1}{16}$ to $\frac{1}{8}$ of a grain,	In pill or mixture.
Sodæ Arsenias,	$\frac{1}{12}$ to $\frac{1}{8}$ of a grain,	In pill or draught.

Hygienic Treatment.—Before concluding, a few words are requisite as to the hygienic measures best adapted for cutaneous diseases. As a general rule, the diet must be, of course, regulated according to the individual requirements of each case; but as these affections are usually evidences of constitutional debility, though so frequently attended with a tendency to local inflammatory or irritative action, it should be nutritious, but not stimulating. Restriction to an almost purely milk and farinaceous diet is attended with the best results in the majority of instances, and should be almost invariably enforced with infants and children. Change of air to a dry, elevated position, is often of great service, but extremes of cold and heat should be avoided as much as possible. For the latter reason, the surface of the body should be kept as far as can be of a uniform temperature by attention to the clothing worn, which, however, should never be such as to check the insensible perspiration, or tend to condense it on the integuments. That worn next the skin should be soft and unirritating, and therefore woollens should be avoided, soft calico or silk being preferred for under-clothing. In referring to change of air I wish to record it as the result of my experience, that a residence at the sea shore usually proves injurious in cutaneous eruptions, the fine saline particles which float about in the atmos-phere appearing to aggravate the disease by exciting local irritation ; the climate of those districts which are situated a short distance inland is, however, well adapted for persons afflicted with them.

Great objections are often raised to the cure of cuta-neous eruptions, particularly those which are attended with a copious secretion, more especially if they have been of long existence, for fear of their sudden removal, or the stoppage of the discharge with which they may be at-tended, causing some grave internal disease ; but I have never seen any ill consequences result when they were removed by constitutional treatment, not even in the case of infants or children who may be teething ; on the con-trary, I have invariably witnessed the general health to be much improved in all respects thereby ; but the sud-den cure by the employment of topical remedies only, such as caustics or powerful astringents or stimulants, is certainly not advisable unless the eruption is of small extent and has been of short duration.

BIBLIOGRAPHICAL INDEX.

ADDISON, THOMAS.—On the Keloid of Alibert, and on true Keloid.— *Med.-Chir. Trans.*, Vol. xxxvii. Lond.: 1854.

ADDISON, THOMAS.—*On the Constitutional and Local Effects of Disease of the Supra-renal Capsules.* Lond.: 1855.

ADDISON, THOS., and GULL, WM.—On a Certain Affection of the Skin —Vitiligoidœa—α Plana, β Tuberosa.—*Guy's Hospital Reports* (N.S.) vii. 265. 1851.

ÆTIUS.—Tetrabiblos. Lat: per Janum Cornarium (in Vol. ii of *Medicæ Artis Principes post Hippocratem et Galenum.* Folio. Paris. Exc. Hen. Stephanus. 1567).

AITKEN, WILLIAM.—*The Science and Practice of Medicine.* 2 vols. Fourth Edition. Lond.: 1866.

ALDERSON, JAMES.—Notice of a Case of Skin Disease, accompanied with Partial Hypertrophy of the Mammary Gland.—*Med.-Chir. Trans.*, vol. xxxvii. Lond.: 1854.

ALFORD, HENRY (Dean of Canterbury).—*Greek Testament.* Lond.: 1859-62. 5 vols.

ALIBERT, JEAN LOUIS.—*Description des Maladies de la Peau.* Folio. Paris: 1825.

ALLEY, GEO.—*Observations on the Hydrargyria, or that Vesicular Disease arising from the Exhibition of Mercury.* Lond.: 1810.

AMERICAN JOURNAL OF MEDICAL SCIENCE. Edited by Isaac Hays. Philadelphia, U.S. Published quarterly.

AMERICAN MONTHLY JOURNAL OF MEDICAL SCIENCES.

ANDERSON, T. M'CALL.—*The Parasitic Affections of the Skin.* Lond.: 1861.

ANDERSON, T. M'CALL.—*A Practical Treatise upon Eczema.* Lond.: 1863.

ANDERSON, T. M'CALL.—Syphilitic Pemphigus in the Adult. Is there such a Disease?—*Glasg. Med. Journ.,* July 1, 1864.

ANDERSON, T. M'CALL.—*On Psoriasis and Lepra.* Lond.: 1865.

ARAN, M.—On Ferruginous Collodion.—*Br. and For. Med.-Chir. Rev.*, July, 1853, p. 277.

ARCHDALL, MERVYN.—*Monasticon Hibernicum; or, an History of the Abbeys, Priories, and other Religious Houses in Ireland.* 4to. Dublin: 1786.

ARCHIVES GÉNÉRALES DE MÉDECINE. Paris. Published monthly.

ARCKEN (VAN) G.—Description of the American Curate, a Non-classified Disease of the Skin.—*Amer. Month. Med. Journ.,* April, 1858.

Aretæus.—Ἀρεταίου Καππαδοκος τὰ σωζόμενα (The extant works of Aretæus. the Cappadocian). Ed. and Trans. by Fr. Adams, LL.D. Lond.: Printed for the Sydenham Society, 1856.

Avicenna.—Avicennæ Medici Arabi Liber Canonis, &c., cum Lucubrationibus Benedicti Rinii, M. D. Folio. Basiliæ: 1556.

Babington. Benjamin Guy.—On an Anomalous form of Eruptive Disease. which it is proposed to designate Rubeola Notha.—Trans. of Epidem. Soc., Lond. Vol. ii. Part I. Lond.: 1865.

Balfour, Geo. W.—Notes from Practice (On Erysipelas—Of its Treatment with Iron).—Month. Journ. Med. Sci., May, 1853.

Banks. John Thomas.—Cases of Ichthyosis.—Dub. Quart. Journ. Med. Sci., N.S., xii. Dublin: 1851.

Barensprung. Dr.—On the Existence of Herpes in Domestic Animals. and its Communication to Man.—Review of in Br. and For. Med.-Chir. Rev., July. 1857, p. 263.

Barensprung. Dr.—On the Treatment of Prurigo.—Dub. Quart. Journ. Med. Sci., May. 1860. p. 492.

Barensprung. Dr.—Herpes Zoster depends on an Affection of the Ganglia on the Posterior Roots of the Spinal Nerves (Dr. Schmidt's case in point).—See Ranking's Abstract, xli. p. 145. (This paper is misquoted in Chap. III of the present work, p. 123. as taken from Br. and For. Med.-Chir. Rev., Jan., 1863.)

Bartholini, Thom.—De Morbis Biblicis Miscellanea.—(Vide Ugalini's Thesaurus Antiquitatum Sacrarum, Vol. xxx, p. 1521. Folio. Venetiis: 1765. Classed Fag. W. 1—30, in Library Trin. Coll., Dub.)

Barton. J. K.—Case of Bronzed Skin, with Disease of the Suprarenal Capsules.—Dub. Hosp. Gaz., 1859, p. 203.

Bastian. H. Charlton.—On the Structure and Nature of the Guinea Worm.—Trans. of Linnæan Society, Vol. xiv, p. 101. Lond.: 1864.

Bateman. Thomas.—Delineations of Cutaneous Diseases. Lond.: 1817.

Bateman. Thomas.—A Practical Synopsis of Cutaneous Diseases. Sixth Edition. Lond.: 1824.

Bazin. M. E.—On Molluscum or Acne.—Journal des Connaissances Médicales. Paris: 1851.

Bazin. M. E.—Recherches sur la Nature et le Traitement des Teignes. Paris: 1853.

Bazin. M. E.—Review of his Researches into the Nature and Treatment of Tinea.—Br. and For. Med.-Chir. Rev., Oct. 1853, p. 416.

Bazin. M. E.—Leçons Théoretiques et Cliniques sur les Syphilides. Recueillées et Publiées par Louis Fournier. Paris: 1859.

Bazin. M. E.—Leçons Théoretiques et Cliniques sur les Affections Cutanées de Nature Arthritique et Dartreuse. Rédigées et publiées par L. Sargent. Paris: 1860.

Bazin, M. E.—Leçons Théoretiques et Cliniques sur les Affections Cutanées Parasitaires. Rédigées et publiées par Alfred Pouquet. Second Edition. Paris: 1862.

BAZIN, M. E.—*Leçons Théoretiques et Cliniques sur les Affections Cutanées Artificielles et sur Lèpre, les diathèses le Purpura, les Difformités de la Peau.* Recueillées et publiées par M. le Docteur Guérard. Paris : 1862.

BAZIN, M. E.—*Leçons sur les Affections Génériques de la Peau.* Recueillées et publiées par M. le Docteur Bandot (Emile). Paris : 1862.

BEALE, LIONEL.—On Contagion.—*Med. Times and Gaz.,* Sept., 1865. See Todd, R. B.

BEGBIE, J. WARBURTON.—On Ichthyosis ; with Special Reference to the Particular Forms in which it Occurs.—*Ed. Med. Journ.,* July, 1861.

BELCHER, T. W.—On the External Use of Starch in Cases of Small-pox and other Skin Diseases of an Inflammatory Nature.— *Dub. Hosp. Gaz.,* 1856.

BELCHER, T. W.—On the Treatment of Psora in Military Hospitals. *Dub. Quart. Journ. Med. Sci.,* vol. xxxiii. Dublin : 1862.

BELCHER, T. W.—*Notes on the Treatment of Continued Fevers, and other Acute Diseases.* Dublin : 1863.

BELCHER, T. W.—A Description of a Bed intended to be Used in protracted Fever Cases. One of the Papers in *Tractatus Medici.* Dublin : 1864.

BELCHER, T. W.—The Hygienic Aspect of Pogonotrophy. One of the Papers in *Tractatus Medici—op. super. cit.;* See also *Ranking's Abstract.* July to Dec., 1864, p. 12.

BELCHER, T. W.—The Hebrew, Mediæval, and Modern Leprosies Compared. — *Dub. Quart. Journ. Med. Sci.,* vol. xxxvii. Dublin : 1864.

BELCHER, T. W.—Brief Considerations Respecting the Weights and Measures, and the Nomenclature of the Pharmacopœia.— *Dub. Quart. Journ.,* vol. xxxviii. Dublin : 1864.

BELCHER, T. W.—Remarks on the Hebrew Catalogue of Skin Diseases.—*Dub. Quart. Journ.,* vol. xxxviii. Dublin : 1864.

BELCHER, T. W.—Cases Treated at the Dispensary for Skin Diseases, Bishop Street.—*Dub. Quart. Journ.,* vols. xxxix and xl. Dublin : 1865.

BELCHER, T. W.—*Memoir of John Stearne, M. and J. U. D., S.F.T.C.D., Founder and First President of the College of Physicians, including the Original Charter of that College, and other Records concerning the Profession of Physic in Ireland, never before published ; with a Review of his writings.* Dublin : 1865.

BELL, G. HAMILTON, and BELL, CHARLES.—The Treatment of Erysipelas by the Muriated Tincture of Iron.—*Month. Journ. Med. Sci.,* June, 1851, p. 497.

BENNETT, JOHN HUGHES.—*The Principles and Practice of Medicine.* Fourth Edition. Edin. : 1865.

BIETT, M. LE DOCTEUR.—See Cazenave et Schedel.

BLAKE, R. H.—*M. Caillault on Diseases of the Skin in Children.* Second Edition. Trans. and Noted. Lond. : 1863.

CAZENAVE, ALPHÉE.—*Traité des Maladies de Cuir Chevelu.* Paris: 1850.

CAZENAVE, ALPHÉE.—*Annales des Maladies de la Peau et de la Syphilis.* Paris: 1851.

CAZENAVE, ALPHÉE, and SCHEDEL.—English Translation.—See Burgess.

CAZENAVE, ALPHÉE.—See Burgess.

CEELEY, ROBERT.—Observations on the Variolæ Vaccinæ (Illustrated).—*Trans. Prov. Med. and Surg. Assoc.*, vols. viii and x. Lond.: 1840 and 1842.

CELSUS.—*De Medicina; ex recensione Leonardi Targœ.* Edin.: 1815.

CHAUSSIT, M.—*Traité Elémentaire des Maladies de la Peau.* Paris 1853.

CHURCH, WILLIAM S.—Report of a Cure of Ichthyosis, with Congenital Malformation of the Aorta.—*St. Bartholomew's Hosp. Reports*, vol. i, 1865, p 198.

COBBOLD, T. SPENCER.—*Entozoa; an Introduction to the Study of Helminthology, with Reference more Particularly to the Internal Parasites of Man.* Lond.: 1864.

CODEX PHARMACOPÉE FRANÇAISE.—Redigée par ordre du Gouvernement par une Commission Compósee de MM. les Professeurs de la Faculté de Médecine, et de l'Ecole Spéciale de Pharmacie de Paris. Paris: 1837.

COLLIS, MAURICE, H.—On the Treatment of Anthrax by Pressure. *Dub. Qu. Journ.*, vol. xxxvii. Dublin: 1864.

COMTES rendus des Séances de l'Académie des Sciences. Paris: 1842.

COPLAND, JAMES.—*A Dictionary of Practical Medicine.* 3 vols. Lond.: 1858.

CORRIGAN, DOMINIC JOHN.—Lecture on Porrigo.—*Dub. Hosp. Gaz.*, Aug. 15, 1845.

CORRIGAN, DOMINIC JOHN.—*Lectures on the Nature and Treatment of Fever.* Dublin: 1853.

CORRIGAN, DOMINIC JOHN.—Treatment of Acute Pemphigus.—*Cyclopœdia of Practical Medicine.* Lond.: 1854. Vol. iii, p. 263.

COTTON, CHARLES.—Case of Bronzed Skin, and Disease of Suprarenal Capsules.—*Med. Times and Gaz.*, July 11, 1857.

COTTON, RICHARD PAYNE.—Report of Some Cases of Molluscum Contagiosum, with Observations on its General History and Pathology.—*Ed. Med. and Surg. Journ.*, vol. lxix. (This paper is misquoted on p. 277 of the present work, as written by Dr. Paterson.)

CRAIGIE, DAVID.—Description of a Case of the Molluscum of Dr. Willan. *Ed. Med. and Surg. Journ.*, vol. lxxv. 1851.

CREMEN, DAVID.—Report on the Epidemic Scarlatina which visited Cork in 1863, &c. Dublin: 1863.

CUMMINS, WILLIAM JACKSON.—On the Use of Arsenic.—*Dub. Qu. Journ. Med. Sci.*, Nov., 1864.

COMMINS, WILLIAM JACKSON.—Remarks on Scarlatia
Jour., Feb. 1865.

CYCLOPÆDIA OF PRACTICAL MEDICINE AND SURGEE
Forbes, Tweedie, and Conolly.—See Corrigan.

DANIELSSEN, D. C., and BÖRCK, W.—Traité de la S₁
Elephantiasis des Græcs. Paris: 1848. Als
original edition, and a Critical Review of it in
For. Med.-Chir. Rev., vol. v, 1850, p. 71.

DEBOUT, M.—The Local Application of Sulphate of
pelas.—Braithwaite, vol. xxxi, p. 275.

DECAISNE.—A New and Speedy Method for the C₁
Braithwaite, li, 275; and Glasg. Med. Journ.,
482.

DELARUE.—Creasote in Erysipelas.—Med. Times
April, 1857, p. 344.

DEVERGIE, ALPH.—Traité Pratique des Maladies
Troisième Edition. Paris: 1863.

DICKSON, STEPHEN.—Observations on Pemphigus.—'
Academy, vol. i, 1787.

DIDAY, P.—A Treatise on Syphilis in Newborn Chi
ham Soc., English Translation. Lond.: 1859.

DOBSON, SIR RICHARD.—On the Treatment of Erys
merous Punctures in the Affected Part.—Med
xiv, 206. Lond.: 1828.

DUBLIN HOSPITAL REPORTS. 5 vols. First publishe

DUBLIN JOURNAL OF MEDICAL SCIENCE. Dublin.
lished quarterly.

DUBLIN MEDICAL AND PHYSICAL ESSAYS. Vol. i. I

DUBLIN QUARTERLY JOURNAL OF MED. SCIENCE.
lished quarterly.

DUCHESNE, DU PARC M.—Nouvelle Prosopalgie. F

DUCHESE, DU PARC M.—On the Treatment of Pruri
xl, 125.

DUCKWORTH, DYCE.—Observations upon some Poin
tomy of the Supra-renal Capsules.—St. Barthe
Reports, vol. i., 1865, p. 224.

DUGDALE, WILLIAM.—Monasticon Anglicanum. 3
London: 1817-30.

DUNCAN, J. MATTHEWS.—See Spence.

DURKEE.—Erythema Tuberculatum.—Boston Me
Journ., April, 1856, p. 189.

EDINBURGH MEDICAL JOURNAL. Edinburgh. Publi

EDINBURGH MEDICAL AND SURGICAL JOURNAL. Edinb₁
published quarterly.

EICHSTEDT.—Discovery of Microsporon Furfur in F
Froriep's Notizen. 39 Band. July–Sept., 184

ELLIOTTSON, JOHN.—The Principles and Practice
Edited, with Notes, &c., by Nath. Rogers. Lo₁

ESMARCH, FR.—On the Use of Cold in Surgery.—*New Sydenham Society's Selected Monographs* (vol. xi, N.S.). Lond.: 1861.

FABRE.—*Bibliothèque du Medicin-Praticien.* 5 vols. Paris.

FAYER, J. (Calcutta).—Elephantiasis of the Leg Treated by Ligature of the Femoral Artery.—*Ed. Med. Journ.*, Nov., 1865.

FOX, TILBURY.—*Skin Diseases of Parasitic Origin; their Nature and Treatment.* Lond.: 1863.

FOX, TILBURY.—*Skin Diseases, their Description, Pathology, Diagnosis, and Treatment.* Lond.: 1864.

FOX, TILBURY.—*Classification of Skin Diseases, with Comparative Tables.* Lond.: 1864.

FRAZER, WILLIAM.—*Treatment of Diseases of the Skin.* Dublin: 1864.

FRAZER, WILLIAM.—Remarks on a Common Herpetic Epizoötic Affection, and on its Alleged Frequent Transmission to the Human Subject.—*Dublin Quar. Journ.*, May, 1865.

FRICKE, CHARLES.—Case of Cirrhosis of the Liver, and Bronzed Skin.—*Br. and For. Med.-Chir. Rev.*, vol. xx, 1857; and *North American Med.-Chir. Rev.*, 1857.

GALEN.—*Hippocratis et Claudii Galeni Opera.* Ex. Editione Renati Charterii, M.D. Folio. 9 tom. Lutetiae. Paris: 1679.

GENDRIN, A. N.—*Histoire Anatomique des Inflammations.* Paris: 1826.

GIBERT, C. M.—*Traité Pratique des Maladies de la Peau, et de la Syphilis.* 3ème Edition. Paris.

GILIBERT, M.—*Monographie du Pemphigus ou Traité de la Maladie Vésiculaire.* Paris: 1813.

GILLETTE, Dr.—*Du Sclérème Simple.*—*Archives Gén. de Médecine,* Dec., 1854. Paris.

GINTRAC, Dr.—*De la Pellagre dans le Department de la Gironde.* Bordeaux: 1863.

GOOD, JOHN MASON.—*The Study of Medicine.* Third Edition. By S. Cooper. 5 vols. Lond.: 1829.

GOOLDEN, R. H.—Sesquichloride of Iron in Erysipelas.—*Med. Times and Gaz.*, 12th Nov., 1853, p. 592.

GOOLDEN, R. H.—The Turkish Bath.—*Braithwaite*, xliii, p. 371.

GRAHAM, THOMAS J.—*On the Treatment of Scarlet Fever and Measles with Susquicarbonate of Ammonia.* Second Edition. London: 1861.

GRANTHAM, JOHN.—The Dermic Application of Medicated Steam in the Treatment of Diseases of the Skin.—*Brit. Med. Journ.*, 20th Aug., 1864.

GRAVES, ROBERT J.—*Clinical Lectures on the Practice of Medicine.* Edited by Neligan, 1848, 2 vols.; and reprinted in 1 vol. Dub., 1864. Also a French Edition by Dr. Jaccoud. Second Edition. Paris: 1863.

GRAVES, ROBERT J.—Contagious Psoriasis and Bucnemia Tropica. —*Dub. Hosp. Reports*, vol. iv, 1827, pp. 53, 54.

... ... the Treatment of ... Diseases;

HANDFIELD JONES. ... On Smallpox and Vaccination.—Med. Times and Gaz. Sept. 1855.

HARLEY, GEORGE. Rats in... with the Supra-renal Capsules had been removed. Med. Times and Gaz. 28th Nov., 1857.

HARLEY, GEORGE. On the Histology of the Supra-renal Capsules. Med. Times and Gaz., 19th Dec., 1857.

HARLEY, GEORGE.—An Experimental Inquiry into the Function of the Supra-renal Capsules, and their Supposed Connection with Bronzed Skn.—*Br. and For. Med.-Chir. Rev.*, vol. xxi, 1858, p. 204.

HARLEY, GEORGE.—Pathology of the Supra-renal Capsules.—*Br. and For. Med.-Chir. Rev.*, vol. xxi, 1858, p. 498.

HARRISON,   .—Addison's Disease of the Supra-renal Capsules. —*Brit. Med. Journ.*, vol. ii, 1861.

HAYDEN, THOMAS.—On Supra-renal Melasma.—*Dub. Quar. Journ.*, Feb., 1865.

HEBRA, FERDINAND.—*Diagnostic der Hautkrankheiten in Tabellairischen Ordnung nach Dr. Hebra's Vorlesungen von Dr. Bendict Schulz.* Wien : 1845.

HEBRA, FERDINAND.—Ueber Kraetze.—*Med. Jahrbücher des K. K. Oester.* Staates : xlvi, pp. 280-292 ; xlvii, pp. 44-54, 163-173.

HEBRA, FERDINAND.—*Hautkrankheiten (Contributions to Virchow's Handbuch der Speciellen Pathologie und Therapie).* Erlangen : 1854-64. Several parts.

HEBRA, FERDINAND.—*Atlas of Cutaneous Diseases.*—Printed for the New Sydenham Society.

HENDERSON.—*Iceland, or a Journal of Residence in that Island.* 2 vols. Edin. : 1818.

HENDERSON, T. A.—Induration of Cellular Tissue in Infants.—*Med. Times and Gaz.*, 14th July, 1860.

HENDERSON, WILLIAM.—Notice of the Molluscum Contagiosum.— *Ed. Med. and Surg. Journ.*, No. 148. Vol. 56.

HENRY, N. E., ET GUIBOURT, G.—*Pharmacopée Raisonnée ou Traité de Pharmacie Pratique et Theoretique.* Tome ii. Paris : 1828.

HIGGENBOTTOM, JOHN.—*A Practical Essay on the Use of the Nitrate of Silver in the Treatment of Inflammation, Wounds, and Ulcers.*—Third Edition. Lond. : 1865.

HILLIER, THOMAS.—*Handbook of Skin Diseases for Students and Practitioners.* Lond. : 1865.

HILLIER, THOMAS.—A Case of Elephantiasis.—*Med. Times and Gaz.*, 1st April, 1865.

HIPPOCRATES.—Τοῦ Μεγάλου Ἱπποκράτους Πάντων τῶν Ἰατρῶν Κορυφαίου τὰ Εὑρισκόμενα. Ed. Anutio Fœsio. Genevæ : 1657. Folio. 2 vols.

HOLMES, T.—*A System of Surgery, Theoretical and Practical, in Treatises by Various Authors.* 4 vols. 8vo. Lond. : 1860-64. See also "Lee."

HOLT, RICHARD.—Remarkable Case of Morbus Addisonii.—*Lancet*, 21st Oct., 1865

HOOD, PETER.—*The Successful Treatment of Scarlet Fever, and Affections of the Throat, &c.* Lond. : 1857.

HORNER.—*Medical Topography of Brazil.*

HUBSCH.—*Gaz. Méd. d'Orient*, 1859.

HUGHES, JOHN.—On Diseases of the Supra-renal Capsules, or Morbus Addisonii.—*Dub. Qu. Journ.*, vol. xl, 1865, Nov.

38

... ... —ases of Erysipelas. with some Re-
... ... 415. Lond.: 1825.
... ... —A ... ... Report on Rodent Ulcer.—
... ... 1851 Aug. 1849. &c.
... ... — ... ... the ... ... and *Prevention of*
... ... Eighth Edition. London:

... ... Yellow. Dr R. J. Graves. Tra-
... ... Paris. 1843. 2 vols.
... ... —... ... as Respecting an Ulcer of a Peculiar
... ... the Eyelids and other parts of the
... ... 1847.
... ... —... ... the Nature and Management of
... ... —Dub. ... 1841.—See *Braithwaite*. xxix,

... ... —in Foreign ... —*Med. Times and Gaz*. Aug.,

... ... —... ... ... of the *Jews*. Whiston's
... ...
... ... de Plantæ. Paris: 1851.
... ... —Report of Cork Street *Fever Hos-*
... ... Dublin: 1846.
... ... —Statistics of the Epidemic of *Scarlatina*
... ... 1834 to 1842. &c. Dublin:

... —a Disease in which a Disease like Measles arose
... ... with some general Remarks.—*Dub. Qu.*
... ... 1848.
... ... Memoir of John Moore Neligan,
... ... Aug. 1848.
... ... Vegetable-*Parasites*
... ... by Edwin Lankester. Printed
... ... 1856-7.

... ... weekly
... ... Opium and Castor Oil.—
... ... and Gaz. 27th Nov.,

... ... —*l'Animalcule qui la*
... ... Paris 1853. See also "Recent
... ... Med.-Chir. *Review*,

... ... on the Nature and Treatment of
... ... Dublin: 1825.
... ... Dublin: 1863.
... ... Nature. Transmission : one of the
... ... See also "Holmes."
... ... London. Fifth

LIVEZAY, Dr.—Local Applications in Erysipelas.—*Med. Times and Gaz.*, 14th March, 1857, p. 269; and *Boston Journ.*, vol. lv, p. 262.

LORRY, D.—*Tractatus de Morbis Cutaneis.* 4to. Paris: 1777.

LUCRETIUS.—*De Naturá Rerum.*

LYONS, ROBERT DYER.—*A Treatise on Fever.* Dublin: 1861.

MACBRIDE, DAVID.—*A Methodical Introduction to the Theory and Practice of the Art of Medicine.* Second Edition. 2 vols. Dublin: 1777.

M'DONNELL, ROBERT.—On Sclerema.—*Dub. Hosp. Gaz.*, 1855–56.

MACLAGAN, J. M'GRIGOR.—On Colchicum Autumnale, Chiefly with Reference to the Growth of the Plant, its Physiological and Therapeutical Actions (In *Cutaneous Diseases*, p. 27).—*Month. Journ. Med. Sci.*, Jan., 1852.

MACLEOD, GEORGE H. B.—*Outlines of Surgical Diseases.* London: 1864.

MACNAMARA, RAWDON.—See Neligan.

MALMSTEN, Prof. (of Stockholm).—On Cod Liver Oil in Eczema.—*Med. Times and Gaz.*, 7th July, 1865.

MARTINEAU, LOUIS.—*De la Maladie d'Addison.* Paris: 1864.

MEAD, RICHARD.—*Medica Sacra; or, a Commentary on the Most Remarkable Diseases Mentioned in the Holy Scriptures.* Translated from the Latin by Thomas Stack. Lond.: 1755.

MEDICAL PRESS. Dublin. Published weekly.

MEDICAL TIMES AND GAZETTE, THE.—London. Published weekly. (Various papers, especially those on "Modern Dermatology," 1865.)

MEDICO-CHIRURGICAL TRANSACTIONS, THE.—Published Annually by the Royal Medical and Chirurgical Society. London.

MEUSCHINIUS, JO. GERHARDUS.—*Nov. Test. ex Talm., &c.* Illustr. 4to. Lips.: 1736. See Rhenferdius.

MILTON, JOHN L.—*On the Modern Treatment of some Diseases of the Skin.* Lond.: 1865.

MOORE, WILLIAM (F.K. and Q.C.P.).—On the more Aggravated Forms of Diseases of the Skin (Pemphigus, Gangrænosus, Pompholyx Diutinus, Herpes Capitis, Eczema Impetiginodes, &c.).—*Dub. Hosp. Gaz.*, 1859, p. 35.

MOORE, WILLIAM (F.K. and Q.C.P.).—On the Sapo Laricis in Cutaneous Diseases.—*Op. cit.*, p. 91.

MOORE, WILLIAM (F.K. and Q.C.P.).—On the Nature and Treatment of some of the more Ordinary Diseases of the Skin (Eczema, Herpes, Porrigo,'&c.).—*Op. cit.*, p. 117.

MOORE, WILLIAM (F.K. and Q.C.P.).—On the Pathology and Therapeutics of Diseases of the Skin (Squamous Diseases).—*Dub. Hosp. Gaz.*, 1860, p. 22.

MOTT, VALENTINE.—Remarks on a Peculiar Form of Tumor of the Skin denominated Pachydermatocele.—*Med. Chir. Trans.*, xxxvii, 155. Lond.: 1854.

MOUFFET.—*On the Acarus Scabiei.* 1650? See p. 156.

....—A Treatise on the Continued Fevers of ..... Britain. Lond. ....

.... Adams—On Eruptive Diseases of the Scalp. ....

.... Adams—Atlas of Cutaneous Diseases. Dublin: ....

.... T...—On Scarlatina Nigricans.—Dub. Quart. ... Jour. .... May. 185..

.... A...—.......... their Uses and Modes of .... Sixth Edition. By Macnamara. Dublin: ....

.... A...—....... Mineral Medicine.—See Graves.

S.... Hugh.—On the External Application of Tincture of Iodine in Erysipelas.—Med. Times and Gaz. II. Dec. 1852. p. 590.

.. .. Prof. Qu. Coll. Cork.—Contagion ....—Dub. Qu. Jour. Med. Sci. Feb. 1864.

. ... A...—On Treatment of Anthrax by Pressure.—Dub. ....

.... V...—Cases of Ichthyosis Sporia vel Sebacea.—Med. ... . Lond.: 1863.

....—The Plague at Athens as Described by ... .—Dub. Qu. Jour. Med. Sci. May. 1858.

....—........ Erythema.—Vide Schilling.

....—Three Cases of Rodent Ulcer.—Med. Times and ....

....—Case of Great Pigment Deposit in the Skin (so-..... Bronzed Skin without Disease of the Supra-renal Cap-sules.—Med. Times and Gaz. 1856. vol. xvii. N.S.

.... R....—Cases and Observations on the Molluscum .... of Bateman. with an Account of the Minute Structure of the Tumors.—Ed. Med. and Surg. Journ. vol. ... . See Cotton Richd. Payne.

Pathological Society. Transactions of.—London. Published Annually.

Pharmacopœia, British.—Published pursuant to the Medical Act, ... Lond. 1864.

Pharmacopœia. Collegii Medicorum Regis et Reginæ in Hiberniâ. Dublin 1849.

Pharmacopœia. The. of the King and Queen's College of Physicians in Ireland. Dublin: 1850. Supplement. Dublin: 1856.

Pharmacopœia. The. of the Royal College of Physicians of Edin-burgh. Edin. 1841.

Pharmacopœia Collegii Regalis Medicorum Londinensis. Lond.: 1841.

Pharmacopœia. Codex. Française.—See Codex.

Pharmacopœia Rossensis.—See Henry et Guibourt.

Plenck. Josephus Jacobus.—Doctrina de Morbis Cutaneis. Edit. Secunda Aucta. Viennæ. 1783.

Pliny.—Plinius (Caius Secundus) Veronensis, Senior.—*Naturalis Historiæ*, 37 Libri. Recensuit et Commentariis Instruxit Julius Sillig. Hambrugi et Gothæ : 1857–8.

Plumbe, Samuel.—*A Practical Treatise on Diseases of the Skin.* Lond. : 1824.

Popham, John.—A Case of Bronzed Skin.—*Dub. Qu. Journ.,* Aug., 1865.

Prosper, Alpinus.—*Ægypti Historiæ Naturalis.* Lugdini Bata-vorum : 1735.

Purser, John M.—Two Cases of Onychomycosis, with Remarks.—*Dub. Qu. Journ.,* Nov., 1865.

Radcliffe.—See Ranking.

Ranking, W. H. and Radcliffe, C. B.—*The Half-yearly Abstract of the Medical Sciences.*

Ranking, W. H. and Radcliffe, C. B.—On Development of the Œstrus. Abstract of a paper in vol. xxix.

Rayer, P.—*Traité Théoretique et Pratique des Maladies de la Peau.* Paris : 1826. 2 vols.

Remak.—On Inoculating with Parasites.—*Medinische Zeitung,* 1842.

Rhazes (Abú Becr Mohammed Ibu Zacaríyá Ar-Rázi).—*A Treatise on the Smallpox and Measles.* Translated from the original Arabic, and Edited for the Sydenham Society by Wm. Alex. Greenhill. Lond. : 1848.

Rhenferdius.—De Leprâ Cutis Hebræorum ; included in *Meuschen's Nov. Test. ex Talm.* Illustr. Classed, D-d, 32, in Library, T.C.D.

Richardson, B. W.—An Anomalous Exanthem, Rosalia Idiopathica.—*Trans. Epidemiological Soc., Lond.,* vol. ii, Part 1, 1862–4. Lond. : 1865.

Ricord, Ph.—*Traité Complet des Maladies Vénériennes.* Paris : 1851.

Riolanus, Johannes.—*Opera cum Physica tum Medica.* Folio. Frankofurti : 1611.

Robin, Ch.—*Histoire Naturelle des Végétaux Parasites, qui Croissent sur l'Homme et sur les Animaux Vivants.* Paris : 1853.

Robinson, Edw. (D.D.).—*Biblical Researches in Palestine.* 8vo. Lond. : 1841.

Rokitansky, Carl.—*A Manual of Pathological Anatomy.* 4 vols. Lond. : 1854. Sydenham Society Edition.

Ross, George.—*On Ringworm, Scall-Head, Baldness, and other Parasitical Diseases of the Head and Face.* Lond. : 1864.

Routh, Charles.—Juniper Tar Ointment.—*Lancet,* 22d Oct., 1853, p. 337.

Russell, James.—Cases of Pemphigus, Apparently Originating in Disease of the Cutaneous Nerves, with Remarks.—*Med. Times and Gaz.,* Oct. 29, 1864.

Russell, James.—Cases of Pemphigus, Urticaria, and Shingles.—*Med. Times and Gaz.,* 21st Oct., 1865.

SALISBURY, J. H. Newark, Ohio.—**Remarks on Fungi**, with an Account of Experiments showing the Influence of the Fungi of Wheat Straw on the Human System, and Some Observations which point to them as the Probable Source of Camp Measles, and perhaps of Measles generally.—*Amer. Month. Med. Journ.,* July and Oct. 1862.

SCHEDEL, .—See Cazenave.

SCHILLING, G. G.—De *Lepri Commentationes.* Recensuit, J. D. Hahn. Lugduni Batavorum : 1778.

SCHMIDT, E.—*Jahrbücher Der in-und Ausländischen Gesammten Medicin.* Leipzig. Vol. ci.

SCOTT, ROBERT.—See Liddell.

SEDGWICK, .—True Keloid.—*Path. Soc. Trans.,* xii. p. 234. Lond : 1861.

SEDGWICK, WILLIAM.—On Sexual Limitation in Hereditary Diseases.—*Brit. and For. Med.-Chir. Rev.,* vol. xxvii. 1861.

SEDGWICK, WILLIAM.—On the Influence of Sex in Hereditary Disease.—*Brit. and For. Med.-Chir. Rev.,* July. 1863.

SEMLER, J. S. SALOMON, S.T.P.—*Historiæ Ecclesiasticæ Selecta Capita.* 3 vols.. 8vo. Hal : 1767–69.

SHAPTER, THOMAS.—*Medica Sacra : or, Short Expositions of the More Important Diseases Mentioned in the Sacred Writings.* 8vo. Lond : 1834.

SIMON, J FRANZ.—*Animal Chemistry, with Reference to the Physiology and Pathology.* Translated and Edited for the Sydenham Society by George E. Day. 2 vols. Lond.: 1845.

SIMON, GUSTAV.—*Anatomical Descriptions of Diseases of the Skin.* Berlin : 1848.

SIMPSON, JAMES Y.—Antiquarian Notices of Leprosy and Leper Hospitals in Scotland and England.—*Ed. Med. and Surg. Journ.,* vols. lvi and lvii.

SMITH, WILLIAM.—*Dictionary of the Bible.* Lond : 1861–63. 3 vols. Articles Leprosy and Medicine.

SMITH, WILLIAM ABBOTTS.—*On Human Entozoa.* Lond : 1863. 8vo.

SPENCE, G. W. and DUNCAN J. MATTHEWS.—On the Occurrence of Bots in the Human Subject.—*Ranking.* xxix.

SQUIRE, BALMANNO.—On Impetigo.—*Med. Times and Gaz.,* Aug. 20. 1864.

SQUIRE, BALMANNO.—On Animal Parasite Diseases of the Skin.—*Med. Times and Gaz.,* 19th Aug.. 1865.

STARTIN, JAMES.—On Cure of Nævus by Subcutaneous Elastic Strangulation.—*Med. Times and Gaz.,* 3d July. 1852.

STEARNE, JOHN.—*Adstruitio Medica : Seu de Bentitudine et Miseria, Horis Essentia, Origine et ad Ipsam Methodo, hujus Natura Causas et Remediis Tractatus.* 4to. Dublin : 1658.

STOKES, WHITLEY.—On an Eruptive Disease of Children.—*Dub. Med. and Phys. Essays,* vol. i. p. 146. Dublin : 1818.

STOKES, WILLIAM.—Solution of Gutta Percha in Chloroform to Prevent Pitting in Variola.—*Braithwaite,* xxvi. p. 374.

SYDENHAM, THOMAS.—*Opera Omnia*, Edidit. Gul. Alex. Greenhill. Lond. (Sydenham Soc. Edit.): 1844.

TACITUS, OPERA.—*A. J. Lipsio Emendata et Illustrata.* Folio. Ant.: 1585.

TANNER, THOS. H.—*The Practice of Medicine.* Fifth Edition. Lond.: 1865.

TREVAN, WILLIAM:—An Account of a Singular Case in which there was a Black Secretion from the Skin of the Forehead and Upper Part of the Face.—*Med.-Chir. Trans.*, vol. xxviii. Lond.: 1845.

THOMSON, ANTHONY TODD.—*A Practical Treatise on Diseases Affecting the Skin.* Completed and Edited by Edmond A. Parkes. Lond.: 1850.

THOMSON, ARTHUR S.—On the Peculiarities in Figure, the Disfigurations, and the Customs of the New Zealanders, with Remarks on their Diseases and on their Modes of Treatment.—*Br. and For Med.-Chir. Rev.*, April, 1854, vol. xiii.

TODD, ROBERT BOWMAN.—*Clinical Lectures.* Edited by Lionel Beale. Second Edition. Lond.: 1861.

TRENCH, RICHARD C. (Abp. of Dublin).—*Notes on the Miracles.* Second Edition. Lond.: 1860.

TROGUS, JUSTIN.—*Historia.*

TROUSSEAU, M.—Elastic Collodion.—*Braithwaite,* xxxii, p. 358.

TWEEDIE, ALEX.—*Lectures on the Distinctive Characters, Pathology, and Treatment of Continued Fevers.* Lond.: 1862.

UGOLINI, .—See Bartholini.

VELPEAU, M.—On the Application of Photosulphite of Iron in Erysipelas.—*Braithwaite*, vol. xxxi, p. 275; and *Med. Times and Gaz.*, vol. i, 1855, pp. 239, 289.

WALSH, ALBERT.—On the Constitutional Origin of Erysipelas, and its Treatment.—*Dub. Qu. Journ. Med. Sci.*, Aug., 1850.

WATSON, THOMAS.—*Lectures on the Principles and Practice of Medicine.* Fourth Edition. Lond.: 1859.

WELLS, SPENCER.—On Ligatures in Nævus.—*Med. Times and Gaz.*, 4th Nov., 1854.

WERTHEIM, Dr. (of Vienna).—On the Nature of Psoriasis.—*Gaz. Hebd. de Méd. et Chir.*, Paris, 1864; and *Med. Times and Gaz.*, July, 1864.

WILDE, Sir WILLIAM ROBERT.—Report on the Status of Disease.—(*Irish Census,* 1851) Bluebook.

WILKS, SAMUEL.—On Disease of the Supra-renal Capsules, or Morbus Addisonii.—*Guy's Hosp. Reports,* N.S., vol. viii. Lond.: 1862.

WILLAN, ROBERT.—*On Cutaneous Diseases.* 4to. Lond.: 1808.

WILSON, ERASMUS.—*Diseases of the Skin.* Fifth Edition. Lond.: 1863. See also First and Fourth Editions.

WILSON, ERASMUS.—*An Inquiry into the Relative Frequency, the Duration and Cause of Diseases of the Skin.* Lond.: 1864.

WILSON, ERASMUS.—On the Phytopathology of the Skin and Nosophytodermata, the so-called Parasitic Affections of the Skin.— *Br. and For. Med.-Chir. Rev.*, Jan., 1864.

WILSON, ERASMUS.—*Students' Book of Cutaneous Medicine.* Part i. Lond.: 1864. Part ii. Lond.: 1865.

WITT, CHARLES.—*An Effective and Simple Remedy for Scarlatina, Fever, and Measles, with an Appendix of Cases.* London (Third Edition): 1862.

GENERAL INDEX

OF

WORDS AND MATTERS.

Acanthia lectularia, 359
Acarus folliculorum, 170
    scabiei, 156
Achorion Schönleinii, 363
Achroma congenitale, 326
    vitiligo, 326
Acne, 168
    indurata, 172
    molluscoides, 275
    punctata, 170
    rosacea, 171
    sebacea, 169, 279
    sebacée cornée, 265
    simplex, 169
    syphilitic, 386
    varioliformis, 275
Acrodynia, 53
Addison's disease, 334
Ætius, 168
Ακμὴ, 168
Albinoes, 325
Albinoismus, 325, 326
Aleppo evil, 292
Alex. III, bull de leprosis, 285
Alibert's classification, 31
Alkaline baths, 419
    cathartic draught, 431
    lotion, 79, 85
        sedative, 423
        stimulating, 423, 424
    mixtures, 431
Alopecia, 408
    areata, 411
    from mental anxiety, 409
    lotions and pomades for, 410
    symptomatica, 410
    unguale, 412
Alterative mixtures, 432

Alum wash (Cazenave's), 424
Anneau herpétique, 128
Anodine lotions, 423
Anthrax, 199
Appendages of the skin, diseases
    of, 405
Area, 410
Arsenic in eczema, 117
    Dr. Cummins on, 118
    ioduretted solution of the
      iodide of potassium and, 247
Artificial classifications, 28
Asiatic pills, 248
Astringent lotions, 424
    ointments, 427
Aussatz der, 230
Author's classification, 40

Bahereth, 295
Bahereth kehe, 298
Bahereth lebhana, 298
Baker's itch, 211
Baldness, 408
Bandages, 416
Baras, 291
Barat lebana, 291
Barbadoes leg, 294
Baths, 417
    alkaline, 419
    ammonia, 418
    gelatine, 418
    iodine, 419
    mercurial, 420
    sulphur, 420
    Turkish, 115
    vapor, 417, 418
Beard, canities of, 406
Bed for cases of exanthemata, 96

Bennett's classification. 40
Beras. 299
Bibliographical index. 437
Blattern. 92
Bieb. 30, 101
Blind boils. 199
Bohak. 298
Boil or furuncle. 198
Bots or gad-fly. 359
Bouten (ecthyma). 192
Bouton d'Alep. 292
Bran ty face. 171
Bricklayer's itch. 109
Bronzed skin. 334
Bull de leprosis. 285
Bulla. 30
Bullae. 101
Burnt holes. 144
Butcher's treatment of elephantiasis Arabum, 296

Caenbay. 293
Callositates. 308
Camp measles. 85
Camphor ointment. 428
Cancroide. 355
Cancroides. 44, 339
Canities. 405
    of beard. 405
    remarkable case of absence of
       in an aged person. 406
Cantharides, tincture of, in psoriasis. 251
Cerate, 334
Carbonate of ammonia in psoriasis. 250
Carbuncle. 199
Carbuncled face. 171
Carnochan's treatment of elephantiasis Arabum. 296
Cataplasms. 420
Caustic of chloride of zinc, 421
    of iodine. 421
    solution. compound, 421
Caustics. 420
Cazenave's classification, 32, 34
    treatment of lupus, 353
    alum wash. 424
Ceratum cucumis. 426
    galeni. 426
Cheloid tumor. 354
Chigoe or chigger). 359
Chionyphe, carteri, 377

Chloasma, 256, 259
Chloride of zinc caustic, 421
Classification, 25
    Alibert's, 29, 31
    artificial system of, 28
    author's, 40
    Bennet's, 40
    Buchanan's, 35
    Cazenave's, 31, 34
    Fox's, 39
    Hardy's, 35
    Hebra's, 35 •
    Lorry's 29
    Mercurialis, 29
    natural systems of, 31, 36
    Plenck's, 30
    regional systems of, 29, 37
    Riolanus', 29
    Turner's, 29
    Willan's, 29
    Wilson's, 31–34
Clavus. 306
Cold cream, 426
Collodion in skin diseases, 416
    use of in erysipelas, 68
    corrosive, 421
    vesicating, 139
Comedones, 274
Condylomata, 308
    syphilitic, 392
Constitutional medication, 415
Copland's pomade for alopecia, 410
Corns, 306
    soft. 307
Corrosive sublimate mixture in syphilides, 390
    soap. 429
Couperose. 171
Cream, cold, 426
    cucumber, 426
Crusted tetter, 179
Cryptogamia of favus, 362
    of sycosis, 371
Cucumber cream, 426
Cyanopathia, 333

Dandriff, 256
Dartre crustacée, 179
    erythemoide. 48
    farineuse, 203
    phlyctenoide. 123
    rougeante, 339

Dartre squameuse humide, 102
   tarmineuse, 253
   vive, 102
Dartrous diathesis, 108, 113
Depilation in ringworm, 139
Dermatophytæ, 44, 358
Dermatozoa, 359
Diaphoretic mixtures, 432
   pills, 431
Diathesis dartrous, 108, 113
Dickson on pemphigus gangræno-
   sus, 144
Donovan's solution, 399
Dracunculus, 359
Draught, alkaline cathartic, 431
Dry scale, 230
   tetter, 230
Dupey's sulphate of copper lotion,
   424

Ear, herpes of, 124
Eating hive, 144
   tetter, 339
Eau de Cologne, 138
Ecchymoses, 312
Ecphyma mollusciforme, 274
Ecthyma, 192
   acutum, 193
   cachecticum, 195
   chronicum, 194
   gangrænosum, 195
   infantile, 194
   luridum, 194
   syphilitic, 388
   vesiculare, 195
Ectozoa, 359
Eczema, 101
   capitis, 107
   chronicum, 105
   Devergie's stages of, 113
   elementary lesions in, 112
   faciei, 105
   fendillé, 104
   impetiginodes, 104, 186
   marginatum, 109
   mercuriale, 109
   rimosum, 104
   rubrum, 103
   simplex, 102
   solare, 109
   syphilitic, 384
   umbilicale, 108
Elephantiasis, 284

Elephantiasis anæsthetica, 291
   Arabum, 294
   Carter on, 290
   Danielssen and Böeck on, 288
   Græcorum, 284
   Italica, 293
   tuberculosa, 291
Elephant skin disease, 284
Ephélides ignéales, 331
Ephelis, 329
   hepatico, 330
   lenticularis, 329
   melaina, 334
   syphilitic, 395
   violacea, 332
Epidemic of erythema, 53
   of pemphigus, 145
'Επφλόγισμα, 56
Erbgrind, 360
Erbsenblattern, 192
Erratic erysipelas, 59
Erysipelas, 56
   contagiousness of, 62
   erratic, 59
   gangrenous, 60
   idiopathic, 57
   metastatic, 60
   phlegmonous, 59
   symmetrical, 59
   traumatic, 60
   treatment of, 63
   true, 57
Erysipèle, 56
Erythema, 48
   circinatum, 50
   fugax, 49
   intertrigo, 50
   leve, 50
   marginatum, 50
   nodosum, 51
   papulatum, 51
   simplex, 49
   syphilitic, 382
   tuberculatum, 51, 52
Esthiomanic scrofula, 347
Esthiomanos ambulans, 341
   serpiginosus, 341
Evanescent urticaria, 74
Exanthema, 30
   hemorrhagica, 317
Exanthemata, 40, 46
   Hillier's tabular diagnosis of,
   98

Exanthemata syphilitic. 382
Exclusion of air. treatment by. 415

Face, acne of. 171
    eczema of. 115
    impetigo of. 183
Favus. 360
    disseminé. 344
    en nexus. 364
Febris erysipelatosa. 5?
    mortificans. 56
Filaria medinensis. 359
Finnen. 148
Fire. sacred. 126
    St. Anthony's. 54
Fischschuppenkrankheit. 264
Fish-skin disease. 264
Flux. sebaceus. 273
Furfur capitorum. 355
Firmus ambulatoria. 129
Fothergill's sore throat. 50
Frambœsia. 291
Freckles. 329
Frusserde dechter. 359
Fungus foot. 375
Furunculi. 195

Gall-fly. 359
Gale. 154
Galen's cerate. 423
Gelatine baths. 116
Glycerine wash. 424
Goolden. Dr.. on Turkish bath in eczema. 115
Graves on gutta percha in skin diseases. 415
    on iodine in ringworm. 140
Gray hair. 405
Grocer's itch. 109. 211
Gruby on mentagra. 373
Guillott. M.. alkaline ointment, 119
Guleet kusta. 291
Guinea-worm. 359
    disease, 359
Gum, 206
    red. 206
    white, 207
Gutta percha in skin diseases, 416
Gutta rosacea, 171

Hæmorrhagiæ, 43, 312
Hair, diseases of, 405
    falling out of, 408

Hair, grayness of, 405
Hardy's stages of eczema, [
    treatment for the itch,
Heat, prickly, 209
Hebra's tincture, 119
Hebrew leprosy, 298
Helmerich's itch ointment,
Hemlock ointment, 423
Herpe dartre, 122
Herpes, 122
    auricularis, 124
    capitis, 130
    circinatus, 128
    erethemoide, 48
    iris, 132
    labialis, 124
    miliaris, 123
    phlyctenodes, 123
    præputialis, 125
    pudendalis, 126
    squamosus, 129
    tonsurans, 129
    zoster, 126
Higginbottom's treatment (
    sipelas. 70
Hillier's table for diagnosis
    anthemata, 98
Honigwabbengrind, 360
Huile de cade, 119
Humid tetter, 102
Hydrargyria, 109
Hydropathic packing in pac
    249
Hygienic treatment of ski
    eases. 496
Hypertrophiæ, 288, 43
    syphilitic, 392

Ichthyiasis, 264
Ichthyose, 264
Ichthyosis, 229, 264
    cornea, 265
    hysterix, 265
    papillary, 267
    scutellata, 265
    sebacea squamosa, 265
    simplex, 265
    spinosa, 265
    squamosa, 265
Idiopathic erysipelas, 57
Ignis sacer, 126
Impetigo, 178
    capitis, 183

Lupoid impetigo, 186
Lupus, 339
    devorans, 343
    exedens, 340
    nonexedens, 340
    serpiginosus, 341
    superficialis, 340
      non-tuberculosus, 341
    vorax, 345
LXX, the, 155, 299

Maclagan, Dr., on the urine in
    urticaria, 78
Macula, 30
Maculæ, 43, 325
    of typhus and typhoid fevers,
    100
    syphilitic, 394
Madura foot, 376
Mark, mother, 309
Marsh's soaps, 429
Masern, 85
Measles, 85
    Babington on, 86
    Kennedy on, 86
    Salisbury on, 87
Measles, Camp, 86
Melasma, 256
Melitagra, 181
Mentagra, 371
    contagiosum, 373
Mermaids, 268
Mercurial baths, 420
    eczema, 109
Microscopical discoveries, 28, 366
Mixtures, alkaline, 431
    alterative, 432
    diaphoretic, 432
Molluscum, 274
    acutum, 275
    chronicum, 276
    contagiosum, 275
    non-contagiosum, 275
    pendulum, 276
Morbilli, 85
Morbus Addisonii, 334
    Taurieus, 292
Morphœe of Brazil, 291
Mother-mark, 309
Mycetoma, 376

Nævus, 309
    araneus, 310

Nails, diseases of, 411
    ingrowing of, 411
    parasitic diseases of, 412
Natural systems of classification,
    31, 36
Nethek, 155
Nettle rash, 72
Ngerengere, 292
Nirles, 123
Nitrate of silver stain, 332
Noli me tangere, 343

Œstrus, 359
Ointment, camphor, 428
    cucumber, 426
    Helmerich's, 163
    hemlock, 428
    scrophularia, 149
    stavesacre, 164
    white hellebore, 164
Ointments, 425
    astringent, 427
    sedative, 427
Onychomycosis, 412
Ophiasis, 411
Order of S. Lazarus, 285
Osborne, Professor, on plague at
    Athens, 324
Ὀυλή, 101

Pachydermia, 295
Packing in psoriasis, 249
Papula, 29
Papulæ, 42, 202
    syphilitic, 389
Papulous scall, 192
Parasites, 359
Parasitic diseases, 358
    germs contagious, 330
    in brewers, 330
    transmissible from animals to
    men, and *vice versa*, 330
Pediculi in Impetigo, 185
Pediculus pubis, 221
Pellagra, 293
Pemphigus, 140
    acutus, 141
    chronicus, 145
    contagiosus, 147
    foliaceus, 146
    gangrænosus, 143
    infantilis, 143
    simultaneus, 141
    successivus, 141

Pemphigus, syphilitic, 385
Pemphigus in children, 144
Petechiæ, 312
Petite verole, 92
Phlegmonous erysipelas, 59
Phlogosis erythema; 48
Phlyzacia, 42
Phthiriasis, 221
    capitis, 221
    corporis, 221
    pubis, 221
Phthirius, 221
Pills, Asiatic, 248
    diaphoretic, 431
Pimples, 29, 42, 202
Pityriasis, 253
    capitis, 256
    diffusa, 254
    labiorum, 256
    localis, 254
    nigra, 255, 282
    oris, 256
    palmaris, 256
    palpebrarum, 256
    plantaris, 256
    præputialis, 256
    pudendalis, 256
    rubra, 254
    versicolor, 255, 358
Plague at Athens, 324
Plica Polonica, 407
Pomade, cucumber, 426
    Helmerich's, 163
    turpentine, 329
    Copland's, for alopecia, 410
Pompholyx, 140
    benignus, 143
    diutinus, 145
    solitarius, 143
Pope Alex. III. de leprosis, 285
Porcupine men, 268
Porrigo, 360
    decalvans, 408
    favosa, 361
    lupinosa, 364
    scutulata, 130
Posological table, 435
Poussée (Lichen), 203
Powders, 428
    dusting, 428
Prepuce, herpes of, 125
Prescriptions, Lucas' act respecting the writing of, 433

Prickly heat, 209
Prima lunago, 168
Prurigo, 217
    formicans, 219
    mitis, 218
    palmaris, 222
    pedicularis, 221
    podicis, 222
    præputialis, 222
    pubis, 222
    pudendi, 221
    scroti, 221
    senilis, 220
    urethralis, 222
    vulgaris, 218
Prurit, 217
Ψώρα, 154
Ψώρα ἑλκώδης, 178
Psoriasis, 230
    aggregata, 233
    annulata, 238
    capitis, 235
    centrifuga, 236
    confluens, 233
    diffusa, 233
    guttata, 231
    gyrata, 233
    infantilis, 238
    inveterata, 234
    labialis, 235
    lepræformis, 236
    nummularis, 239
    orbicularis, 238
    palmaris, 235
        centrifuga, 236
        syphilitic, 390
    palpebrarum, 235
    præputialis, 235
    pudendalis, 235
    punctata, 232
    rupioides, 239
    scrotalis, 235
    syphilitic, 390
    unguium, 235
    Psoriasis, vulgaris, 23.
    hydropathic packing in, 249
Psydracia, 42
Pudendum, herpes of, 126
Pulex irritans, 359
    penetrans, 359
Purples, 313
Purpura, 313
    cachectica, 317

Purpura contagiosa. 317
    febrilis hæmorrhagica, 317
        simplex. 315
    hæmorrhagica, 315
    senilis. 315
    simplex. 314
    urticans. 314
Pustula maligna. 209
Pustule. 42, 147
    syphilitic. 386
Pustules. 42, 147

Ralledrge. 289
Rainbow ringworm, 132
Rash. 30
    nettle. 73
    rose. 80
    tooth. 204
    typhoid. 100
    typhus. 100
    wildfire. 207
Red gum. 204
Red precipitate soap. 429
Regional classifications. 29, 37
Rheumatism and urticaria, 76
Ringworm. 128
    of the scalp. 130
    rainbow. 132
    depilation in, 140
Robin's description of porrigo. 362
Rodent ulcer. 345
Rosalia. 82
Rose rash. 80
Roseola. 80
    æstiva. 81
    annulata. 81
    autumnalis. 81
    cholerica. 83
    febrilis. 83
    idiopathica. 80
    infantilis. 81
    miliaria. 83
    punctata. 82
    symptomatica. 82
    syphilitic. 383
    vaccina. 83
    variolosa. 83
Rosy drop. 171
Routh. Dr., juniper ointment, 120
Rubeola. 85
    maligna, 86
    nigra. 86
    notha, 86

Rubeola, reference to writers on, 88
    sine catarrho, 86
    sine exanthemate, 86
    vulgaris. 86
    Witt's treatment of, 88
Ructa kusta, 291
    pitia, 291
Rugeole. 85
Rupia, 150
    escharotica, 144, 151
    prominens, 151
    simplex, 151
    syphilitic, 385

Sacred fire, 126
Sahafati. 230
Sappachath, 230
Saltwater bathing, 418
Sapo laricis (Moore's), 430
Sarcoptes hominis, 156
Satyriasis, 284
Scabies, 154
    cachectica, 159
    lymphatica. 159
    papuliformis, 159
    purulenta, 159
    Col. Jebb on, 165
    King James I. on, 158
Scald head, 360
Scale, 30, 228
    dry, 230
Scall, 102
    head. 360
    papulous, 192
Scalp, eczema of, 107
    herpes of, 130
    impetigo of, 183
    psoriasis of, 236
    ringworm of, 130
Scarlatina, 89
    anginosa, 90
    levigata. 89
    maligna, 90
    milliformis, 89
    papulosa. 89
    phlyctenosa, 89
    plana, 89
    pustulosa, 89
    references to writers on, 92
    simplex, 89
    sine exanthemata, 90
    vesicularis, 89
Scarlatine, 89

Scarlet fever, 89
Scharlach fieber. 89
Schuppen, 253
Schwindfluken. 203
Scorbutus. the plague described
  by Thucydides, 324
Scotch fiddle, 155
Scrofulide pustuleuse. 155
Scrofula. esthiomanic. 347
Scrophularia ointment, 149
Sebaceous flux, 279
Seborrhea sicca, 265
Secondary eruptions, 378
Sedative alkaline lotions, 423
    ointments, 427
Sedgwick's case of ichthyosis, 270
Seeth, 101
Shell-fish, urticaria caused by, 75
Shvet kusta, 291
Shingles, 126
Silver, nitrate of, stain from, 322
Skin, diseases of appendages of,
  405
Smallpox, 92
Soap of corrosive sublimate, 429
    juniper tar, 430
    red precipitate, 429
    sulphur, 429
    white precipitate, 429
Soaps, 429
    Hendrie's, 430
    juniper tar, 430
    Marsh's, 429
    Moore's, 430
Soft corns, 306
Solution of iodide of potassium
  and arsenic, 247
Sore throat, 90
    Fothergill's, 90
    putrid, 90
Spedalskhed, 288
Squama, 30
Squamæ, 42, 228
    syphilitic, 390
St. Anthony's fire, 56
Stains, 30
    syphilitic, 394
Stavesacre ointment, 164
Stearne's case of alopecia from
  mental anxiety, 409
Stearrhœa, 278
    flavescens, 279
    nigricans, 281

Stearrhœa simplex, 279
Steatozoön folliculorum, 170
Stimulant wash, 423, 424
Stokes. Whitley, on pemphigus, 143
Strophulus. 206
    albidus, 207
    candidus, 207
    confertus, 206
    intertinctus. 206
    volaticus, 207
Sudamina, 110
Suintement, 186
Sulphur baths, 430
    soap, 429
Sulphurous lotion, 424
Sunbahiree, 291
Sunburn, 329
    rash, 108
Supra-renal capsules, disease of, 334
Sycosis, 371
    mentis, 371
Syphilide squameuse cornée, 392
Syphilides, 44, 378
    Zittmann treatment of, 403
Syphilitic acne, 386
    condylomata, 392
    ecthyma, 388
    eczema, 384
    ephelis, 395
    eruptions, 378
    erythema, 382
    exanthemata, 382
    herpes, 384
    hypertrophiæ, 392
    impetigo, 387
    lepra, 390
    lichen, 389
    maculæ, 394
    papulæ, 389
    pemphigus, 385
    psoriasis, 390
    pustulæ, 386
    roseola, 383
    rupia, 385
    squamæ, 390
    tubercles, 392
    urticaria, 382
    vesiculæ, 384
Syphilization, Böeck on, 402

Table for diagnosis in exanthemata, 98
Table, posological, 435

Terminthus, 192
Tetter, 122
   crusted, 179
   dry, 230
   eating, 339
   humid, 102
Therapeutics, 415
Sudamina, 155
Tinctura Saponis viridis cum pice, 71
Tinea 380
   capitis, 129
   favosa, 81
   tonsurans, 129
Tooth-rash, 208
Topical medication, 415
Traumatic erysipelas, 61
Trichophyton sporuloides, 405
Trichosis capitis, 129
   tonsurans, 129
Tubercular lichen, 208
Tubera, 84
[illegible], 325, 295
Tumour, 3, 305
Tubercles and mild films, 282
Turgescence, 293
Turpentine ointment, 354
Turkish bath, Dr. Goolden on, 417
Typhus in nomade, 326
Ulcerative rash, 140

Urticaria, 142
Urticaria, tuberosa
[several illegible lines]

Vaccination, 18
Vaccinia, 19

Vapor baths, 417
Varicella, 97
Variola, 92
   confluens, 93
   discreta, 93
   sine exanthemate, 94
Varioloid, 94
Varus, 168
Velpeau's treatment of erysipelas, 71
Venereal eruptions, 378
Verrucae, 305
Vesicating collodion in ringworm, 139
Vesicle, 30, 101
Vesiculae, 41, 101
   syphilitic, 336
Vesicular ecthyma, 185
Vibices, 312
Vienna Paste, 421
Vitiligo, 326
Vitiligoidea plana, 282
   tuberosa, 282

Warts, 305
Washerwomen's itch, 109, 211
Water-blebs, 140
White gum, 207
   hellebore ointment, 164
   leprosy, 290
   precipitate soap, 429
White rash, 207
Willan's classification, 29
Wilson's classification, 31–34
Wolf, the, 342

Yuck, 174

Zinc, 215
Zinc oxide, 173
Zittmann's treatment in syphilides, 465
Zona, 124
Zoster, 124
Zoonic diseases, 6

ATLAS OF CUTANEOUS DISEASES.

BY J. MOORE NELIGAN, M.D., M.R.I.A., &c.

With beautiful Colored Plates, presenting nearly one hundred elaborate representations of disease, colored after nature.

In one very handsome 4to. volume, extra cloth, price $5 50.

A compend which will very much aid the practitioner in this difficult branch of diagnosis. Taken with the beautiful plates of the Atlas, which are remarkable for their accuracy and beauty of coloring, it constitutes a very valuable addition to the library of a practical man.—*Buffalo Med. Journal.*

The lithographs are so colored as to be true and faithful representations of these ninety varieties of a class of diseases whose exact diagnosis is thus made plain and easy, and which, in the absence of such aid or a long and attentive study, is so difficult that very few practitioners seriously attempt it. The work is cheap, and no practitioner ambitious of a high professional status can afford to dispense with such helps.—*Nashville Journal of Medicine.*

Neligan's Atlas of Cutaneous Diseases supplies a long existent desideratum much felt by the largest class of our profession. It presents, in quarto size, 16 plates, each containing from 3 to 6 figures, and forming in all a total of 90 distinct representations of the different species of skin affections, grouped together in genera or families. The illustrations have been taken from nature, and have been copied with such fidelity that they present a striking picture of life; in which the reduced scale aptly serves to give, at a *coup d'œil*, the remarkable peculiarities of each individual variety. And while thus the disease is rendered more definable, there is yet no loss of proportion incurred by the necessary concentration. Each figure is highly colored, and so truthful has the artist been that the most fastidious observer could not justly take exception to the correctness of the execution of the pictures under his scrutiny.—*Montreal Med. Chronicle.*

The diagnosis of eruptive disease, however, under all circumstances, is very difficult. Nevertheless, Dr. Neligan has certainly, "as far as possible," given a faithful and accurate representation of this class of diseases, and there can be no doubt that these plates will be of great use to the student and practitioner in drawing a diagnosis as to the class, order, and species to which the particular case may belong. While looking over the "Atlas" we have been induced to examine also the "Practical Treatise," and we are inclined to consider it a very superior work, combining accurate verbal description with sound views of the pathology and treatment of eruptive diseases. It possesses the merit of giving short and condensed descriptions, avoiding the tedious minuteness of many writers, while at the same time the work, as its title implies, is strictly practical —*Glasgow Med. Journal.*

Dr. Neligan deserves our best thanks for this attempt to supply a want which has been long felt. For a small sum he here presents us with an Atlas containing some ninety plates of the more common and rarer forms of affections of the skin; and, for the benefit of those who possess his useful Manual, he supplies with each illustration a reference to the chapter of that work where the disease receives special attention. Great care has evidently been taken to procure proper subjects for the artist and the daguerreotype, which has been employed in several of the plates "to secure correctness in the design."—*Edinburgh Med. Journal.*

The art of Chromo-lithography has, in the present instance, achieved a very satisfactory result in the production of colored illustrations of cutaneous diseases. Great credit is due to Dr. Neligan in supplying to the student so useful a work. Some of the drawings are particularly close representations of nature. We would instance the first plate, giving the various forms of erythema, and an admirable one of erysipelas of the face; the forms of herpes (plate 4); of impetigo (plate 7), &c. Plate 13 gives a most artistic representation of purpura, which cannot fail to impress the student so that he would at once recognize the disease at the bed-side. Nor are the illustrations of lupus and porrigo favosa less characteristic. We need scarcely add that we recommend the work.—*British and Foreign Medico-Chirurg. Review.*

Rayer in France, and Erasmus Wilson in England, have given us admirable illustrations of this interesting class of diseases; and Dr. Neligan has now contributed to the medical pictorial literature of Ireland a most creditable volume, which may vie with the others in fidelity and finish.—*Medical Times and Gazette.*

HENRY C. LEA, Philadelphia.

NAME	DATE DUE

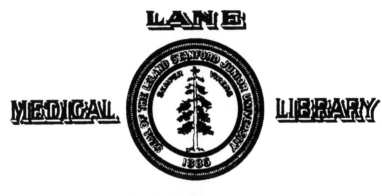

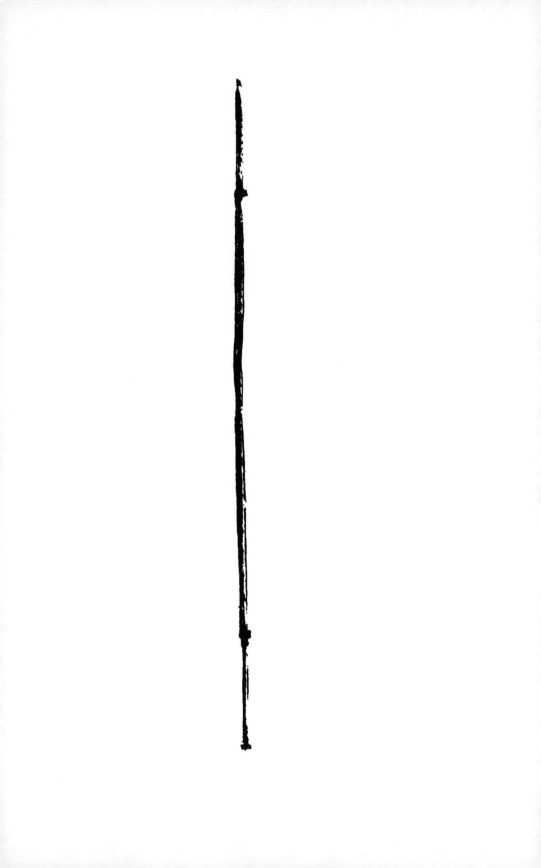

SKIN DISEASES,

INCLUDING THEIR

DEFINITION, SYMPTOMS, DIAGNOSIS, PROGNOSIS,
MORBID ANATOMY, AND TREATMENT.

A MANUAL FOR

STUDENTS AND PRACTITIONERS.

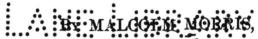

BY MALCOLM MORRIS,

JOINT LECTURER ON DERMATOLOGY AT ST. MARY'S HOSPITAL MEDICAL SCHOOL,
AND FORMERLY CLINICAL ASSISTANT, HOSPITAL FOR DISEASES OF THE
SKIN, STAMFORD STREET, BLACKFRIARS.

WITH ILLUSTRATIONS.

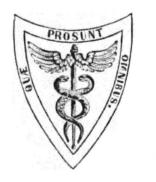

PHILADELPHIA:

HENRY C. LEA.

1880.

PREFACE.

In undertaking this little work, my object has been to supplement, not to supplant, existing treatises upon a subject which it is difficult to condense and arrange, and one, therefore, which has proved tedious to the student.

Commenced some months ago, to assist not only the students, but myself also, in the delivery of a course of Lectures at St. Mary's Hospital Medical School, it has by degrees so far exceeded its original limits as to have suggested the second half of its present title; for, while its simplicity will, it is hoped, adapt it to the wants of the student, its conciseness may commend it to the general practitioner.

To Mr. Jonathan Hutchinson and Mr. Warren Tay I am especially indebted for the useful knowledge which I obtained from them whilst acting as Clinical Assistant at the Hospital for Diseases of the Skin, Blackfriars; and to my friend and colleague, Dr. Cheadle, I owe my sincere thanks for kind assistance and for special opportunities of observing many interesting cases.

Moreover, I have not hesitated in the process of compilation to make constant requisition upon numerous authorities on Dermatology, both British and Foreign.

The Anatomy of the Skin in the first chapter is founded chiefly upon Biesiadecki's article in Stricker's "Manual," and Klein and Noble Smith's "Atlas of Histology." The plates which have been placed at my disposal by Dr. Klein form but a part of the kindness I have received at his hands, and which I here heartily wish to acknowledge. For the skilful execution of the woodcuts, I think I am justified in speaking in no measured terms of the able work of Mr. Noble Smith.

I must also express my thanks to my friend, Dr. Alfred Sangster, for much valuable assistance.

M. M.

63 MONTAGU SQUARE, HYDE PARK, W.
November, 1879.

CONTENTS.

CHAPTER I.

Anatomy and Physiology, ... 13

CHAPTER II.

Morbid Anatomy, ... 31

CHAPTER III.

Classification, ... 40

CHAPTER IV.

Scarlatina—Morbilli—Rötheln, ... 46

CHAPTER V.

Variola—Varicella—Vaccinia, ... 61

CHAPTER VI.

Typhus—Enteric—Diphtheria, ... 74

CHAPTER VII.

Equinia—Pustula maligna—Verruca necrogenica—Framboesia
—Erysipelas—Septicæmic rashes—Surgical rash, . . 85

CHAPTER VIII.

Syphilis—Infantile syphilis—Vaccino-syphilis, . . . 97

CHAPTER IX.

Erythema simplex, læve, fugax, intertrigo; multiforme, including papulatum, tuberculatum; annulare, iris, gyratum—Erythema · nodosum—Roseola—Urticaria—Pellagra, ... 117

CHAPTER X.

Lichen simplex, ruber, planus, marginatus, scrofulosorum—Prurigo— Prurigo infantum—Relapsing prurigo, ... 129

CHAPTER XI.

Herpes febrilis, gestationis, iris—Hydroa—Pemphigus vulgaris, foliaceus, ... 142

CHAPTER XII.

Eczema simplex—Acute: Eczema erythematosum, squamosum, papulatum, vesiculosum, pustulosum, fissum seu rimosum, rubrum, Ecthyma — Chronic: Eczema capillitii, faciei, articulorum, manuum et pedum, crurale, genitale, corporis—Intertrigo—Porrigo or Impetigo contagiosa, ... 150

CHAPTER XIII.

Pityriasis rubra—Psoriasis vulgaris—Pityriasis, . . . 168

CHAPTER XIV.

Furunculus—Anthrax—Delhi boil—Ulcers, ... 177

CHAPTER XV.

Hyperæmia—Anæmia—Hæmorrhages of the Skin—Purpura simplex, papulosa, rheumatica, hæmorrhagica—Scorbutus—Hæmatidrosis, ... 187

CHAPTER XVI.

Zoster—Cheiro-pompholyx—Pruritus—Dystrophia cutis, . 197

CHAPTER XVII.

Ephelis — Lentigo — Melanoderma — Morbus Addisonii—Chloasma uterinum — Ichthyosis — Xeroderma —Morphœa—Scleroderma —Sclerema neonatorum—Elephantiasis Arabum—Elephantiasis teleangiectodes—Dermatolysis, ... 209

CHAPTER XVIII.

Albinismus—Leucoderma—Atrophia cutis, ... 226

CHAPTER XIX.

Clavus—Tylosis—Verruca — Cornu cutaneum—Keloid—Fibroma— Xanthoma—Lupus vulgaris—Lupus erythematosus — Rhinoscleroma—Nævus—Angioma—Lymphangioma, . . 230

CHAPTER XX.

Lepra maculosa, tuberosa, anæsthetica—Carcinoma—Epithelioma— Ulcus rodens—Sarcoma, ... 255

CHAPTER XXI.

Seborrhœa oleosa, sicca, Ichthyosis sebacea neonatorum—Acne punctata, comedo, milium—Acne vulgaris—Acne sycosis—Acne rosacea — Molluscum contagiosum — Hyperidrosis — Anidrosis — Bromidrosis—Chromidrosis—Sudamina, ... 269

CHAPTER XXII.

Hirsuties—Lichen pilaris—Nævus pilosus—Canities—Alopecia— Alopecia areata—Trichorexis nodosa—Onychia—Onychogryphosis — Onychauxis — Onychatrophia — Changes in the nails during general diseases, ... 285

CHAPTER XXIII.

Pediculosis—Scabies—Eruptions produced by fleas, bugs, &c.—Tinea tonsurans—Kerion—Tinea sycosis—Tinea circinata—Eczema marginatum—Tinea versicolor—Tinea favosa. . . . 294

CHAPTER XXIV.

Eruptions produced by drugs, ... 314

INDEX, ... 317

MANUAL

OF

SKIN DISEASES.

CHAPTER I.

ANATOMY AND PHYSIOLOGY.

ANATOMY.

THE skin is the covering of the body which protects the more delicate tissues from injury, and joins the mucous membrane at the various orifices. The surface is not smooth, but consists of elevations, grooves, and depressions. The elevations form in places, such as the palm of the hand and sole of the foot, lines and wrinkles. The smallest elevations are caused by the prominence of the papillæ of the true skin. The grooves correspond to the lines or wrinkles, and lie between them. The depressions or pores of the skin are produced by the openings of the hair follicles, sebaceous and sweat glands,

The skin consists of two parts :

> The Epidermis,
> The Corium, or true skin,

together with more or less subcutaneous connective tissue. Besides these two layers there are certain structures to be described, viz., adipose tissue, sweat glands, sebaceous glands, hair follicles and hairs, muscular tissue, nails, bloodvessels, nerves, and lymphatics.

2

EPIDERMIS.

The epidermis is composed of four different layers or strata :

1. Rete Malpighii, or rete mucosum.
2. Granular layer.
3. Stratum lucidum.
4. Stratum corneum.

1. *Rete Malpighii.*—This is made up of a stratified pavement epithelium. The cells of the deepest layer are columnar in form, with oval nuclei; above, there are several

FIG. 2.

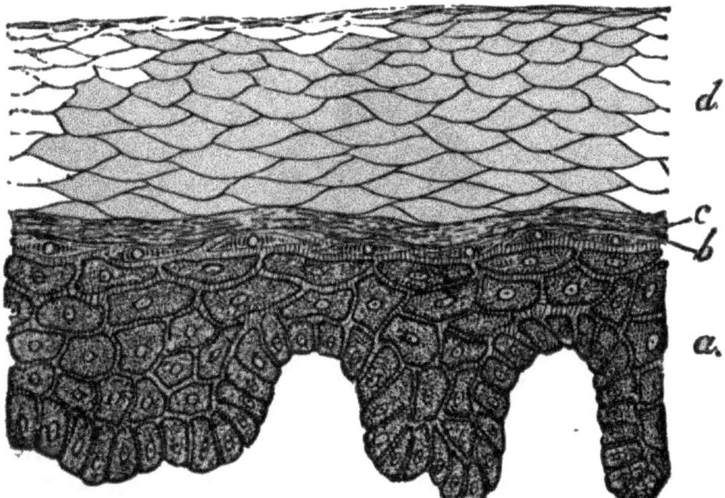

THE EPIDERMIS.

a, rete Malpighii; *b*, granular layer; *c*, stratum lucidum; *d*, stratum corneum.
(From Klein and Noble Smith's " Atlas of Histology.")

layers of polyhedral cells, with more or less spherical nuclei. The most superficial cells and their nuclei are flattened. The polyhedral and the columnar-shaped cells are joined together by fine fibrils, the so-called prickle cells of Max Schultze; these fibres are simply the prolongation of the mass of fibrils that constitutes the chief structure of the cells themselves. Thus the cells are composed of a delicate network, called the intracellular network, and a hyaline interfibrillar substance. Between the cells are the intercellular spaces, which are occupied by a clear semi-albuminous substance, the intercellular cement. In the spaces are seen branched connective tissue corpuscles, and the termination of nerves extending from the corium.

In dark colored skins the deepest cells contain pigment granules. The rete rests upon the true skin, and adapts

Fig. 3.

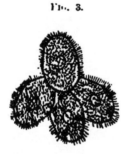

THE STRUCTURE OF CELLS. (Klein.)

itself to the elevations of the papillæ, the prolongations passing between them being named the interpapillary processes.

Secondly. There is a layer of flattened cells, shaped in vertical section, situated on the surface of the proper cells of the rete Malpighi. Each cell contains a nucleus from the end of which rodlike granules radiate. The granules have been seen at the mouths of the sweat ducts and in the cells.

Thirdly. The cells are homogeneous or finely granular, and are closely packed

4. *Stratum Corneum.*—This consists of many layers of horny non-nucleated scales. In various parts of the body this 'layer alters considerably in thickness, being very dense on the palms and soles.

CORIUM.

The corium is composed of connective tissue elements, in which are imbedded various important organs, such as the glands of 'the skin and their ducts, hairs, bloodvessels, and nerves. This connective tissue occurs as a dense felt-work, formed by bundles of fibres, which divide and cross each other repeatedly. Each bundle is formed of fine fibrils that yield gelatin, and are held together by an albuminous fluid cement substance. This substance is also found between the bundles themselves, each of which probably possesses a hyaline sheath as well: acids or boiling cause the bundles to swell up. On account of the difference in density, the corium is said to be divided into two parts; the superficial is known as the papillary body, in which the bundles of connective tissue are very thin, less dense, and hence more transparent. Between the groups of bundles, or trabeculæ, are spaces called lacunæ, which anastomose with one another by means of narrow channels. These lacunæ and channels form the lymph canalicular system, and contain flattened, nucleated, branched connective tissue corpuscles, the nucleated parts lying more particularly in the lacunæ, while the branched processes extend into the channels. There are certain elevations on the surface of the corium, of various sizes and shapes, called papillæ, between which are processes of the rete Malpighii. The largest are found on the palm of the hand and fingers. Some only contain vascular loops, others also nerve fibres and tactile corpuscles. A thin basement membrane lies between the corium and the rete Malpighii.

etween the lobes. Adipose tissue has characters in com-
1on with gland tissue; thus to each lobe and lobule there
1 an afferent artery and one or more efferent veins, with a
etwork of capillaries encircling the fat cells, either indi-
idually or in groups of two or three.

SWEAT GLANDS.

A sweat gland is a tube, composed of a membrana pro-
ria and of a lining epithelium, which consists of a single
ayer of columnar epithelial cells. The gland proper is

FIG. 4.

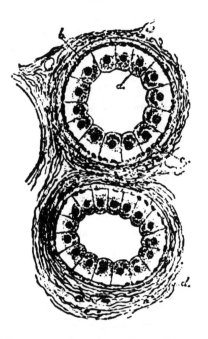

TRANSVERSE SECTION OF SWEAT GLAND.
lium; b, muscular coat cut transversely; c, nucleated membrana
propria; d, connective tissue. (Sangster.)

in the subcutaneous tissue, and is formed by the
on of the deep part of the tube. The duct passes

from the gland proper in an oblique and vertical direction
through the corium and epidermis to open on the surface.
The epidermic portion is called the mouth of the duct; in
it there is no membrana propria or special epithelium, and
in consequence it is surrounded only by the cells of the
epidermis.

The duct is lined at the commencement by a continuation
of the rete Malpighii, the cells of which are stratified, but
gradually, as the deeper parts are reached, the epidermis is
reduced, first to two layers of pavement cells and then to a
single layer of short columnar cells, which at the lowest
portion become elongated.

The tube of the gland proper, in some parts of the body,
contains a single layer of thin longitudinal unstriped muscle fibres, which is situated between the membrana propria
and the columnar epithelial cells. The glands that have
this muscular coat are usually larger in size than the variety
without it, and are especially well developed on the volar
side of the hand and foot, axillæ, scrotum, labiæ, and
scalp. They also occur by the side of the smaller glands.
The ceruminose glands of the external ear passage are of
the same structure as the larger variety, with the addition
of yellowish-brown pigment granules in the epithelial cells.
Sweat glands occur on all parts of the surface, but are
more numerous on the palms and soles.

Sebaceous Glands.

The sebaceous glands are situated in the corium, and consist of gland substance and excretory ducts, which open
usually at an acute angle into hair follicles, but occasionally
upon the surface. The gland substance is composed of lobules, filled with polyhedral cells, which open into the excretory ducts. A lobule is therefore a sac containing cells.
The sac is a transparent and colorless nucleated membrane
destitute of structure, and the cells are epithelial cells, the

are found at the entrance of the nose, the lips, the labia externa, and the scrotum.

HAIR FOLLICLE.

This is a depression in the corium which has a blind inferior dilatation and a funnel-shaped excretory duct. The

FIG. 6.

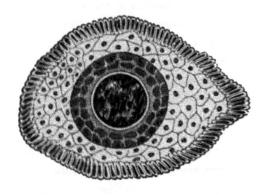

TRANSVERSE SECTION OF HAIR AND HAIR FOLLICLE.

neck is the contracted part below the duct where the sebaceous follicle opens. The follicle itself consists of two parts:

1. The hair sac.
2. The root sheath.

The hair sac consists of three layers,—external, middle, and internal.

The external layer is composed of fibres of connective tissue which run parallel to the axis of the hair and join the fibres of the corium above, whilst below they encircle the dilated extremity of the follicle.

The middle layer is formed of transverse fibres of connective tissue, between which is a homogeneous, slightly granular material that contains numerous rod-shaped, transversely arranged nuclei. This layer is highly contractile. Between these two layers are situated two or more longitudinal blood-vessels, which by their free anastomoses form a network around the follicle. The papilla of the hair protrudes into the cavity of the follicle, and is constituted of connective tissue fibres derived from this layer. The constricted portion of the papilla is the neck, and the thicker part the body, which has a conical extremity. The length is generally double the breadth.

The internal layer, thin and transparent, is a continuation of the basement membrane of the corium, and is called the vitreous membrane; the outer surface is smooth, whilst the inner is covered with prickles.

The root sheath consists of two layers:

1. The external root sheath.
2. The internal root sheath.

The external root sheath is a continuation of the rete Malpighii, which dips into the follicle, but terminates usually at a level with the apex of the papilla. The external layer of cells, viz., those that are in contact with the basement membrane, are columnar in shape, with nuclei at the inner extremity; the cells of the next layer are polyhedral, and the most internal are flattened. The sheath is thinnest at the neck of the follicle, but becomes thicker towards the bulb, where in the hairs of embryos and children small, simple or compound, budlike prolongations of the cells are seen.

The internal root sheath consists of two layers:

1. The outer or Henle's layer.
2. The inner or Huxley's layer.

1. *The outer or Henle's layer* is a thin, transparent membrane, which commences at the neck of the follicle and ex-

tends as far as the external root sheath. The membrane is composed of oblong, non-nucleated, highly refractile scales in immediate contact with one another, which run parallel to the long axis of the hair.

2. *The inner or Huxley's layer* consists of flattened, fusiform, nucleated cells filled with small refractile granules. At the lower part of the follicle, and also towards the neck, the two layers are indistinguishable. The follicles of lanuginous hairs are so small that the relations between them and the sebaceous glands are reversed, and they appear merely appendages of the relatively large gland.

MUSCULAR TISSUE.

Striated muscular tissue is present in the skin of the face, where it terminates in the corium.

A small involuntary muscle, called *arrector pili*, arises in the upper part of the corium, passes obliquely through it, and is inserted into the inner sheath of the hair follicle below the sebaceous gland; but some hair follicles have two muscles, which encircle the gland, and have a twofold action—to erect the hair and to compress the gland. There is, however, other involuntary muscular tissue in the corium, which runs either horizontally, as in the scrotum (dartos), or circularly, as in the nipple and in the areola around it.

HAIR.

A hair is divided into the shaft, which projects beyond the skin, and the root, which lies imbedded in the hair follicle. The structure of a hair consists of cortical substance, with addition, in some of the larger hairs, of a central medulla, composed of granular polyhedral cells.

A cuticle of homogeneous, transparent, non-nucleated scales, overlapping one another at their margins, incloses the cortical part. The root, which terminates in the bulb, .

surrounds a papilla projecting from the corium at the bottom of the follicle, and is composed of nucleated cells resembling the deeper cells of the rete Malpighii. The outer of these cells are flattened, and the inner are columnar in form and rest upon the surface of the papilla. In the root there is, besides the above-mentioned cuticle, another layer of flattened cells, which fits into spaces between these, and is continuous with Huxley's layer. The cortical substance, which is colorless in gray hairs and contains various colored pigment granules in other hairs, is, in the main portion, composed of longitudinal fibres, which, towards the bulb, appear as fusiform cells with rod-shaped nuclei, and which, at the transition into the bulb, become shorter and shorter until the polyhedral cells constituting the bulb are reached.

Hairs grow by the multiplication of the cells of the bulb lying next to the papilla. These new cells are gradually pushed outwards by the formation of yet newer cells, and become more fusiform as they leave the papilla. They also become more elongated, owing, perhaps, to the pressure of the internal root sheath. Hair are dissolved by strong solutions of potash.

NAILS.

The nails are horny, elastic, transparent, concavo-convex laminæ imbedded in the skin on the dorsal surface of the last phalanges, and are composed of nucleated epidermic cells firmly cemented together. They have an anterior, a posterior, and two lateral borders, an upper convex and a lower concave surface, the latter of which is situated on what is called the bed of the nail. This bed is formed by the rete Malpighii, the corium, and the subcutaneous tissue below it.

The last contains no fat, and its fibres pass in separate bundles from the periosteum of the phalanges backwards to the posterior border or root of the nail. The anterior part surface is lined by an endothelial membrane, formed of a single layer of flattened nucleated cells. The corpuscles are connected with medullated nerve fibres, which form the stalk, and are found most frequently in the subcutaneous tissue of the volar side of the hand and foot. The central clear mass is the axis cylinder of the nerve fibre, which usually divides into two or more branches, that terminate in pear-shaped or irregular bodies, called buds, and are composed of a dense network of minute fibrils. In some instances the corpuscle appears to have a second stalk, which is really an artery, that ultimately divides into branches, that give rise to a capillary plexus between the capsules.

B. *End Bulbs of Merkel.*—These are situated in the tissue of the papillæ or amongst the epithelium, and occur as single large and slightly flattened transparent nucleated cells inclosed in a capsule of connective tissue, and are in direct connection with the medullated nerve fibres.

C. *Tactile Corpuscles.*—These are oval bodies found in some of the papillæ, more particularly at the ends of the fingers. They, like the end bulbs, consist of a capsule, which contains a soft core composed of several small cells, and the termination of a medullary nerve fibre.

LYMPHATICS.

The lymphatics of the skin are grouped into two systems, the superficial and the deep.

The superficial resemble lymphatic capillaries, as their walls are composed of a single layer of endothelial plates. They form a network in the superficial part of the corium in immediate vicinity to the rete Malpighii and parallel to the surface, and into it branches of varying length enter from the papillæ.

The deep lymphatics also form a network, which lies in the subcutaneous tissue, but the meshes are larger and possess the character of tubes to a greater degree than in the superficial plexus.

These two systems communicate by means of branches that are in immediate association with the bloodvessels. The adipose tissue contains numerous lymphatics.

PHYSIOLOGY.

The skin serves some more or less important services in the economy, such as secretion, absorption, and tactile perception.

Secretion takes place in the form of perspiration by means of the sweat glands, which are continually carrying on their functions.

Perspiration is a clear, colorless, acid fluid, with a distinctive odor, that differs in various parts of the body. In a healthy man about thirty ounces is secreted in twenty-four hours, but this amount may be easily increased according to circumstances. For instance, more is secreted in summer than in winter, and more in consequence of exercise; certain foods and drugs also increase the flow, while at times mental emotion does the same. The perspiration that is perceptible to the sight is called sensible, and the portion that evaporates insensible. Perspiration consists chiefly of water, the average amount of solids being 1.81 per cent.

Constituents of Solids.

1. Sodium chloride and traces of other salts.
2. Fatty acids, such as formic, acetic.
3. Neutral fats and cholesterin.
4. Ammonia (urea), and possibly other nitrogenous bodies.
(Foster.)

The amount of carbonic acid given off in twenty-four hours is from four to ten grams, and the oxygen that is absorption is rather easy; however, the chief substance lost is water.

Animals that have been varnished soon die, and the use of some form of poisoning due to the absorption of some of the constituents of the perspiration. The skin has the power of absorbing, as is seen in the action on the system of certain drugs, like mercury and arsenic, after they have been well applied to the surfaces in a greasy form. The body also increases in weight by prolonged immersion in fluids.

For a description of the laws concerning the sense of touch the student is referred to the textbooks of Physiology.

CHAPTER II.

MORBID ANATOMY.

THE morbid processes which take place in the skin show themselves on its surface as certain discolorations, elevations, etc. ·These have received the name of the primary lesions. Enumerated, they are as follows:

1. Macule.
2. Papule.
3. Tubercle.
4. Wheal.

5. Vesicle.
6. Bulla.
7. Pustule.

Hebra's definitions are:

1. *Macule.*—Any change in the normal color of the skin, arising from disease, and not uniformly distributed over the whole surface of the body.

2. *Papule.*—Any morbid change in the skin which forms a solid projection above the surface, in size between a millet seed and a lentil, and containing within it no fluid.

3. *Tubercle.*—Any solid swelling of the skin, caused by disease, which contains no fluid, is as large as a lentil, bean, or hazelnut, and covered with epidermis.

4. *Wheal.*—A solid form of eruption slightly raised above the surface of the skin, of which the superficial area greatly exceeds the thickness.

5. *Vesicle.*—An elevation of the horny layer of the epidermis by transparent or milky fluid, corresponding in size to papules.

6. *Bulla.*—An elevation of the epidermis, in size between

a lentil and a goose's egg, containing transparent or yellow purulent fluid.

7. *Pustule.*—A small abscess, covered only with epidermis.

The process of ordinary inflammation of the skin is the sole mode of production of such lesions as the wheal and bulla, and is also the commonest cause of the other primary lesions.

In considering inflammation of the skin, it is necessary to bear in mind a few facts as to its anatomy. There is the deep plexus of vessels lying close beneath the level of the hair follicles, giving off branches, which in their turn break up to form anastomotic networks round the follicle and sweat glands. From it also communicating branches pass upwards to join the superficial plexus. The latter is situated beneath the papillæ, which are freely supplied with branches from it. Owing to this distribution of bloodvessels in the skin, the papillary body, the hair follicles, and the glands are the most vascular parts of the integument, and as such are the first to give evidence of the inflammatory process.

Thus during the early stages of inflammation the dilatation of the vessels and the increased blood flow give rise to hyperæmia of the part, which becomes visible through the epidermis. The surface becomes red, and inflammatory macules are produced, which, according to their shape and distribution, constitute the eruptions known in this country as rashes.

Examples.—Roseola, measles, erythema.

When the inflammatory process is confined to a minute area, as round the orifice of a hair follicle, and when in addition to the hyperæmia, there is a further stage of inflammation present, viz., exudation into the substance of the papillæ, the inflammatory papule is formed.

Examples.—Lichen, papular stage of eczema.

If the above condition extends to an area larger than that of a lentil, it is termed an inflammatory tubercle.

Example.—Erythema tuberculatum.

A similar state produces the wheal, but the inflammatory. œdema of the papillary body is quite peculiar. The process is very acute, and the exudation readily reabsorbed ; so that wheals are characterized by their transitory duration. In size they are, if discrete, about as large as the finger-nail, or somewhat smaller, but may become much larger by confluence. They vary in color according to circumstances, but for the most part are usually violet-red. The presence, however, of the exuded fluid sometimes forces the blood from the vessels, and the wheal then becomes white. As this first takes place in the centre, it is not unusual to see white wheals with red margins. Wheals are generally irregular in outline. The process which gives rise to them is neurotic in origin, probably causes vaso-motor spasm.

In the lesions hitherto considered the inflammatory exudation has not advanced beyond the true skin. In the vesicle, however, the serum transudes the boundary line between the rete mucosum and the papillæ, and making its way in the intercellular spaces, pushes the moist Malpighian cells asunder, and finally upheaves the horny layer of the epidermis. According to the extent of the area of epidermis raised by the exuded serum, a vesicle or bulla results.

Examples.—Vesicles, in herpes, vesicular stage of eczema ; bullæ, in pemphigus.

The transition from the vesicle to the pustule is merely the passage of the inflammatory process from a simple serous exudation to one accompanied by migration of leucocytes. Thus the fluid of vesicles is often seen to become milky, and afterwards straw-colored, as the serum becomes richer in cells.

Example.—Impetiginous eczema.

Sometimes the inflammatory process subsides rapidly after having given rise to one or more of the primary lesions, such as papules and vesicles, and generally leaves behind it vestiges which may be traced for some time afterwards.

Whether the inflammation be transitory, whether it per-. sists and becomes chronic, or is so by its nature from the beginning, certain secondary changes are set up in the tissues. As is well known, the epidermis derives its nourishment from the papillary body; consequently, congestion of the latter structure leads to a disturbance of nutrition of the epidermic cells; they do not pass through their chemical and physical changes, and are prematurely shed in larger or smaller masses as flakes or branlike scales. This is known as desquamation. It accompanies almost every inflammatory process, whether it be one which is of passing duration, as in measles, or whether it be chronic, as in psoriasis.

The next secondary change in the tissues resulting from inflammation is excessive deposit in the pigmentary layer of the epidermis, causing more or less brownish staining of the part, especially common in chronic inflammations. This change is known as pigmentation. There is another variety, not so permanent, which may accompany acute inflammatory conditions, and probably arises from the changes taking place in the exuded coloring matter of the blood, analogous to those seen in bruises.

An example of the first variety of pigmentation is well seen in chronic eczema, and of the second in some forms of old-standing urticaria.

A third change results from the increase in the cellular elements in the true skin, whether they be migrants from the blood or proliferated from the connective tissue corpuscles already existing in the part. It seems that they ultimately lead, by a process of fibrillation, to an increase of fibrous tissue. Thus the corium and subcutaneous tissue become hypertrophied. The fold of skin thus affected is pinched up with difficulty from the subjacent tissues, and, on being compared with a fold of sound skin, the increase in substance is at once apparent.

This infiltration of the skin is well marked in chronic eczema. It is always accompanied by pigmentation and desquamation.

There are certain changes, some of which affect the primary lesions themselves, which have received the name of secondary lesions; they are:

1. Scale.   4. Fissure.
2. Excoriation.   5. Scar.
3. Crust.

The scale (*squama*) has already been discussed in connection with the process of desquamation.

The excoriation (*excoriatio*) is produced by the exposure of the moist rete by the removal of the horny layers of the epidermis. This happens when vesicles burst, or are ruptured by the violence of scratching or rubbing. It is not uncommon to see whole areas denuded of horny epidermis and exuding drops of serum from the exposed rete. This exudation soaks into linen in contact with the part and stiffens it, or it dries on the surface and gives rise to the secondary lesion known as the crust (*crusta*).

According to the character of the discharge crusts vary in appearance. Simple serous exudation gives rise to grayish leathery crusts; when there is pus the crusts are yellow, and may be brown, or even black, owing to a mixture of blood with the exudation.

The crusts that form on the head and face often have a peculiar honeylike appearance, due to the presence of sebaceous matter. Sometimes the affected surface, after having ceased to exude and commenced to desquamate, again becomes moist; the crusts and scales thus formed alternately, remaining adherent, are called *lamellated crusts*.

Crusts are best seen in eczema.

The fissure (*rhagas*) is nothing more than a crack in the skin. It may extend only to the epidermis, but more frequently involves the corium. Fissures occur in skin which is rendered brittle by infiltration, and especially in parts which are subjected to much movement, such as the hands and flexures of joints.

The scar (*cicatrix*) replaces lost tissue. Scars indicate that the inflammatory process has been of the gangrenous variety—that is to say, it has been so severe that the cell production in the papillary body has caused strangulation of the vessels and consequent death of the part.

This variety of inflammation is characteristic of the disease variola, but it may occur spontaneously or as a result of continued irritation of the part in other affections—herpes, for example. Scars are white, smooth, devoid of hair follicles or glands. The appearance of a single scar furnishes no information as to its cause.

It has been shown how the process of ordinary inflammation of the skin may produce the so-called primary and secondary lesions, how its severity may cause loss of tissue, and how, when chronic, it leads to more or less permanent changes in the tissues.

Although the primary lesions, for the most part, correspond to certain types of inflammation, they cannot be regarded in any other light than that of evidencing so many stages in the inflammatory process, and as such they naturally pass from one into the other. Thus a disease which is generally characterized by the development of macules may present tubercles, or even bullæ, from the fact that an inflammation, which ordinarily stops at simple hyperæmia, has passed into one accompanied by exudation. Again, the eczematous inflammation commences in a papular eruption. Here it may cease; but more frequently the papules develop into vesicles, and these perhaps later on into pustules.

A want of appreciation of the manner in which one type of inflammation passes imperceptibly into another has led to much confusion in dermatology.

There are certain specific inflammations of the skin, associated with diathetic conditions, such as syphilis, struma, and leprosy. These inflammations all commence in the substance of the true skin as small rounded cells, which are deposited in groups in the spaces of a fine recticulum, and are richly supplied with delicately-walled bloodvessels. From the great similarity of these deposits to ordinary granulation tissue, Virchow includes them all under the head of granulation growths. The deposits give rise to elevations on the surface, which, according to their size, are termed papules or tubercles ; or they may be so superficial and diffuse as to appear like a simple macule. After a time the disturbance of the nutrition of the epidermis causes desquamation, and the tubercles are seen to be covered with scales. Unless interfered with by treatment, the tendency of these deposits of new growth is to increase until a point is reached at which their proper nutrition can no longer be maintained ; they then break down and ulcerate ; as they heal cicatrices are left, the result of the destruction of tissue which perishes with the new growth.

Some other modes of production of the primary lesions must now be briefly noticed.

A macule is defined as "any change in the normal color of the skin." Besides the inflammatory macule we must include the discoloration caused by the escape of the coloring matter of the blood into the surrounding tissue, as seen in purpura. These purpuric macules are distinguished from the inflammatory by the fact that the color does not disappear on pressure. Occasionally one variety passes into another. Small dotlike purpuric macules are called petechiæ. When once the coloring matter of the blood has entered the tissues, the part undergoes a characteristic series

4

of changes in color, as seen in bruises. There are white
macules, due to absence of pigment in the skin, as in leucoderma, and brown, due to excessive deposit of pigment,
as in liver-spot and freckle, or to parasitic growth, as in
tinea versicolor.

Papules arise from many causes besides that already
pointed out as resulting from inflammatory œdema of the
papillæ. There are, for instance, the papules arising from
minute lupus or syphilitic deposit in the corium. They are
also formed by a heaping up of the epidermis at the mouth
of the hair follicle (*lichen pilaris*). There are conditions
of the sebaceous glands which lead to the production of
papules, as when they degenerate and form little white solid
bodies protruding above the level of the skin, especially in
the neighborhood of the eyelids (*milium*).

A very important mode of forming papules is seen in
lichen ruber, in which an overgrowth of the cells of the
external root sheath of the hair is said to take place, and
ultimately produces the flat-topped, umbilicated papule.
There are also other less important varieties of papules.

All that applies to the papule may be said of the tubercle,
the distinction between them being only the very artificial
one of size. Tubercles either result from deposits of new
growths (syphilis, lupus), or from a further development of
smaller papules, as in the variety of erythema multiforme,
known as erythema tuberculatum.

The wheal has already been discussed. Besides the vesicle
of ordinary inflammation, which is best seen in eczema, it
is said that there is another variety, produced in connection
with the sweat duct in the condition known as sudamina.
Vesicles which occur in situations where the epidermis is
thick, as on the hands, acquire a peculiar sodden appearance at their margins, and are now known as the sago-grain
vesicles.

Under the head of pustule must be included the catarrhal

pustule, which often occurs as a further development of the vesicle, and also those suppurations round the hair follicles which result in small abscesses. Although the latter commence deep in the substance of the corium, the pus makes its way to the surface, and they ultimately appear as minute abscesses covered only with epidermis (acne).

The inflammatory bulla is seen in pemphigus. Other conditions give rise to the formation of bullæ, but chiefly as the result of accident (erysipelas, erythema multiforme). What may be termed false bullæ, as sometimes seen on the hands, are produced by the confluence of vesicles.

The foregoing remarks on the general pathology of the skin will serve to show that for purposes of diagnosis the so-called primary lesions are, according to their definition, wholly useless:

First, because they may be caused by totally distinct conditions.

Secondly, because they may change as the process which gives rise to them becomes modified.

CHAPTER III.

CLASSIFICATION.

NEARLY every author who has written on skin diseases has suggested a new method of classification, based on some theory of supposed utility. The first system of any importance was founded by Willan, whose idea was to class the diseases under the heads of the more important external manifestations: thus he employed nine orders, each named after some particular symptom of an eruption, without paying any regard to the general character of the disease. For instance, varicella, herpes, and eczema are included in the order vesiculæ.

The next classification to be noticed is that of the French school, which is called the natural system, because the nature of the disease, and not the symptoms, forms its basis. This was introduced by Alibert, and modified later by Hardy, but has not been used to any great extent in this country.

The anatomical system was proposed by Erasmus Wilson, who grouped skin diseases into four principal classes:

1. Affections of the corium.
2. Of the sudoriparous glands.
3. Of the sebiparous glands.
4. Of the hair and follicles.

These classes are divided into several sub-classes.

The classification introduced by Hebra, and most frequently made use of in this country and in America, is founded on anatomico-pathological principles. He defines twelve classes:

1. Hyperæmiæ cutaneæ.
2. Anæmiæ cutaneæ.
3. Anomalies of the cutaneous glands.
4. Exudations.
5. Hæmorrhagiæ cutaneæ.
6. Hypertrophiæ.
7. Atrophiæ.
8. Neoplasmata.
9. Pseudoplasmata.
10. Ulcerationes.
11. Parasites.
12. Neuroses.

Classification by cause would undoubtedly be the best, if sufficiently correct information could always be obtained; but in the present state of our knowledge of the subject such a plan is only partially possible. However, it will be seen that the last two classes in the following system are classified on this principle.

The system in this work is, in the first place, somewhat similar to Erasmus Wilson's in having two anatomical divisions; and, further, with certain slight modifications it resembles Hebra's in subdividing them into pathological classes.

DIVISION I.—DISEASES OF THE SKIN PROPER.

Class I.—EXUDATIONES.

Sub-class A.—*Induced by Infection or Contagion.*

1. Scarlatina.
2. Morbilli.
3. Rötheln.
4. Variola.
5. Varicella.
6. Vaccinia.
7. Typhus.
8. Enteric.
9. Diphtheria.
10. Equinia.
11. Malignant pustule.
12. Verruca necrogenica.
13. Framboesia.
14. Erysipelas.
15. Septicæmic rashes.
16. Surgical rash.
17. Syphilis.

Sub-class B.—*Of Internal or Local Origin.*

Erythematous,	1. Erythema	Simplex, læve, fugax, intertrigo, multiforme, nodosum.
	2. Roseola	
	3. Urticaria	
	4. Pellagra	
Papular,	1. Lichen	Simplex. Ruber and pianus. Scrofulosorum.
	2. Prurigo	Of Hebra. Infantum, of Hutchinson. Recurrens,
Vesicular and bullous,	1. Herpes	Febrilis. Gestationis. Iris.
	2. Pemphigus	Vulgaris. Foliaceus.
Eczematous and pustular,	1. Eczema	Simplex. Rubra. Varieties local.
	2. Impetigo contagiosa porrigo.	
Squamous,	1. Pityriasis rubra.	
	2. Psoriasis.	
	3. Pityriasis.	
Phlegmonous and ulcerative,	1. Furunculous.	
	2. Anthrax.	
	3. Delhi boil.	
	4. Ulcers (varieties).	

Class II.—VASCULAR.

Hyperæmiæ, Anæmiæ, Hæmorrhagiæ,	Purpura simplex. " rheumatica. " hæmorrhagica. Scorbutus.

Class III.—NEUROSES.

Zoster.
Cheiro-pompholyx.
Pruritus.
Dystrophia cutis.

Class IV.—HYPERTROPHIÆ.

Pigmentary, ...
{
1. Ephelis, lentigo.
2. Melanoderma.
3. Morbus Addisonii.
4. Chloasma uterinum.
}

Epidermis and papillæ, ... Ichthyosis, xeroderma.

Connective tissue, ...
{
1. Morphæa.
2. Scleroderma.
3. Sclerema neonatorum.
4. Elephantiasis arabum.
5. Elephantiasis teleangiectodes.
6. Dermatolysis.
}

Class V.—ATROPHIÆ.

Pigmentary, ...
{
1. Albinismus.
2. Leucoderma.
}

Connective tissue, ... Atropia cutis.

Class VI.—NEOPLASMATA.

Sub-class A.—*Benign.*

Papillomatous, ...
{
1. Clavus.
2. Tylosis.
3. Verruca.
4. Cornua.
}

Of connective tissue, ...
{
1. Keloid.
2. Fibroma.
3. Xanthoma.
}

Of granulation tissue, . . .
{
1. Lupus, . . { Vulgaris.
Erythematosus.
2. Rhinoscleroma.
}

Of bloodvessels, ...
{
1. Nævus.
2. Angioma.
}

Of lymphatics, ... Lymphangioma cutis.

Sub-class B.—*Malignant.*

1. Lepra, . .
{
Maculosa.
Tuberosa.
Anæsthetica.
}
2. Carcinoma.
3. Epithelioma.
4. Ulcus rodens.
5. Sarcoma.

Division II.—DISEASES OF THE APPENDAGES OF THE SKIN.

Subdivision A.—*Of the Sebaceous Glands.*

1. Seborrhœa.
2. Acne punctata. . . . . . . { Nigra (comedo).
   { Alba (milium).
3. Acne vulgaris.
4. Acne sycosis.
5. Acne rosacea.
6. Molluscum contagiosum.

Subdivision B.—*Of the Sweat Glands.*

1. Hyperidrosis.
2. Anidrosis.
3. Bromidrosis.
4. Chromidrosis.
5. Sudamina.

Subdivision C.—*Of the Hair.*

1. Hirsuties.
2. Lichen pilaris.
3. Nævus pilosus.
4. Canities.
5. Alopecia.
6. Alopecia areata.
7. Trichorexis nodosa.

Subdivision D.—*Of Nails.*

1. Onychia.
2. Onychogryphosis.
3. Onychauxis.
4. Onychatrophia.
5. In general diseases.

Class A.—PARASITIC AFFECTIONS.

Animal, ...

1. Pediculosis, . . . { Corporis. Capitis. Pubis.
2. Scabies.
3. Eruptions from fleas, etc.

Vegetable, . . .

1. Tinea tonsurans.
2. Kerion.
3. Tinea sycosis.
4. Tinea circinata.
5. Eczema marginatum.
6. Tinea versicolor.
7. Tinea favosa.

Class B.—ERUPTIONS PRODUCED BY DRUGS.

It will be noticed that although, in the main, we have followed Hebra, yet there are certain alterations in arrangement, due chiefly to the more recent researches in pathology. Much assistance has been gained from Dr. Bulkley's article on the subject in the "Archives of Dermatology" for April, 1879, and many of his suggestions and names have been adopted.

ACUTE INFECTIOUS DISEASES

The acute infectious diseases agree in certain broad features. As a rule, each occurs but once in the history of an individual, one attack protecting the patient from a subsequent attack if he be exposed to the virus.

They are run an acute course, and are characterized, first, by an incubation period, or period of latency, from the time when the poison is received to the appearance of the first symptom of the disease; secondly, by the presence of symptoms of constitutional disturbance; and, thirdly, during some period of the disease by the existence of an eruption on the skin.

Each of these diseases reproduces itself in any susceptible person exposed to its poison, and never causes any of the other acute infectious diseases.

Varieties of the same disease, however, do not necessarily produce the same variety, for these modifications are due not to any special properties of the poison, but to some condition in the constitution of the person who receives it.

Although some epidemics are known to be more fatal than others, the difference between them is due not to any special virulence of the disease, but depends altogether on the condition of the community into which the disease is introduced. Occasionally it is found that the members of a family are all attacked by a very severe form of scarlatina, contracted from the same person, but this occurrence must not be regarded as a proof of anything but a special susceptibility of the family to the influence of the disease.

When large numbers of persons are attacked, as in the case of schools, where family susceptibility can be eliminated, it is not found that the character of the disease is the same in all cases, although it may be derived from the same source.

Finally, it must be pointed out that, having regard to the infectiousness of the diseases in this category, their early recognition is a matter of great importance, in order that persons suffering from them may be isolated and the necessary steps be taken to disinfect the articles they have infected.

SCARLATINA—SCARLET FEVER.

Definition.—Scarlatina is an acute infectious disease characterized by the presence of a red rash on the body and extremities, and of redness and swelling of the fauces, accompanied by symptoms of constitutional disturbance.

Symptoms.—Between twenty-four hours and seven or eight days after the reception of the poison the patient is attacked by shivering, vomiting, headache, and sore throat. The soreness of the throat rapidly increases, and from twelve to thirty-six hours after the beginning of the constitutional symptoms a rash commences to appear on the chest, neck, and wrists, whence it may extend over the whole body. The rash is generally at its height about the third or fourth day of the disease, then begins to fade, and disappears in about a week or ten days. This disappearance is followed by desquamation of the cuticle, which generally begins in

the latter part of the second week, but may commence as
the rash fades or not until the end of the sixth week. Desquamation occurs over the whole body, particularly on the
hands and feet, and is by no means limited to the site of the
eruption.

During the continuance of the rash the condition of the
fauces is characteristic; the whole mucous membrane is
highly injected, the papillæ of the soft palate are bright
red and prominent, and the whole of the parts are more or
less swollen. Occasionally ulceration of the tonsils takes
place, and the glands of the neck are nearly always somewhat enlarged, and sometimes suppurate. The tongue at an
early stage of the fever is covered with a white fur, through
which the papillæ, which have become red and swollen,
show themselves, particularly at the edges, thus giving the
strawberry appearance well known as a symptom of the
disease. Later on, as the fever subsides and as the rash
fades, the tongue commences to desquamate, the fur is gradually removed, leaving it of a bright-red color, with its papillæ considerably enlarged, and gradually the bright redness fades to a normal hue, the papillæ cease to be swollen,
and it recovers its usual appearance.

From the first symptoms of the disease the temperature
is higher than normal, and becomes still higher on each subsequent day until the third or fourth day, when a temperature of 103° to 104° is reached, the evening temperature
being usually higher than the morning by about a degree.
At the end of a week the temperature gradually falls, and by
about the tenth or fourteenth day has again become normal.
The pulse is considerably quickened, especially at night,
when in adults 120 pulsations often occur in the minute.
During the course of the disease the patient suffers from pain
in the throat, particularly in swallowing; he has severe
headache, and frequently some delirium. At the height of
the fever albumen is often present in the urine, but disap-

pears as the fever subsides; at a later stage, however, especially about the end of the third week, there is a tendency for it to reappear.

These are the symptoms of an average attack of scarlatina, but it must be borne in mind that they are liable to considerable modification—that the rash may be absent, or may appear only in a few dark patches or as a bright efflorescence over the whole body; that the constitutional disturbance may be almost absent or may be of the severest character; that the condition of the throat varies with the severity of the attack from a simple injection to a condition ending in sloughing of tonsils, uvula, and cervical glands; and that the delirium may be altogether absent, or present at night only in a mild form or in the most violent type.

It is now necessary to describe more particularly the varieties of rash which are present in the different forms of scarlatina.

In an attack of average severity the rash first appears on the chest and neck as minute red points, which are slightly raised, the skin intervening between them being of the normal color. Later on they become brighter, and the redness which is at first limited to them extends over the intervening skin. If examined carefully, they can still be distinguished by the fact that they are redder than the surrounding skin. At this stage the skin is found to be rough on passing the hand over it. As the rash becomes more fully developed the identity of the red points is lost in the general hyperæmia; but this stage is not always reached, and in the milder form of scarlatina this identity is not lost until the rash commences to fade, while in some rarer forms the eruption does not become confluent during its whole course. The distance between the spots varies in different parts of the body. On the chest, neck, and face they are so close as usually to become confluent, while on the wrists, backs of the hands, and dorsum of the feet they are farther apart, and more frequently remain separate than when situated on the chest and neck. In some cases the intense hyperæmia of the red spots causes minute vesicles to be formed at these points. These vesicles last but twenty-four or forty-eight hours, and when they dry up the skin desquamates freely.

In the most severe forms of scarlatina an entirely different eruption is present. Instead of bright-red points appearing there is at once an escape of coloring matter from the capillaries into the superficial layers of the skin. This happens within twenty-four or thirty-six hours from the first symptom. A purple mottled appearance is thus produced, which but partially fades on pressure. There is slight general hyperæmia of the skin, but the rash is of a dusky red, which betokens an unfavorable termination. Accompanying this form in children there is the most intense restlessness and partial unconsciousness, while in adults complete consciousness sometimes remains, but there is constant vomiting of brown liquid from the stomach, a feeble, rapid, and compressible pulse, and a sense of extreme prostration. Between this and the milder forms of scarlatina there is every gradation, but it may be accepted generally that the tendency to hæmorrhage and the dusky color of the rash is an indication of a severe form of the disease. In the most severe forms the tongue is spongy; later it becomes dry, glazed, and red, and finally cracks and bleeds.

The temperature in the hæmorrhagic form is not always specially high, often not reaching above 103°; but its chief characteristic is irregularity, a considerable fall often preceding the fatal termination, while in the death agony it rises, and even after death continues to rise.

Occasionally later in the disease, even as long as a month after the first symptom, the patient again suffers from sore throat, the fauces again become swollen and injected, albumen appears in the urine, and a rash once more is developed on the chest. This varies much in appearance, but usually

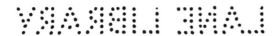

begins as a number of minute red points, which are soon lost in a general hyperæmia. The rash lasts sometimes but twelve hours, sometimes two or three days, and is, in all probability, due to some septic condition.

During desquamation an occasional simple injection occurs on the chest, without the presence of any constitutional symptoms. It is not uncommon, also, during convalescence, to find the legs covered with a mottled rash, which does not fade on pressure, due to the escape of blood coloring matter into the surrounding tissue. This lasts but a few days, and is also not attended by any constitutional symptoms.

Finally, it must be remembered that in all these rashes there is no tendency to œdema of the skin, except occasionally slight fulness or puffiness about the eyes, and that, with the exception of those specially mentioned, all fade on pressure.

Diagnosis.—Care is often required in the diagnosis of scarlatina, although in an attack of moderate severity its symptoms are sufficiently well marked to make its separation from other diseases a simple matter. It will not be necessary to refer to all the symptoms already described, but it will be sufficient to point out that at any period of the rash the disease may be recognized not only by the character of the eruption, but by the sore throat, the injected fauces, the strawberry character of the tongue, the pyrexia, and the constitutional symptoms.

In the most severe form, when no rash is present, the diagnosis of scarlatina is almost an impossibility. Vomiting and high temperature, succeeded by restlessness, delirium, and coma, are symptoms which are rather suggestive of poisoning than of a specific fever; but, as a rule, cases such as these do not occur singly, and other cases of less severity occurring immediately afterwards in members of the same family often throw light upon the first case.

In the hæmorrhagic forms the same difficulty also exists,

but to a less degree, for in them the condition of the throat
is often sufficient to aid the diagnosis.

From the hæmorrhagic form of variola,—the disease for
which it is likely to be mistaken during small-pox epidemics,—it may be distinguished, first, by the implication of
the throat; secondly, by the absence of pain in the back in
scarlatina, an almost constant symptom of variola; and,
thirdly, by the absence of the abortive papules and vesicles
which can usually be found among the hæmorrhages in the
latter.

From roseola it may be distinguished, first, by the smaller
size of the red points in the rash of scarlatina, and by the
fact that in scarlatina the skin intervening between these
points soon becomes injected. The condition of the throat
and tongue, as well as the presence of pyrexia, makes the
diagnosis between the erythemata and scarlatina a simple
matter. Between a very mild form of scarlatina, in which
the space intervening between the red points does not become injected, in which the temperature is but slightly
raised and the throat but little affected, and roseola there
is often much difficulty in diagnosis; but it must be noted
that in scarlatina a larger extent of the soft palate and
fauces are injected than in roseola, and that the enlargement of the papillæ of the tongue covers a larger surface
than in the latter disease; moreover, the papules of roseola
are more raised than the red points of scarlatina.

The accompanying table (p. 53) shows the distinctive
symptoms of scarlatina, measles, and rötheln.

Prognosis.—The termination of a case of scarlatina can,
as a rule, be correctly predicted after the rash has existed
for twenty-four hours. Until this time a guarded opinion
should always be given. When the rash is fully developed
and of a bright-red color; when the throat affection is characterized more by injection than by swelling of tonsils and
enlargement of cervical glands; when the pulse is not in-

Rash,	SCARLATINA.	MEASLES.	RÖTHELN.
	Consists of minute red points close together on a bright-red hyperemic ground.	Consists of papules of larger size, arranged somewhat in crescentic manner on a white ground of normal skin. The skin intervening between the spots is slightly reddened, but later on the patches become confluent.	Consists of slightly raised patches, varying in size, but usually about the size of a pea.
	First appears on chest, neck, and face.	First appears on forehead and face, and extends downwards.	First appears on chest.
	Appears after about twenty-four hours' illness.	Appears after about seventy-two hours' illness.	Appears first, or is preceded for a few hours by slight catarrh.
	Attended by marked injection of fauces, increase of temperature, strawberry tongue, slight suffusion of eyes.	Only slight sore throat and but little injection, high temperature, furred tongue, papillæ sometimes enlarged, but to a less extent than in scarlatina. Marked coryza.	Fauces injected, but less so than in scarlatina. Temperature slightly increased. Tongue furred.
	Followed by desquamation of skin in large flakes. Glands of throat enlarged.	Occasionally by desquamation of skin in very small scales. Glands, as a rule, not enlarged.	No desquamation, or only in the shape of small scales. Glands enlarged at different portions of body, and especially at back of the sterno-mastoid muscle.

5

creased in adults to above 120 at night, recovery may be
expected. When, however, the rash is badly developed and
of a dark color or hæmorrhagic, the pulse very rapid, and
a tendency for the temperature to be very irregular, the
mortality is very high.

In giving an opinion on the probable termination of a
case of scarlatina, it should be borne in mind that the mortality is inversely proportionate to the age of the patient,
children of two or three years of age dying in much larger
proportion than those older. It may also be noted that
rickety children, as a rule, have much more severe attacks
than others, and that they are more liable to suffer from
severe throat affection and suppuration of glands.

Morbid Anatomy (abridged from Klein's " Report to the
Privy Council ").—In scarlatina the morbid changes which
take place in the skin are mainly those of hyperæmia and
slight exudation, with consequent nutritive changes in the
epidermic layers.

1. The rete Malpighii, as a whole, is thickened, its cells
separated by more or less fluid effusion, and leucocytes to a
considerable extent are present. In some of the cells the
nuclei are seen to be enlarged and constricted or double, indicating fission of the rete cells.

2. In later stages the rete is less thickened, but here and
there local thickenings of the stratum lucidum, the cells of
which are full of granules, and partial loosening of the stratum corneum are found, preceding the separation of large
masses by desquamation. In the hair follicles the epithelium of the external root sheath is often thickened, has its
nuclei dividing, and contains some scattered leucocytes.
The inner root sheath is also thickened, more nucleated
and granular. The epithelium of the sweat glands shows
signs of germination, and is sometimes found loose in
the tubes, having been detached by inflammatory exudation, which sometimes contains blood. Occasionally in S.

maligna hæmorrhages occur into both the cuticle and the corium. The corium in early stages presents signs of inflammatory œdema, its papillæ are enlarged, the lymphatics and bloodvessels well filled, and leucocytes present in abundance. In the bloodvessels there is multiplication of the endothelial nuclei and of the muscle cells in the walls of the arterioles.

Treatment.—Inasmuch as scarlatina is an acute disease running a rapid course, the treatment consists in putting the patient under circumstances most favorable to his recovery. Thus a well-ventilated room of moderate temperature, the careful regulation of diet,—which should consist simply of milk, beef tea, etc., during the pyrexial period,—attention to the bowels, and, if. necessary, in severe cases, when the strength is failing, the administration of stimulants, are as a rule sufficient. Delirium and sleeplessness, when present, are best treated with chloral hydrate and bromide of potassium. The frequent sponging of the body with water, vinegar, etc., is extremely useful. Severe pyrexia should be treated with cold baths. The patient should remain in bed for three weeks from the beginning of the disease, with a view to preventing kidney complication. Albumen, after two or three weeks' illness, should be constantly looked for, and the treatment regulated accordingly.

MORBILLI—MEASLES.

Definition.—Measles is an acute infectious disease characterized by the production of an eruption of red papules, accompanied by symptoms of coryza and general constitutional disturbance.

Symptoms.—From ten to fourteen days after the reception of the poison the patient becomes ill and feverish, shivers, sometimes vomits, and complains of headache. The skin becomes dry and hot, the tongue coated with white fur,

through which a few large papillæ may show themselves;
the eyes become suffused, the eyelids swollen, the fauces injected, and sneezing, pain in the frontal sinuses, and all the
symptoms of a severe catarrh appear. The temperature
rapidly increases, the pulse is quickened, and the rash appears on the fourth day, first on the forehead and face, and
thence extends over the rest of the body and extremities,
about one or perhaps two days being occupied in its complete development.

As the rash makes its appearance the face becomes more
swollen, the coryza increases, and an exacerbation of the
constitutional symptoms, together with some amount of
bronchitis, nearly always appears. After the rash has existed for two or three days it gradually fades, and the constitutional symptoms subside.

The rash first presents itself as a number of small red spots
irregularly scattered over the skin, which rapidly become
raised, forming dark-red colored papules from $\frac{1}{16}$ to $\frac{1}{4}$ of an
inch in diameter.

On the face especially, and on all parts of the body where
the papules are closely aggregated together, they coalesce
and form patches of various sizes and of a crescentic shape;
as the rash fades a temporary staining of the skin remains,
which disappears after some days. The rash fades on pressure, but at once reappears on the removal of the finger,
and its disappearance is often followed by desquamation of
the skin in small scales.

Several varieties of the rash are described.

1. *Morbilli Læves.*—In this variety healthy skin intervenes between the maculæ, which are but slightly raised.

2. *Morbilli Papulosi.*—The papules are more raised and of
a dark-red color; they are situated at the mouth of hair
follicles, and closely resemble the papules of small-pox.

3. *Morbilli Vesiculosi.*—The mouths of the hair follicles
are filled with fluid, and small vesicles are thus produced.

4. *Morbilli Confluentes.*—Occur when the maculæ are crowded so closely together that they coalesce and no healthy skin intervenes between them.

5. *Morbilli Hæmorrhagici.*—This form of rash results from hæmorrhage into the maculæ, which of course do not then fade on pressure.

Diagnosis.—There are four diseases for which measles may at first sight be mistaken,—scarlatina, rötheln, roseola, and variola.

The following table will show the difference between these diseases in the early stages; at a later stage the difference in the appearance of the rashes become more marked, the different constitutional symptoms more fully developed, and the diagnosis consequently easier :

MORBILLI.	SCARLATINA.	RÖTHELN.
Rash appears on the fourth day.	Rash appears on the second day.	Rash appears on the first day.
Slight sore throat Tongue furred, few papillæ enlarged.	Considerable sore throat and injection of fauces. Tongue furred, many papillæ enlarged.	Slight sore throat. Tongue furred ; papillæ slightly enlarged, chiefly at edges.
Severe catarrhal symptoms.	No catarrh.	Slight catarrh.

ROSEOLA.	VARIOLA.
Rash appears on the first day.	Rash appears on the third day.
Slight sore throat. Tongue very slightly furred, only few papillæ enlarged at edges.	Slight sore throat. Tongue furred, papillæ not enlarged.
No catarrh.	Suffusion of eyes only. Severe lumbar pain.

Prognosis.—Usually favorable, but at times dangerous, owing to the long complication.

Morbid Anatomy.—On examining the measles eruption in

its earliest stages, we find usually slight hyperæmia round the orifice of a sebaceous follicle, with slight swelling from effusion of plasma. Occasionally swelling alone is present, and more rarely the hyperæmia only. Round the minute hyperæmic papule thus formed (often with a hair in its centre) a roseolar patch, due to hyperæmia of the papillary body, soon appears. Slight exudation of plasma, with a few corpuscles, usually follows, and causes elevation of the papule itself. The pale brownish stain seen after the fading of the rash is due to changes in the escaped red corpuscles, and is deeper in proportion to the intensity of the previous congestion.

During the process of retrogression single or multiple reddish points, minute extravasations, may occur on the site of previous spots, or the hæmorrhages may appear more diffusely over the whole spot and have definite margins. These are due to local weakness of the bloodvessels, allowing an easy escape of red corpuscles.

Occasionally the extravasations take place at the height of the rash, and remain after the papules have faded. Minute vesicles sometimes are seen in the centre of the spots, but they are met with chiefly in cases where profuse sweating is present; they are probably sudamina.

Treatment.—This consists in putting the patient on a proper regimen and paying careful attention to the bowels, etc. The lung complication may require the administration of an emetic and the application of warm poultices to the chest. Local treatment of the rash is not required, but sponging the body with aromatic vinegar and water is useful in allaying irritation.

RÖTHELN—GERMAN MEASLES.

Definition.—Rötheln is an acute infectious disease characterized by an eruption of red blotches on the skin, and attended by slight sore throat, slight coryza, and but little constitutional disturbance.

Symptoms.—After an incubation period, usually of about fourteen days, an eruption of oval or round spots, of a lighter red color than those of scarlatina or measles, appears on the chest, afterwards extending over the rest of the body, which vary in size from a pin's head to a threepenny piece. If the spots be large they are generally irregular in their shape; if small, they are more crowded together, and give an appearance more resembling scarlatina. The spots are generally discrete, but the rash is more often confluent on the face than on any other part of the body. The rash lasts about two days, and then fades, leaving a slight brown stain, which gradually dies away; it is rarely followed by desquamation, and, if at all, only in the form of minute scales. In rare cases the spots have been known to become vesicular. The constitutional symptoms which accompany the appearance of the rash are chiefly those of catarrh, and occur at the same time as the rash, or precede it by less than twelve hours, and not by some days, as in measles. The fauces are somewhat injected, and the tonsils may be even slightly swollen. The tongue is coated with white fur, through which a few large papillæ can be seen, more often at the tip than elsewhere. An important symptom which accompanies the others is the tendency of the lymphatic glands to become enlarged, which is more constantly the case in the neck, especially in those situated behind the sterno-mastoid muscle, but the glands of other parts of the body are not always exempt. Increase of temperature is rare in rötheln, or is limited to the first few hours of the disease.

Diagnosis.—Rötheln may be confounded with three other affections,—scarlatina, morbilli, and roseola. The chief characteristic points between rötheln and scarlet fever and measles are shown on p. 53 under the head of Scarlatina;

from roseola it can be best distinguished by the absence of coryza in the latter disease, and by the glandular enlargement which occurs in the former. See also table, p. 57.

Prognosis is always favorable.

Morbid Anatomy.—The light-red spots are due to capillary hyperæmia of the papillary layer, which very rarely goes on to slight exudation into the rete Malpighii, causing slight elevation of the spots. As they fade a very faint and transient pigmentation may remain, and minute epidermic flakes may be shed. The vesicles occasionally seen on the back are probably miliaria.

Treatment.—No special treatment is required.

CHAPTER V.

Class I.—EXUDATIONES—*continued.*

VARIOLA—VARICELLA—VACCINIA.

VARIOLA—SMALL-POX.

Definition.—An acute infectious disease characterized by the existence of a rash, which passes through the successive stages of papules, vesicles, and pustules, accompanied by symptoms of considerable constitutional disturbance.

Symptoms.—On the fourteenth day after the reception of the poison, headache, nausea, feverishness, severe lumbar pain, and general *malaise* are experienced. After forty-eight hours—that is, on the third day of the disease—an eruption of red papules appears on the face, especially its upper part, and on the wrists, then extends over the chest and back and the limbs generally; about two days are occupied in the gradual appearance of the rash.

The actual site of the spots is round a hair follicle or the orifice of sebaceous or sweat glands. The papules are frequently arranged in threes and fives in a crescent shape, two crescents often coming together to form a circle. A few hours after the first appearance of a red spot it gradually becomes elevated, increases in size, assumes a dark-red color, and is hard or "shotty" to the touch; on the third day of the eruption the summit of the elevation becomes vesicular, and gradually, as the whole elevation takes this

character, the summit becomes depressed, till on the fourth
or fifth day of the eruption an umbilicated vesicle is formed,
containing clear fluid.   All the vesicles are not, however,
umbilicated, this condition apparently depending on their
being formed round the opening of a hair follicle.   The
contents of the vesicles gradually become more turbid, and
by about the sixth day of the eruption become pustular.
The base of the pustule then becomes hard, and the whole
of the skin, especially about the face, becomes œdematous.
About the eighth or ninth day of the eruption the pustules,
which in the meantime have largely lost their umbilication,
burst, and crusts or scales form on the surface.   After a
variable time, of from a few days to five or six weeks, the
crusts are shed, and a depressed purple stain alone remains
to indicate the position of the former pustule ; from this a
succession of fine scales are frequently shed.   The color
may persist for some weeks, but gradually fades, and the
depression contracts, leaving a cicatrix, the well-known
"pitting" of small-pox.

If the pustules have been numerous the skin of the face
rarely recovers its normal pink, transparent appearance,
but remains permanently of a uniform pasty white color.
During convalescence small abscesses frequently form in
the skin, chiefly on the thighs and legs.

During the whole course of the disease the constitutional
symptoms are severe.   The temperature is increased to
about 104°, 105° Fahrenheit, the tongue is covered with
thick creamy fur, severe pains in the head and limbs, and
especially in the back, are constantly present, while delirium, sometimes of the most violent character, and intense
itching of the skin during the whole course of the eruption,
prevent sleep, which is much required.   As the crusts are
formed the fever decreases until the temperature becomes
normal.   The severity of the constitutional symptoms de-

pends altogether on the amount of rash. It has been stated that considerable variation exists in the different forms of small-pox; these will now be described.

1. *Variola Discreta.*—The pustules remain separate from each other during the whole course of the disease.

2. *Variola Semi-confluens.*—A few pustules run together on the face.

3. *Variola Confluens.*—The pustules run together all over the body.

4. *Variola Corymbosa.*— The pustules are arranged in groups, the skin surrounding which is free from eruption. This is a rare and fatal form of the disease.

5. *Variola Hæmorrhagica.*—In this, the most severe form of variola, there is a bruised appearance.

The character of the bruises is such that it would be impossible to distinguish them from those produced by blows. But at the same time there is hæmorrhage beneath the conjunctivæ, and bleeding from nearly all the mucous membranes of the body. In this form, although there is great prostration, the mind is clear. The tongue is thickly covered with white fur, and the lumbar pain is severe. Often the attack is fatal before the appearance of the rash, but if not the papules appear rather as small hæmorrhages into the skin with ill-defined margins.

If the vesicular stage be reached the vesicles have irregular margins, which are obscured by the hæmorrhage, and the fluid which they contain becomes black from the presence of coloring matter from the blood.

The characteristic papules of small-pox may be preceded by a petechial rash. This consists of a quantity of minute petechiæ, closely aggregated together, which do not fade on pressure; their most frequent site is the lower part of the abdomen and the inner side of the thighs, the axillæ, the upper part of the arms, and the skin over the clavicle.

The whole of the surface affected presents a dark and mottled appearance.

This rash must not be confounded with the true variola hæmorrhagica; often, however, the two are combined, and in these cases dark-purple or rather blue bruises appear among the petechiæ; if there be no bruises—that is, if the rash be purely petechial and not hæmorrhagic—the petechiæ in a few days gradually fade, and are replaced by the true papules of variola, which appear while the petechiæ are still present. Sometimes the papules are preceded by a hyperæmia of the skin, which may be diffuse or in separate spots, and the disease then presents an appearance closely resembling scarlatina, which is sometimes called variola roseola. The site of this rash is not limited, as in the petechial variety, but may occur over the chest and arms. It is not uncommon to see the roseolous and petechial rashes combined in the same individual, but they more often appear separately; both usually commence on the second day of the disease.

Finally, it must be remembered that small-pox often occurs in persons who have been previously vaccinated, and that under these circumstances the course of the disease is greatly modified. The successive stages of development of the rash are more rapidly completed, the rash is far less abundant, and the constitutional symptoms are less marked.

Diagnosis.—The diagnosis of variola in the early stage is not so easy as in the latter.

The roseolous rash may be mistaken during the first forty-eight hours both for scarlatina and roseola. Other symptoms, arranged in the following table, assist even at this early period in distinguishing between these diseases.

Symptoms during First Forty-eight Hours.

VARIOLA.	SCARLATINA.	ROSEOLA.
Very slight sore throat.	Severe sore throat.	Very slight sore throat; redness limited to edge of soft palate.
Tongue furred.	Tongue furred.	Tongue slightly furred.
Papillæ not enlarged.	Papillæ enlarged.	Papillæ enlarged only at edges.
Rash of short duration.	Rash may last some days.	Rash of short duration.
Severe pains in back.	No marked pains in back.	No marked pains in back.
Pyrexia and constitutional symptoms.	Pyrexia and constitutional symptoms.	Pyrexia and constitutional symptoms subside with appearance of rash.

On the third day, when the papular rash is appearing, it may be mistaken for measles, but it must be remembered that the rash appears on the third day in small-pox, and on the fourth day in measles, and that in the latter the chief constitutional symptom is coryza, whereas in the former there is only slight suffusion of the eyes and the usually well-marked lumbar pain. In a few hours the characteristic feeling of shotty papules, observable in passing the hand over the rash, makes the diagnosis of small-pox more simple.

A not uncommon mistake is to confuse acne, when accompanied by a pyrexial attack, with small-pox. Simple as the diagnosis apparently is, the two diseases are occasionally confounded, and it is well, therefore, to point out that the date of the appearance of the acne and the absence of the special constitutional symptoms of small-pox must be borne in mind. The same rule will enable small-pox to be dis-

of the stratum lucidum, which undergo swelling and segmentation.

In the vesicular stage it is seen, on examining sections under the microscope, that the pock presents a chambered structure, most marked in its upper portion. It probably arises, according to Rindfleisch, through the serous infiltration of the epidermis not raising the horny layer *en masse*, as in a simple vesicle, but forcing its way gradually in between the lamellæ. It thus pushes asunder and displaces them from a horizontal to an oblique or vertical position. The fine filaments seen in the lower part of the vesicle may possibly be the remains of the cementing substance of the epidermis. The umbilicus seen in the centre of many of the vesicles is usually obviously due to the presence of hair follicles or the ducts of sweat or sebaceous glands, the tissues of which, being more resistant, act as bridles holding down the centre of the pock. It is not met with in every vesicle, and usually disappears at the stage of suppuration.

In the suppurative stage the papillary layer and the subjacent part of the corium are richly infiltrated with leucocytes, which escape freely into the vesicle. When mature, the umbilicus and most of the septa in the centre have melted away, and the pock consists of a somewhat irregular cavity filled with pus, mingled with epithelial debris.

In the process of drying up, or scabbing, the hyperæmia and exudation diminish; the rete cells at the margins and base of the pustule begin to cornify, and gradually form a fresh horny layer, which covers the papillæ, denuded, but not destroyed, and forms a closed capsule round the little pus mass; this dries up and is cast off. In some cases, however, the exudation of leucocytes, being excessive, separates the fibres of the papillæ widely, and pressing on the vessels cuts off their blood supply and produces necrosis. Hence the base of the pock is formed by a pale slough, which has to be cast off by the suppuration around it. The tissue thus destroyed is replaced by granulations, which heal by second intention and leave a permanent scar.

In variola hæmorrhagica the hæmorrhages affect all the layers of the skin, and often the subcutaneous tissue also; they are probably due to transudation of corpuscles rather than to rupture of vessels, as no morbid condition has been detected in the latter. The hæmorrhages proceed not from the capillary plexuses round the hair follicles and glands, but from the loops in the papillæ at their apices or in their substance, as well as in the subjacent cutis.

During the stage of desiccation, since the centre of the pustule begins to dry up before the margin, an umbilicus is again formed even in pocks where it was at first absent.

Treatment.—This consists in putting the patient upon a suitable diet, placing him in a well-ventilated room, attending to his bowels, seeing that he gets sufficient sleep, and, when necessary, administering stimulants. With a view to prevent pitting, many applications and methods have been used; solution of nitrate of silver, carbolic acid solutions, painting with collodion, powdering with fuller's earth, pricking and emptying the vesicles, have all in turn been resorted to without any favorable result.

The application of oil to the surface is, however, useful in allaying the intense itching which accompanies the rash, and care should be taken to prevent the patient wounding the vesicles by scratching.

When the scabs form, if they be large, they will often retain pus; they should then be softened with a poultice and removed. Abscesses should be opened early.

VARICELLA—CHICKEN-POX.

Definition.—Varicella is an acute infectious disease, characterized by the production on the body of small round vesicles, appearing in successive crops. These dry up and form scabs, which fall off, sometimes leaving cicatrices.

Symptoms.—About a fortnight after the reception of the poison a crop of small roseolar papules, varying in number from a dozen or so to several hundred, appear first on the upper part of the body,—usually the face,—and are scattered irregularly over the surface, but not in twos and threes, as in variola. Within a few hours the papules become vesicular, and the rash is then usually described as having at this period the appearance of having been produced by a number of small drops of scalding water thrown on the skin.

The vesicles are of small size, usually less than one-fifth of an inch in diameter, filled with clear fluid, giving them a bright, glistening appearance, and seldom have a central depression. After twenty-four hours the vesicles become slightly turbid, and at the end of two or three days are covered with scabs. Later these separate, occasionally leaving pitting of the skin. On the first day of the rash about a dozen or fifteen vesicles appear, on the second day there may be as many as 100 to 150, and successive outbreaks occur during the first four or five nights. The rash is never confluent, but occasionally two vesicles may coalesce.

The eruption is generally attended with considerable itching and some constitutional disturbance, which is never severe. The temperature rarely rises above 100° Fahrenheit. The constitutional symptoms seldom precede the rash by more than a few hours, and usually occur simultaneously with it.

Diagnosis.—There is only one disease for which varicella can ever be mistaken, and that is variola. The differences between the eruptions will be found on p. 66. It may be well to mention that a vesicular syphilide has been occasionally mistaken for varicella, but to distinguish the two diseases it will only be necessary to point out that the syphilitic eruption rarely appears without other syphilides being present. The history and course of the two affections will serve to confirm the diagnosis.

Prognosis.—Favorable.

Morbid Anatomy.—On a small roseolar papule, due to superficial hyperæmia of the cutis, a small loculated vesicle soon forms. On examining this microscopically the cells of the upper layer of the rete are found filled with numerous refracting globules, scattered through the protoplasm and undergoing vesicular transformation. These cells, opening into one another, give rise to an irregularly loculated cavity, situated between the horny and the deeper layers of the rete, containing serous fluid, in which leucocytes and multinucleate epidermic cells float. As the cells undergo fatty degeneration, the clear serous fluid soon becomes turbid, and is absorbed, leaving a small brownish crust. On the separation of the scab there is left merely a slight depressed stain, which fades in time, leaving no trace unless suppuration and superficial ulceration of the papillary layer have taken place.

Treatment.—No specific treatment is required; the constitutional symptoms may be treated on general principles. The irritation of the skin is relieved by the application of oil. If suppuration occurs beneath the scab, the pus should be set free by poulticing.

VACCINIA—VACCINATION.

Definition.—An acute infectious vesicular disease of the cow, communicable to man, and which has the effect of protecting the latter from attacks of small-pox.

Symptoms.—With the disease in the cow we have here no concern, and therefore shall only describe the rash produced in the human subject by the inoculation of the cow-pox in a person who has not previously been vaccinated. If a puncture be made in the skin of such a person with a lancet, and the vaccine matter be inserted with care, after two days, during which nothing appreciable occurs, a papular elevation is produced. On the fifth or sixth day this becomes a pearl-colored vesicle of a round or oval form, depressed in the centre and with its edges raised. On the eighth day the vesicle is more distended, but the depression in the centre still remains. On the seventh or eighth day a red ring is formed round the vesicle, which may be two or three inches in diameter. The redness fades on pressure, but the area is harder and more tender than the surrounding skin. About the tenth day the redness begins to disappear, and the lymph in the vesicle is seen to become thick and purulent, while the umbilication is less marked. At the end of a fortnight a scab forms, which remains adherent till about the end of the third week, when it falls off, leaving in its place a somewhat circular depression, which is foveated. These pits correspond with the cells of the vesicles. The cicatrix contracts somewhat, but otherwise, as a rule, remains for life.

Two or three days after the operation considerable itching of the part is experienced, and about the seventh or eighth day there is usually, especially in young children, some amount of constitutional disturbance, such as shivering, loss of appetite, and general *malaise*. At this period the temperature is somewhat slightly increased; sometimes also the axillary glands become enlarged.

Although this is the course of by far the majority of the cases of vaccination, some are, from time to time, found which do not run through quite the same symptoms as described above. Thus, occasionally a rose rash (*roseola vaccinia*) makes its appearance between the third and eighteenth day after inoculation, commencing most often in the neighborhood of the irritation and extending over other parts of the body. This rash consists of very slightly raised spots of a red color, varying in size from a quarter of an

inch to three or four inches in diameter. It lasts but a day
or two, and is not followed by desquamation or deposit of
pigment.

In *Variola vaccinia herpetica* a crop of vesicles appears
on the third day after the operation, and is preceded by an
attack of shivering. They soon burst; the fluid which
escapes irritates the adjoining skin, and an eczematous
condition of the part is produced, the skin becoming hard
and œdematous. Intense itching accompanies this outbreak,
and the axillary glands often become enlarged.

In *Variola vaccinia bullosa* a bulla of variable size, with a
red edge, takes the place of the ordinary vesicle. It contains a clear liquid, which soon escapes, leaving a crust,
which is shed without producing a scar, unless ulceration
takes place, when the cicatrix is of considerable size.

In *Variola vaccinia furunculosa* red tubercles are formed,
which subsequently suppurate.

Occasionally *Erysipelas* appears about the seventh to the
tenth day round the vesicle, and spreads over the arm. It
does not differ from ordinary erysipelas, and is accompanied
by œdema, pain, and considerable constitutional disturbance.
In some cases the pustules, instead of drying up and forming scabs, burst, and ulceration takes place. The ulcers
are attended by itching, pain, and constitutional disturbance. This condition rarely results from lymph which has
passed through the human subject, but occurs more frequently after inoculation direct from the cow.

But one other variety has to be described,—that in which
perfect vesicles are never developed, but scabbing occurs
after a little fluid has been formed. It may be well also
to mention that revaccination produces vesicles the typical
characters of which are less marked, appearing earlier and
running a more rapid course than in primary vaccination.

Syphilis will be noticed under "Syphilis," p. 114.

-A favorable result always follows vaccination, except in the rare cases when erysipelas occurs among young children.

Morbid Anatomy.—The structure of the vaccinal exanthem, in its successive stages of papule, vesicle, and pustule, is much the same as in variola.

The umbilicus of the vesicle is formed at the point of puncture, and is said to be due to the inflammation excited by the scratch, causing adhesion of the corium and epidermis, so that the subsequent serous effusion separates the cuticle around the band thus formed. The vesicle is loculated, and, like that of variola, its umbilicus may disappear when suppuration sets in. Scabbing takes place in the centre and extends to the margin of the pock.

Treatment.—Vaccination requires but little treatment. The vesicles should be carefully protected from injury, and oil should be applied to allay the itching. On the eighth day, if the vesicles be much distended, a few punctures into them is useful to relieve tension. If there should be any tendency to retention of pus or ulceration beneath the scabs, they should be removed by a poultice, and the wound treated according to the rules for treating ulcers. If the erythema be great, or if erysipelas occur, the arm should be kept in a sling and lotio plumbi should be applied to the part.

Finally, it should be borne in mind that lymph should never be taken, for the purpose of vaccination, from any but a perfect vesicle, with a proper areola, in the person of a healthy child vaccinated for the first time.

CHAPTER VI.

Class I.—Ex<small>U</small>DATION<small>ES</small>—*continued.*

TYPHUS—ENTERIC—DIPHTHERIA.

TYPHUS FEVER.

Definition.—Typhus is an acute infectious disease characterized by the production of a mottled rash, which becomes petechial, and which is accompanied by considerable constitutional disturbance.

Symptoms.—Thirteen or fourteen days after the reception of typhus poison there is a sense of chilliness and headache, accompanied occasionally by vomiting, and general pyrexial symptoms. On the third day, more often on the fourth or fifth, the mulberry rash of typhus makes its appearance. The rash can be described as consisting of two parts. The one which is simply an indistinct dark mottling appears as if it were a little distance beneath the surface of the skin, and is described as the "subcuticular" mottling. The other consists of a quantity of small purple maculæ scattered over the surface of the skin, and appear to be altogether on the surface. When they first appear they are very slightly raised, but in a few hours become perfectly flat. The subcuticular mottling may exist by itself, but the maculæ are usually present as well. The rash is fully developed in less than forty-eight hours from its commencement, and no rash is ever produced after this period. For the first few days the spots fade on pressure, but later on a yellow stain is left, and still later pressure produces no effect on the spot, which has then become petechial; the petechiæ remain, appearing like minute hæmorrhages, and often last as long as three weeks, but the mottling disappears earlier. The rash appears first on the wrist, upper part and sides of abdomen, and about the edges of the axillæ; later it gradually extends over the whole abdomen and chest. The constitutional symptoms steadily increase, especially the delirium, which is often of a violent character. The tongue, which is first coated with white fur, becomes dry, brown, and sometimes black, and great difficulty is experienced in protruding it, on account of sordes collecting about the mouth. Later the tongue begins to moisten at the edges, and the appetite rapidly returns, even before the tongue has cleaned. During the whole course of disease the temperature is raised constantly to 104° or 105° Fahr. The maximum temperature is usually reached on the fourth day, when a slight fall takes place; a further fall occurs about the seventh day, and although at the beginning of the second week it is slightly lower than during the first, it rises until the crisis occurs. This takes place generally between the twelfth and seventeenth days. The temperature then falls rapidly, and becomes normal within three or four days of the crisis, unless some complication be present.

Occasionally erysipelas and glandular swellings, especially of the parotid, occur during the course of the fever.

Diagnosis.—Typhus is frequently mistaken for brain disease, pneumonia, measles, and enteric fever. In the first two it is only necessary to point out that no rash exists; from measles, however, the diagnosis is not always an easy matter. In both the rashes appear on the same day, but differ in certain essential particulars (see table).

The diagnosis of typhus from enteric fever is a perfectly easy matter, and a mistake should never be made between these two diseases (see table).

Prognosis.—The chances of recovery depend altogether upon age. The young nearly always recover, while among

Typhus.	Measles.	Typhus.	Enteric.
Rash not very often present on the face.	Rash commonly present on face.	Commences suddenly. Rash on fourth or fifth day.	Commences insidiously. Rash at end of first week.
Macules smaller than measles, separate from each other, and not raised.	Macules often coalesce and are raised.	Dark, mottled, non-elevated rash.	Group of lenti dar ro-seolous papules.
Subcuticular mottling present.	Subcuticular mottling not present.	Rash fully developed in forty-eight hours.	Rash apprs in successive crops, aeh spot lasting two or three days.
Suffusion of eyes, but no coryza.	Coryza.	Rash becomes petechial. Diarrhœa less common than in enteric.	No ise. Diarrhœa common.
		Flat abdomen.	Full, tender abdomen.
		Heavy, dull expression of face.	Flushed cheeks, glistening eyes.

those of middle or advanced life the mortality is very high. Fat, heavy persons are more likely to die than those who are more spare. A large amount of rash, which soon becomes petechial, especially if it be of a dark color, an absence of fall of temperature at some period during the first week, a sudden rise of temperature during the third week, a very rapid pulse, much delirium, coma, convulsions, and suppression of urine, are all unfavorable signs.

Morbid Anatomy.—The rash of typhus is due to superficial hyperæmia of the cutis, but, as exudation is absent, the spots remain on a level with the rest of the skin. At a later stage the darkening of the spots is produced by tho escape of red corpuscles from the vessels, and actual petechiæ sometimes form. These subsequently undergo the same changes as purpuric spots.

Treatment.—This should be regulated on general principles.

ENTERIC OR TYPHOID FEVER.

Definition.—Enteric or typhoid fever is an acute infectious disease characterized by swelling and subsequent ulceration of the Peyer's and solitary glands of the ileum, usually accompanied by successive crops of rose-colored papules, chiefly on the abdomen, together with abdominal symptoms and considerable constitutional disturbance.

Symptoms.—From ten to sixteen days after the reception of the poison, headache, chilliness, and occasionally shivering, followed by a little delirium, are experienced. With these symptoms there is increased temperature, a furred tongue, and sometimes diarrhœa, or more often irregularity of the bowels, a few days of constipation being followed by purging. On the seventh, or from that to the twelfth day, in cases where a rash is present, a crop of rose-colored papules, from half a line to two lines in diameter, make their ap-

pearance ou the abdomen, chest, and back. These are
slightly elevated, aud disappear on pressure, but reappear
the moment the finger is removed. There number varies
from two or three to a hundred or so, but usually not more
than about half a dozen are present at a time. Each crop
lasts from three to six days, and is usually followed by subsequent crops. When the papules fade, no discoloration·of
the skin remains, and the rash is never permanent. The
duration of the rash is from one to three weeks, but occasionally recurs at a later date if there is a relapse.

During the course of the disease the abdomen becomes
prominent, and often tympanitic and tender on pressure,
especially in the right iliac fossa, where it often produces
gurgling.

The constitutional symptoms increase in severity after
the first week, and sometimes the delirium is violent in
character. The tongue becomes drier as the fever progresses, and towards the latter part of the second week is
dry, very red, and glazed. Diarrhœa becomes a more common symptom in the second week, and is sometimes very
severe. The stools are liquid and of a yellow-ochre color.
If allowed to stand, the more solid portion settles to the
bottom, and is then found to consist of shreds of undigested
food mixed with sloughs and debris from the ulcers in the
intestines. Often they contain a little blood. In some cases
severe hæmorrhage occurs from the ulcers, and the stool
then consists almost wholly of blood.

At a later stage of the fever the ulceration of the intestinal glands occasionally extends through the peritoneum,
and perforation of the intestines, with its accompaniments
of extravasation into the peritoneal cavity and consequent
peritonitis, results. The temperature in enteric fever is
always increased during the first week; it rises higher and
higher until a temperature of 104° Fahr. is frequently

reached. The morning temperature is lower than the evening, and during the second and third week this is maintained. Later, however, usually in the third week, as the recovery begins, the difference between the morning and evening temperature is much more marked. Occasionally a sudden fall of temperature takes place, due usually to hæmorrhage from the bowel; but if any rise be observed, it is due to some complication, often of the lung. The pulse is always increased in enteric fever, often 120 at night, but less frequent in the morning.

In the mild cases the patient begins to recover at the latter part of the second week, and in more severe cases at a later date. Convalescence is always slow. Among the complications are hæmorrhage from the intestine, perforation of intestine, peritonitis, and pneumonia.

Occasionally two or three days before the lenticular spots make their appearance they are preceded by a scarlet rash, which spreads over the whole body. It is a mere temporary hyperæmia, and fades on pressure.

In rare cases petechiæ and purpuric spots occur during the course of the fever; they are in no way associated with the lenticular spots.

Taches bleuâtres are sometimes observed. They consist of blue patches, from two or three to eight lines in diameter, of irregular shape, usually separate, but sometimes coalescing. They are not raised, and give an appearance somewhat resembling the typhus spots, but they do not pass through the same changes as the latter. They are usually situated on the abdomen, thighs, and back.

Sudamina frequently occur, and are followed by desquamation.

Diagnosis.—The diagnosis of enteric fever is usually not a difficult matter. The high temperature, the prominent abdomen, the dry red tongue, the diarrhœa, and, when present, the lenticular spots, conclusively point out the disease. It can be recognized by the flushed cheeks, glistening eyes, and parched lips, which contrast strongly with the heavy, dull, leaden appearance of typhus, and by other symptoms, which are given in a tabular form on p. 76.

Prognosis.—Young children rarely die of enteric fever, but as age progresses mortality increases. A very high temperature which is not attended with morning remissions, much diarrhœa, hæmorrhage, tympanitis, delirium of a violent character, much muscular tremor, are unfavorable indications. The amount of rash is not prognostic of a favorable or unfavorable termination.

Morbid Anatomy.—The enteric papule begins as a small, circumscribed pink spot, due to hyperæmia of the papillary layer. In a day or two it becomes slightly raised, owing to the exudation of plasma into the papillæ and rete, and in some cases a minute vesicle, due to further collection of serum, forms at its apex. As the spot fades the plasma is absorbed, and the faint brown stain left by it soon disappears. The anatomy of the *taches bleuâtres* has not been investigated.

Treatment.—Considerable care is necessary in the treatment of enteric fever. The patient should not be permitted to leave his bed until convalescence has well advanced, should be fed on fluids only, and should be given no vegetable food. The diarrhœa should be carefully controlled, and constipation treated by enemata.

For tympanitis, peritonitis, etc., opium is the best remedy. Hæmorrhage should be treated with astringents and ice. Finally it may be stated that antipyretic treatment, both by cold bathing and the administration of quinine, has proved very successful on the Continent and in England when it has been systematically carried out.

DIPHTHERIA.

Definition.—Diphtheria is an acute infectious disease in which there is a tendency to the formation of false membrane on mucous and abraded surfaces, chiefly of the fauces and respiratory tract, accompanied by considerable constitutional disturbance.

Symptoms.—After an incubation period, which varies greatly, but which is probably from twenty-four hours to ten days, shivering and vomiting set in, and the temperature becomes increased. The throat becomes sore, and there is some amount of stiffness about the neck. The fauces become of a dark-red color, the tonsils swollen, and at the end of two days from the beginning of the disease a quantity of minute white points appear on the surface of one or both sides of the fauces. As these spots increase in number, they coalesce and form a thick yellowish-white membrane. This sometimes consists of a single piece, but is often scattered over the surface in separate patches. The cervical glands become enlarged, the tongue coated with white or brown fur, the pulse and temperature increased, and the urine albuminous.

In the next stage the membrane separates, often leaving unhealthy sloughing ulcers.

In this stage recovery may take place, or death may result from exhaustion; during any period of the illness asphyxia, resulting from the production of false membrane in the larynx or bronchial tubes, may be fatal. In the course of the disease a roseolous rash may appear over the body. This is not different from the roseola which appears with other acute diseases.

Convalescence after diphtheria is very slow; often paralysis of groups of the muscles shows itself within six months from the beginning of the attack.

Diagnosis.—Diphtheria may be confounded with (*a*) scarlatina, (*b*) tonsillitis, (*c*) herpetic sore throat. The points of difference between these diseases is shown in the following table:

DIPHTHERIA.	SCARLATINA.
Throat of deep red, which is not uniformly distributed.	Throat of bright red, which is uniformly distributed.
Patches of thick yellow membrane on any portion of fauces.	Large white, thin, irregularly shaped exudations on fauces.
Tonsils unequally swollen.	Both tonsils equally swollen.
Tongue coated with white fur.	Tongue furred, with large papillæ.

HERPETIC SORE THROAT.	TONSILLITIS.
Throat less red than in scarlatina or diphtheria.	Throat less red than in scarlatina or diphtheria.
Small white points on tonsils.	Small, thin, yellow exudation points over surface of tonsils.
Tonsils unequally swollen.	Tonsils unequally swollen.
Tongue furred.	Tongue furred.

Prognosis.—Diphtheria, under any circumstances, is a disease in which a guarded prognosis should be given. During the whole course of the disease symptoms may arise which are the precursors of a fatal termination.

Those cases are most serious which occur in young children, when there is a tendency to extension of the membrane, when an alteration in the voice betokens affection of the larynx, or when the powers of the patient begin to fail early.

Morbid Anatomy.—The diphtheritic poison, as it affects the mucous membrane, may give rise to two degrees of morbid changes:

1. The catarrhal stage, representing affection of the epithelial layers only, the disease not undergoing any further

2. The fibrinous stage, where, either with or soon after the catarrhal stage, there sets in an exudation of plasma, which gives rise to a fibrinous pseudo-membrane.

In the catarrhal stage, on making a section through the grayish-white, slightly raised patch, the epithelial layer is not obviously thickened, and the grayish change extends only here and there into its substance. Numerous masses of micrococci are found on and in the superficial epithelial layers, forming somewhat flattened deposits. From these, processes of micrococci extend down into the rete Malpighii, spreading out here and there into roundish aggregations or colonies. The rete cells themselves are swollen, and have their nuclei more distinct.

Leucocytes next invade the diseased patch more and more, filling up all the space in the epithelium not already occupied by micrococci. Mingled with them there are large young cells, three or four times the size of leucocytes, and some multinuclear cells. This cellular or purulent infiltration helps to check the extension downward of the fungus growth, and finally leads to the casting off of the patch of epithelium.

In the fibrinous stage, either soon after the appearance of the fungoid growth or after some pus formation, an exudation of plasma into the epithelial and subepithelial tissue lifts up the portion already infiltrated with numerous forming a thick false membrane which soon undergoes necrosis. The surface consists of granular debris and masses of epithelium. Mixed with numerous cells in the deeper layers are loosened up tissue elements, swollen and disintegrating, converted into fine filaments, with at first a few scattered nuclei, and later exudations of fibrin fill up the interspaces already previously formed. Examining the later stages and, on microscopic examination fine in the subsequent as the surface is approached. After twenty-four to forty-eight hours the rupture of the capillaries in the papillary layer gives rise to slight hæmorrhages, which are surrounded and shut off by subsequent fibrinous exudation. The cords of micrococci, extending gradually downwards towards the subepithelial layers, are thus being constantly pushed off towards the surface; but as the exudative process slackens, some of them extend into the lymphatic spaces of the tissue, filling them and the lymphatic vessels as well.

As the exudation of plasma finally ceases, the purulent infiltration forms a line of demarcation, and with the increased secretion from the mucous glands either floats off the membrane *en masse* or checks the downward growth of the micrococci from the latter, which then slowly breaks down on the surface and is washed away.

Treatment.—The removal of the false membrane is of no avail; antiseptic applications are, however, very useful, and the patient's powers should be most carefully supported. The internal administration of the tincture of the perchloride of iron is valuable, both for its local action as an antiseptic and for its hæmatemic properties. If the larynx becomes affected, and there be much local obstruction to breathing, tracheotomy should be at once resorted to, for it is of no use to wait until the patient's powers are almost exhausted. The operation is itself a trivial one, and should therefore not be postponed.

CHAPTER VII.

*Class I.—*Exudationes—*continued.*

Equinia—Pustula Maligna—Verruca Necrogenica—Frambœsia—
Erysipelas—Septicæmic Rashes—Surgical Rash.

Equinia—Glanders—Farcy.

Definition.—An acute infectious disease of the horse, ass,
or mule, communicable to man by inoculation of a wound
or abraded surface, and it is said by the prolonged contact
of infected matter with the unbroken skin or mucous membranes, or by inhalation of air impregnated with the poisonous particles. It produces severe constitutional symptoms,
and usually a pustular rash.

Symptoms.—The disease as it occurs in animals need not
be discussed, except to remark that there is no essential
difference between glanders and farcy. They are both
caused by the same virus, both equally contagious, and
differ only in certain clinical and anatomical details. The
"farcy buds" are merely one of the manifestations of
"glanders," as a gumma or tubercular syphilide is of syphilis. According to the course and duration of the disease,
an acute, subacute, and chronic form of glanders may be
described. In acute glanders, after an incubation period of
three to five days, or even of two or three weeks, *malaise*,
loss of appetite, and obscure pains in the joints and muscles
of the extremities are experienced. At the same time the
skin round the wound or excoriation which has been inoculated becomes red, painful, and slimy; the lymphatics and

8

glands become enlarged, red, and painful, and there is often an erysipelatous redness or cellulitis extending for a considerable distance round. The ulcer enlarges, its base and sides become corroded and grayish-white, with a foul discharge; there is great prostration, with severe pain in the joints and muscles, and high fever is often present. Rigors are rare unless the disease is complicated with septicæmia.

If the attack be produced by inhalation of the poison, it commences with general symptoms only, and the first definite sign is the eruption. This consists of red spots,—at first small papules, but soon enlarging into little indurated tubercles about the size of a pea,—scattered over the face and more or less over the rest of the body. Pustules, and occasionally vesicles, soon form on their apices, burst, and leave foul ulcers. Sometimes larger nodules—farcy buds—at first form along the course of the lymphatics of the skin and subcutaneous tissue, but soon break down and suppurate, leaving deep irregular ulcers with sloughing surfaces. Similar nodules and abscesses in the intermuscular tissue, and suppuration in and around the joints, are often met with, also hæmorrhages into the swellings. In the affection of the mucous membranes, especially of the nose, either at the beginning, if the disease has been inoculated there, or after the previous phenomena, there is severe pain and swelling with a mucous discharge, clear and viscid at first, but later brownish, offensive, and sanguineous. Tumors and ulcers may be found in the nose. Severe cough, pain in the chest, and expectoration of matter resembling the nasal discharge mark the implication of the lungs with the diseased growths. The pulse is small and frequent, headache is often severe, and delirium is not uncommon.

In subacute glanders the symptoms are, on the whole, the same, only less intense and more protracted. The pain and the retarded suppuration caused by the ulcers usually produce a condition of hectic.

In chronic glanders there is, as in the acute forms, at first redness and swelling round the inoculated spot, with inflammation of the lymphatics, glandular enlargement, and some fever. - The general symptoms subside for a time, but the ulcers go on slowly spreading in some places, healing in others. After a time nodular tumors or farcy buds, red spots, and pustules may arise, producing abscesses and ulcers on the skin, in the muscles, joints, and viscera. The nasal and other mucous membranes become affected, as in the acute form, and tubercles or ulcers about the larynx give rise to hoarseness or sudden œdema of the glottis. Bronchitis and pneumonia are frequently met with.

The fever may be high if there is much suppuration and rapid formation of abscesses, or may assume a hectic type.

Even in the event of a favorable course recovery is very slow, and often incomplete; the abscesses and ulcers gradually heal, the nasal discharge lessens and finally ceases, and the gastric and respiratory symptoms disappear. It is necessary to add that at any time the chronic variety may become acute and rapidly fatal.

Diagnosis.—The inoculation wound may be at first mistaken for the result of cadaveric poisoning, but is distinguished when the rash, nasal affection, and other symptoms set in. When acquired by inhalation, or where no wound is present, the early symptoms may lead to confusion with enteric fever if there is much pyrexia, *malaise*, headache, and delirium, or with rheumatic fever if the joint and muscular pains predominate. The appearance of the rash and nasal complication soon makes the diagnosis clear.

The papules may at first resemble those of variola, but they are larger and not "shotty;" they soon develop into pustules and ulcers, instead of drying up into scabs; and abscesses, usually absent in variola, are almost constant in glanders.

Chronic glanders may be mistaken for syphilis; the history of contact with horses or persons suffering from the former, and the absence of the usual signs of the latter, will suffice to distinguish between the two diseases.

Prognosis.—Acute glanders is nearly always fatal, usually in seven or ten days from the onset of the attack. In the subacute forms of the disease death does not occur till after the second or third week, and about twenty-five per cent. recover.

In the chronic form the usual duration is about four months, and fifty per cent. recover.

Morbid Anatomy.—In acute glanders the cutaneous and nasal tubercles—farcy buds—so often met with in the horse, are frequently absent in man, and the morbid changes resemble those of pyæmia. As regards the skin, there are found, after death, scattered over the body, especially on the face and extremities, the red spots observable during life, with vesicles or pustules in some places and abscesses or ulcers in others. The vesicles containing caseo-purulent or bloody fluid have often a gray sloughy base. In the small cutaneous abscesses the pus is often of a viscid nature, and mixed with blood and shreds of tissue. Œdema, erysipelatous or phlegmonous changes, may also be present in the surrounding skin. The cutaneous nodules or tubercles are found to consist of localized deposits of small round cells in the sub-papillary layer of the corium, which at a later stage give rise to infiltration of the papillæ with leucocytes. The papillæ being thus disorganized, pus collects beneath the epidermis, forming a small abscess, which on bursting leaves a foul ulcer.

In the internal organs, such as in the mucous membranes of the nose, pharynx, and trachea, in the lungs, muscles, bones, and abdominal viscera, nodules, ulcers, abscesses, and hæmorrhages are frequently found.

Treatment.—No treatment is of any avail in the acute forms of the disease. In the chronic little can be done beyond keeping up the strength with a liberal and stimulating diet.

Pustula Maligna—Malignant Pustule.

Definition.—A disease produced by the poison of animals suffering from charbon, characterized by the formation of a pustule, by subsequent gangrene, and by severe constitutional disturbance.

Symptoms.—It first appears as a small dark-red patch, on which an elevation soon grows ; a small pustule forms on this and bursts. The inflamed area rapidly extends, becoming hard, and sloughs. Symptoms of severe constitutional disturbance accompany the local affection, and death frequently takes place in four or five days from the beginning of the disease. It is produced in man by direct contact with the diseased animal, but there is also some evidence that it can be conveyed by flies.

Diagnosis.—There is no disease for which malignant pustule can be mistaken.

Prognosis.—Usually fatal.

Morbid Anatomy.—Sections of the developing malignant pustule show that the central black spot is produced by hæmorrhage into tissue which has already undergone gangrene. There is acute inflammatory œdema around, and as the process of hæmorrhage and gangrene spreads gradually from the centre, we get finally the fully developed dark-red or blackish spot covered with a vesicle containing blood-stained purulent fluid. The pustule is usually surrounded by extensive phlegmonous inflammation of the adjacent skin and subcutaneous tissue. The hæmorrhagic infiltration is seen to extend deeply into the substance of the corium, sending out reddish radiating branched processes. There is also more or less scattered hæmorrhage in the œdematous tissue, and in the corium in isolated patches.

The fluid of the vesicle contains enormous quantities of slender, rod-shaped bacteria (*Bacillus anthracis*) aggregated in masses in the substance of the rete. As the disease advances they infiltrate the papillæ, hair follicles, sebaceous glands, and the deeper layers of the corium, finally making their way into the blood and infecting the body generally. An excess of leucocytes and plasma is present in the corium and papillæ. These bacilli have been cultivated out of the body, and after several generations had been obtained were found to produce anthrax when introduced into the bodies of animals.

Treatment.—In an early stage destruction of the affected part by caustics, or its entire removal by the knife, is advisable. If this be impossible, warm poultices should be applied, and attention should be directed to sustaining the patient's powers.

Verruca Necrogenica.

Definition.—A disease occurring among those who are engaged as butchers or in making post-mortem examinations, and consisting of warts produced by infection from dead animal matter.

Symptoms.—The warts consist simply of patches of morbid growths, having somewhat the appearace of epithelial cancer.

Diagnosis.—The occupation of the patient readily enables the character of these growths to be recognized.

Prognosis.—They have a tendency to recur, but are otherwise innocent.

Treatment.—Removal by the knife or by caustics.

Frambœsia—Yaws.

Definition.—A contagious disease of the West Indies and Africa, rarely seen in this country, characterized by the appearance of a pustular eruption, which is replaced by a series of ulcers and attended by considerable constitutional disturbance.

Symptoms.—It commences with feverishness, and soon after small papules are produced, which are most numerous on the face and the extremities, and gradually grow until they reach the size of a sixpence. At the end of a few days a pustule forms on the elevation, and bursts, leaving a thick crust, beneath which ulceration takes place; on this ulcer large granulations grow, giving an appearance which has been compared to a raspberry, but eventually these cicatrize and heal. This condition may go on for months, during which successive crops of the pustules may be produced. The constitutional symptoms are feverishness, sore throat, and sometimes dropsy.

Diagnosis.—There is no disease for which this can be mistaken.

Morbid Anatomy.—The morbid changes have not been investigated.

Treatment.—No specific treatment is known; the ulcers must be treated with stimulating applications, and the strength must be kept up with stimulants and a generous diet.

ERYSIPELAS.

Definition.—An acute contagious disease, characterized by the production of a local inflammatory condition of the skin, and attended with symptoms of constitutional disturbance.

Symptoms.—There is still room for doubt whether an ordinary inflammation of the skin of itself can become erysipelatous, or whether a specific contagion is required for the production of the disease. It is certain, however, that wherever there is abrasion of the surface, the skin at this point is likely to be attacked by erysipelas if the patient be exposed to unhealthy conditions—such, for instance, as a current of air escaping from a foul water-closet, or contact with decomposing matter. When once generated, the inflammation spreads by extension to contiguous surfaces, and is easily conveyed by the hands of the attendants to other patients. It is the opinion of some that two forms of this disease exist,—viz., a traumatic and an idiopathic erysipelas,—and that the latter is not communicable. Evidence on this is, however, unsatisfactory; the belief probably arises from the fact that in hospitals the so-called idiopathic variety is usually treated in medical and not surgical wards, and that the patients therefore present no broken or absorbent surface for the reception of the poison.

The disease usually commences with a feeling of chilliness, headache, and often with vomiting. The tongue becomes furred, the pulse rapid, the temperature rises, and in severe cases the vomiting remains constant. There is a sensation of pain and itching at the seat of inflammation. When the part is first attacked the skin becomes red, shining, and slightly swollen, but the redness disappears temporarily on pressure. As the disease extends to the surrounding parts, the skin becomes of a darker red and the swelling increases, and at the end of about three days the redness may fade and the swelling subside, while the cuticle over the part desquamates.

In some cases the cuticle is raised into vesicles or bullæ, giving rise to the different varieties of erysipelas, to be described as follows:

Erysipelas Vesiculosum.—While the inflammatory condition exists, a crop of small vesicles appears on the affected surface, which last a day or two, then burst, and leave small brown scabs.

Erysipelas Bullosum.—In this form, in which there is considerable swelling of the part after the inflammation has existed a few days, bullæ appear, which last a few days and then burst, leaving scabs.

Erysipelas Pustulosum.—The contents of the vesicles or bullæ become purulent.

Erysipelas Crustosum.—Simply a later stage of the former, characterized by the crusts which are formed (Hebra).

Erysipelas Fugax.—The variety in which the inflammation moves from place to place, and is of short duration in each locality. In some cases the inflammation passes through some or even all the forms just mentioned above. In the majority of instances the area of redness is bounded by a well-defined line; but this is not always present, and it is sometimes difficult to determine the exact point where the inflammation ends and the healthy skin begins. The extent of surface covered is also very variable, being in some cases very limited, in others extending over the greater part or whole of the body, but the latter condition is very rare. The locality of the inflammation, to some extent, affects the course of the disease. Thus in *erysipelas faciei* there is considerable œdema of the skin over the orbits, cheeks, and lips. This does not extend beyond the forehead, nor laterally beyond the ears; the rest of the surface is red but not swollen. The attack may be limited to one side of the face, but it usually extends to both, although its starting-point is on one side. It frequently arises from local breach of surface, due to some previously existing disease, such as otorrhœa, decayed tooth, or some skin eruption, such as eczema.

This variety is attended with considerable constitutional disturbance, often delirium. Other varieties of erysipelas are usually mentioned, being named after the parts of the body attacked; there is little to be said about them beyond the fact that the amount of swelling varies according to the denseness of the part. In those cases where the swelling is great, suppuration and sloughing often result, preceded by a dark-purple appearance of the skin.

Diagnosis.—The local inflammation in erysipelas is distinguished from the more extended rashes of the acute specific diseases; from erythema it may be recognized by the absence of symptoms of constitutional disturbance, of swelling, and of desquamation in the latter, as well as by the rapidity with which the erythemata pass through their various stages.

Prognosis.—This depends upon the constitutional symptoms and the condition of health of the patient at the time when attacked. If the fever be high, if there be much delirium, if vomiting be constant, or if there be signs of exhaustion, the opinion must be guarded, as a fatal issue may occur rapidly. The facial variety is the most serious on account of brain complications. In the majority of cases recovery takes place.

Morbid Anatomy.—On cutting through the thickened and somewhat indurated portion of skin, the surface of the section shows the corium thickened, gelatinous-looking, and juicy, merging into the subcutaneous fatty tissue, with which it is in a manner blended. From the cut surface a sero-fibrinous fluid, containing leucocytes and a few red corpuscles, exudes.

Thin sections, under the microscope, show an abundant effusion of leucocytes throughout the whole of the affected tissue. The bloodvessels especially are surrounded by thick cords of accumulated leucocytes, most marked in the marginal spreading part, where there are comparatively few connective tissue spaces. Towards the centre the leucocytes are more diffusely spread, and are present in great numbers in and around the lymph spaces and lymphatic vessels. The endothelium of the latter is often swollen and granular, and sometimes is found desquamating. The epidermis, as well as the sweat and sebaceous glands and the hair follicles, becomes similarly affected with sero-fibrinous and cellular infiltration. The epidermic cells, especially those of the upper layer of the rete, are swollen, and as serum transudes, it gradually separates the layers in the stratum lucidum and produces vesicles or bullæ. As the inflammatory process extends to the subdermic tissue, the fat cells, the blood and·lymphatic vessels, become surrounded by lines of effused leucocytes. During the subsidence of the process the epidermis, owing to the alteration of the cells of the stratum lucidum having interfered with the conversion of their protoplasm into keratin, desquamates, and the degeneration and gradual absorption of the effused white and red corpuscles gives rise to a reddish-brown stain.

Treatment.—At the onset of the attack a brisk purgative is necessary; and, indeed, during the whole course of the disease attention must be paid to the bowels. Iron in some form, and in large doses, is the most useful drug to be given. Locally, the application of cold to the part is agreeable, and is probably of benefit; dusting with flour may be tried. Hebra recommends the application of mercurial ointment. Care should be taken to remove scabs retaining pus by means of poultices; suppuration should be treated with free incisions. It it believed by some that a superficial erysipelas in an early stage can be localized by drawing a ring round the affected part with a stick of caustic, but in practice this is often found to fail.

SEPTICÆMIC RASHES.

Definition.—Rashes occurring during septicæmia.

Symptoms.—During the septicæmic condition it is not uncommon to find rashes develop. They may appear as a simple hyperæmia, or consist of slightly raised patches or papules, which may be distinct from each other or may be confluent. The skin intervening between the papules may be normal in appearance or may be more or less injected. The papules, as a rule, fade on pressure, but return to their previous condition as soon as the finger is removed. Sometimes hæmorrhages take place from the edges of the papules, and give rise to a mottled appearance of the skin; these, of course, are not affected by pressure. In some cases, in addition to this rash, a quantity of vesicles or bullæ form; but these seem to be due to some neurotic condition, and more often follow an injury to the spinal cord. The papular rash usually first shows itself on the backs of the hands, wrists, the olecranon, and patella; on the chest and abdomen the patches frequently are larger than on the extremities. The appearance of the rash is always, for a variable time, preceded by considerable constitutional disturbance, in nearly every case commencing with a severe rigor. The temperature is much increased, and the usual symptoms of septicæmia are present. These rashes may occur at any time when the patient is suffering from septicæmia.

Prognosis.—This is almost always unfavorable.

Treatment.—No local treatment is required.

Surgical Rash.

Occasionally, a few days after an operation, a roseolar rash appears over the body, attended with sore throat, high temperature, and other constitutional symptoms. Although mention of the affection has not been made under Scarlatina, there are many who believe it to be identical with this disease. The symptoms, it is true, have not been distinguished from those of scarlatina, to which it bears the closest resemblance, but sufficient evidence to prove their identity has not yet been adduced.

CHAPTER VIII.

Class I.—EXUDATIONES—*continued.*

SYPHILIS—INFANTILE SYPHILIS—VACCINO-SYPHILIS.

SYPHILIS—POX.

Definition.—A chronic infectious disease, produced by contagion or by inheritance from an affected parent, characterized by a train of definite symptoms, occurring in a definite order. According to Hutchinson it is a prolonged exanthem ; hence the position it occupies in this classification.

Symptoms.—Inoculation of the virus is followed by an interval during which no signs are manifested of its presence. This is the incubation period.

Occasionally a slight redness indicates some local irritation at the point where the poison was introduced, which, however, speedily subsides, and, unless the chancroidal virus has been mixed with that of syphilis, nothing as a rule is seen.

The primary sore makes its appearance between the fourteenth and thirtieth day after exposure to contagion. It is doubtful whether a shorter period than ten days ever elapsed between infection and development of the chancre ; on the other hand, it is unsafe to decide that syphilis has not been contracted because six weeks have not passed since the last known risk was incurred.

It is usual to divide the manifestations of syphilis into three classes or stages,—primary, secondary, and tertiary.

The following table shows the period to which the chief symptoms and lesions are usually referred:

PRIMARY.	SECONDARY.	TERTIARY.
	Constitutional Phenomena.	
Local Phenomena.		*Remote Phenomena.*
The chancre.	Induration of remote	Arterial system :
Induration of the	glands.	Aneurism.
chancre.	Pyrexia.	Nervous system :
Induration of near	Sore throat.	Paralysis, etc.
glands.	Pain in limbs, etc.	Respiratory system :
	Alopecia.	Ulceration of lar-
	Iritis.	ynx.
	Syphilides :	Phthisis.
	Roseola.	Osseous system :
	Lichen.	Caries, etc.
	Psoriasis.	Liver
	Acne.	Periosteum
	Vesicles.	Testicle Gummata.
	Condylomata.	Cellular
	Mucous tubercles.	tissue
		Late syphilides :
		Rupia.
		Impetigo.
		Ecthyma.
		Tubercles.
		Lupus.
		Ulcers.

Mr. Hutchinson has made the following convenient division of the course of the disease:

A. *Incubation.*—From "exposure" to induration of chancre and neighboring glands; rarely less than ten days or more than six weeks; usually from three to five weeks.

B. *Development.*—From induration to appearance of rash, sore throat, and fever; two to four weeks.

c. *Exanthem Stage.*—So-called secondary symptoms. Very variable in extent, and dependent much on treatment; may exist for two years from infection, or even more.

D. *Post-exanthem Stage.*—A period of latency; sometimes with occasional relapses.

E. *Tertiary Stage.*—Period of " remote sequelæ." Symptoms proper to this stage rarely occur before six months from infection, or they may never manifest themselves at all. They may appear at any time throughout life, and are specially prone to do so when the patient is exposed to depressing influences, such as long, exhausting illness or privation.

The primary sore, or chancre,—the initial lesion of syphilis,—may present a great variety of appearances; it may exist by itself, or be complicated by the presence of a so-called " soft chancre," thus constituting a " mixed " sore. It is rare to find more than one true chanrce upon the same individual; yet exceptions to the rule are at times met with, notably in vaccino-syphilis. The seat of the sore is always at the point of inoculation; hence in the majority of cases it makes its appearance on some part of the genitals. It may, however, be accidentally produced on the fingers, eyelid, tonsils, lip, tongue, navel, or anus. The most typical though by no means the most common form of primary sore is the " true Hunterian chancre." This commences as a small, almost painless papule, dusky red in color, and slowly increases in size till it attains the proportions of a tubercle; when fully developed its dimensions vary from the size of a split pea to that of a sixpence; its outline, usually circular, may be modified by its situation: for instance, on the finger it may creep round the nail. After this, ulceration takes place upon the summit, with the formation of a grayish slough, often compared to moist washleather. The secretion is slight in amount, and consists of serum and epithelial debris, not of true pus. By the removal of successive sloughs the ulcer gradually deepens, and an excavated or crater-shaped depression is produced. Soon after the appearance of the chancre—generally within a week—a peculiar induration may be observed in the edges, base, and for a little distance in the surrounding tissues. It is of a tough consistency, much resembling cartilage and harder than ordinary inflammatory effusion, and is due to the presence of fibro-plastic elements, which infiltrate the layers of the corium and subcutaneous tissue. This condition, which to the touch feels like a coin or ring, may persist for some time after complete cicatrization of the sore, but finally disappears by a process of fatty degeneration. It is most typical in parts where the connective tissue is abundant, such as the prepuce.

A far more common form of chancre is first noticed as a mere abrasion of the cuticle, which, instead of healing, increases in size, becomes slightly eroded, or in some cases elevated, is covered by a scanty non-purulent secretion, undergoes induration, and finally heals with little or no contraction of tissue. In another variety a simple crack or fissure, which at first presents no appearance indicative of syphilis, obstinately refuses to heal, becomes indurated, and is followed by signs of constitutional infection. The amount of inflammation accompanying a primary sore varies much; it is generally slight, but when irritation is set up by caustics it may become excessive, and in delicate subjects may result in destructive phagedænic process. The duration of a primary sore is seldom less than two weeks and rarely more than three months.

Indolent enlargement of the glands nearest to the sore is usually observed within a week from the first appearance of the pimple or abrasion, but is attended with little or no pain. Suppuration occurs only in rare instances, where there has been much irritation of the primary sore.

Secondary Symptoms.—At a variable period after inoculation—generally between the eighth and eleventh week—signs of constitutional infection make their appearance. The primary sore by this time may have healed, but this is by no means the rule; and even in cases where the ulcer has disappeared the hard mass of induration will be easily felt. The first constitutional symptom is fever, which usually precedes the appearance of the rash on the body by twenty-four hours; it is not always well marked, and is said by Fournier to be more common in women than in men. In spite of the elevation of temperature there is, according to some, a craving appetite peculiar to this stage. The other symptoms are severe neuralgic headache, worse at night; great pain in the limbs, more especially in the joints; enlargement of the lymphatic glands throughout the system, particularly those of the occiput and axilla; sore throat; and an eruption on the skin. The sore throat may commence as a simple erythema, but soon small shallow ulcers are seen scattered over the tonsils, root of the tongue, and upper part of the pharynx. Following the classification, and to a great extent the description, of Bäumler, we may divide the phenomena as seen on the skin into the following groups:

I. Circumscribed hyperæmia with but slight infiltration—muscular syphilide; roseola.

II. Marked infiltration of the papillary body.

A. In the form of papules—papular syphilide.
B. In large patches—squamous syphilide.

On mucous membranes, or at favorable points on the cutis—moist papules (condylomata lata).

III. Especial implication of the immediate vicinity of the follicles (hair and sebaceous).

A. Simple infiltration with scanty or no exudation in the follicles—lichenous syphilide.

B. With acute suppuration in the follicle—acne syphilitica.

C. Exudation into small, markedly infiltrated groups of follicles with rapid formation of crusts—impetigo syphilitica.

IV. Infiltration with sub-epithelial suppuration and superficial ulceration—pustular syphilide (pemphigus syphiliticus, ecthyma syphiliticum, rupia syphilitica).

V. Infiltration with disintegration to a considerable depth (gummous)—tubercular syphilide.

Macular Syphilide—Roseola Syphilitica.

This form of the exanthem is the first and most common. It consists of rose-colored spots of a roundish or irregular shape, varying in size from a pin's head to that of a pea, disappearing on pressure and coming out in crops. The site varies with the severity of the attack. Sometimes but few spots are to be found on the chest, and in other cases the whole body may be covered. As a rule the eruption, if not treated, lasts for weeks, when it gradually fades, leaving slight coppery stains, which ultimately disappear. Occasionally roseola syphilitica relapses, when the spots differ somewhat from their original character, being paler in color, fewer in number, and very often assuming an annular form.

Papular Syphilide.

When a case has been neglected this form of syphilide is often the first to appear, but it may be developed from the preceding variety. The papules vary in size from a grain of wheat to a pea, and are at first red in color, gradually becoming darker. They are hard and usually smooth, but occasionally covered with small scales. The eruption may occur on any part of the skin, but its favorite sites are the borders of the scalp, the forehead,—where it forms a band called the corona veneris,—on the palms and soles, on the back of the neck, either in depressions or wrinkles, or on the flexor surfaces of the joints. If the papules are situated on the moister parts, such as the female genitals, or about the anus, or beneath the breasts, they may resemble the characters of condylomata. Relapses may take place late in the disease, when the papules are arranged in an annular form, often attacking unsymmetrically the palms and soles. The papules persist for a longer or a shorter period, according to circumstances, and finally disappear, leaving a deeply pigmented stain.

Moist papules, or condylomata lata, are found on the mucous membranes as well as on the parts already mentioned, in the form of superficial white spots, in which there are abrasions of the membranes and a circumscribed thickening of the epithelium. They thus resemble the effect produced by nitrate of silver. The condylomata at times, and especially on the surface, will ulcerate, when the condylomatous ulcer is produced, but more frequently they spread rapidly, owing to the contagion of the secretion, and then appear in large masses.

Squamous Syphilide.

This form of syphilide arises either from a gradual enlargement of a single papule or from the coalescence of several papules, when the infiltration is excessive, causing desquamation on the surface. The appearance is somewhat that of common psoriasis, but the scabs are dirty in color, quite different to the white transparent scales of the common disease. It may occur on any part of the body, but when, as is often the case, it appears late, it may show itself as a single patch of crescentic outline.

Lichen Syphiliticus.

Occurs in the form of papules, which closely resemble simple milium, and consist of hard granules, like gum, found in the epidermis, which, when scooped out, leave small pits. They are at first red, but gradually become yellow, and are situated in groups of a dozen or more. When the inflammatory process that gives rise to them is severe, vesicles, or even pustules, may result.

Acne Syphilitica.

In all respects, with perhaps the addition of a slightly coppery areola, this variety resembles acne vulgaris. The situation of the disease is the same in both, and the only point which can assist in the diagnosis is the presence of other syphilides on the skin. If the acne spots become pustular, with the rapid formation of crusts, syphilitic impetigo is produced.

Pemphigus Syphiliticus.

Occasionally vesicles, large enough to deserve the title of bullæ, are seen, chiefly on the hands, and to them Bäumler has given this name. It is most common in hereditary syphilis.

Ecthyma Syphiliticum.

Ecthyma is one of the later eruptions, occurring in the tertiary stage. It is unsymmetrical, altogether irregular, and characterized by pustules situated on inflamed bases. The pustules are caused by an infiltration into the epidermis of a fluid that rapidly becomes purulent. They soon burst, and so produce ulcers, which extend at the edges in a serpiginous manner, and when healed leave scars that may be pigmented.

Rupia.

This is the severest form of the pustular variety. It commences as a hard papule, which softens in the centre into a deepseated pustule, which soon dries, and forms a conical-shaped scab, having the appearance of a limpid shell. When the scab falls off a foul circular ulcer is left, that ultimately circatrizes, leaving a permanent scar. It usually begins on the face, and extends to other parts of the body, chiefly the extremities. Rupia is generally unsymmetrical, and therefore a tertiary symptom, but in badly nourished persons it may occur comparatively early in the disease.

Tubercular Syphilide.

Tubercles are described as hard, flat, elevated bodies of a copper color, which usually attack the face, tongue, penis, and limbs late in the disease. They commence as small papules, which enlarge and become scaly or scabby on the surface. Beneath the scales ulceration may take place.

Tertiary Symptoms.—Under the head of secondary symptoms all the syphilodermata have been briefly mentioned, it being impossible to divide them correctly into secondary and tertiary manifestations, because the numerous exceptions to the rule destroy the rule itself. The truth is, that all these varieties may occur more or less at the same time, or that they may overlap each other in such a way as to interfere with the conventional arrangement into fixed periods. Still it is useful, clinically, to retain the three divisions; and, more than that, there are certain general characters connected with the tertiary stage which help us to decide whether a symptom is a remote sequela or one of the acute phenomena of the disease.

Certain characteristics of the tertiary stage:

1. Great obstinacy in healing and proneness to recur.

2. General absence of symmetry.

3. Invasions of deep organs and tissues as well as the superficial.

The late syphilides are most commonly of the pustular or tubercular type. The term syphilitic lupus is applied to a tubercular syphilide of the face, resulting in severe ulceration and extensive destruction of the bones and tissues; the name is ill-chosen, as it is apt to cause confusion with lupus vulgaris, which is not syphilitic. Ulcers are very common in this stage, and may arise as a result of boils, pustules, or tubercles. They are usually circular, with well-defined edges, looking as if they had been punched out with an instrument. They spread slowly, and destroy the deeper tissues in the process. A list of the other tertiary lesions has been given at the commencement of the chapter, and it is not within the scope of this work to do more than mention them.

Diagnosis.—The primary sore, or true chancre, has to be distinguished from the non-syphilitic chancre, or chancroid. The following are the chief points to be considered in deciding between them:

1. *Site.*—It is extremely rare for the non-infecting sore to exist upon any part except the genitals. The true chancre, though affecting the same locality, may be found elsewhere.

2. *Number.*—The soft sore has a tendency to multiplicity. The chancre, or hard sore, is usually solitary.

3. *Time of Appearance.*—The soft sore nearly always appears within three days of contagion. The hard rarely shows itself before the tenth day.

4. *Induration.*—Very slightly marked in a soft sore that has not been treated by caustics; well defined and cartilaginous in a chancre.

5. *Secretion.*—The soft sore secretes pure pus; the hard chancre, serum and epithelial debris.

6. *Bubo.*—The bubo resulting from a soft sore has a tendency to swell, be painful, and suppurate. The whole group of glands become glued together, and cannot be moved under the skin, whereas in the case of a true chancre the glands rarely suppurate unless the sore is irritated, or unless it takes on a phagedænic character. The ganglia become hard, are not glued together, remain freely movable under the skin, and are only slightly tender.

Herpes præputialis is sometimes mistaken for a chancre, but this mistake can only occur after the rupture of the vesicles, when the ulcer that is left resembles the "simple abrasion" of primary syphilis. The history of a crop of vesicles, the smarting pain, the absence of induration, the date of appearance, and the rapid subsidence under simple treatment, are the main points to note in forming a diagnosis.

Syphilides, or Syphilo-dermata.

The general characteristics of skin eruptions due to syphilis are:

1. Tendency to present several types simultaneously. The macular, papular, and squamous forms constantly occur together, and may present every variety of intermediate stage.

2. A tint generally compared to "copper" or "raw ham," and especially well marked in inveterate eruptions.

3. The general color of the skin becomes yellow or earthy, implying the presence of a special cachexia.

4. Less itching than non-specific eruptions.

5. Tendency to leave brown stains, and to produce other pigmentary changes, such as leucoderma.

6. A disposition on the part of the ulcerative forms to spread in a characteristic serpiginous manner.

...e eruptions is where the parts of the body are usually affected by the non-syphilitic eruptions, such as the flexor surfaces of the limbs, the palms and soles.

Cutaneous syphilide or syphilitic erythema presents the following peculiarities:—

1. The production of scales is less profuse than in common psoriasis.

2. The more gleaming appearance of the patches is ... marked, and there is a tendency to an ulcerative condition ... the formation of ..g-colored scale.

3. The inner sides of the arms and thighs suffer more than the elbows and knees.

4. A marked tendency to affect palms and soles.

Syphilitic Iritis.—The ...c effusion is seen in the form of patches ... nodules, especially at the margin of the iris, instead of appearing as a film covering the whole organ. There is ... no pain than is the case with the traumatic and rheumatic varieties.

Syphilis of the Tongue, as a result of a gumma which has ... down, produces an obstinate, ragged ulcer, which has often the appearance of cancer. The history and the presence of other symptoms of syphilis will assist the diagnosis, while the scrapings, placed under the microscope, would indicate the presence or absence of the characteristic elements. Erichsen says: "The syphilitic ulcer is elongated, irregular, and does not rapidly extend . . . . while the cancerous ulcer is of a more circular shape, has hard everted edges, and spreads with great rapidity." Syphilis and cancer may both produce a hard, non-ulcerating tubercle in the tongue, but here, in addition to the history, we must bear in mind that cancer usually attacks the tip and edges, while syphilis affects the deep substance, of the organ. (Erichsen.)

Prognosis.—The prognosis as regards absolute cure in a case of syphilis is most uncertain. It is true that many patients, after one or two attacks of secondary symptoms, if properly treated and of sound constitution in other respects, may never again be troubled by any manifestations of the disease. It is also, no doubt, true that the chance of immunity from fresh symptoms increases with the time that has elapsed since the disappearance of the last. Still, it is never safe to announce that we have seen the last of it. Any depressing influence, any severe illness, great privation, or overwork may excite the disease to renewed activity. Cases in which syphilis has reappeared after an apparent quiescence of twenty years are by no means rare. The important question, When may a man marry who has had syphilis? is one which ought to be considered under the head of prognosis. Much might be said upon the subject, but it will be sufficient here to assert that it is absolutely unsafe to marry until all constitutional signs of the disease have disappeared for at least twelve months. With the exception of infantile syphilis, which often destroys the child within a few months, it is only as a result of old-standing tertiary mischief that the disease is ever fatal.

Morbid Anatomy.—On examining under the microscope a *hard chancre* which has become fully developed, an infiltration of small round cells will be observed throughout the whole substance of the corium or mucous membrane, imbedded in an amorphous or slightly granular substance, and specially numerous around the bloodvessels, the walls of which are usually somewhat thickened and contain numerous round cells. As the cellular infiltration extends into the rete Malpighii, it produces impaired nutrition of the epidermis and subsequent scaling. In the later stages the conversion of the exuded cells into connective tissue maintains the induration, especially in the marginal part of the chancre.

The *roseolar syphilide* consists in a mere localized hyper-æmia of the papillary layer, going on gradually to slight effusion of plasma, with accumulation of cells around the capillaries and a slight increase of nuclei in their walls.

In the *papular syphilide* the papillary layer is the seat of a cellular infiltration, identical in appearance with that of the hard chancre. The epidermis covering the little nodules becomes thinned or scaly, and occasionally a very slight subepithelial exudation gives rise to a shallow vesicle.

In "*mucous tubercles*" the same essential changes take place, but under the influence of warmth and moisture the papillary body hypertrophies, and the epidermis being macerated, a molecular ulceration of the exposed papillæ occurs. "Mucous tubercles" that are kept dry assume the appearance of ordinary papular syphilides.

The *squamous syphilide*, due to the enlargement of a syphilitic papule or to the coalescence of several, presents similar anatomical changes.

In the simplest cases of *lichenous syphilide* there is an infiltration of small round cells just outside the hair and sebaceous follicles, combined with hyperæmia of the follicu-lar plexus. In more acute cases there is slight exudation into the follicles, forming minute discrete vesico-pustules, which soon dry up, and, falling off, leave small dark, de-pressed, slowly-fading scars.

Occasionally the intervening skin between the papules becomes affected, and the papillary layer being infiltrated, the little group of lichenous spots becomes converted into a scaly eruption.

If the process be still more acute, leading to suppuration in and round the follicles, the *acneiform syphilide* is pro-duced; and if the skin intervening between the follicles becomes affected, an aggregation of closely-packed pustules on an inflamed base is formed, which soon becomes covered with a greenish-yellow granular crust, producing the *impetiginous syphilide*.

In the *vesicular* and *bullous syphilides* the serous effusion into the epidermis, separating the cells of the stratum lucidum, gives rise to vesicles, the contents of which, often turbid and blood-stained from the first, soon become purulent. The crusts formed by the drying up of the contents leave only a slight scar on falling off. If the base of the vesicle becomes red and inflamed, and the rete with the papillary layer be more or less destroyed, the so-called *ecthymatous syphilide* is produced. Owing to the loss of tone, the scars left after separation of the scabs and healing of the ulcers are depressed, and often deeply pigmented.

By an extension of the infiltration round the periphery of the scab, successive layers are added from below, and a conical prominence, seated on a purplish-red ulcerated surface, is gradually formed, termed the *rupial syphilide*.

In the *tubercular syphilides* there is a formation of gummata in the substance of the true skin. In the deeper layers of the corium there are seen small nodules, grayish-red and homogeneous on section, and merging gradually into the surrounding tissue, so that they cannot be enucleated.

Microscopically they consist of masses of round cells closely aggregated together in a meshwork of fine fibres. The marginal portions in older nodules, and the whole mass in the younger ones, are pretty freely supplied with vessels; but in process of growth these get gradually obliterated in the centre, which then undergoes mucous or caseous degeneration. The margin, on the other hand, may undergo condensation from partial conversion of the round cells into spindle cells and connective tissue. As the nodule extends towards the surface, the swelling, which at first has presented the appearance of a colorless papule, becomes redder, and, slowly involving the papillary layer, causes irritative changes in the epidermis. These may result in desquamation only, or, by the exudation of a little serum, in the formation of a thin yellowish crust. Sometimes, also, a vesicle is formed, which dries up to produce a crust, beneath which ulceration of the tubercle slowly takes place. If the tubercle be large and softened in the centre, when it reaches the skin a bluish-gray furuncle-like body is formed, which on bursting discharges a yellowish material, and in consequence a deep, slowly-spreading ulcer is produced.

Infantile or Inherited Syphilis.

A child may inherit syphilis from either parent, but in the majority of cases the mischief may be traced to the father. This arises from the fact that a woman whose constitution is infected at the time of conception, or becomes so during gestation, is particularly liable to abort. When delivery takes place at full term, the child rarely survives it more than a few weeks. It should be mentioned here that some deny the possibility of direct contamination of the foetus by the father, and maintain that the mother is always intermediately infected. Nothing is known with certainty of the means by which the disease is transmitted, but it is certain that the placenta not uncommonly shows traces of the malady. (Virchow.)

Infantile syphilis may either appear at or soon after birth, or may not give any signs of its presence till several weeks have elapsed. The former cases are the more serious, and usually terminate fatally. They are characterized by a bullous or pustular eruption, which never appears later than the first week. The first seat is generally on the palms and soles, spreading thence to the trunk, limbs, and occasionally to the face. Dirty-red, circular spots, of variable size, are first seen, and effusion beneath the cuticle converts these into blebs, which after a time rupture and produce unhealthy excoriations, obstinately resisting treatment.

Fresh crops of blebs appear, some of which at times attack the mouth and nose. The nails fall off, and finally the child becomes a mass of ulcerating sores, and succumbs in less than a month. The name pemphigus neonatorum was applied to this form of the disease before its nature was understood, but it is more correct to call it pemphigus syphiliticus.

In the more numerous class of cases the child may be apparently healthy at birth, or merely somewhat undersized. After a period, varying from a fortnight to two months, it becomes emaciated, delicate, and irritable; the skin is shrivelled, rough, dry, and of a peculiar earthy color. Mucous tubercles, accompanied by catarrh of the nasal mucous membrane, make their appearance, and give rise to much swelling and profuse thin secretion. The characteristic noise produced by the child's efforts to remove the obstacle to respiration has obtained for this symptom the name of "*the snuffles*." At about the same time as the coryza an eruption appears, usually commencing about the anus and buttock, whence it may extend to any or every part of the surface, more especially over the face. Macules, papules, and scaly patches, in varying proportions, make up a rash of a mixed character, which it is impossible to refer to any one form. The color, however, presents the copper tint of syphilis.

Condylomata about the anus cause much trouble, and "rhagades" are found in that situation, and about the mouth, where they leave scars.

In addition to these symptoms the infant usually suffers from severe diarrhœa, stomatitis, and loss of flesh and hair, and in consequence assumes the aspect of an old man. At the end of twelve months, if properly treated, all these symptoms subside. Tertiary manifestations make their appearance between the ages of four and fourteen. As in the adult, they appear in the bones and deeper tissues as well as in certain eruptions, such as rupia and ~~ecthyma~~. Besides these there are certain lesions which are specially characteristic of the inherited form of the disease.

A. Cloudiness and opacity of the cornea, known as "interstitial keratitis."

B. Certain changes in the teeth, probably the result of early stomatitis. These changes are most marked in the permanent set, but may be observed to a less extent in the milk teeth. The incisors, especially those of the upper jaw, suffer most, the median being first attacked. They are small in size and pegged, rapidly wear away, and present a notch in the centre of the edge and a wide interval between them. The canines suffer, but to a less extent. (Hutchinson.)

C. Depression of the nasal cartilages produces the remarkable flattening of the bridge of the nose.

D. Less common than any of the preceding is an enlargement of the lower end of the humerus and sternal end of the clavicle.

Vaccino-Syphilis.

The series of carefully observed cases reported by Mr. Hutchinson in this country, and the report by Dr. Pacchiotti, of Turin, who was specially employed to observe an outbreak of the disease in the Rivalta valley in 1861, leave no doubt that syphilis is occasionally produced in healthy persons by careless vaccination with lymph taken from infected children. Under these circumstances the disease runs precisely the same course and exhibits the same symptoms as when inoculation takes place in other ways.

Treatment.

Primary Sore.—There is considerable doubt whether any good is gained by the vigorous cauterization of the primary sore, which is so strongly recommended by some surgeons; at all events, if the plan is adopted, it must be done early and with the strongest form of caustic, such as pure nitric acid. The usual and best local application is black wash. When a case is decided to be one of syphilis, no time should be lost in giving the antidote, which is undoubtedly mercury. Some authorities recommend waiting till the secondary symptoms have shown themselves before using the remedy, but it is better to try and lessen their severity by its early use.

In administering the drug we may select from a large number of methods, of which the following are the most important:

A. *By the Mouth.*—One drachm of the solution of corrosive sublimate three times a day; four or five grains of blue pill, with a little opium, night and morning; one grain of the green iodide three times a day, or five grains of Plummer's pill as often, as the best preparations to be used.

B. *By the Rectum.*—Bryant advises the use of mercurial suppositories.

C. *By Hypodermic Injection.*—Four grains of the perchloride in an ounce of water; fifteen minims for a dose.

D. *By Vapor Baths.*—Using from ten to thirty grains of calomel for each bath.

E. *By Inunction.*—A drachm of mercurial ointment may be rubbed into the axillæ or groin night and morning.

Two or more of the preceding modes may be used together, and it is sometimes an advantage to vary during the treatment the mode of administering the drug. In a mercurial course attention should be paid to the following points:

1. Avoid profuse salivation. The gums must be carefully watched, the teeth being cleansed twice or three times daily with an aromatic or astringent wash.

2. Warn the patient against catching cold.

3. Continue the treatment for some time after the disappearance of the symptoms, and discontinue the use of the drug gradually rather than suddenly.

4. Give a simple and nutritious diet, with a moderate amount of good wine and beer. Avoid fruits of all kinds.

5. Stop the use of the drug, or give it very cautiously, if the patient is cachectic, and substitute for it iron, cod-liver oil, and other tonics.

Secondary Symptoms.—They should be treated on a similar plan—that is, by the administration of mercury, if it has not been already commenced during the primary stage. Ulcers in the mouth and throat should be lightly touched with nitrate of silver or with a solution of perchloride of mercury.

Condylomata about the anus, etc., are best treated by dusting them with calomel.

Tertiary Symptoms.—Mercury by the mouth, with only a few exceptions, should be avoided in this stage, especially when the deeper tissues are involved. In its place the drug to be relied upon is iodide of potassium, which should be given in full doses of ten to thirty grains three times a day.

Gummatous deposits in the skin should be treated locally, by means of mercury ointment, or the oleate of mercury. In this stage good food, wine, change of air, and general tonics are of great importance.

Infantile syphilis must be treated by mercury. The usual modes of administering it are by the mouth, in the form of one or two grains of gray powder, night and morning, or by the inunction of mercurial ointment, which is most easily applied on the child's abdominal binder.

CHAPTER IX.

Class I.—EXUDATIONES—*continued.*

Sub-class B.—*Of Internal or Local Origin.*

1. *ERYTHEMATOUS GROUP.*

Erythema simplex, læve, fugax, intertrigo; multiforme, including papulatum, tuberculatum; annulare, iris, gyratum—Erythema nodosum—Roseola—Urticaria—Pellagra.

ERYTHEMATA.

Definition.—The erythemata are characterized by the existence on the skin of dusky-red, slightly raised patches of various sizes, which occasionally vesicate, run an acute course, and are attended with little or no constitutional disturbance.

Symptoms.—When the patches first appear, they are surrounded by a hyperæmic zone, which prevents their margin being clearly defined; at the end of a few hours this zone disappears without leaving any pigment, and the erythematous papules can be distinctly recognized. After lasting a few days the papules fade, and are usually followed by desquamation, which is limited to the site of the eruption. In some cases, during the height of eruption, a small vesicle or bulla may be produced. There is no itching, and but little, if any, constitutional disturbance. The papules are most frequently found on the back of the hands and the dorsum of the feet, where, as a rule, they commence even when they extend to other parts of the body. They occur less often on the arms and legs, and seldom extend to the face and

trunk of the body, never without implicating the limbs.
A large number of varieties of this rash have been described
by different writers, depending on differences noticeable in
the character of the eruption itself, in its site, and in the
amount of constitutional disturbance it produces.

With one exception, to be afterwards mentioned, they are
attended by but little if any increase of temperature; indeed, but for the appearance of the rash there is nothing in
the patient's condition, either local or constitutional, which
would attract attention to the disease.   They all agree
in the rash being unilateral; when the trunk is implicated,
both sides of the body are affected at the same time.   The
duration of the disease varies greatly, and it often has a
tendency to return to parts which have been attacked in the
first instance, and from which the eruption has already
faded.

Erythema læve occurs as the result of venous obstruction,
and is a mere hyperæmia of the skin; it frequently is a
consequence of some general condition, such as dropsy, and
is more often seen on the legs.   The redness is preceded by
œdema of the skin, and may not progress further than the
stage of hyperæmia, but occasionally bullæ form on the surface.

Erythema fugax is a simple hyperæmia of the skin, which
is due to gastric disturbance or local irritation.   It consists
of patches of redness of irregular shape, which appear in
different parts of the body, frequently on the face and upper part of the trunk.   The patches are of very short
duration, come and go rapidly, and in most cases itch and
tingle while present.

Although these diseases are usually described as erythemata, it is doubtful whether they should not, as Hebra suggests, be excluded on the ground that they are only hyperæmiæ of the skin.

Erythema intertrigo is a local erythema, produced by the

friction of opposed surfaces of the skin, and occurs in fat persons, more particularly children. It soon becomes moist, when it assumes the nature of eczema, under which head it will be again noticed.

Of the other varieties described by different writers, such as Wilson, Rayer, and Fuchs, only those included by Hebra under the name of erythema multiforme will be noticed. Hebra looks upon these varieties as merely different stages of development of the same eruption; thus E. papulatum and E. tuberculatum differ from each other simply in the size of the patch, in the former being about the size of a pin's head or larger, in the latter about the size of a four-penny piece. They occur generally on the backs of the hands and feet, and occasionally extend to the arms and legs, and rarely to the face and body. In both forms they are of a dusky-red or violet color, and when they first make their appearance are surrounded by a zone of redness, which lasts but a few hours. At the end of three or four days they fade, occasionally leaving a temporary yellow stain, due to escape of coloring matter of the blood into the skin. A slight desquamation follows the fading of the papules. The papules are succeeded by others, but the whole course of the eruption is limited to a few days. The young are most frequently affected by this form of erythema, most often in the spring and autumn of the year. A difference of opinion exists as to which sex is most frequently attacked.

Erythema annulare results when the erythematous patch begins to fade in its centre, leaving a red ring surrounding a pale surface.

Erythema iris is produced when a second or third ring is formed outside the inner, due to a fading of the redness in the circumference of the patch. In this, as in all varieties, vesication may take place.

Erythema gyratum is said to occur when portions of the rings of E. iris fade, and in consequence of several patches being close the rings run together, forming a serpentine eruption.

The circular form of erythema differs only from the papular in the appearance of the eruption. They present themselves on the same parts of the body, last but a few days,—never beyond a month,—and cause almost no constitutional disturbance.

ERYTHEMA NODOSUM.

This variety of erythema differs widely from the preceding forms in the character of the eruption,—in its site, in its symptoms,—and, in fact, it is not a skin disease at all. It consists of oval swellings, at first hard, but at a later stage soft, from a half to four or five inches in length. At the commencement the swellings are pale red, but gradually become of a dark-red or violet color. After a few days, as the color fades, it is replaced by a yellow discoloration, which persists for some time after the disappearance of the swelling. These swellings occur in crops of rarely less than a dozen in number, most frequently on the front of the lower extremities, but are by no means limited to this site. A second, sometimes even a third, crop makes its appearance, invading parts which in the first attack have escaped, and thus the eruption extends over other parts of the body. This form of erythema is not attended by any itching, but is characterized by considerable pain at the seat of eruption, and great general debility, anæmia, and gastric disturbance.

Diagnosis.—Simple erythema can only be confounded with prurigo, from which, however, it can be distinguished by the extreme itching and blood crusts of the latter, and by the limitation of the rash of prurigo to the back and extensor surfaces of the arms and legs; while erythema attacks the anterior surface as well. The varieties of erythema multiforme can hardly be mistaken for any other disease, with the exception, perhaps, of the gyrate form, which may be taken for ringworm of the body. The rapidity of the appearance and disappearance of the former, and the absence of microscopical evidence, are points to guide us in our diagnosis.

Erythema nodosum can be readily distinguished from all other eruptions by the tenderness of the patches, the pain they occasion, and by the constitutional and gastric symptoms which accompany it, as well as by the gradual alteration in color from day to day, resembling a bruise.

Prognosis.—Always favorable, although the period of duration varies. Death after E. læve results not from the erythema, but from the disease during which it occurs. The length of an attack of E. nodosum depends on the number of crops which appear; five or six weeks is, however, an outside limit. Like the rest of the erythemata, the symptoms disappear spontaneously.

Morbid Anatomy.—The changes in the skin may be due to—

1. Simple hyperæmia of the superficial layer of the cutis.
2. Hyperæmia followed by exudation.

The former exists in E. simplex and E. intertrigo.

On examining the affected portion of the skin with a simple lens, magnifying about twenty diameters, a great number of minute red dots are seen, which are the tops of the capillary loops in the papillæ, especially in the region of the hair follicles. As the turgescence of the minute vessels passes off readily, no morbid appearances are to be found after death.

In the latter condition, in addition to the simple hyperæmia of the papillary layer, there is exudation of plasma, of pale and then of red corpuscles, according to the severity of the process, followed often by various secondary inflammatory changes. In E. papulatum, following on the hyperæmia, there is slight effusion of plasma in the substance of the papillary layer, giving rise to slight elevation of the little spots. An excess of serum, transuding into the epidermis, and collecting in the stratum lucidum, may give rise to minute vesicles. In E. nodosum a number of pale, together with a few red, corpuscles, as well as a large amount of plasma, are effused. The exudation pressing on the vessels, gives rise, as in a wheal, to the pallor in the centre of the patch, and the breaking-down and pigmentary changes in the red corpuscles produce the purplish, greenish, and yellow discoloration in the same way as in a fading bruise.

Treatment.—In the treatment of E. læve every care should be taken to assist the circulation of the part ; the limb should be raised, carefully supported, and warm fomentations applied. Often acupuncture by means of Southey's trocars becomes necessary to relieve the œdema. Bathing the part with an astringent lotion is recommended.

In E. fugax the diet should be carefully regulated. Often this eruption is due to the use of soap, which should of course be avoided. Local treatment is unnecessary, not only in this form but in all the varieties of erythema, on account of the short duration of the eruption. In E. intertrigo attention should be paid to keeping the part dry and clean ; a weak tar lotion is of use. The constitutional treatment of all the erythemata should consist in regulating the bowels and in the subsequent administration of acid and bitter tonics.

Roseola.

Much difference of opinion exists among dermatologists concerning the diseases usually classed under this heading. Willan has described, under the name of roseola, a variety of rashes which are not recognized by all writers, and Hebra especially doubts their existence. There may be some difficulty in agreeing with Willan in the correctness of describing as separate affections R. infantilis, R. æstiva, R. autumnalis, R. annulata, but we shall mention a rash under the name of roseola which is by no means limited to one period of the year. A roseolous rash, occurring in association with some of the acute infectious diseases, has been described under the head of these diseases.

Definition.—Roseola is an acute disease characterized by the production on the body of small rose-colored papules, and attended by very slight constitutional symptoms, which make their appearance at the same time as the rash.

Symptoms.—The rash consists of minute red and slightly elevated spots, scattered over the chest and neck, less often extending over the face and arms. They disappear temporarily on pressure, last but a few days, and fade, leaving a discoloration of the skin, but are sometimes followed by slight desquamation. Feverishness, headache, and occasionally vomiting are present at the commencement of the rash.

The constitutional symptoms are, however, slight; the temperature is seldom as high as 102° Fahr., and more often only just above normal. The fauces are frequently a little injected, but the redness does not extend beyond the edge of the soft palate, and the tonsils are not swollen. The tongue is slightly furred, and the papillæ along its edge are often prominent.

Diagnosis.—Roseola is often mistaken for scarlatina, and the diagnosis between the two affections is frequently a matter of considerable difficulty. They differ in the fact that the papules in the former are more widely separated from each other than those in the latter, and the skin intervening between the papules does not become red in roseola, as it does in scarlatina. The constitutional symptoms in roseola appear at the same time as the rash, while in scarlatina they precede it. Roseola is not infectious, and occurs

more frequently among young women and children than
other persons. Also see table, p. 57.

Prognosis.—Roseola always ends in recovery in a few
days.

Morbid Anatomy.—The changes are the same as in the
milder forms of erythema, the processes usually stopping
short at hyperæmia only, but sometimes going on to slight
exudation of plasma. The vascular plexuses round the
hair follicles, sweat and sebaceous glands, are the regions
specially involved.

Treatment.—Nothing is required beyond rest for a day
or two.

URTICARIA—NETTLE RASH.

Definition.—A disease the chief symptoms of which is the
production of wheals on the skin, causing great irritation,
usually unattended by any constitutional symptoms, but
sometimes by fever, pain in the epigastrium, and headache.

Symptoms.—The eruption makes its appearance at the
same time as any constitutional symptoms which exist, and
consist of a quantity of wheals. These vary greatly in size,
in quantity, in shape, and in color; but the difference in
the variation in color is due to their being in different
stages of development. As a rule they appear first as red
elevations, which increase in size, becoming white in the
centre with red margins. They may occur on any part of
the body, and although each individual wheal does not last
many hours, a succession may make their appearance for
weeks or months. They are accompanied by a severe itching or stinging sensation of the part, and constitutional
symptoms may or may not be present.

In some individuals a condition of skin exists which may
fairly be considered to result from an urticarial diathesis.

Several forms of urticaria are recognized.

Urticaria Febrilis.—In this form the eruption is preceded

by shivering, headache, furred tongue, and vomiting. Soon
a number of slightly raised wheals appear over the greater
proportion of the body, and usually begin on the wrists and
neck. These come and go rapidly, and the itching is intolerable, so much so that it is impossible not to rub or
scratch them. Wherever the skin is touched fresh wheals
appear, till in this way the surface is more or less covered.
From the scratching the skin becomes excoriated, but desquamation does not occur at any time. The irritation is
always worse at night.

Urticaria conferta is a chronic variety of the disease in
which the wheals are abundant but limited to one or two
localities.

Urticaria evanida is also a chronic form, in which the
wheals come and go rapidly.

Urticaria perstans is a variety in which the eruption continues without changing for some weeks, and may perhaps
be the same form which has been well called by Dr. Alfred
Sangster Urticaria pigmentosa, in which the wheals last for
years, leaving a deposit of pigment, which causes a mottled
appearance on the skin.

Urticaria tuberosa is rarely seen; in it the wheals are of
a larger size than in the others, and it occurs in persons of
weak constitution.

Urticaria miliaris, U. vesicularis, U. bullosa, are described
and so called because vesicles or bullæ form on the surface
of the wheal. They are extremely rare.

In *Urticaria papulosa* the wheals are so small as to resembles papules. Hebra says that they increase in size,
but later in the disease diminish again.

Diagnosis.—Urticaria is easily distinguished from the
erythemata by the more diffused character of the eruption
and the difference in the site, by the absence of local irritation in erythema, by the urticarial wheals being white in
the centre with red margins, and more raised than the ery-

thematous patches; from measles and scarlatina by the absence of coryza and sore throat in urticaria, and its lowness of temperature, and by the different courses these diseases run; from erythema nodosum by the presence of itching in urticaria and heat and pain in the former.

The ease by which the rash is excited in certain varieties of urticaria by the slightest irritation of the skin is often a useful diagnostic sign.

Urticaria often arises from the ingestion of some special article of food, such as mussels, oysters, cucumber, mushrooms, etc., and even cold water; but in many persons it arises without any apparent cause. It is undoubtedly affected by season, in some being worse in cold than in hot weather. The young are more liable to it than the old, and it is occasionally associated with irregularities of menstruation, pregnancy, the presence of parasites in the alimentary canal, and arises very frequently from the irritation caused by the bites of fleas, bugs, etc.

Prognosis.—Urticaria is not a fatal disease. As a rule an attack passes off in a few days, but it may be extremely obstinate and resist all forms of treatment.

Morbid Anatomy.—On examining a vertical section of an urticarial wheal we find the connective tissue bundles of the corium separated by effused plasma. The capillaries and small vessels are dilated, especially in the marginal zone of the wheal, full of blood, and surrounded by lines of effused leucocytes, which are present in larger numbers than normal throughout the whole corium. The lymphatics of the skin are widely dilated and full of lymph. In some cases escape of red corpuscles by transudation, or actual rupture of the vessels, gives rise to pigmentary and other color changes in the wheal.

Each wheal usually corresponds with the area of distribution of a terminal arteriole, and is supposed to be produced by paralysis of the vasomotor nerves supplying the branch; but opinions differ as to the way in which this can give rise to exudation.

Treatment.—If a cause, either internal or external, can be found for its existence, it should be at once removed.

In acute urticaria it is well to begin with an emetic or purgative, or both. In both acute and chronic forms it is important to diet the patient carefully, paying particular attention to avoid his having indigestible food, salt meat, pork, etc. The bowels should be regulated, and the patient kept cool. With a view to allay irritation, sponging the skin with cold water should be adopted. Saline baths and lotions are useless, but washing with weak vinegar is agreeable, and should be persisted in if the irritation be severe. Aconite has been given internally with doubtful benefit, but arsenic is certainly of value in some of the more persistent forms of the disease.

PELLAGRA—ITALIAN LEPROSY.

Definition.—Pellagra is a serious disease, occurring endemically in Northern Italy and Southern France, one of its chief characteristics being an erythema of the skin. This appears on those parts of the body most exposed to the sun, such as the hands and arms, neck and chest. Women suffer from it on the face, owing to the fact that their head dresses do not protect them from the sun's rays, while among men, whose faces are screened by large hats, this part is more rarely affected.

Symptoms.—It commences as a mere erythema of the skin, which is accompanied by a sense of irritation. During the winter this subsides, but a deposit of more or less pigment remains. Vesication does not occur, but the erythema is followed by desquamation. On the return of the summer the erythema again makes its appearance, and each year the skin is left more stained with pigment. At first the patient simply complains of lassitude, but gradually becomes melancholic; later on suffers from marked cerebral symptoms, which terminate in insanity.

Prognosis.—The length of the disease—that is, from first symptom to death—varies from a few to ten or twelve years, usually about five. Although it generally proves fatal, this is not always the case; but even when recovery takes place it is only partial. Complete restoration to health is rare.

The causes of pellagra are not well understood. It is a disease altogether confined to the poor, and to those who work in the sun. It has been attributed to the character of the food which these people eat, and has been thought to be associated with maize, their chief article of diet. In the damp seasons maize is attacked with a parasitic fungus, which is supposed by Bellardine to be the origin of pellagra. When maize is supplemented by other food, as in the large towns, the disease does not exist. Pellagra is not contagious, nor is there any evidence that it is hereditary, although members of the same family who are exposed to the same conditions are often attacked with it together.

Treatment.—The treatment of the local inflammation is simple. Protection from the rays of the sun always leads to a subsidence of the symptoms. As has been explained, a nourishing and varied diet in the early stages of the disease will often restore the patient to health.

CHAPTER X.

Class I.—EXUDATIONES—*continued.*

2. *PAPULAR GROUP.*

Lichen simplex, ruber, planus, marginatus, scrofulosorum—Prurigo
—Prurigo Infantum—Relapsing Prurigo.

LICHEN.

UNDER the title of lichen a considerable number of diseases have been described, many of them presenting appearances which differ very widely from each other. Willan
includes not only those conditions which will shortly be
described, but others which differ in their course as well as
in their appearance; thus "Lichen pilaris" of Willan is
more fitly described as a disease of the hair follicles, and is
apparently the disease which Devergie called Pityriasis
pilaris, while the Lichen agrius and Lichen tropicus of
Willan are believed by Hebra to be varieties of eczema.
Hebra, indeed, objects to Willan's Lichen simplex, on the
ground that it is an acute disease of the skin, but in the
following account L. simplex will be retained for the reason
that, with this exception, its appearance and course are such
as necessitate its association with the other forms which are
accepted by Hebra as true lichens. We shall therefore
limit ourselves to describing three forms,—L. simplex, L.
ruber of Hebra or L. planus of Wilson, and L. marginatus,
including scrofulosorum.

Definition.—Lichen may be defined as a papular disease
of the skin, with more or less local irritation.

LICHEN SIMPLEX.

Lichen simplex is characterized by a group of minute papules, that appear more frequently on the back of the neck and upper extremities, but often on other parts of the body. The papules are acuminated and of a red color, and last a variable time, usually about five or six days. They gradually disappear, and are followed by trifling desquamation. Occasionally slight signs of constitutional disturbance accompany the local symptoms, such as feverishness and headache. Locally an itching or tingling sensation is present at the site of the eruption.

LICHEN RUBER (*Hebra*), LICHEN PLANUS (*Wilson*), LICHEN PSORIASIS (*Hutchinson*).

Lichen ruber of Hebra is comparatively rare in this country. Hebra describes it as "an eruption of miliary papules which are at first distinct from one another, and covered with thin scales." The papules remain the same size during the whole course of the disease. Successive crops of the eruption appear, and thus the papules become aggregated together; eventually they are so closely placed that they come in contact with each other, and in this way are formed "continuous patches of variable size and shape, red, infiltrated, and covered with scales." As the disease progresses the patches extend over different parts of the body, the skin becomes greatly thickened, and when this condition .exists over joints their movement is interfered with. Frequently in the folds of the skin over the joints of the fingers fissures occur and extend into the corium, becoming filled with black crusts of blood. The natural lines and wrinkles about the face disappear, the nails become either greatly thickened, brittle, and of a yellowish-brown, or thin and of a light color. The hair of the head, pubes, and axillæ is never affected. This variety itches but little.

Under the names of Lichen planus and Lichen psoriasis Wilson and Hutchinson describe diseases which are probably the same as the Lichen ruber of Hebra. Mr. Hutchinson, in his "Lectures on Clinical Surgery," 1879, says: "Under slightly different names Hebra and Wilson have independently described this disease, and have agreed most closely as to all its main features."

This disease usually presents itself in the form of patches of a round or oval shape, or running in lines, and consists of an aggregation of small round flat-topped papules, some of which may have a minute central depression, which is the opening of a hair follicle. In the earlier stages of the disease the papules are more scattered, but as the eruption develops they increase in number, and have a tendency to become confluent, often forming patches resembling common psoriasis; this, however, never results from the increase in size of the individual papules. The papules are of a livid red, or violet tint, and each is covered with a small thin scale. Often the eruption has at first sight an appearance like herpes, which on closer observation is found to be due to the shiny character of the scales. The patches never are moist, and have no tendency to become ezcematous; but they are aggravated by such forms of local irritation as tight garters. The rash is usually symmetrical, is first noticed on the limbs, but subsequently extends to the trunk, and in many cases attacks the tongue. It is occasionally accompanied by scaliness of the palms and soles. Itching is nearly always a constant symptom, and when present is very severe. The pruriginous condition resulting from the scratching often changes the character of the eruption. A tendency to constant relapses characterizes this variety, and a history of previous attacks is often an important aid to diagnosis. Persons affected with this dis-

ease are generally about forty years of age, and are very
rarely under twenty. As a rule there is little or no constitutional disturbance, but the general health may suffer
as a result of repeated attacks.   •

Lichen Scrofulosorum, Lichen Circumscriptus, Lichen Marginatus.

Although Hebra describes under the name of L. scrofulosorum a variety of lichen which he believes to occur
only in scrofulous subjects, there is reason to doubt whether
the limitation thus indicated is altogether advisable; at all
events, in this country we are accustomed to see cases which
answer generally to this description, occurring also in others
than scrofulous persons, and differing in certain characteristics to be mentioned hereafter.

In Hebra's variety all the papules appear about the same
time in groups; they may vary greatly in color, from that
of the normal skin to a deep brownish-red. The shape of
the groups is usually circular. The papules undergo no
change, and are attended by but little local irritation. The
eruption differs in its site from the other forms of lichen in
being usually confined to the trunk and seldom attacking
the limbs.

The English forms of Lichen scrofulosorum,—viz., L. circumscriptus and L. marginatus,—occur, as has already been
pointed out, in persons who cannot be called scrofulous.
The papules are grouped together in rings or patches, and
a tendency to the former is very common. On the outer
side of the rings the skin is normal, but within the circle
is often slightly yellow, whilst the papules themselves are
usually red. The eruption grows by extension of the rings,
which as they increase in size meet other rings, and the papules disappearing at the point of contact, the so-called gyrate variety is produced. As the papules fade the skin is

left stained with pigment. The usual site of this form of lichen is the back and chest. Some amount of itching is always present, which is aggravated by flannel vests.

Diagnosis.—The lichenous eruptions have to be distinguished from each other, from psoriasis, eczema, pityriasis rubra, tinea tonsurans, and pityriasis versicolor.

In the early stage it must be noticed that while lichen ruber begins with the development of red papules, which are scattered on any part of the body, but usually on the limbs, and are surmounted by small scales, the papules of lichen marginatus are of a lighter color, are collected together in groups or rings, and appear more frequently on the trunk. Psoriasis begins with the formation of minute papules covered with white shining scales, situated mostly on the extensor surfaces of the limbs, and not aggregated together. Eczema begins with an eruption of small papules and vesicles, the latter containing clear fluid. The papules are never scaly, and are scattered irregularly, usually on the flexor surfaces of the limbs.

Later lichen ruber appears as red patches, consisting of aggregated papules, covered with thin scales. The patches never become moist. In lichen scrofulosorum and marginatus the papules appear in groups, that fade in the centre. In the more advanced stage of psoriasis large patches are formed by the coalescence of the original small spots through growth at their periphery ; they are all covered with white glistening, transparent scales, and in eczema the oozing from the surface gives rise to crusts, which are a most important diagnostic sign.

Pityriasis rubra at this stage can be diagnosed by the absence of infiltration, and by the fact that it extends uniformly over the greater part of the surface of the body. In the most advanced stage the eruption of lichen ruber consists of red patches covered with thin scales, the individual papules having disappeared. The skin is thickened,

12

and the nails are affected. Lichen scrofulosorum never attacks the whole surface in the same manner as lichen ruber, and patches or rings rarely become scaly.

In the most advanced stage psoriasis can be distinguished from lichen ruber by the smaller amount of surface affected, and by the fact that healthy skin intervenes between the patches ; from lichen marginatus it can be easily diagnosed by the tendency of the rash in the latter to form rings with simply stained skin in the centre. Old-standing eczema can always be recognized by the crusts.

The eruption of pityriasis rubra can only be confounded with that of lichen ruber in the late stage, and can be distinguished from it by the absence of infiltration of the skin and severe constitutional symptoms of the former.

Lichen marginatus may be mistaken for ringworm of the body, but a microscopic examination of some of the epidermis will at once settle the doubt; the same disease may also bear some resemblance to pityriasis versicolor, but this can only occur when the rash is fading, and can be easily distinguished in the same way.

Prognosis.—There is comparatively little danger attending the lichenous diseases seen in this country, although some of them are very intractable, and last a long time on account of frequent relapses.

Morbid Anatomy—Lichen Ruber.—On examining vertical sections of skin affected with lichen ruber, the epidermis is seen to be thickened and dried, especially on the hands and feet, but thin and scaly on other parts. The corium is also thickened and denser than normal, if the case is of old standing. The hyperæmia seen in life disappears after death. Under the microscope thin sections of the papules when first formed show merely enlargement of the root sheath at the base of the hair follicle, with numerous nodular outgrowths from it into the corium. Later the upper part of the root sheath may become enlarged, being, according to Hebra, pointed towards the hair follicle and expanded above, forming a series of concentric funnel-shaped envelopes round the hair. In the fully developed papules changes are found in other portions of the skin. The epidermis is thickened, and the rete·Malpighii contains small round cells. The papillæ are enlarged, contain more round cells than normal, and have their fibrous tissue increased. The vessels in the papillary body and corium are enlarged and surrounded by small round cells. The root sheaths of the hair are thickened, as described above, and the arrectores pili are usually hypertrophied. The sebaceous and sweat glands do not seem to be primarily affected, but undergo degenerative changes as the disease progresses.

Lichen Scrofulosorum.—On examining thin sections of the small papules at an early stage, the tissue round the vessels of the sebaceous and hair follicles affected is found to contain numerous leucocytes. This infiltration gradually extends upwards, and in the fully developed papules not only the follicular wall but the papillæ round the orifice of the hair follicle are filled with small round cells. In the later stages the exudation invades the hair follicle and sebaceous glands, and masses of cells are found between the root sheath and the follicular wall, in the substance of the root sheath itself, and in the rete Malpighii around the orifice of the follicle.

Treatment.—The treatment of lichen must be both local and constitutional. With regard to the former, the chief aim must be to allay the irritation, so as to afford rest, to remove all sources of irritation, such as flannel, and to apply soothing lotions and ointments composed of such drugs as hydrocyanic acid and weak preparations of tar. It is also necessary to pay great attention to cleanliness. In lichen scrofulosorum the local application of cod-liver oil is stated by Hebra to be of great value, but in applying this remedy care should be taken to keep it in constant contact

with the skin.   As regards internal remedies for lichen ruber or planus, there are no drugs so valuable as the various
preparations of arsenic, but to produce any good result they
must be taken in full doses and continued for a long period.
It must be borne in mind that the use of this remedy must
not be abandoned during the intervals of apparent cure, but
must be continued with a view to prevent a relapse.   If
there is any proof of a scrofulous habit, cod-liver oil and
iron must be given.

Prurigo.

Definition.—Prurigo is a chronic papular disease of the
skin, accompanied by intense irritation.

Symptoms.—The severe form of this disease described by
Hebra as seen on the Continent is happily very rare in this
country, only one or two cases having been reported.

The milder conditions known in England are prurigo
mitis, occurring among children, and the relapsing prurigo
of Hutchinson.   Inasmuch as the prurigo of Hebra has
many peculiarities in which it differs from the disease we
understand by the same name, a short *résumé* of Hebra's
description will therefore first be noticed.

Prurigo of Hebra.—The eruption first appears in the
shape of subepidermic papules of the size of hemp seeds;
they are but slightly elevated above the surface, of the same
color as normal skin, and are recognized more by the touch
than the sight.   They are always isolated, and may come
out on all parts of the body, but, however severe, leave intervals of healthy skin.   They are attended by intense itching, which causes the patient to scratch, giving rise to excoriations of the surface and the formation of small blood
crusts on their summits.   After this has lasted for some
time the whole of the skin affected becomes hard, brawny,
and darker in color, owing to the deposit of pigment.   As
the disease progresses the normal furrows of the skin are

seen to become deeper and farther apart; this is especially observable on the backs of the hands, the fingers, and the wrists. To the more severe form, which lasts the whole of life, the name of prurigo ferox is given. The parts most frequently attacked are the front and back of the chest, the whole of the back, loins, abdomen, and particularly the extensor surfaces of the limbs. The rash is less commonly present on the arms and thighs than on the forearms and legs, and on the whole more often attacks the lower than the upper extremities. Even in the most severe forms the flexor surfaces of the joints, the genitals, scalp, and face escape. Frequently eczema is produced as the result of the irritation, and in consequence the lymphatic glands become enlarged. Although the disease is never absolutely cured, at times the symptoms are so mitigated that it appears to have disappeared. Weather apparently has some effect on its intensity, for it is always more severe in cold than in warm seasons. Prurigo is not congenital, but nearly always commences soon after birth.

Prurigo Mitis.—Prurigo, as we understand it, is, as compared with the above disease, a simple malady. Although the objective symptoms in both varieties resemble each other, the English disease does not run such a protracted course as the German, and is in fact limited almost entirely to early life. The delicate skin of infants is usually in the first instance irritated by some local cause, such as flannel or the bites of parasites; as a result a papular eruption, together with some amount of urticaria, is developed, chiefly on the back and the extensor surfaces of the limbs. This is accompanied by severe itching, and when the child is old enough to scratch blood crusts are formed, which constitute an important characteristic of the disease. On passing the hand over the back the whole skin feels rough like a nutmeg grater.

Prurigo mitis usually occurs in delicate and badly-nour-

ished children, and is certainly more common among the
poor, probably owing to their being more exposed to the
causes above mentioned. The disease does not usually last
longer than a few years, and is rarely seen in persons above
the age of ten years.

Mr. Hutchinson has recently paid considerable attention
to the prurigo of infants, and has made several important
and interesting observations on its causation. He points
out that there is considerable difference in the appearances
of the ordinary eruption, which depends on the size of the
papules and the amount of urticaria accompanying them,
in some cases the papules being "hard, rough, and dry, like
a nutmeg grater, while in other cases they are of larger
size, like half-developed wheals of urticaria, with perhaps
even some tendency to vesication," and that there are besides two other distinct varieties to be distinguished. In
one of these positive vesication takes place, and the palms
and soles are affected. The history of the case leads to the
belief that the child has in the first instance suffered from
varicella. He states that it is not uncommon to find that
the skin eruption commenced with a sudden outbreak of
disease, which rapidly changed its character, and that, inasmuch as abortive varicella undoubtedly occurs, the first
outbreak was probably due to this disease, which was not
then recognized.

The ordinary prurigo eruption begins more gradually
and varies in severity, being better in winter and worse in
summer, and is due to the irritation produced by fleas or
other parasites, which are more abundant in the warm than
in the cold weather.

A pruriginous condition of skin may, however, also be
induced by varicella or vaccination, which is not developed
until the skin is subsequently irritated by fleabites or some
other local cause.

Prurigo may therefore be produced in one of three ways:

1st. By the local irritation of fleas, or by wearing flannel, etc.

2d. By these local causes acting on a skin which has been previously made susceptible to their influence by a previous attack of varicella or vaccination.

3d. By the direct irritation of varicella itself without the intervention of any other exciting cause.

Relapsing Prurigo.—This disease, first described by Hutchinson, differs from the other forms of prurigo,—first in the age at which it occurs, having a tendency to commence about puberty; and secondly, in the color of the papules, which are in this variety red. Together with the papular rash, which attacks most frequently the face, neck, and upper extremities, there is often an erythematous blush. Sometimes the rash leaves scars. Relapsing prurigo is attended with less itching than is the case in the other varieties, and does not produce the same hardness of skin as in Hebra's prurigo; its distribution is the same as in the latter, inasmuch as it never attacks the palms, soles, genitals, or flexures of the joints.

Diagnosis.—Prurigo may under some circumstances be mistaken for scabies, phthiriasis, eczema, urticaria, pruritus, and erythema.

From scabies it may be distinguished by the different sites of the two diseases. The presence of the rash on the genitals and on the flexures of the joints will serve to eliminate prurigo. If a burrow can be discovered and the acarus produced, the diagnosis is of course easily settled; besides, pustules and constant itching are points in favor of scabies.

From pediculosis it may be diagnosed by the absence of pediculi.

From eczema it is often difficult to distinguish it, especially when the two diseases are combined. The character

of the skin near the eruption assists the diagnosis, the reddening which accompanies eczema being entirely absent in
prurigo. The scattered eruption, the blood crusts, and the
tendency of the papules to bleed in prurigo are points of
difference from eczema.

From urticaria and pruritus it can be recognized by the
absence of papules in these two diseases.

From erythema (see Chapter IX, p. 120).

Prognosis.—The prognosis of Hebra's variety is unfavorable, and although the patient may live for years, his life
is made utterly miserable by the intense itching. The prurigo of infants, due to a local cause, is curable when the
cause is removed, but the duration of the disease is often
protracted. The relapsing prurigo of Hutchinson is always
a most obstinate form, lasting, in consequence of so many
relapses, for years.

Morbid Anatomy. — On microscopic examination the
changes found in Hebra's variety are described as follows:

The epidermis is thickened considerably, especially in the
rete Malpighii, where numerous small round cells are found.
The papillary layer shows the papillæ enlarged, full of
young cells, and their vascular loops dilated. Leucocytes
are also found pretty freely scattered in the hair papilla and
also the root sheath, and in the corium around the follicle.
In chronic cases spindle-shaped cells are found in the
corium, and especially round the vessels.

Treatment. Beyond attempting to alleviate the patient's
condition by attending to his general health and procuring
sleep, nothing can be done to cure the variety described by
Hebra. Since prurigo of children is often due to a local
cause, this must be sought for and carefully removed;
children, as a rule, outgrow prurigo, but considerable relief
can be obtained from the use of tar baths, consisting of two
or three or more teaspoonfuls of liquor carbonis detergens

to a gallon of warm water. In such a bath the child should
be kept for at least half an hour twice a day, and in the
interval should be well anointed with a soothing ointment.
For cachectic or strumous children cod-liver oil and steel
wine should be prescribed. In the relapsing variety arsenic
is of value.

CHAPTER XI.

Class I.—Exudationes—*continued.*

3. *VESICULAR AND BULLOUS GROUP.*

Herpes febrilis, gestationis, iris—Hydroa—Pemphigus vulgaris, foliaceus.

HERPES.

Definition.—Herpes is an acute vesicular disease of the skin, which runs a rapid course and is accompanied by local irritation and sometimes by symptoms of constitutional disturbance.

Of the many varieties usually mentioned under this title only three are important enough to need special description : herpes febrilis, herpes gestationis, and herpes iris.

Symptoms.—*Herpes febrilis* may be described as a neurotic disease, and commonly occurs as a symptom of catarrh or of pneumonia, but may be due to any condition producing a rigor, such as the passing of a catheter. Whatever may be its cause, it always appears to be produced through the influence of the nervous system, and in all its forms the temperature is slightly increased, and the patient complains of headache and *malaise.* The eruption often precedes any constitutional symptom, and may occur on almost any part of the body, but its most common sites are the lips, tonsils, uvula, mucous membrane of the mouth, palate, and more rarely the face, ears, and tongue.

The eruption appears in groups, and lasts about seven or eight days. It consists of small papules, which become vesicular and which contain a clear fluid. After lasting two or three days this fluid becomes turbid, and is generally absorbed, though in some instances the vesicle bursts and crusts are formed. The vesicles themselves are situated on inflamed bases, and an itching or burning sensation always accompanies, and sometimes precedes by a few hours, the appearance of the eruption.

When herpes occurs on the lips, the vesicles are few in number, and rapidly coalesce and dry up into scabs, but when it appears on the mucous membrane of the mouth, they soon burst and leave a superficial ulceration. Again, when the vesicles form on the tonsils, uvula, or soft palate they also burst, but leave white patches on the mucous membrane, which are liable to be mistaken for diphtheria and this mistake is rendered more probable by a swelling of the tonsils, which is occasionally seen at the same time. Although this disease usually occurs in isolated cases a whole family is sometimes found to be attacked by it.

As a sub-variety of herpes febrilis may be mentioned herpes progenitalis, in which the vesicles are developed on the prepuce, glans, or dorsum of the penis in the male and on the labia or mons veneris in the female. The vesicles are generally few in number and form small clusters, last but a short time and then drop off leaving healthy skin; when, however, the vesicles are broken by scratching, small superficial ulcers result, which, as a rule, speedily heal and, further, it must be noticed that when there is some induration of the part, it is difficult to distinguish the herpetic ulcer from the syphilitic chancre. Frequently, also there is some amount of swelling, and the appearance of the eruption is often preceded by pain.

Herpes gestationis occurs in pregnant and puerperal women, but is rarely seen in England. It was first described by Bulkley and Bulkley. It is not always vesicular, but consists of papules ...

sizes, from a pea to a bean, which appear in groups over
the body, chiefly on the extremities. The eruption is preceded by and accompanied with severe itching, which continues after its disappearance, and by slight symptoms of
constitutional disturbance and considerable pains in the
limbs. Pigmentation is often left after the eruption disappears. This variety lasts some weeks, and is often prolonged
by relapses.

Herpes iris, described by Willan as a separate variety, is
characterized by the arrangement of the vesicles in rings
round a single vesicle, and two or even three rings may be
seen outside each other. They do not make their appearance simultaneously, but in successive circles, and those
vesicles nearest the centre often subside during the growth
of fresh vesicles at the periphery. It must not, however, be
expected in herpes iris that all the vesicles are to be found
arranged in this orbicular manner; it is sufficient to characterize the disease if some only are arranged in rings, whilst
others appear in irregular crops; and it must be noticed
also that, though they are usually discrete, they may coalesce and form bullæ. The disease itself lasts a variable
time, usually from one to four weeks, according to the number of rings formed, and is not accompanied by any constitutional symptoms. Hebra points out the tendency of
herpes and erythema to behave in a similar manner in producing multiform varieties, and that herpes circinatus results from herpes iris in the same way that erythema iris
results from erythema annulare. The erythematous and
herpetic rashes select the same sites, for they both occur
most frequently on the backs of the hands and feet, at times
on the limbs, in some instances as high as the arms or thighs,
but hardly ever on the trunk. Hebra, indeed, goes so far
as to say that, taking into consideration the similarity of
the mode of development, the course and the seat of the two

diseases, he is tempted to regard them as modifications of one and the same disease.

Diagnosis.—Herpes is not likely to be mistaken for any other disease, for the vesicles are larger than in eczema, and do not spread from the periphery, and are smaller than in pemphigus. The inflamed bases on which the vesicles are seated, the rapid course of the disease, and the sense of irritation which accompanies it, are sufficiently marked characteristics to prevent mistakes.

Prognosis.—The prognosis is always favorable, although the disease is occasionally protracted in the ringed variety.

Morbid Anatomy.—The morbid appearances are identical with those found in pemphigus, and are therefore included in the description of the latter disease.

Treatment.—No local or constitutional treatment is known to affect the course of the disease.

HYDROA.

Definition.—In addition to these varieties of herpes, some mention must be made of a rare disease of a kindred nature, termed hydroa by Bazin, who divides it into vesicular hydroa, vacciniform hydroa, and bullous hydroa. It is defined as a chronic disease of the skin, occurring in arthritic subjects, and characterized by groups of vesicles or bullæ.

Symptoms.—Vesicular hydroa first appears as small, round, deep-red spots, with well-defined edges, varying in size from a lentil to a threepenny piece, and sometimes surrounded by a rose-colored area. The next day a vesicle forms in the centre of the spot, filled with a transparent yellow fluid, which in a day or two is absorbed from the centre, when the vesicle itself becomes a black scab.

Sometimes, especially during the cold weather, the fluid in the vesicle is so rapidly absorbed that there is only to be seen a white or yellow macula, formed by loose epidermis

round, but may lose their shape by becoming confluent.
The fluid in the bullæ is at first clear and alkaline, but in
a short time becomes turbid and acid. A bulla may terminate by absorption of its fluid, when nothing but the
dried-up cuticle remains, or it may burst, when it leaves
an ulcerated surface, more or less covered with crusts. A
dark stain remains for some time to mark the site of a
bulla, and as the disease has a tendency to appear in successive crops, the skin gradually becomes more and more
stained. The bullæ may be scattered irregularly over the
body, or may be grouped together in circles or semicircles,
from the circumference of which fresh bullæ grow at the
same time as those in the centre disappear. In other but
rare cases red patches of skin are found, in which the bullæ
are badly defined or even absent. All parts of the surface
may be attacked with pemphigus, even the vagina and the
rectum, but the head, palms, and soles are almost always
exempt. At the conclusion of the disease the skin becomes
dry, and desquamation, often over a larger area than the
actual site of the eruption, takes place. As a rule constitutional symptoms are not severe, depending solely on the
amount of the eruption, but when the bullæ are of large
size, and crops rapidly succeed each other, the itching becomes intolerable.

Pemphigus foliaceus differs from the preceding variety in
color, situation, and character of the blebs. The bullæ are
of a red or yellow tint, and the vessels of the base can be
seen through the fluid, which in this variety is small in
quantity and does not distend the bulla. Around the first-
formed bullæ others are developed, which eventually coalesce, while the fluid escapes and leaves crusts, the appearance of which is compared by Cazenave to that of flaky
pie-crust. Although this condition is at first limited in area,
it gradually spreads over the surface; and as there is no
disposition for the part originally attacked to heal, a large

attached to the roof and floor of the vesicle. The fluid in pemphigus consists at first of clear serum, in which numerous pale and only a few red corpuscles are found, but as the leucocytes soon undergo fatty degeneration, the contents assume an opalescent and then a more purulent appearance. Occasionally a large mixture of red corpuscles gives the serum a distinct sanguineous character.

Treatment.—This consists in improving the general condition, while local applications appear to exercise no influence on the course of the disease. A generous and nourishing diet is necessary, and for medicine arsenic in full and repeated doses is as important as quinine is in ague. Much relief also is afforded by frequent bathing, removing the crusts, and keeping the ulcers clean.

Little, however, can be done in pemphigus foliaceus but to combat the symptoms as they arise.

CHAPTER XII.

*Class I.—*EXUDATIONES—*continued.*

4. *ECZEMATOUS AND PUSTULAR GROUP.*

Eczema simplex, Acute: Eczema erythematosum, squamosum, papulatum, vesiculosum, pustulosum, fissum seu rimosum, rubrum—Ecthyma, Chronic: Eczema capillitii, faciei, articulorum, manuum et pedum, crurale, genitale, corporis—Intertrigo—Porrigo or Impetigo contagiosa.

ECZEMA—MOIST TETTER.

Definition.—Eczema is an acute inflammatory disease of the skin, characterized by an erythematous papulo-vesicular or pustular eruption, which usually gives rise to a moist, reddened surface, and from which a serous discharge that stiffens linen exudes freely. In the latter stages it takes the form of a dull-red or brownish surface covered with scales. A sensation of burning or marked itching accompanies it.

Symptoms.—The eruption may present various appearances, as the disease, instead of going through the typical course above indicated, may stop short at any one of the stages mentioned, or may pass over or abbreviate some of them and then remain stationary. In this way, instead of the red, excoriated, weeping surface most commonly seen, a condition which is almost entirely erythematous, papular, vesicular, pustular, or squamous, may be met with, and, according as one or other condition is most prominent, several varieties have been described.

Various secondary changes may affect the portion of skin

suffering from eczema. Infiltration of the cutis and sub-cutaneous tissue, cracks and fissures, abundant pus formation, superficial ulceration, and the production of scabs are some of the phenomena most frequently met with. Scratching, in consequence of the intense itching, often excites a renewed attack, and contributes materially to the extension and persistence of the eruption. Eczema may occur without any obvious cause in persons otherwise healthy; it may be excited by various local irritants, chemical, mechanical, thermal, etc.; it may affect those who are gouty, syphilitic, or strumous, and in some instances it may be hereditary.

Digestive, uterine, and nervous disorders may predispose to or aggravate an attack of eczema, and should be taken into account in the treatment.

According to its course and duration, eczema may be divided into the *acute* and the *chronic* type, the latter being far the most commonly met with; but local varieties, differing in appearance according to their site, require special description. Eczema occurs in males more frequently than in females; of 6798 cases recorded by Hebra, McCall Anderson, and others, 4467 were males, and only 2331 females.

Acute eczema is characterized by the occurrence of inflammatory redness and swelling of the skin, followed usually within forty-eight hours by the eruption of numerous minute vesicles containing clear yellowish serum, and accompanied with a sensation of burning and tension. Within a week the vesicles either dry up and desquamate or burst, leaving red oozing points, or rapidly become pustular, giving rise, from desiccation, to thin brownish or yellow crusts, which in separating leave a reddish scaly surface, that itches slightly. A feeling of chilliness or slight pyrexia is usually the only constitutional symptom, and within a fortnight the whole eruption may disappear. More frequently, however, fresh crops are seen, either round the first or on different parts of the body, attended by severe itching, which causes violent scratching and produces excoriations. Successive acute attacks may thus prolong the disease, or it may pass into a chronic form.

According to situation, the appearances vary somewhat. On the face the redness and œdema of the skin are well marked, and may resemble erysipelas; the surface is, however, irregular and granulated, not uniformly smooth and shiny, as in the latter, and the disease is very prone to relapse and become chronic. On the hands and feet the eruption appears as a collection of smally watery vesicles, with swelling and little or no redness at first, but they soon coalesce, and later on dry up; pain and tension are severe if the disease is extensive, but give place to itching as the eruption subsides. On the genitals swelling and redness form the main phenomena, the vesicles being usually small. Hebra states that in the male, while the penis remains dry and the vesicles rarely exceed a pin's point in size, on the scrotum they are larger, and on bursting give rise to an abundant discharge.

Repeated attacks usually cause the disease to become chronic

Universal acute eczema is a rare variety, attended, according to Hebra, with but little constitutional disturbance besides a feeling of great chilliness. Different appearances are presented by the eruption, according to its site. On the face it produces the changes already described, on the trunk it resembles scarlatina which is beginning to desquamate, on the flexures of the limbs vesicles and raw weeping surfaces are more common, while on the scalp the abundant scabs which are produced by the secretion from the vesicles, and retained by the hair, form a foul-smelling, offensive-looking mass.

Chronic eczema presents appearances of the same nature as those met with in the acute disease,—viz., papules, vesicles, pustules, crusts, and extensive red, moist, and weeping, or dry scaly surfaces.

The frequent relapses and the persistence of the disease cause a more abundant serous discharge, and the prolonged infiltration of the skin often gives rise to hypertrophy of the papillary body, with sclerosis of the cutis and subdermic tissues.

According as one or other lesion predominates, we may have *eczema erythematosum*, with simple inflammatory redness of the skin, followed by desquamation; *eczema squamosum* (often described as pityriasis rubra), with abundant formation of scabs on a reddened, infiltrated basis, with little or no discharge; *eczema populosum* (frequently termed lichen eczematodes, etc.), with an eruption of small red aggregated papules; *eczema vesiculosum*, the vesicles being either small and rapidly bursting, or larger and by confluence forming bullæ where the skin is thick and dense, as on the hands and feet; *eczema pustulosum*, where, either from the beginning or soon after their appearance, the vesicles become pustular, and, drying up, give rise to brownish, yellowish, or black crusts, conditions which have been raised to the rank of a new and separate disease under the name of impetigo contagiosa; *eczema fissum seu rimosum*, where numerous cracks of varying depth in an erythematous dry or moist surface occur in places where the skin is normally thrown into folds; and *eczema rubrum*, where the red, infiltrated, excoriated surface, usually discharging profusely, is well developed. This last form is accompanied by severe burning heat, and later on by intense itching; constitutional symptoms—fever, headache, and digestive derangement—are well marked, and the surface presents numerous bright-red points of hyperæmia, from which fluid keeps continually exuding, like the drops of water on the surface of salt butter (Hutchinson). The disease described as *ecthyma* consists of an eruption of large flattened pustules on a red,

indurated, slightly raised base, giving rise frequently to
dark-brown, dense crusts, and unhealthy, sloughy ulcers ; it
is merely a form of pustular eczema occurring in debilitated
cachectic persons living under bad hygienic conditions.

Of the local varieties of chronic eczema the following
will now be described :

1. Eczema capillitii.
2. Eczema faciei.
3. Eczema articulorum.
4. Eczema manuum et pedum.
5. Eczema crurale.
6. Eczema genitale.
7. Eczema corporis.

1. *Eczema Capillitii.*—In eczema of the scalp, owing to the
presence of the hair, which becomes glued together by the
sero-purulent discharge, a dense matted crust may be produced if the disease is left to run its course unchecked, until
the entire scalp is affected. Pus, mingled with sebaceous secretion from the numerous glands, forms beneath the crusts,
and pediculi, their ova, and even maggots may find a rest-
ing-place in the filthy, stinking mass. When occurring in
discrete spots and in clean people the discharge and crusts
are constantly removed, and the disease is easily recognized.

In the later stages, when the crusts have separated and
the discharge is less in quantity, a red, infiltrated surface
covered with numerous scales adherent to the hairs is seen.

This variety is usually pustular, occurs most often in
children, and may persist for years if neglected. Subcutaneous abscesses and glandular enlargements are not unfrequently met with, especially in strumous children. In
chronic cases there is some loss of hair, speedily renewed,
however, when the disease is cured, except in neglected cases
where profuse suppuration under the scabs has destroyed
the hair follicles.

2. *Eczema Faciei.*—Eczema of the face, when it affects the hairy parts, resembles the former variety in the liability to the production of shallow pustules with a hair passing through them, which dry up and form yellow, greenish, or brown crusts. On removal they leave a red, moist, or scaly surface. In chronic cases the hair follicles become more deeply involved, as in sycosis; the skin is dusky red and thickened, and permanent alopecia is apt to follow, from the destruction of the hair bulbs. Pain and burning heat, with later on some itching, accompany the eruption.

Eczema of the eyelashes, or tinea tarsi, frequently confounded with inflammation of the Meibomian glands, is merely a local eczema implicating the hair follicles and glands, and is always accompanied by itching. Redness, swelling, and excoriations, and scabbing of the margins of the lids, with partial or complete loss of the eyelashes, may be produced by it.

Eczema of the nostrils usually terminates in the formation of a thick scab, which felts together the margins and blocks up the orifice. The continual pus formation under it causes often an erysipelatous swelling of the mucous membrane or skin of the nose.

On the smooth parts of the face eczema is usually symmetrical, unless produced by purely local causes.

Eczema of the ears may occur merely as a moist fissure at the reflection of the auricle from the mastoid process, or as a weeping or crusted red surface at the back of the auricle, on the lobule, or elsewhere. The skin is prone to excessive swelling and discharge, which either drips away constantly or dries up, forming stalactiform crusts. Hearing, always somewhat impaired, is made much worse when the meatus is affected and blocked up more or less completely by crusts and ceruminous discharge.

Eczema of the lips may present either a red, scaly, infiltrated or a moist surface. There is often marked œdema, with painful fissures or large yellow crusts.

On the cheeks and forehead large yellow crusts, looking like dried honey,—which gained for the disease in this site the names of crusta lactea and melitagra flavescens,—are most commonly seen.

3. *Eczema articulorum* occurs on the flexor surfaces of the limbs, and leads to slight contraction, with great pain on moving the subjacent joint. The skin, red, much infiltrated, and oozing or crusted, is traversed by numerous fissures, following the lines of the normal folds of skin, causing the application of the name eczema fendillé. Eczema rubrum occurs most frequently in these situations.

4. *Eczema Manuum et Pedum.*—The fissured variety of eczema is here most common, especially on the palms and soles, where the skin presents a dry, inelastic, thickened appearance, itches considerably, and is traversed by numerous deep, painful fissures. The vesicular form, with large blebs, pustules, crusts, or moist surfaces, may also occur. Local irritants—water, sugar, lime, soda, soap, dyes, etc.—are the most common causes of eczema restricted to the hands or feet ; hence the so-called " grocer's itch," " baker's itch," etc., are merely local varieties of eczema.

5. *Eczema crurale* is often modified, and its typical features concealed, by conditions peculiar to its site, such as varicose veins, ulcers, scars, pigment patches, and œdema, leading to chronic dermatitis.

The disease hence arises sometimes around a varicose ulcer or scar, sometimes on a pigmented patch, and at others the œdema appears as if secondary to the skin affection ; but in all cases eczema, whether as simplex, rubrum, or squamosum, is easily recognized.

6. *Eczema genitale*, occurring in the chronic form, affects in the male the scrotum and penis either together or separately. On the penis it appears as raised red transverse

lines; on the dorsum it is most marked when the skin is stretched, with a moister red area on the under surface of the organ. Though itching is severe, and induces much scratching and excoriation, there is but little discharge. On the scrotum it may occur as an abraded red surface, comparatively free from infiltration, or as an irregular fissured or greatly hypertrophied elephantoid mass in inveterate cases, exuding an abundant sticky discharge, which, as it decomposes and dries up, becomes extremely offensive.

On the female genitals the disease affects the labia majora chiefly, and may extend to the nymphæ and vulva or to the adjacent parts of the thigh and abdomen, and takes usually the form of eczema rubrum. When affecting the mucous membrane it causes an abundant blennorrhagic discharge, resembling that of gonorrhœa, and there is usually much burning and itching. Appearing about the anus, it leads to the formation of painful itching fissures in the direction of the normal radiating folds of skin. There is often slight prolapsus ani, and the discharge is abundant and offensive.

7. *Eczema corporis*, presenting the general characters of the disease as described on p. 151, has some special peculiarities when it attacks the navel and nipples. The nipple and the adjacent areola are denuded of epidermis, red, swollen, moist, and painful; and crusts may form, under which either healing goes on or increased secretion, which oozes under or through the scab, and is accompanied by severe itching and pain. It may spread gradually to the surrounding skin, and is very obstinate; but, once cured, it leaves but little permanent damage behind.

On the umbilicus it takes either the ordinary form of eczema rubrum or impetiginosum, or that of an œdematous projecting red surface denuded of epidermis, and discharging freely or covered with a yellowish or greenish-brown scab.

Eczema intertrigo occurs in the axillæ, between the nates,

14

between the mammæ and chest, and in other places where folds of skin secrete much moisture and rub together, and appears as a moist, red, and tender surface, sometimes slightly excoriated.

The so-called *eczema marginatum*, formerly held to be a special variety of eczema, has now been shown to be merely one of the manifestations of ringworm of the body.

Diagnosis.—Eczema in one or other of its forms may sometimes be mistaken for the following diseases : erythema, erysipelas, lichen ruber, herpes febrilis, miliaria, scabies, pemphigus foliaceus, psoriasis, pityriasis rubra.

In *erythema* the smooth isolated spots which generally appear on the backs of the hands, the sharply defined edges, the absence usually of vesicles, discharge, and crusts, and the slightness of subjective symptoms, form a ready means of separation from eczema erythematosum or papulatum, which have a rough—often vesiculate—surface shading off into the surrounding skin.

Erysipelas is separated from acute eczema by the marked pyrexia, which begins usually with rigors, by the smooth surface with well-defined edge, and the rapid spreading of the patches, by the affection of the lymphatics, and the greater severity of the burning heat and pain. Erysipelas may, however, supervene on an attack of eczema.

Lichen ruber, which in aggregated patches may resemble eczema papulatum or squamosum, never becomes at any stage vesicular, and the isolated, flat-topped, shiny, solid papules that are found round the margin of the patch are quite characteristic.

Herpes febrilis, which occurs most commonly on the lips and prepuce, is distinguished from eczema of the same parts by the larger size and longer duration of the vesicles, and the absence of infiltration and itching. The vesicles dry up in a few days, and are not succeeded by fresh crops, as in eczema.

Miliaria differs from eczema in the fact that the vesicles occur in groups, usually on the abdomen and thorax, in the course of some febrile disorder. The eruption is of short duration, and is unattended by itching. In eczema, on the other hand, there is little or no constitutional disturbance, the vesicles are aggregated on a red base, there is marked itching, and the disease tends to become chronic.

In *scabies* the vesicles, pustules, and scabs which are produced by the irritation of the parasite, or the itching and scratching that it excites, are undistinguishable from those of eczema. Careful examination will usually show near the pustules the little dark lines of the burrows, with a terminal dilatation from which the acarus can often be extracted. The appearance of the disease on the hands and feet, wrists and abdomen, is also a suspicious circumstance.

Pemphigus foliaceus presents an appearance that is often difficult to distinguish from general eczema which discharges only slightly and is becoming scaly. The peculiar cachexia, the diarrhœa and marked weakness, and the pigmentation of the skin, together with the tendency of pemphigus foliaceus to begin on the front of the trunk, contrast markedly with the absence of cachexia and pigmentation, the itching and the tendency to infiltration and sclerosis of the skin, in eczema.

The condition known as eczema squamosum may sometimes be mistaken for *psoriasis*. The latter affects mainly the extensor surfaces instead of the flexors, as in eczema. The scales, thick, adherent, and silvery, are seated on abruptly defined, dark-red patches, while in eczema the scales are thin, loose, not silvery, and the bright-red patches merge more gradually into the adjacent skin. Psoriasis is dry throughout, while chronic eczema always discharges at one period of its existence.

Pityriasis rubra, regarded by some as merely a variety of eczema, differs, according to McCall Anderson, in the uniform redness and defined margin of the eruption, extending gradually to cover the whole surface, in the rapid exfoliation of large scales, in the burning heat and comparatively slight itching, and in the absence of any considerable infiltration, while the punctate appearance of the skin, the papules, vesicles, and crusts are quite wanting.

Eczema of the hands and feet may, by the confluence of several vesicles under the thick palmar cuticle, acquire bullæ, which resemble those of *pemphigus*. Small vesicles and a definite eczematous eruption are usually present in the neighborhood, and prevent the possibility of error.

Both *psoriasis* and a *tertiary squamous syphilide* affecting the palms and soles may be indistinguishable from eczema, and only the discovery of evidences of these diseases on other parts of the body can determine the diagnosis.

The diagnosis of the principal diseases of the scalp is given in the following table.

DIFFERENTIAL DIAGNOSIS BETWEEN ECZEMA CAPITIS AND SEBORRHŒA, PSORIASIS, VESICO-PUSTULAR SYPHILIDE, TINEA TONSURANS, AND FAVUS OF THE SCALP.

ECZEMA.	SEBORRHŒA.	PSORIASIS.	VESICO-PUSTULAR SYPHILIDE.	TINEA TONSURANS.	FAVUS.
1. Most frequent in children, in the debilitated or strumous.	1. Usually in adults.	1. Most often in healthy persons, rarely in strumous.	1. Usually in adults only.	1. Frequent in children.	1. No special proneness in strumous.
2. Often attacks the whole scalp. Ulcers, if any, superficial; crusts thick, yellowish, brittle; pus, epithelium, and granular matter. Seated on red, infiltrated, moist, often excoriated surface, which itches excessively.	2. Crusts are thin, oily, can be kneaded into masses; consist chiefly of sebum and epithelium on a smooth, only surface; nor, or only slightly, red, and non-excoriated or indistinct; itching only slight.	2. Eruption usually white, scaly, and silvery; dry from onset and throughout course; red base, only slightly infiltrated, and itching only slight.	2. In small patches usually; often deep ulcers with sloughy bases.	2. Patches usually circular, deficient in hair; crusts, etc., not necessarily present; itching slight.	2. Round, dry, sulphur yellow, cup-shaped crusts, penetrated by dull brittle hairs, with abrupt edges and often bald patches.
3. Syphilitic history and phenomena only accidental, if present at all.	3. Usually no specific phenomena.	3. Usually no specific history.	3. Usually a history of primary syphilis, and presence of alopecia, etc.		
4. Distinct eczema often on other parts of body, on flexor surfaces or behind the ears.	4. Usually only slight, oily crusting on face near scalp.	4. Well-marked scaly patches, usually present on extensor surfaces of elbows and knees.	4. Syphilides, squamous, pustular, tubercular, etc., with coppery color, usually present on body.	4. Ringworm of body (tinea circinata) often present.	4. Cupped yellow crusts may be found on hairy parts of the body.
5. Hair healthy, occasionally falling out; no parasite.	5. Hairs often drop out.	5. Hairs only slightly affected.	5. Hairs fall out freely, and incurable alopecia may result.	5. Hairs twisted, thickened, whitish, broken or short, easily extracted; filled with trichophyton tonsurans.	5. Hairs dull, dry, brittle, easily extracted, loaded with achorion Schönleinii.
6. Non-contagious.	6. Non-contagious.	6. Non-contagious.	6. Communicable by inoculation, which produces a hard chancre, followed by	6. Contagious.	6. Contagious.

Prognosis.—In itself the disease alone is never fatal. An ordinary attack of acute eczema runs through its various stages and subsides, leaving little or no trace within a week or ten days. Fresh crops of eruption arising near the original patch, or on distant parts of the body, may appear in succession, and prolong the disease for many weeks, verging gradually into the chronic form. The latter, with alternations, retrogressions, and relapses, may persist for months or even years.

Among the local varieties of chronic eczema the more limited the area of the patch the more obstinately does it persist in spite of treatment.

Morbid Anatomy.—Microscopic examination shows that the papular and vesicular stages are produced as follows : Abundant transudation of plasma and cells gives rise to an enlargement and elongation of the papillæ, which contain numerous leucocytes. Biesiadecki describes a numerous plexus of spindle-shaped cells between the ordinary rete elements which they inclose in their meshes. The cells of the stratum lucidum next enlarge and burst, and fluid collecting between the rete and horny layers produces a vesicle containing serum and leucocytes. The vascular plexuses of the papillary layer, and of the hair and gland follicles, are hyperæmic. In chronic cases there is more or less cell infiltration of the cutis, most dense around the vessels, which gradually extends down into the subcutaneous tissues, and, by the production of spindle cells and new-formed fibrous tissue around the fat cells and capillaries, causes a sclerosis of the skin resembling that met with in elephantiasis. The columnar rete cells contain brown pigment, and in the corium thin strands of pigment mark the sites of obliterated vessels.

Treatment.—In the constitutional treatment the main indications are—first, to remove or modify any condition which predisposes to the occurrence of the disease ; and, secondly, to give sufficient nutritious, easily digested food, and to forbid the use of stimulants.

Hence the action of the bowels must be regulated by occasional doses of the aperient mineral waters, such as Carlsbad or Hunyadi Janos. Gouty symptoms must be combated by colchicum and alkalies, and for strumous children cod-liver oil and iron is required.

In the acute forms antimony is of the greatest value, and, according to Dr. Cheadle, often does good when all other remedies fail. It should be given in doses of $\frac{1}{12}$ to $\frac{1}{6}$ of a grain two or three times a day. In the chronic forms arsenic, iron, quinine, and strychnine are of use as tonics, but none of them have any specific action on the disease.

In local treatment the indications are :

1. To use sedatives only, or mild unirritating applications during the acute stages, or in acute exacerbations of the chronic form.

2. To remove thoroughly all scales or scabs before applying local remedies.

In the stage of heat and tension dressing with simple cold soft water, or with a lead and opium lotion, is the best remedy to apply, but soap of all kinds should be avoided. Dusting powders of starch, oxide of zinc, or chalk may be tried. Crusts should be removed by softening them with oil or a bread-and-water poultice, and then scraping them off gently. After cleaning the part with oatmeal paste, or with simple water, the surface is ready for local applications. The best are *mild* solutions of tar or weak preparations of mercury; of the former the most convenient form is Wright's liquor carbonis detergens. It is an alcoholic solution of coal tar, and mixes well with water; ʒij to the eight ounces of water is the strength which should be used at first, and should be gradually increased if the lotion is nate cases Hebra recommends the thorough application of a strong potash solution as a last resource.

PORRIGO—IMPETIGO CONTAGIOSA.

Definition.—A local disease of the skin, communicable by inoculation, excited most commonly by accidental irritation, and characterized by an eruption of flat vesicles, which rapidly change into pustules and dry into yellow friable crusts.

Symptoms.—From scratching or from any accidental irritation of the skin there arises, usually on the face or head, but sometimes on the hands, an eruption of isolated small vesicles, which soon become pustular and then dry into yellow scabs. These scabs vary in size from a split pea to a shilling, and appear as if "stuck on," since there is no inflammatory areola around them. Dr. Tilbury Fox, who first distinguished the disease as a separate affection, states that the eruption is generally preceded by a slight pyrexia, and by *malaise* and sensations of chilliness; also that it is accompanied by severe itching, which is particularly troublesome at night.

On removing the scabs a reddened base secreting a gummy, purulent fluid, which does not stiffen linen like that of eczema, is seen, and as the disease abates the scabs fall off from the erythematous base and the red spots gradually fade.

When the head is affected the posterior cervical glands are apt to enlarge, and if the disease be neglected pediculi may be present among the scabs. The disease is spread from one part of the body to another, and from one person to another, by the direct inoculation of the pus.

Diagnosis.—The eruption of discrete vesicles, which soon become pustules and scabs, the absence of serous discharge and the presence of pus, the inoculability, the contagiousness and the slight pyrexia which precedes it, are the points which are supposed to separate porrigo from eczema.

Prognosis.—The disease runs an acute course, and usually lasts about a fortnight. It may be prolonged by successive eruptions, but is never dangerous to life.

Morbid Anatomy.—The conditions met with resemble those of eczema. Fungous elements have been found in the crusts, but not in the contents of the vesicles, so that they are probably accidental.

Treatment.—The removal of the scabs by oiling and poultices, and the subsequent application of a mild mercurial ointment, or a carbolic acid lotion (1 in 20), to destroy the infective character of the pus, are the remedies that are needed to effect a cure.

iasis rubra both in the reddening of the skin and the production of epithelial scales, but the former is limited to the face, and is attended with "enlargement of the mouths of the hair sacs and sebaceous glands, which are also plugged with masses of hardened sebum."

Prognosis.—The prognosis in this disease is very unfavorable, and the majority of cases terminate fatally.

Morbid Anatomy.—In early stages the microscopic examination shows little besides scaling of the horny layer, with moderate serous and cellular infiltration of the rete and of the papillary layer. In other cases there is marked atrophy of the whole skin, the rete and the papillary layer are atropied, the horny layer thin and scaly, the connective tissue fibres of the corium thickened, and elastic fibres more numerous. There is also considerable deposit of pigment, and the hair follicles, sweat and sebaceous glands are much wasted.

Treatment.—No treatment has been found of any material use in checking the course of this disease, but the employment of tepid baths and the application of oil and emollient ointments is recommended by Hebra.

Psoriasis Vulgaris.

Definition.—Psoriasis is a chronic disease of the skin, characterized by the production of white silvery scales on hyperæmic bases.

Symptoms.—The eruption begins with congestion of the papillæ of the skin, giving rise to an increased production of epidermic cells in the form of a quantity of minute elevations, which increase in size, and are separated from each other by healthy skin. When these are of the size of pins' heads, the name *psoriasis punctata* is given to the eruption; as they develop they have the appearance of drops of mortar, and it is then known as *psoriasis guttata;* a further in-

crease by growth of the periphery brings them to the size
of coins, when the rash is described as *psoriasis nummularis.*
While the patches first formed in this way develop in size,
others are continually beginning, until patches of all sizes
are to be seen. These patches of diseased skin have a tendency to heal in their centres, while extension takes place
at their margins, and as a result rings are formed, the cir-
cumferences of which vary in thickness according to the
size of the patches, since the healing process in the centre
takes place more rapidly than the growth at the margins.
To this variety the name of *psoriasis circinata* or *lepra* is
usually given. Frequently two rings come in contact with
each other at the edges, thus forming the figure 8; or three
rings will meet, producing a trefoil. Often, however, the
circles are not complete, and as a result a quantity of wavy
lines are formed. This variety is known as *psoriasis gyrata*
or *figurata.* The rings never overlap each other, each presenting an impenetrable barrier to the extension of contiguous rings. The name of *psoriasis universalis* is given to the
eruption when the patches increase in size, coalesce, and
cover the whole of the body. This is very rarely met with,
and even when it does occur a considerable portion of
healthy skin remains unattacked and intervenes between
the diseased patches. When the thickening of the skin
and the growth of epidermic cells is very marked, the eruption is called *psoriasis inveterata.* A further form has been
described by McCall Anderson under the name of *psoriasis
rupioides,* owing to the special prominence of the patches,
which are usually larger than in psoriasis guttata. "The
accumulation of the epidermis takes place to an unusual
extent, so that on many of the patches it assumes the shape
of large conical crusts marked by concentric rings." When
the crusts are removed no ulceration remains, but "a slightly
elevated dusky-red surface is exposed to view, which sometimes bleeds a very little."

Although when psoriasis first appears there is little discoloration of the skin, it soon becomes raised and of a
marked red color, which as time goes on grows darker. At
a later stage the scales are shed, leaving the red patches
still raised but bare. At a further period, when the disease
commences to heal, the patch becomes less and less elevated,
and the color lighter and lighter, till eventually the eruption fades, leaving the skin perfectly normal and not stained
with pigment.

Psoriasis, as a rule, is attended by some amount of local
irritation, and the scratching which results leads to the
formation of small blood crusts. Hebra has pointed out
that these will always be found on the edge of the patch as
well as in its centre, and states that the older patches only
itch at their margins, and concludes therefore that the itching only occurs while the eruption is growing.

Psoriasis may occur on any part of the body, but the tips
of the elbows, the fronts of the knees, and the head are especially liable to be affected. It may be limited to the knees
and elbows without attacking other parts, but if the rest of
the body is implicated these regions are but rarely exempt.
When the head is attacked, the eruption extends beyond
the part covered with hair and forms a ring round the forehead and ears. Often the disease penetrates into the meatus of the ear, and thus produces deafness. Psoriasis is
never seen on the mucous membranes or the red margins of
lips, and but rarely on the palms and soles. The nails are
sometimes subjected to the action of the disease, and then
become thick, friable, and of a brown color.

Psoriasis of the scalp produces no changes either in the
color or structure of the hair, although it causes it to be
shed more freely than is naturally the case.

Although much difference of opinion exists regarding the
conditions that lead to the production of psoriasis, there is
no reason for believing that climate, habits of life, special

occupations, exposure to cold, uncleanliness, diathesis, temperament, pregnancy, mental emotion, syphilis, gout or other diseases, or even sex, race, or age, have any influence on its origin. It is undoubtedly hereditary, and it is comparatively rare to find psoriasis in one member of a family without finding it in another.

Diagnosis.—Psoriasis may be confounded with seven diseases :

1. Squamous syphilide (see Chap. VIII, p. 108).
2. Lichen ruber (see Chap. X, p. 133).
3. Eczema squamosum (see Chap. XII, p. 154).
4. Pityriasis rubra (see p. 170).
5. Pityriasis can be distinguished from psoriasis by the contrast of the thick white scales of the latter with the thin dark scales of the former, and by the absence of thickening of the skin in pityriasis.
6. Ichthyosis is easily recognised by the absence of the redness of the skin and the white silverlike scales peculiar to psoriasis, and by the fact of the disease affecting the whole surface and being congenital.
7. Tinea circinata occasionally bears a rough resemblance to psoriasis, but it does not attack the knees and elbows, its scales are not silvery, and microscopic examination will enable the parasite to be distinguished.

Prognosis.—Psoriasis is not a fatal disease, but is exceedingly obstinate, though to some extent amenable to treatment, and it is liable to relapse.

Morbid Anatomy.—Thin sections from a patch which has not lasted long show the epidermis much thickened, especially the rete, which is soft and contain many leucocytes. The papillæ also are infiltrated with numerous leucocytes, which fill up the connective tissue meshwork, and the vessels are dilated, while their adventitia is thickened and loaded with cells.

15

Old patches often show thickening and induration of the whole corium, with vascular dilatation, serous and cellular infiltration, and some deposit of pigment in the branch cells as deep as the subcutaneous fatty tissue.

In psoriasis inveterata the papillæ on the back of the sacrum, and over the olecranon and upper part of the tibia, become enlarged and sclerosed, forming hard warty masses as in ichthyosis. The scales are made up of masses of cells from the stratum lucidum, which, as in other conditions producing inflammatory overgrowth, have not undergone the usual horny transformation, but have simply dried up and become pervaded with air. To this their friable consistency and their silvery color, as well as the readiness with which they separate from the hyperæmic papillary layer, are due.

Treatment.—The treatment of psoriasis consists in the use of constitutional and local remedies. Of the constitutional remedies no drug has proved of such service as arsenic, which should be given in increasing doses until the eruption begins to disappear, and then continued in small quantities for a great length of time.

The alkaline treatment has been said to be attended with success, but it is of doubtful value. It is given in the form of liquor potassæ, in doses of twenty or thirty drops three times daily. McCall Anderson has seen much benefit derived from the use of carbonate of ammonia, which should be given in doses increasing from ten to forty grains.

The internal administration of tar is also stated to be beneficial when other remedies fail, but it is by no means a drug to be relied upon.

The local treatment of psoriasis is most important, but though the employment of it without any internal remedy does remove the external appearance of the disease, a real cure is not effected on account of its liability to return. Both modes of treatment should, therefore, be adopted at the same time, and the internal should be continued for a considerable period after the apparent cure.

When the inflammation is excessive the continuous application of cold water is of great benefit in removing the scales and limiting their production.

This may be carried out by means of baths or by local cold packing; the former should be done thoroughly by immersion of the whole body or one limb for many hours at a time.

Before applying local remedies it is necessary first to endeavor to remove the scales. This is best carried out by means of soft soap, and so effectual is this plan sometimes that no further application is required.

Of local remedies those of a stimulating character are the most suitable, such as preparations of tar. The huile de cade, or common tar itself, or better still the liquor carbonis detergens, ought to be tried, but no drug has proved so successful in such a large proportion of cases as chrysophanic acid, which may be used in the form of an ointment consisting of ten to thirty grains of the acid to one ounce of vaseline or lard. Chrysophanic acid is the active principle of Goa powder, the Indian remedy for ringworm, and was first recommended in psoriasis by Mr. Balmanno Squire. The chief objection to this drug is the amount of irritation it produces, not so much in the patch to which it has been applied, but in the neighboring skin. Sometimes this irritation is very severe, when the use of the remedy should be immediately suspended.

PITYRIASIS.

Definition.—Pityriasis is a chronic squamous disease of the skin, in which the scales are branny and are seated on a non-infiltrated surface.

Symptoms.—The eruption consists of the production of a quantity of fine scales, which are continually being shed and reproduced. The skin of the affected part may be slightly red, but there is no effusion into or thickening of the epidermic layer. There is but slight itching of the part, and, unless the skin be delicate, excoriations rarely result from scratching. Any portion of the body may be affected with pityriasis, but the most common sites are the hairy parts, more particularly the scalp. The ordinary condition, known as pityriasis capitis, has been shown by Hebra to be due to an increased secretion of the sebaceous glands, and is in no sense of the word a pityriasis.

Diagnosis.—Pityriasis may be confouded with:

1. Psoriasis (see p. 173).
2. Tinea tonsurans. The only certain mode of diagnosis is by the use of the microscope, which shows the characteristic fungous elements in tinea; in addition, to the naked eye the hair is seen to be broken off short, and is easily extracted.

Prognosis.—Pityriasis is a chronic and often intractable disease, but is never attended with any serious result.

Treatment.—It is usually treated locally by the application of alkaline lotions. The best are carbonate of potash, ʒj to the half pint; or liquor potassæ, ʒij to ℥viij of water. Ointments containing either a little sulphur or mercury, or both combined, are useful. In very protracted cases arsenic may be tried.

CHAPTER XIV.

Class I.—EXUDATIONES—*continued.*

6. *PHLEGMONOUS AND ULCERATIVE GROUP.*

Furunculus—Anthrax—Delhi Boil—Ulcer.

FURUNCULUS—BOIL.

Definition.—A boil is an acute localized inflammation of the true skin, which usually terminates in necrosis and discharge by suppuration of a central portion or "core."

Symptoms.—The ordinary follicular boil begins as a small, hard, painful spot in the true skin, which soon becomes red on the surface. Inflammatory swelling, heat, and pain rapidly occur, and in the course of a day or two a small subconical elevation, which throbs and is acutely sensitive, is produced. A minute yellow spot next appears at the apex of the swelling, the cuticle thins and ruptures, and pus is gradually discharged from a small orifice. As the orifice enlarges, within it is seen a grayish or yellow slough, called the "core." This becomes loosened and finally cast off, together with shreddy pus; and as the inflammatory redness and swelling subside, the little cavity fills up with granulations and heals, leaving a slightly depressed, often pigmented scar.

In the "blind" or subcutaneous boil the starting-point is in the deeper layers of the cutis; the tumor is therefore less prominent, and pus is slower in reaching the surface. The process is, however, the same in both varieties.

Boils are most frequently excited by local irritants, such

as the undue use of hydropathic bandages and poultices, or from post-mortem virus, etc.; but in certain states of the system there appears to be a special predisposition to their occurrence. Persons suffering from diabetes or convalescent from acute diseases, especially enteric fever, seem specially liable to them. Though single boils cause little or no disturbance of the general system, yet when they are numerous and extensive, and occur in weakly and irritable individuals, there may be considerable fever.

Diagnosis.—The circumscribed, painful swelling, going on to suppuration with the discharge of a "core," cannot well be mistaken for any other skin affection.

Prognosis.—The course of a boil is usually towards recovery after suppuration has set in, but occasionally it may disappear spontaneously, or under treatment, without breaking. They are prone to recur, and successive crops may last for weeks.

Morbid Anatomy.—This is included under Anthrax.

Treatment.—In the early stage mercury with belladonna and glycerin, or the application of belladonna or soap plaster, is said to check the development of a boil. When more advanced, frequent poulticing, to relieve pain and to promote the discharge and separation of the sloughs, is the proper treatment. Yeast, in doses of a tablespoonful two or three times daily, is said to be of use in preventing fresh attacks; but the most appropriate internal remedies are quinine and iron or ammonia and bark. The diet should be generous and liberal, with a fair amount of beer and good port wine; and, in addition, change of air may be recommended.

ANTHRAX—CARBUNCLE.

Definition.—An acute localized inflammation of the true skin, differing from that in furunculus by the multiplicity of the cores and by the liability of the intervening skin and the subjacent tissues to slough. The constitutional symptoms are usually severe.

Symptoms.—Carbuncle begins as a flattened, slightly elevated swelling of the true skin, slightly red in color, and attended with severe pain and marked fever. Usually there are several points of intense inflammation, that lead to necrosis of the tissues and the formation of "cores." Considerable inflammatory infiltration surrounds the little nodule. As in a boil, suppuration soon commences; but, as the cores usually form only the superficial indications of more extensive subcutaneous sloughs, it has to continue a long time before they are separated, during which lymphangitis, cellulitis, and septic absorption, giving rise to pyæmia, may occur.

Carbuncles appear most frequently on the nape of the neck, buttocks, and external surfaces of the limbs; they occasionally arise on the face and lips, in which situations the liability to phlebitis and fatal septicæmia is very great. They are usually solitary, but sometimes are multiple, and not infrequently a succession of them appears in different parts of the body.

Diagnosis.—Carbuncle can only be mistaken for a collection of boils which have become confluent. The more intense pain and constitutional symptoms, the more extensive subcutaneous necrosis, and the greater proneness to sloughing of the skin will serve to distinguish it.

Prognosis.—Carbuncle, always an affection of serious import, is especially grave in those suffering from exhausting diseases or in a cachectic condition, however produced. The intense pain, causing sleeplessness, and the nervous exhaustion, the severe fever, the prolonged suppuration, with the special liability to septicæmia, in carbuncle of the face and lip, are all elements which intensify the danger in proportion as they are well marked.

Morbid Anatomy.—Both of these affections, boil and car-

buncle, may be considered together, the essential feature
being the formation of necrosed masses of tissue, which are
solitary in the former and form the "core." A carbuncle
containing several "cores" may be considered anatomically
as formed by the confluence of several boils. The morbid
anatomy has not been thoroughly made out; it is stated,
however, that there is an acute inflammation either in the
connective tissue passing from the base of a hair follicle
down into the subcutaneous fatty tissue, or around one or
more sebaceous glands, as the primary phenomenon. The
hyperæmia and abundant exudation of plasma into the
loose subcutaneous tissue form the large swelling round the
central spot. The accumulation of cells and plasma being
excessive, the blood supply is either cut off from the central
core, or the vessels round become thrombosed, and in consequence the mass dies. A "line of demarcation" soon
forms, and the "core" becomes loose and can be removed.

In anthrax the process is the same; the "cores," however,
are multiple, there is much more œdema of the cellular tissue, and the intensity of the inflammation may cut off the
blood supply from the intervening tissue, causing a grayish
slough or black gangrenous mass.

Treatment.—An abundant, nutritious, and easily-digested
diet, with stimulants in proportion as the patient is depressed
or debilitated, are essential parts of the general treatment.
Iron and quinine, or ammonia and bark, as for boils, should
be given. As measures of local treatment the free crucial
incision, the subcutaneous incision of the nodule, and cauterization with potassa fusa have been advised and practiced.
In the early stages Hebra recommends the application of
cold, by means of ice bladders, to check the extension of
inflammation and subsequent suppuration. Poultices and
warm poppy fomentations, with some antiseptic, such as
carbolic acid or thymol, to lessen the risk of septic absorption and to promote the separation of the sloughs, are un-

doubtedly useful. These measures are probably quite as efficacious as the more active treatment mentioned above.

Delhi Boil.

Definition.—A chronic endemic disease met with in India, characterized by the production of a small flattened nodule, which undergoes slow ulceration and heals with loss of substance, leaving a whitish, depressed scar.

Symptoms.—Delhi boil is said to begin as a small reddish spot with a central papule, gradually enlarging to form a smooth, reddish-brown, flattened nodule, which then begins to desquamate and ulcerate. Yellowish-white points, which are the altered hair and gland follicles, soon become covered with a thin scab, under which suppuration slowly goes on. An indolent sore, with hard edges and base of flabby granulations, is present under the scab. After lasting two or three months the sore usually begins to heal, and leaves a whitish, irregular scar.

The disease attacks the exposed parts of the body, and does not seem materially to affect the general health. It is said to be communicable by inoculation.

Morbid Anatomy.—This is described as follows: Microscopic examination of the papule, before ulceration has begun, shows the connective tissue of the corium infiltrated with masses of cells, oval or roundish in shape, yellowish-brown, and with one or more nuclei. The glands and papillæ appear to be destroyed by this growth, and the hair follicles become enlarged, while here and there these cystic dilatations are observed in the hairs themselves. After ulceration has commenced, in the purulent discharge pigmented bodies, resembling the ova of distomata, are said sometimes to occur.

Treatment.—Local treatment only is necessary, consisting in the thorough application of strong nitric acid if the nod-

ate we in an early stage, or if process has if an ulcer have
formed, which converts the disease into a simple ulcer that
soon heals.

ULCERS.

The following brief account of ulcers and their treatment
has been contributed by Mr. Edmund Owen:

An ulcer is well defined as being a solution of continuity
with loss of substance. The common cause of ulceration of
the skin is suppuration in the dermal connective tissue.
The collecting pus, in its escape to the surface, destroys the
superimposed dermal layer, and the epidermis, being thus
deprived of its nutritive supply, dies and is shed.

Now, whatever conditions interfere with the nutrition of
the skin necessarily predispose to the formation of ulcers.
Thus, when the function of the veins of the leg becomes
impaired from a failure of the valves to check the downward fall of the blood, stagnation in, or rather congestion
of, the cutaneous capillaries results, and from the distended
vessels the serum oozes, so that the tissues become œdematous, pitting on pressure.

In this sodden and unhealthy skin a comparatively slight
irritation, or trivial injury, is frequently attended by lesions,
troublesome out of all proportion. And thus the chafing of
a badly-fitting boot, or the fretting of a dirty or rough stocking, or a knock against a stair, may determine the formation of an ulcer, which will persistently refuse to yield to
ordinary therapeutic measures.

As a rule varicose ulcers are associated with eczema, an
attack of eczema often preceding and determining their
onset.

Common-sense, with a little practice, will soon enable the
student to select with great promptness the adjectives best
describing the varicose ulcer, but the term "chronic" only
too often denotes its chief characteristic.

The following is a list of the different kinds of ulcers usually met with:

The *healthy* ulcer, which is circular and is generally covered by a little thick pus; the granulations red and even with the surface of the part; the edge of the sore is covered by a slightly depressed, bluish-white film of new epidermis, which gradually loses itself in sound tissue. The treatment, whatever it may be, is evidently well chosen, for the sore is healing.

The *weak* ulcer is covered by large and pale granulations, which are heaped up on the surface but are painless. The local treatment best adapted will be rest, aided by the pressure of a pad of dry lint and a bandage or strapping. Stimulating lotions may be of use, also resinous and other ointments. A change of application is often attended with such good results that the weak ulcer is converted into one of the preceding class.

The *indolent* ulcer is gray and glazed, and is surrounded by an unyielding mass of tissue, which has been rendered thick and discolored from long-continued congestion. The discharge is thin, and often of a most foul odor.

Blistering fluid applied around the margin may sometimes effect much good by causing absorption of plastic deposit, but the poor and ill-fed can rarely submit to such treatment as out-patients. With in-patients two semi-elliptical incisions on the side of the sore will relieve much tension and promote a healthy condition.

The *inflamed* ulcer is recognized by placing over it, but not in contact with its raw and painful surface, the palm of the hand. The parts around are livid, hot, and tense. Poulticing affords great relief by diminishing the heat and pain.

The *phagedænic* or *gangrenous* ulcer is, as the former term implies, a sore which extends by eating its way into the neighboring skin. It shows no attempt at healing; on the contrary, the discharge is thin and bloody, and the surrounding parts are livid and swollen.

Opium given internally with quinine and acid, poultices and cleansing lotions, and the hot leg-bath will be required.

The *irritable* ulcer is to be distinguished from the inflamed ulcer by the absence of heat when the hand is held over it, as well as by the watery nature of the fluid thrown off from its surface. It is exceedingly painful, and its essential pathological character depends, according to Hilton, on the exposure of a nerve upon its surface. The exquisitely tender spot is to be made out by searching over the granulations with a probe; the treatment will consist in the division of the twig above the spot indicated by the examination. Opium and tonics may be required.

Although the leg and ankle are the most frequent seats of ulcers, on account of the unfavorable influence with which the force of gravity continually acts upon the venous blood, still it is hardly necessary to remark that there may be other than varicose ulcers even on the surface of the lower extremity. Any part of the body may be the seat of an ulceration which is the result of the destructive influence of neoplastic deposits. Thus are begotten the *tubercular*, the *lupoid*, and the *syphilitic* ulcers.

But to give a description of all these varieties of sore would be to write an essay on pathology, which, in the small space which can be devoted to the subject, is manifestly impossible. So we must content ourselves by concluding with a few general remarks which may be found of service to the student in his early practice.

First, then, when ulcers are found in regions where one is not accustomed to see them, as upon the knee, calf, thigh, trunk, arm, or face, they are not unfrequently of syphilitic origin.

Of course the integument of these areas may be attacked by ulcers which are not the result of syphilis. But if the sores are multiple, clean-cut, with rounded or crescentic margins, and appearing in successive crops, there is quite enough to justify the suspicion of the student, and even, it may be, to induce him to commence the treatment of the patient with the internal administration of iodide of potassium in full doses. But we will venture here to offer him two cautions,—firstly, not to place too much faith in what is known as a " coppery stain " about an ulcer; and, secondly, not to conclude that, because an ulcer has healed whilst the iodide is being taken, therefore the sore was the result of a breaking down of a deposit left as the result of syphilitic infection.

A last word concerning the treatment of those numberless ulcers which are the result of dilated veins. They occur chiefly in laundresses, ironers, hostlers, and others who stand much during the day, and who drink freely, whether of tea or beer. Rest is more easily enjoined than enforced; but the amount of vascular fulness may be diminished by regulating the amount of fluid absorbed. The veins require support; but this cannot often be obtained in the shape of the costly elastic stocking, nor, if there be eczema present, could that useful aid be tolerated, for the moisture from the vesicular eruption would soon render the webbing hard, irritating, and worse than useless.   .

Martin's india-rubber bandages are useful in some cases, but their application requires more care and manipulative skill than these patients usually possess, whilst their cost often puts them beyond the reach of most of these sufferers. Considerable success may be obtained by applying a piece of strapping firmly, but not too tightly, around the limb, *above* the ulcer and below the dilated veins, leaving the sore exposed for the application of lotions or ointments. Theory might perhaps suggest that such a method of treatment is unscientific, as it would offer another barrier to the easy return of the venous stream. But practice shows that the strapping so applied generally affords the greatest comfort by cutting off the weight of the downward-pressing column of venous blood, in the same way that the application of a truss affords relief in a bad case of varicocele. The strapping is best applied by the patient before he gets out of bed in the morning; its use may be dispensed with at night. In some cases of varicose eczema also the wearing of a garter below the knee affords great relief.

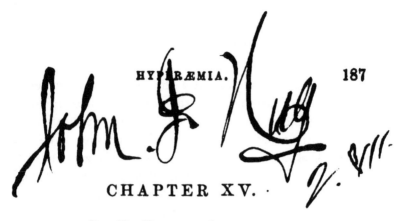

CHAPTER XV.

Class II.—Vascular Affections.

Hyperæmia—Anæmia—Hæmorrhages of the Skin—Purpura simplex, papulosa, rheumatica, hæmorrhagica—Scorbutus—Hæmatidrosis.

In the class of Vascular Affections of the Skin the subdivisions Hyperæmia, Anæmia, and Hæmorrhages are included.

In themselves the two first are of slight importance and do not endanger life; but as the manifestations or symptoms of graver conditions, or as the early stages of further changes in the skin, they require a more complete description. Cutaneous hæmorrhages are similarly of slight moment if not symptomatic of variola, scarlatina, typhus, etc., and of the so-called purpura hæmorrhagica, which is more properly a general vascular disease than one of the skin.

HYPERÆMIA.

The hyperæmic affections, characterized in general by an undue injection of blood into the capillaries, small veins, and arterioles of the superficial layer of the skin, fall conveniently into the two subdivisions of active and passive.

In the former of these the skin has usually a brighter red color, and the appearance is accompanied by a feeling of irritation, as of burning or itching, by moderate swelling, and sometimes by slight elevation of temperature; while in the latter the hue is more livid, the temperature lowered or only normal, and a feeling is experienced of numbness or even anæsthesia. The division between these

Symptomatic hyperæmia may be excited by physical causes, such as anger, shame, etc.,—*i. e.*, in the form of a blush or of a more diffuse and slighter injection—or it may arise in the course of dentition or gastric disturbances in infancy, when it has been termed erythema, roseola infantilis, strophulus, etc., or vaccinia, variola, enteric fever, cholera, rheumatism, and other diseases, when it has been variously named erythema or roseola vaccinia, etc.

Passive hyperæmia may be either general, under the influence of heart or lung disease, causing mechanical congestion, or local, from pressure on the veins or deficient arterial *vis a tergo*. The two latter, which have been termed livedo mechanica and livedo calorica respectively by Hebra, will now be described.

Livedo mechanica, arising under the influence of pressure from tight clothes, garters, varicose veins, etc., appears as a purplish-red, bluish, or grayish-black discoloration of the skin, disappearing under pressure, with slight swelling if there be no œdema. When the cause is removed it gradually subsides.

Livedo calorica is the name applied to the bluish-red or purplish tint seen on the nose, ears, etc., of persons exposed to the cold, and to the dark lines about half or three-quarters of an inch wide which form serpentine figures on the extremities and trunk. The latter are chiefly visible on the extremities, and, but less obviously, on the trunk, and though fading on pressure, disappear only when the patient is warm. Occasionally in the midst of the purplish background vermilion-red patches are observable, varying in size from ⅛ to ¼ of an inch, and sometimes surrounded by a pale zone.

If the action of cold be prolonged, it may in weakly, chlorotic persons give rise not only to congestion, but to exudation and an eczematous condition to which the name chilblain has been applied.

Morbid Anatomy.—The active hyperæmia leave little or

no traces for examination after death beyond slight pigmentation of the rete cells. The experiments of Auspitz lead him to a very probable explanation of the persistence after removing the ligature of the brown pigmentation subsequently left by the vermilion-colored spots noticed in passive hyperæmia. He ascribes it to the admixture with the transuded serum in the tissue of red corpuscles, which subsequently give rise to hæmatoidin crystals and yellow or brown pigment. The pale streaks are due to the shutting off from the circulation of certain tracts of vessels which are empty or contain only clear serum, as in embolism, etc.

ANÆMIA.

Anæmia of the skin may be general, as in chlorosis, after loss of blood, exhausting discharges, etc.; or local, under the influence of cold, undue action of local vasomotor nerves, pressure, etc.

It is of importance only so far as it modifies the appearances of eruptions, and produces apparent retrogression in such as are characterized by hyperæmia. Thus the exanthems of scarlatina and measles may fade if exposed to cold, or an old psoriasis be lost sight of after severe hæmorrhage, only to reappear as the former vascularity of the skin returns.

Treatment.—The application of cold water, spirit lotion, or lotio carbonis detergens, to relieve the burning and itching in active hyperæmia, is all that is necessary.

HÆMORRHAGE OF THE SKIN.

A. Traumatic, . . . From wounds, bruises.

B. Symptomatic, .
  1. Purpura,
    Simplex.
    Papulosa.
    Rheumatica.
    Hæmorrhagica.
  2. Scorbutus,
  3. Hæmatidrosis.

Extravasations of blood in the skin take the form of:

1. *Petechiæ*—round or irregular, bright or livid-red spots, not raised, varying from $\frac{1}{18}$ to $\frac{1}{2}$ an inch in size, appearing as if splashed on the skin.

2. *Vibices*—long streaks, either branching or parallel to one another.

3. *Ecchymoses*—dark-red irregular patches, varying in diameter from 1 to 3 inches.

They do not fade on pressure, but undergo a series of changes from red to brown, greenish, or yellow before they disappear.

A. *Traumatic.*—The ordinary appearances of a bruise, or ecchymosis, produced, for instance, by a blow on the skin, and the minute petechiæ due to flea or bug bites, are familiar to every one.

B. *Symptomatic.*

PURPURA.

Definition.—Extravasation of blood occurring as puncta, petechiæ, vibices, or ecchymoses, either spontaneously or in the course of various diseases.

Symptoms.—The following varieties have been described:

a. Purpura simplex consists in the occurrence of numerous petechiæ, or vibices, irregularly scattered over the body, usually most markedly on the legs, where there is a tendency to symmetry of the eruption. The disease is said to occur in debilitated persons, but is attended by little or no subjective trouble, and is not dangerous to life. When small papules appear between the hæmorrhages the affection is termed *purpura papulosa*.

b. Purpura rheumatica, or *peliosis rheumatica*, first described as a separate disease under the latter name by Schönlein, is characterized by rheumatic pains in and about the joints, together with an appearance of a rash, which is at first erythematous but soon becomes hæmorrhagic. Though provisionally classed with purpura, it ought rather to be considered a variety of erythema papulatum or nodosum, with which, according to Bazin and others, it is identical. According to Hebra it arises with dragging pains in the joints and some fever, followed in a few days by the eruption near the joints, or more especially on the abdomen and breast. The spots, round and flat, are only slightly raised, gradually fade, with the usual changes of color, and disappear, without desquamation, in a week.

The disease usually attacks strong and healthy persons between the ages of twenty and thirty, and more frequently males than females. It has never been seen in children or aged persons.

c. *Purpura hæmorrhagica* is a severe constitutinal variety, in which the cutaneous extravasations are abundant and large, and accompanied by hæmorrhages into various organs and from mucous surfaces. Marked anæmia and asthenia are induced by the severe losses of blood, and death is not an infrequent result.

The so-called purpura fibrilis is usually only a purpuric rash that appears in the course of one of the acute infectious diseases.

Diagnosis.—A petechial rash, not occurring in the course of one of the exanthemata, may be mistaken for:

1. Fleabites.   2. Scurvy.

Fleabites are most abundant where the folds of the clothes are thick, as on the neck, wrists, waist, and ankles; while purpura affects the lower limbs pre-eminently, and has no special predilection for other sites. It is also hæmorrhagic from the beginning, and does not appear as a roseolar spot, or wheal, with a central red dot.

The following table will show the points of difference from scurvy.

SCURVY.	PURPURA.
1. Is due to privation from vegetables and to depressing circumstances, and is cured by lime juice and fruit.	1. Is not produced by want of vegetables, and lime juice has no influence on its course.
2. Affects usually many persons at the same time.	2. Occurs sporadically.
3. The gums become spongy, the teeth loose, and painful subcutaneous ecchymoses, prone to suppuration, may occur.	3. No affection of gums or painful ecchymoses.
4. Is attended with great prostration and a peculiar dusky pallor of skin.	4. Prostration only proportionate to loss of blood; skin anæmic.
5. Death occurs rarely from hæmorrhage, usually from serous effusions or septicæmia.	5. Death results from asthenia or syncope, the result of hæmorrhage.

Prognosis.—Purpura simplex and rheumatica are affections of slight gravity, and as a rule tend towards spontaneous recovery. Purpura hæmorrhagica is serious in proportion to the amount of internal bleeding; it often resists treatment, and proves fatal by anæmia and exhaustion or syncope.

Morbid Anatomy.—The skin, after death, of a person who during life has had purpura shows—

1. Recent hæmorrhagic spots in the form of subarticular or interstitial puncta, or striæ of a dark-purplish color.

2. Small crusts of dark color, due to the drying up of the petechiæ.

3. Brownish or yellowish stains, marking the position of former hæmorrhages of which the fluid portions have become absorbed and the blood corpuscles more or less altered.

In a section of a recent petechial spot, either in the fresh condition or after hardening, the effusion of blood is seen to be mainly limited to the papillary layer of the corium and the overlying rete Malpighii. On microscopic examination blood corpuscles, the majority of which are more or less broken down, are seen surrounding the hair follicles, having apparently proceeded from the capillary network round the latter. Should the effusions take the form of vibices, the blood corpuscles are found in and around the papillæ of the corium and in the rete, raising the horny layers of the epidermis as in a vesicle.

Microscopic examination of the older spots shows the blood corpuscles broken down and converted into pigment, reddish-brown masses and granules of which are found lying in the meshes of the connective tissue of the corium, and sometimes staining the branched cells a brownish-yellow color.

In the majority of cases of purpura simplex in which a microscopic examination of the blood capillaries has been made, no obvious morbid changes have been found.

Dr. Wilson Fox described albuminoid or lardaceous changes in the capillaries in the vicinity of purpuric spots as traceable in some cases, and in the cutaneous hæmorrhages occurring in certain instances of phosphorus poisoning acute fatty degeneration has been found in the arterioles and capillaries, to the rupture of which the extravasations are ascribed.

Where no alteration of the capillaries has taken place the escape of the red corpuscles is supposed to be due to simple diapedesis, the resistance of the capillary walls being so diminished as to allow the passage through them of red corpuscles when, from any slight exertion, as in standing, strain is thrown upon them.

Treatment.—In the milder forms of purpura, rest in bed, nutritious diet, and tonics are all that is needed.

In purpura hæmorrhagica various drugs, chiefly metallic astringents and those which act on the bloodvessels, have been used; of these, tinctura ferri perchloridi, in doses of xx to xxx drops three times a day, either alone or with ergot and digitalis, gives the best results.

Scorbutus—Scurvy.

Definition.—Scurvy is a general disease of the body characterized by progressive anæmia, severe mental prostration and asthenia, impairment of nutrition and a tendency to the occurrence of hæmorrhages from mucous membranes and into the skin, muscles, and viscera. It is due to privation from, or an insufficient supply of, fresh vegetable food.

Symptoms.—The patient presents at first a dirty, pallid, or earthy-looking complexion, accompanied by languor and *malaise*, mental apathy and depression, and rheumatic pains in the back and the muscles of the limbs. The gums swell, forming deep-red spongy masses round the teeth, which are prone to bleed and ulcerate, giving great fetor to the breath. The teeth may loosen and drop out. Petechiæ appear at first on the lower limbs, followed by ecchymoses and subcutaneous extravasations, which spontaneously, or on slight irritation or injury, are liable to suppurate and give rise to unhealthy, painful, bleeding ulcers. Progressive anæmia, sudden syncope on slight exertion, sanguineous effusions into the pleura and pericardium, gangrene of the lungs, or diarrhœa may lead to a fatal result.

Diagnosis.—From purpura (see p. 193).

Prognosis.—It is serious and often fatal if untreated. Death results most frequently from asthenia or sudden syncope. Cases of moderate severity almost always recover if fresh vegetables be added to the dietary.

Morbid Anatomy.—The cutaneous changes resemble those met with in purpura, already described.

Treatment.—The essential point in the treatment is the restriction of the diet of vegetable food in the form of fresh green vegetables, turnips, carrots, onions, lemon, or lime juice.

The skin affection should be treated by antiseptic and astringent washes. The tendency to syncope should be averted by rest in bed, stimulants, and digitalis.

HÆMATIDROSIS.

Hæmatidrosis, or "bloody sweat," is an affection of rare occurrence. It is a hæmorrhage on the surface of the skin in parts where the cuticle is thin and delicate, and it is produced by rupture of capillaries in the plexus round the mouths of the sweat ducts.

The "stigmata" on the forehead, hands, and feet, stated to occur in the persons of religious fanatics, have proved in most cases, when submitted to a careful scientific examination, to be fictitious.

CHAPTER XVI.

Class III.—NEUROSES.

Zoster—Cheiro-pompholyx—Pruritus—Dystrophia cutis.

ZOSTER—HERPES ZOSTER—SHINGLES.

Definition.—Zoster is a disease of acute and typical course and benign nature, characterized by the eruption of groups of vesicles or erythematous papules, which correspond in situation with the peripheral distribution of a cutaneous nerve—usually on one side of the body—and are produced through the influence of irritative lesions of the nervous system.

Following the classification of Hebra, zoster is divided into the following varieties:

1. Zoster capillitii.
2. Zoster faciei.
3. Zoster nuchæ et colli $\begin{cases} \text{occipito-collaris.} \\ \text{cervico-subclavicularis.} \end{cases}$
4. Zoster cervico-brachialis.
5. Zoster pectoralis.
6. Zoster abdominalis.
7. Zoster femoralis.

Symptoms.—Usually after a few days, sometimes a few weeks, of neuralgic pains, either over the whole region which becomes subsequently affected, or at certain fixed spots corresponding with points of division or emergence from the deeper tissues of cutaneous nerves, the eruption appears

17

...tinity. It consists of an efflorescence of bright-red papules about the size of millet seeds, on an erythematous surface, and is accompanied usually by a burning sensation. Within a few hours, or in a day or two, the papules become vesicles, from the size of a pin's head to that of a pea, filled with a clear serous fluid; they are either quite isolated or closely aggregated, and sometimes by confluence form an irregular bulla. Successive crops of vesicles may prolong the eruptive stage for a week, but each series has all its vesicles at the same stage of development: thus one group may be papular, another vesicular, and a third already desiccated.

After a day or two the contents of the vesicles become opaque and purulent; they then dry up, forming yellow scabs, which usually, about a fortnight after the onset of the affection, fall off, leaving reddish-brown stained patches. Successive efflorescences may, however, prolong the total duration of the disease to three or four weeks, but they always appear upon adjacent portions of skin, *never on that implicated by the first eruption.* The vesicles may be few in number, and confined to a circumscribed area, or closely aggregated along the whole course of a nerve; in the latter case the pain and constitutional symptoms are somewhat severe, and the duration of the attack more prolonged.

As zoster is not usually a fatal disease, cases in which the cause has been ascertained by autopsy are rare. Bärensprung, Charcot, Wagner, Kaposi, and others have found as the most frequent cause hæmorrhage and inflammation of the intervertebral or Gasserian ganglia.

New growths, carcinomatous, tubercular, or purulent collections, causing irritation of the adjacent nerve trunks, or ganglia; traumatic lesions, causing irritation of the peripheral, sensory, or mixed nerves, and meningitis; caries of the vertebræ or locomotor ataxy, causing irritation of the posterior roots—are frequently attended with eruptions of zoster. It has also been noticed after poisoning with carbonic oxide gas, and occasionally during the administration of arsenic (Hutchinson). Hebra and Kaposi, on whose descriptions this account is mainly based, consider as abnormal the following variations in the course and consequences of zoster:

1. Cases in which some part or all of the eruption remains papular and aborts or forms bullæ or pustules, the latter causing destruction of the dermis and giving rise to lasting cicatrices.

2. Cases in which blood appears in the contents of the vesicles, or bæmorrhagic infiltration of their bases occurs. In the latter the vesicles burst, the infiltrated tissue of their bases slowly necroses, and extremely painful ulcers, which take weeks or months to heal, and which leave permanent scars, are produced.

3. Cases in which neuralgia does not abate with the efflorescence, but persists during and long after the eruption. This is rare in the young, more common in the aged.

4. Cases where muscular atrophy, anæsthesia, alopecia, or loss of teeth or atrophy of the alveolar process occurs after the zoster.

5. Bilateral symmetrical zoster.

Zoster usually occurs but once in a lifetime; it rarely passes the middle line before or behind, and then only slightly; it appears at all ages and in both sexes; it affects either side of the body indifferently, being, according to statistics, slightly more common on the right. The groups of vesicles formed are, according to Hebra, always nearest the nervous centres, the subsequent crops lying more towards the periphery of the corresponding nerves.

1. *Zoster capillitii*, best seen in bald persons, occurs on the scalp in the peripheral distribution of the supraorbital and great occipital nerves, and sometimes forms an arch over one parietal bone, terminating near the coronal suture.

2. *Zoster faciei* presents the greatest variety of appearances. Groups of vesicles, limited accurately by the middle line, may appear on the forehead along the course of the supraorbital nerve; at the inner angle of the orbit and root of the nose along the supratrochlear; on the cheek, ala nasi, and lower eyelid along the infraorbital; and in the mouth, palate, and pharynx from implication of the palatine branches of the superior maxillary. Vesicles may appear on the gums, associated with violent toothache, loosening and loss of the teeth, and atrophy of the alveolar process when the superior dental is affected. The eruption may also appear in the region of the auriculo-temporal, on the temple, pinna and meatus of the ear, on the chin, the mental branch, and on the side of the tongue in the course of the lingual. When the whole region of distribution of the ophthalmic branch of the fifth nerve is affected, in addition to the zoster frontalis, there are vesicles, very often hæmorrhagic, on the nose and nasal mucous membrane, from affection of the infratrochlear and ethmoidal twigs; vesicles on the temple and malar prominence, from the zygomatic and lachrymal branches; and conjunctivitis, corneal ulcers, and iritis, from affection of the long root of the lenticular ganglion. Ophthalmitis, thrombosis of the ophthalmic vein, septicæmia, death may thus result from zoster ophthalmicus.

3. *Zoster Nuchæ et Colli.*—The variety occipito-collaris presents vesicles on the back of the neck from the great and small occipital nerves, on the posterior surface of the pinna and lobule (great auricular), and on the side of the neck and beneath the chin. The variety cervico-subclavicularis occurs in the region of distribution of the ascending and descending cutaneous branches of the cervical plexus, on the region of the neck below the scalp back as far as the shoulder, and downwards as far as the skin between the clavicle and nipple.

4. *Zoster cervico-brachialis* affects the brachial plexus, and

presents groups of vesicles on both sides of the arm and forearm as far as the little finger, and on the second and third intercostal spaces as far as the sternum.

5. *Zoster pectoralis* occurs:

a. As a continuous band of vesicles, occupying one to three intercostal spaces, running from the spine to the sternum; to this the terms *zona* and *shingles* were originally applied. The vesicles not unfrequently coalesce, and are sometimes hæmorrhagic; in the latter case the pain is excessive.

b. As patches of vesicles, one usually near the spine, corresponding to the hinder branches of the dorsal nerve; one on the side of the thorax, where the twig of the intercostal nerve penetrates the muscles; and a third near the sternum, at the termination of the nerve. The spinal and sternal groups may pass the middle line about half an inch, and even in bilateral zoster the groups never coalesce to form a complete girdle, as the ends overlap. One group only may be present.

The intense pain in the side and the dyspnœa may sometimes lead to a suspicion of pleurisy.

6. *Zoster femoralis* presents groups of vesicles, appearing usually first on the buttock, to which region they may be confined, or on the front or on the back of the thigh, and they may extend downwards to the ham or calf. On the penis *zoster pudentalis*, from affections of the pudic nerve, may occur, but is sharply restricted to one side of the organ (Kaposi).

Diagnosis.—The sudden appearance, usually preceded by neuralgic pain, of a group of vesicles situated on the peripheral distribution of a cutaneous nerve, and the course of the affection, are sufficient, even in abortive cases, to distinguish zoster from any other vesicular disease of the skin.

Prognosis.—Zoster is a benign disease. An extensive efflorescence of the hæmorrhagic form, with slow healing,

painful ulcers, or severe neuralgia, may wear out an aged,
weakly person, but death rarely results except from some
intercurrent malady.

Morbid Anatomy.—In the intervertebral ganglia undue
vascularity of the surrounding fatty tissue of the ganglion
itself and intracapsular hæmorrhages have been found.
Under the microscope the capillaries of the ganglion are
found loaded with blood, the ganglion cells separated and
destroyed by hæmorrhage, and sometimes surrounded inside their capsules, and numerous leucocytes are scattered
throughout the tissue. When due to affections of the peripheral nerves, at a distance from the ganglion, the condition
is usually one of subacute neuritis. The nerve is grayish,
slightly injected, thickened, adherent to its sheath and adjacent parts, and on microscopic examination an excess of
spindle cells are found in it, causing granular degeneration
of the medullary sheath and the axis cylinders. The vesicles present no essential difference from those of herpes
febrilis or eczema. The acute neuritis of the peripheral
nerves found by Haight near the vesicles resembles that
met with in many other inflammations of the corium, and
is not peculiar to zoster.

Treatment.—No internal or local remedies have yet proved
of the slightest use in cutting short an attack of zoster; all
that remains to be done, therefore, is to palliate the severity
of the symptoms, and to let the disease run its natural
course, avoiding, as worse than useless, any attempt, by cauterization or otherwise, to check the formation of the vesicles. Dusting with powder, and covering with cotton-wool
and a bandage to prevent the clothes rubbing the vesicles,
and, if ulcers form, dressing in the usual way, is all that is
needed locally. Should the pain be intense, narcotics by
the mouth, or better still hypodermically, ought to be used.
The subsequent neuralgia, which is often severe in the aged,

is best treated by quinine and arsenic in full doses, and by the repeated application of the continuous current.

CHEIRO-POMPHOLYX (*Hutchinson*).

Definition.—A disease of the skin characterized by the appearance of small clear vesicles or bullæ on the hands, and sometimes on the feet, usually symmetrical, running a short course, and liable to constant relapses.

Symptoms.—The disease, in its milder forms, is not very uncommon, but the more severe cases, in which large bullæ are produced, are extremely rare.

In persons of nervous temperament, when out of health or worried and depressed, the disease begins by burning and itching between and along the sides of the fingers, followed in a few hours, or on the next day, by the appearance of irregular groups of small, round, deepseated, flat-topped vesicles, containing clear serum, having no inflammatory areola around them, and resembling boiled sago grains. These vesicles usually dry up in a few days, and are followed by slight desquamation; in some more severe cases, however, they enlarge, and by their confluence produce bullæ, which vary in size from a pin's head to $\frac{1}{2}$ or $\frac{1}{3}$ of an inch in diameter, and are scattered over the whole palm or sole. They also dry up in a few days, and the cuticle subsequently desquamates, but occasionally the bullæ burst and then desiccate, leaving red dry patches like psoriasis. The serum, at first clear, may become, if the bullæ last a few days, opalescent and slightly yellowish, but never purulent, and it always remains alkaline.

Frequently the nails are undermined and broken near the root.

Diagnosis.—The rapid and symmetrical development, the short course and tendency to spontaneous cure, the liability to recur, and its occurrence in those of nervous temperament and the worried and overworked, suffice to distinguish it from eczema.

The spontaneous cure and the absence of burrows separate it from scabies.

It differs from sudamina in the fluid being alkaline,—not, as in sweat, acid from the beginning,—a fact which is against the theory of the dependence of the disease on obstruction of the sweat ducts.

Prognosis.—The disease runs a favorable course in a few . days, and is only troublesome through the itching and burning sensation it excites and from its unsightly appearance.

Treatment.—The application of lotio carbonis detergens (℥ij to ℥vj), of vaseline, or of vaseline and liquor plumbi (℈xxx to ℥j), will usually relieve the itching. To combat the general nervous symptoms tonics may be given, of which iron, quinine, and nux vomica are the best, combined with change of air and rest.

PRURITUS.

Definition.—Pruritus is a functional disorder of the skin, arising either spontaneously or as a symptom in the course of various diseases, attended with intense itching. The scratching which it induces may cause excoriations, eczematous or pustular eruptions, and other secondary changes in the skin.

Symptoms.—Pruritus itself is usually merely a symptom produced by :

1. Local irritants, pediculi, acaria, ascarides in the rectum, etc.

2. Consititutional conditions, such as jaundice, diabetes, intestinal, uterine, and genito-urinary disorders, senile decay of the skin, rheumatism, gout, etc.

The chief varieties described are :

a. Pruritus senilis, occurring in old people in association with atrophic changes in the skin. The itching, often intense, induces scratching, from which papules, excoriations, pustules, etc., result. It may be excited by pediculi corporis, in which case the marks of scratching are most distinct on the neck and shoulders.

b. Pruritus ani is a frequent and distressing accompaniment of piles, gout, uterine and other disorders.

c. Pruritus genitalium is most frequent in women, and is usually a symptom of local disease, eczema, etc., of utero-ovarian irritation, or of general diseases, such as diabetes and gout.

Diagnosis.—The intense itching, unattended by special morbid changes beyond those that are the result of scratching, suffices to distinguish it from other diseases of the skin.

Prognosis.—Pruritus, though not fatal, is often obstinate, and causes great distress.

Morbid Anatomy.—No special changes have been found in the skin or cutaneous nerves.

Treatment.—The indications are:

1. To remove or mitigate any local irritation exciting the affection, and to treat constitutional symptoms or diseases of adjacent organs.

2. When no obvious causes can be found, to give tonics, iron, quinine, cod-liver oil, and locally to apply sedative lotions, such as lotio calaminæ, lotio boracis with hydrocyanic acid or dilute carbonis detergens.

When the itching is general, alkaline baths often give great relief, after which an ointment of chloral camphor ℨss. to vaseline ℨj may be used with advantage. Scratching must be strictly forbidden.

18

DYSTROPHIA CUTIS.

Definition.—Certain changes in the skin, other than zoster, usually of an atrophic, inflammatory, or gangrenous nature, which arise under the direct influence of lesions of the nervous system.

Symptoms.—The appearance met with may be arranged under the heads:

1. Atrophic or "glossy skin."
2. Œdematous.
3. Eruptive, erythematous, papular, vesicular, or bullous.
4. Ulcerative or gangrenous, "acute bedsore."

1. "*Glossy skin*" is the term applied by Paget and Weir Mitchell to a peculiar condition, somewhat resembling scleroderma, which supervenes after irritative lesions of the peripheral nerves. It sometimes follows a clean cut, entirely dividing the nerve; but more commonly a partial division, contusion, laceration, or compression in a cicatrix, callus, etc., is the cause. The skin is smooth, pale, and anæmic, or pinkish and blotched, as if by chilblains, glossy, and its natural wrinkles effaced. The epidermis is often fissured, the nails are cracked and distorted, the hair is shed, and the sweat glands are atrophied, and their secretion diminished. The affected part is usually extremely tender and the seat of neuralgic pain, and its temperature is often lowered.

2. *Œdematous.*—There is often slight œdema of the skin and subcutaneous parts in paralyzed limbs, which lasts for a considerable time, and gradually disappears as recovery takes place. Peculiar pale or slightly erythematous localized swelling of the skin and subcutaneous tissue, resembling chilblains, are also met with, appearing after neuralgic attacks at the sites of pain. They are sometimes described as urticarial, but are attended by intense shooting or burning pain, and not by itching.

3. *Eruptive.*—The "lightning pains" of locomotor ataxy, and the neuralgic attacks met with in pachymeningitis, caries, or cancer of the vertebræ, and other affections in which there is compression and irritation of the posterior nerve roots, are often accompanied by an eruption on the painful points of skin, erythematous, papular, vesicular, pustular, or bullous in character. The patches correspond in situation, as in zoster, with the distribution of cutaneous nerves, and in their course and duration resemble that disease.

4. *Ulcerative and gangrenous* patches may occur as the sequelæ of the last-mentioned changes, or as an independent form in the "acute bedsore," to which special attention has been directed by Charcot. This lesion, of grave and usually fatal import in the prognosis of cerebral or spinal diseases, appears, according to this authority, a few days, or occasionally only some hours, after the onset of the nerve symptoms, as an erythematous patch of variable extent and irregular shape, seated, in spinal disease, over the sacrum, in cerebral usually on one of the buttocks. The color, at first light red, or somewhat bluish, fades on pressure, and in some spinal cases there is a phlegmonous-looking infiltration, attended sometimes with anæsthesia, at other times with severe pain. After a day or two vesicles or bullæ, containing clear brownish or sanguineous fluid, appear in the centre of the patch ; these soon burst, exposing a bright-red base, dotted with purplish·black spots of cutaneous hæmorrhage, which often extends as deep as the subcutaneous tissue or muscles. The purple spots soon become confluent, necrose, and form a black slough surrounded by a margin of erythema. Patients rarely live long enough for the slough to be cast off, but in more chronic cases septicæmia and gangrenous meningitis soon prove fatal. These patches appear even when the most scrupulous care is taken

to avoid pressure or any irritation of the skin from the urine or fæces.

Diagnosis.—The occurrence of these phenomena in connection with severe diseases of the nervous system, their restriction to certain special sites, usually related to the cutaneous distribution of nerves, and the presence, before or throughout their course, of neuralgic pain, will clearly indicate their nature.

Prognosis.—As these skin manifestations are merely symptomatic, their prognosis is that of the diseases in which they occur.

"Acute bedsore" is, according to Charcot, an omen of a fatal result.

Morbid Anatomy.—The cutaneous appearances in the erythematous, vesicular, and other eruptions are the same as those in the simple diseases. In "acute bedsore" there is an exudation into the whole corium, with leucocytes and plasma, resembling phlegmonous erysipelas, which is followed later on by hæmorrhagic infiltration and gangrene.

Treatment.—This falls beyond the scope of this work. In "acute bedsore" keeping the part clean, the frequent application of some antiseptic lotion or powder to diminish the risk of septicæmia, and poultices to promote the separation of the sloughs should be employed.

CHAPTER XVII.

Class IV.—HYPERTROPHIÆ.

Ephelis — Lentigo — Melanoderma — Morbus Addisonii—Chloasma uterinum — Ichthyosis — Xeroderma — Morphœa—Scleroderma —Sclerema neonatorum—Elephantiasis Arabum—Elephantiasis teleangiectodes—Dermatolysis.

Pigmentary.

1. Ephelis and Lentigo. 2. Melanoderma. 3. Morbus Addisonii. 4. Chloasma uterinum.

EPHELIS AND LENTIGO—FRECKLES.

FRECKLES are light or dark brown spots, varying in size from a pin's head to a lentil, occurring on the skin of fair or red-haired people. They are found usually on the more exposed regions of the body, such as the face, neck, and backs of the hands and wrists, but appear also on other parts. They are greatly influenced by light, and are always darker in summer than in winter. Some doubt exists whether they can be produced by the sun's rays, but there is reason to believe that many spots otherwise imperceptible are only then visible. Exposure of the limbs to heat will often produce a similar discoloration as the result of a deposit of pigment in the rete. The appearance of the spots is entirely unattended by itching, or indeed any local or constitutional symptom. When the stains are larger, more persistent, and are not influenced by exposure to heat and cold, they are termed *lentigines*.

MELANODERMA.

This term includes all cases in which dark stains are produced through some special condition of the body, such as pregnancy, intemperance, etc.

MORBUS ADDISONII.

In the course of this disease, which is an affection of the suprarenal capsules, a remarkable bronzing of the skin takes place. After the disease has been progressing for some time, the skin is noticed to be of a darker tint than normal, a change often attributed to jaundice. The upper part of the body is usually affected earlier than the lower, but the entire surface becomes eventually involved, the color becoming gradually darker, and—although the shades of color vary in different cases from a light to a dark brown—in the majority of fatal cases the color deepens markedly as death approaches. In parts where pigment is usually deposited, such as the axillæ, flexor surfaces of joints, genitals, nipples, freckles, etc., the shades will be found to be of a darker brown, or even black, making the rest of the skin appear white by contrast.

CHLOASMA UTERINUM.

This term is applied to the pigmentary deposits occurring in women suffering from uterine disease, or as a result of pregnancy. It usually appears in the form of crescentic patches on the forehead and below the hair.

Epidermis and Papillæ.

ICHTHYOSIS AND XERODERMA.

Definition.—Ichthyosis is a congenital hypertrophic disease of the skin, characterized by increased growth of the papillary layer with thickening of the true skin and the production of masses of epidermic scales.

Symptoms.—Some doubt exists whether ichthyosis is always a congenital disease. The characteristic appearance of the skin is sometimes not developed until some years after birth; it is, however, impossible to say that some abnormal condition or tendency did not exist at birth, although it may not have become apparent until a later period, and this view is supported by the fact that ichthyosis is hereditary.

There are many degrees of ichthyosis, ranging from a mere roughness of the skin to a condition resembling that of the skin of the shark. In a case of average severity the growth of the papillary layer is greatly increased, and the whole skin thickened. The natural furrows of the skin are, as the result of this growth, much deepened, and the surface is mapped out into polygonal tracts, presenting an appearance similar to a crocodile's hide. Surmounting the ridges are collections of epidermic scales, which at first are limited in quantity, but as time progresses increase in size. Masses are formed in the centre of a patch, either thin and pearl-colored or of varying shades of color, from green to brown or black, and may also cover the enlarged papillæ, forming projections from the surface. There is a complete absence of perspiration from the parts attacked with the disease, but the unaffected regions, such as the head, usually perspire freely.

Ichthyosis simplex, or *xeroderma*, is the form most frequently met with. It usually becomes apparent in the child at about two years of age, when it is nothing more than a general roughness of the skin, especially marked over the knees and elbows. At a later period the epidermis is shed in flakes and the general roughness is greatly increased, but certain regions, such as the inside of the extremities and the palms and soles, differ from healthy skin only slightly, while the face is dry and furfuraceous. With the exception of these regions the skin is covered with the irregular-shaped patches above described, limited by the natural folds of the skin. On the knees and elbows, on the fronts of the ankles and margins of the axillæ, and, indeed, on all parts exposed to friction, the masses become so thick and black from dirt that the disease is far more marked than on the other regions.

Ichthyosis cornea occurs less frequently than the simple variety. It consists of a growth of hard, horny prominences, often standing out a quarter of an inch, which, being aggregated together, form patches somewhat resembling the condition found on the knees and elbows in ichthyosis simplex. They are believed to be due to an alteration of the lining of the sebaceous follicles into horny material. This first distends the follicle, and then passes through its orifice to the surface, where it protrudes. The exposed end is broken away, and with it a part of the material in the follicle, and a cup is thus left, which is again filled by further growth of the horny substance. When these are thrown off, the skin of the part is left in a normal condition.

Diagnosis.—With the exception of psoriasis there is no disease for which ichthyosis could be mistaken.

For diagnosis from psoriasis see Chapter XIII, p. 173.

Prognosis.—Ichthyosis is a very intractable disease, but is never fatal. It can be somewhat benefited by remedies, but only temporarily. Occasionally, after a prolonged and severe general illness, the disease has been observed to disappear, and has not again returned.

Morbid Anatomy.—Vertical sections show a dense accumulation of horny epidermic cells, containing frequently a considerable quantity of fatty matter; the rete cells, especially between the papillæ, are more numerous and sometimes pigmented, and the papillæ themselves are greatly enlarged and elongated, and contain dilated vessels and numerous cells. In severe cases the hair follicles are more or less atrophied, the sweat and sebaceous glands are wasted, and there is induration and sclerosis of the corium and atrophy of the adipose tissue.

Treatment.—Any local application likely to soften and remove the accumulated epidermis is the proper treatment, and for this purpose alkaline lotions, and soaps of various kinds, the one recommended by Hebra being composed of iodide of sulphur, oil, glycerin, have been tried. Absolute cleanliness is most essential, and the constant and prolonged soaking of the body in water will often lead to a diminution of the ichthyotic condition. Various internal remedies have been tried, but with no benefit.

Connective Tissue.

1. Morphœa. 2. Scleroderma. 3. Sclerema neonatorum. 4. Elephantiasis Arabum. 5. Elephantiasis teleangiectodes. 6. Dermatolysis.

MORPHŒA—ADDISON'S KELOID.

Definition.—Morphœa is a rare chronic affection of the skin, characterized by the occurrence—most often on the face—of roundish or oval pale-pink or ivory-colored patches, which are firm and inelastic, and therefore are not easily pinched up into folds.

Symptoms.—Patches of one to three inches in diameter appear on the skin in the course of some cutaneous nerve, with a pale-yellowish or ivory-like centre, smooth surface, and a well-defined violet or lilac-tinted margin. The corium, apparently dense and thickened, appears to be bound down to the subcutaneous tissue. A feeling of burning or tingling sometimes attends the development of the patches, and there may be slight pain on pressure, but usually no alteration in cutaneous sensibility.

When the patches appear on the face they are sharply limited by the middle line, and may occur in the area of distribution of the supraorbital nerve or other branches of the fifth, but on the trunk and limbs they are arranged in a somewhat similar manner as in herpes. Pigment is occasionally deposited in the skin around the patch, and its absence or presence distinguishes the varieties morphœa alba and morphœa nigra. Owing to the infiltration and rigidity of the skin, the movements of the facial muscles and of the joints, when the skin of these parts is the seat of the disease, are much impaired, so that the fingers remain semiflexed and cannot be either bent or extended, and the expression of the face becomes stony and fixed, like that of a frozen corpse. The sweat and sebaceous secretions, and the growth of hair on the hide-bound patches, are frequently deficient, and the temperature is usually 2° to 3° Fahr. lower than that of the healthy skin, but there is no special trophic change in the parts affected.

The morphœa patches slowly extend, and having reached their acme may, in the course of years, gradually fade, and leave the skin perfectly normal or only slightly pigmented. However, occasionally sclerosis takes place, and the thin, rigid skin acquires a shrunken, parchmentlike appearance, which has been termed morphœa atrophica.

Diagnosis.—Patches of morphœa differ from leucoderma, which they resemble in color and definition, by the hard, infiltrated, and inelastic consistence of the affected skin.

The pale patches of lepra maculosa differ from those of morphœa by being anæsthetic in their centre and usually symmetrical in their distribution, while the former disease is accompanied by affections of the nerves, cutaneous tubercles, etc., which never occur in morphœa.

Keloid can hardly be mistaken for morphœa, so forcible is the contrast between the raised, pinkish, clawlike nodule of the former and the level, pale, smooth patches of the latter.

Prognosis.—Morphœa is never fatal. The disease in some cases tends slowly towards involution, and the normal elastic condition of the skin is restored ; but when sclerosis and atrophy have occurred, permanent deformity is the result.

Morbid Anatomy.—See SCLERODERMA.

Treatment.—No local treatment has proved of any avail, but as general remedies tonics, such as iron, quinine, and cod-liver oil, are indicated if the case is complicated by anæmia or struma.

SCLERODERMA—SCLERIASIS.

Definition.—A rare disease of the skin, in which diffuse infiltrated and rigid areæ are met with over comparatively large portions of the surface of the body.

Symptoms.—Scleroderma begins most frequently on the back of the neck or upper extremities as a slightly raised brownish-red or pale waxy-colored patch, and may spread more or less rapidly over the face, arm, or even over the whole body, or it may take the form of long ribbonlike streaks or patches scattered over the body and limbs. As in morphœa, the skin is thickened, inelastic, and adherent to the deeper tissues, so that it cannot be pinched up, and feels both colder and dryer than the normal skin. Irregular spots of pigment are sometimes met with on or round the patches. Sensibility is sometimes slightly impaired, and the temperature of the part is diminished 1° or 2° Fahr. The epidermis is normal, but may desquamate, and vesicles or other eruptions can appear upon it as on healthy skin. The secretions of the sweat and sebaceous glands are usually, but not invariably, diminished.

When scleroderma is first developed there is a slight localized raised swelling, produced by œdema in the subcutane-

ous tissue, pitting on pressure, and gradually becoming sclerosed. But as the disease progresses the patches become
level with or slightly depressed below the surface of the adjacent skin, and in the variety characterized by the presence
of long hands the healthy skin rises on each side of them.
The indurated patches subsequently, like those of morphœa,
either undergo complete resolution or sclerosis and atrophy.
The mucous membrane of the mouth, the tongue, and the
pharynx sometimes present similar hard white patches.
Patches of morphœa may precede or accompany the development of scleroderma, and the edge of a scleroderma-
tous patch not unfrequently presents an appearance identical with morphœa. The differences in form and color are
comparatively unimportant in view of the resemblances in
the rigid, infiltrated condition of the skin, the similarity, if
not identity, of the anatomical changes, the chronic course
ending in atrophy or resolution of the affected-portions of
skin, and the retention of the cutaneous sensibility observed
in both affections. Hence morphœa and scleroderma, if not
merely stages of the same disease, are certainly due to variations in the intensity and exact localization of the same
morbid process, and bear the same relation to one another as
lupus erythematosus does to lupus vulgaris. In morphœa
the unsymmetrical character of the patches, their abrupt
limitation by the middle line, their arrangement along the
course of cutaneous nerves, as in zoster, in lines or clusters,
the occasional check to the development of the bones of a
limb, and the slow course, unaffected by treatment, are points
which strongly support the theory advocated by Mr. Hutchinson, that, like zoster, the primary cause of the disease is
an affection of the nervous system.

When scleroderma attacks the face, the countenance becomes fixed, the normal folds of the skin disappear, the lips
and eyelids are rigid and sometimes everted, and the move-

ments of the jaws and neck are interfered with, owing to the want of elasticity of the skin.

In the extremities the firm, tendinous bands stiffen the joints, which then become semiflexed and almost immovable, and sometimes deepseated pains are left in the fasciæ and bones. When atrophy of the skin has set in the subcutaneous tissue and muscles waste away, the thin, shrivelled, smooth, and reddish band of pigmented cutis appears to be in direct contact with the bones, and the wasted limb has a dried-up, skeleton-like appearance, which is persistent.

Diagnosis.—Morphœa differs from scleroderma in the form of its patches, which are round or oval and usually small, instead of being ribbonlike and covering a large area, and in their color, which is violet or lilac colored at its sharply defined margin, surrounded usually by a deeply pigmented ring, and yellowish in its central portion as compared with the pale white of scleroderma.

Prognosis.—Like morphœa, scleroderma never causes death, though helplessness and great deformity may result from it. The patches occasionally undergo spontaneous resolution, and the skin resumes its normal character.

Morbid Anatomy.—Sections of the skin in this disease show a general thickening and induration of the corium, which passes gradually into and is fused with the subcutaneous fatty tissue. Microscopically examined, the epidermis is found to be normal, excepting that the rete cells contain some granular pigment. The papillæ are unchanged in shape, but their connective tissue stroma is much more condensed, and forms a narrow meshwork of condensed fibrous bundles. The connective tissue fibres of the corium are much thickened, form a compressed feltwork, and invade the subdermic fatty tissue, broad, dense bundles replacing the thin fibrils between groups of fat cells and compressing them firmly. Cords and networks of round and spindle cells are also found surrounding the fat cells. The vessels in many

places are narrowed and surrounded by round and spindle
cells, but are not usually obliterated or deficient in number.
Sebaceous and sweat glands and hair follicles are but little,
if at all, altered, and the arrectores pilorum are distinct.
In extreme cases the sclerotic changes extend throughout the
subcutaneous tissue, which is much atrophied, even down to
the fascia of the muscles, and there is considerable increase
in number of the elastic fibres.

The disease is considered to begin in the cellular deposits
round the vessels, and in the stage of infiltration to spread
thence in cords along the connective tissue bundles. As the
cellular infiltration becomes converted into fibrous and
elastic tissue the sclerosis of the skin observed in the latter
stages is gradually developed.

The anatomical changes in morphœa have not yet been
completely investigated, but are probably analogous to those
in scleroderma.

Treatment.—No specific internal remedy or local treatment has any effect on the disease, but nutritious diet, good
hygiene, and tonics are recommended.

Sclerema Neonatorum.

Definition.—An acute œdema and induration of the skin,
occurring in young children.

Symptoms.—The cause of this disease is not well understood, but it is believed to be due to some alteration in the
condition of the capillaries, resulting from some previously
existing disease, such as affections of the intestines, lung, or
brain, or some congenital defect. It may also result from
impaired nutrition or syphilis.

It commences with swelling of the lower extremities, following œdema and induration of the skin of the part, which
is itself tense, shining, pits on pressure, and of a red, white,
or livid color.

After a time, varying from a few hours to two or three days, the swelling subsides, leaving the skin wrinkled; sometimes, however, the advanced stage of wrinkling of the skin is the first symptom, and is not preceded by the earlier stage of œdema. The general condition of the child is much altered, and it shows but few signs of vitality, while the temperature is lowered by two or three degrees. The disease gradually spreads upwards till the skin of the face is affected, when the features become immovable and neither the eyes nor mouth can be opened. The reduction of temperature and the loss of vitality continue till death results after from two to ten days' illness.

Diagnosis.—This disease resembles no other. A local œdema cannot be mistaken for it for more than a few hours, and the general condition then suffices to distinguish between the two.

Prognosis.—It is usually fatal.

Morbid Anatomy.—Few changes have been found beyond a more or less œdematous infiltration of the whole skin and a rigid condition of the subcutaneous connective tissue. A slight increase of connective tissue in the deeper corium layer, and nodules and cords of embryonic tissue in the panniculus adiposus between the fat cells, have also been described by some authors.

Treatment.—This consists in first removing the primary cause, when it can be ascertained, and afterwards in restoring, when possible, the circulation through the capillaries of the affected part.

ELEPHANTIASIS ARABUM.

Definition.—Elephantiasis Arabum is an enlargement of some part of the body, usually a limb, due to hypertrophy of the whole of the connective tissue, following an inflammatory condition of the part.

Symptoms.—Under the name of elephantiasis several entirely distinct diseases have been included, and much confusion has resulted from the indiscriminate use of the word; thus, elephantiasis Græcorum is simply leprosy, and elephantiasis Italica is another name for pellagra. It is especially common in hot climates, such as the west coast of Africa, Barbadoes, and Malabar. Its prevalence is not confined to any particular sex, age, or race, but various conditions have been suspected to be concerned in its etiology. It has been attributed to injuries of the veins and lymphatics, which have caused compression, and to lupus, and apparently with some reason to the gummata of syphilis. Elephantiasis Arabum begins with an erysipelatous inflammation of the skin, usually of the leg, which is accompanied with or preceded by feverishness and symptoms of general constitutional disturbance resembling intermittent fever. These symptoms gradually subside, but some amount of swelling of the skin remains. After a variable interval the inflammation of the skin, with redness, swelling, and pain, returns again, accompanied with or preceded by symptoms of constitutional disturbance. The same subsidence takes place, but the local effects last longer than in the previous attack, and leave a greater amount of permanent œdematous swelling behind them. These attacks are repeated from time to time during a series of years, and thus a gradual enlargement of the limb takes place until it has attained huge proportions.

The skin is greatly thickened, shiny, stretched, and of a color varying from light brown to purple. Desquamation may be present, or the skin may be smooth and frequently fissured, when the natural furrows are greatly exaggerated, owing to the thickening of the skin, and when the epidermis is heaped up and macerated by perspiration. The surface may be surmounted with tubercles, the result of growth of fibro-cellular tissue, or with large papillæ, which may or may not be covered with epidermis. Sometimes the whole limb is covered with eczema, and occasionally the skin ulcerates, forming sores of varying size, from which a foul discharge exudes. Enlargement of the lymphatics causes them to stand up on the surface like vesicles, and when they burst or are punctured the milky lymph escapes. Each attack is accompanied by stabbing pains in the limb, but they are more severe at the beginning than at any subsequent period. Severe pain is, however, always felt if the limb be allowed to be in a dependent position for any length of time. Diminution of the sensibility of the surface also results from the disease. The enormous increase of the leg and foot when that part is affected causes the obliteration of the instep and upper part of the foot, and makes it resemble the foot of an elephant, whence the peculiar name.

Elephantiasis of the genitals differs slightly from that of any other part, and affects the scrotum, penis, labia, and clitoris. It commences "in the form of a hard kernel under the skin, usually at the bottom of the left side of the scrotum." From this point the disease spreads, and the skin over it becomes thickened and wrinkled, while the shape of the abdomen undergoes alteration. The penis is also increased in size, but lies partially imbedded in the enlarged scrotum. The skin of its lower surface is pushed forwards, and is only connected with the penis round the glans. The hypertrophied scrotum becomes covered with dilated lymphatics, which at a later stage burst and permit lymph to exude.

The regions usually affected are the lower extremities and the genitals, but the upper extremities and ears may also be the seats of the disease.

Diagnosis.—Simple œdema is the only condition which bears the slightest resemblance to elephantiasis, but never leads to hypertrophy of the tissues.

19

Prognosis.—Elephantiasis may last a lifetime, and although it has no tendency to spontaneous recovery, it is, while life lasts, amenable to treatment.

Morbid Anatomy.—Sections of a limb affected with elephantiasis show the corium thickened and much indurated, the subcutaneous connective tissue greatly increased, in some parts dense and glistening, in others soft and gelatinous: the muscles wasted, soft and yellowish: the fasciæ, intermuscular tissue and periosteum much thickened: and the bones hypertrophied, increased in both length and thickness, and presenting frequently irregular exostoses, which sometimes unite together adjacent bones. Caries and necrosis may also be present. A clear, yellowish, coagulable lymph exudes freely from the cut surface. The veins are dilated, and in places plugged by clots, and here and there may be observed irregular spaces filled with clear lymph.

Microscopically examined the epidermis and papillary layer are seen to be raised into rugose, prominent masses, resembling ichthyosis. In these masses the epidermic horny layers are much thickened, the rete cells pigmented, and the papillæ greatly increased in size. The corium bundles of connective tissue are increased in thickness, present a swollen, gelatinous, and glistening appearance, and are closely felted together. Fusiform and stellate cells are seen between them in places. The subcutaneous connective tissue is occasionally more than an inch thick, in some places dense and fibrous, and fused with the corium, in others soft and gelatinous, consisting of loose areolar and embryonic connective tissue, pervaded with lymph, and in the latter case it merges into the fascia and areolæ, which themselves present similar changes. The muscles, from atrophy and fatty degeneration, become pale, and often seem to lose their true striated fibres, which are apparently replaced by fatty and granular debris, while the nerves are also compressed, indurated, and atrophied. The bloodvessels present their normal arrangement, except that they are more widely separated, owing to the increase of connective tissue. The veins, dilated and thickened in places, are sometimes thrombosed, and in later stages are indicated only by pigmented fibrous cords. The lymphatics are in places much dilated and form small cysts, the walls of which, though usually thickened, are sometimes thin and friable. The interstitial lymph spaces and canaliculi are also enlarged, and here and there form cysts filled with clear yellow lymph or gelatinous embryonic connective tissue.

When the lymphatics are ruptured they discharge abundantly, and the discharge, which consists of lymph or chylous fluid, has been found in some cases to contain filaria sanguinis hominis. The dilatations are ascribed by some authors to the irritation excited by these parasites and the obstruction caused by them in the lymph channels.

The hair follicles, sweat and sebaceous glands, much elongated and widely separated, but otherwise little altered, in the early stages of the disease, becoming later compressed and atrophied.

Treatment.—The first thing to be done is to allay the inflammation by complete rest and, if possible, the elevation of the part affected, and by the application of warm poultices. After the inflammation has been reduced Hebra recommends the use of baths, poultices, and ointments to remove the accumulation of epidermis, and subsequently inunction with blue ointment. Bandages must next be applied to reduce the size of the limb, and Martin's elastic bandage is probably the best for the purpose. Ligature of the main vessel of the limb has been recommended, but with such slight success as hardly to warrant its general adoption.

ELEPHANTIASIS TELEANGIECTODES.

Definition.—This disease is closely related to elephantiasis Arabum, but differs from it in that it may arise without any previous inflammation and is usually congenital.

Symptoms.—This disease is either congenital or appears soon after birth, and is due to some obstruction of the lymphatics. The skin of a limb becomes hypertrophied, and hangs down in rolls or flaps, which vary in color, owing to the enlargement of the vessels, but if pressure be steadily exerted on one of these flaps its size becomes considerably reduced. Although the thickening of the skin which hangs from the lower part of a limb produces an apparent increase in the size of the limb, the upper part has really wasted, and this atrophy is not confined to the skin, but includes the muscles and bones. After a time a quantity of vesicles appear, which may be arranged in groups or lines or may be scattered irregularly, and when these are ruptured the lymph which they contain exudes.

Morbid Anatomy.—In elephantiasis teleangiectodes the essential morbid process is a new formation of connective tissue, at first embryonic, but later on dense and fibrous, in the subcutaneous tissue. The growths next present changes in the skin and subcutaneous tissue analogous to those in elephantiasis Arabum; they are, however, pervaded by slits, gaps, and cysts filled with lymph, and by numerous bloodvessels, which are dilated, communicate freely, and sometimes become cavernous.

Treatment.—Is identical with that suggested for elephantiasis Arabum.

DERMATOLYSIS.

Definition.—Dermatolysis is a growth of the skin, causing it to hang in folds.

Symptoms.—The disease may occur in any part of the body, but according to Alibert it most frequently attacks the eyebrows, face, neck, abdomen, and labia, and is due to a pathological change in the skin, causing an increase of the fibro-cellular tissue. The skin hangs in folds, but no other symptom is present beyond some loss of sensibility in the part.

CHAPTER XVIII.

Class V.—ATROPHIÆ.

Albinismus—Leucoderma—Atrophia cutis.

Pigmentary.

1. Albinismus. 2. Leucoderma.

ALBINISMUS.

Definition.—Albinismus is a congenital absence of pigment from the skin, hair, iris, and choroid, which may be either general or local.

Persons suffering from general deficiency or absence of pigment are termed albinos.

Symptoms.—In albinos the skin is dull white and of delicate texture, the hair is fine and yellowish or white, the iris is pink, and the choroid being devoid of the normal dark pigment, the pupil appears red instead of black. Persons thus affected are stated to be usually of delicate health, and their skins are more prone to suffer from exposure to heat and cold.

The affection is more frequently met with in the tropics, and is more noticed in the dark races.

In the partial form of the disease patches resembling leucoderma are found scattered about the body, giving the person, if dark, a piebald appearance.

Morbid Anatomy.—Microscopic examination of the skin of albinos shows absence of the normal pigment from the deeper rete cells.

Treatment.—No treatment is of any avail.

LEUCODERMA—WHITE LEPROSY.

Definition.—A local deficiency or absence of pigment from the skin and hair, developed after birth and slowly spreading, but causing no constitutional disturbance.

Symptoms.—Leucoderma begins by the appearance of one or more round white patches on various parts of the body, generally near brown moles or warts. The patch has a defined margin, bordered by a ring of excessive pigmentation, which gradually merges in the healthy skin, and the hair on the patch is also white, but the affected skin in every respect except the absence of pigment presents no structural or functional difference from healthy skin. As the patches gradually enlarge they become oval, and by confluence form large pale tracts with convex margins bounded by deeply pigmented rings. As time goes on and the white patches spread, more and more of the skin is affected, till finally only a few brown patches with concave edges are left to represent the normal skin. The disease may originate at any age, but most frequently after puberty, and is almost always bilateral, though exact symmetry is rarely found.

Diagnosis.—The pale patches of lepra maculosa or lepra anæsthetica may be distinguished from those of leucoderma in that their edges are more shaded, the skin often infiltrated and anæsthetic in the centre as well as scarred, and that they often have a purplish raised hyperæsthetic border, whereas those of leucoderma have a sharply defined border and a dark pigmented ring. The structure and functions of the skin also in the latter are normal.

The concave edges of the dark patches which represent normal skin will enable extensive leucoderma to be distinguished from abnormal development of pigment in a healthy skin.

Prognosis.—Leucoderma causes no pain or inconvenience to the person affected, but the white patches, though they

sometimes become stationary, have no tendency to disappea
spontaneously or under treatment.

Morbid Anatomy.—The only change that has been de
tected is an absence of pigment from the deeper layers o
the rete and from the hairs and their bulbs.

Treatment.—No remedies have yet been found to remov
the white patches.

Of Connective Tissue.

ATROPHIA CUTIS.

Atrophy of the skin, besides occurring as a result of vari
ous inflammatory affections or new growths of the skin, is
met with as an independent disease, both in a general and
a partial form.

The first condition is usually a result of retrogressive or
degenerative changes in old persons, and has been called
senile atrophy.

In it the skin becomes dry, wrinkled, rough, less supple
and more or less pigmented. The epidermis is smooth, o
in places branny, the cutis and its papillæ are thinned and
wasted, and the subcutaneous fatty tissue is usually atro
phied. Hairs are scanty or wanting, and the sebaceou
glands either atrophied or presenting degeneration in th
form of milium granules. Anatomically the tissues may
be found either in a condition which is mainly that of *simple
atrophy*, or, in addition, more or less marked *degenerative
metamorphoses* are present.

In the former condition of simple atrophy the cuticle i
thin and the papillæ either wanting or projecting very
slightly above the level of the corium. The corium meshe
are thin, narrow, and contain few small corpuscles and very
little interstitial fluid, while granular pigment, diffuse or in
masses, is abundant. The fat cells are wasted, and contai
vacuoles in places instead of oil globules. The vessels are
thin, atrophied, and pigmented in some places, but varicos

in others, and the hair follicles, though present, have their papillæ wasted and contain no hairs, or only their lanuginous filaments.

In the degenerative conditions, in addition to the simple atrophy, the skin, in tracts of varying extent, becomes brittle and extremely thin, while its connective tissue bundles become converted into a vitreous or gelatinous mass, in which no vessels or nerves are visible. The hair and glandular follicles are also degenerated. The process is supposed to begin in the arterioles, like albuminoid degeneration, and to spread thence to the other tissue.

Partial atrophy of the skin is observed in the form of white scarlike parallel bands, a half to two lines broad and several inches long, or in scattered round maculæ, a quarter to two lines in diameter.

The striæ (*linear atrophy*) which are the most common have a glistening bluish-white appearance, and the skin forming them is unduly thin and depressed. They usually occur on the pelvic brim, the glutei, and the trochanters, and less frequently on the fronts of the thighs or the arms. Under the microscope the papillary layer is found atrophied, the corium much thinned, with its bundles delicate and its vessels fewer in number, and the subcutaneous fatty tissue and appendages are wasted.

The maculæ are much less frequently observed, but Dr. Liveing has found the following changes to occur in them: The spots, at first somewhat reddish, raised above the skin, hard and fibrous, passed on into the ordinary atrophic condition, appearing as discrete round or oval pitlike scars, covered by a thin membrane, and all about the size of a threepenny-piece. Finally a stage of contraction or obliteration sets in, and the spots become less apparent, as if encroached upon by the surrounding healthy tissues. Liveing believes this disease to be allied to scleroderma and morphœa, with which it has been several times associated.

20

CHAPTER XIX.

Class VI.—NEOPLASMATA.

Sub-class A.—*Benign.*

Clavus—Tylosis—Verruca—Cornu cutaneum—Keloid—Fibroma—
Xanthoma—Lupus vulgaris—Lupus erythematosus—Rhinoscleroma—Nævus—Angioma—Lymphangioma.

Papillomatous.

1. Clavus and Tylosis.   2. Verruca.   3. Cornu cutaneum.

CLAVUS AND TYLOSIS.

Definition.—Tylosis, or tyloma, is merely an undue accumulation of horny epidermis, which appears usually on
the extremities, on parts exposed to pressure. The thickened epidermis merges gradually on each side into the normal, and there is little or no affection of the corium.

Clavus, or "corn," is the name applied to an epidermic
accumulation, resembling that in tylosis, in the centre of
which is a conical plug, the apex being situated on, and
pressing down, the corium.

Symptoms.—Tylosis causes usually little or no inconvenience, unless the accumulation be very thick and horny.
Under these circumstances, when affecting the palm, it interferes much with the movements of the hand. When
irritated, a vesicle may be formed, which spreads into a
bulla, the fluid, on account of its long retention, becoming
purulent, and thus a subepidermic abscess may be produced.

The horny crust is loosened and cast off, leaving, after the ulcerated base heals, a perfectly normal surface.

A "corn," on the other hand, causes usually depression, and atrophy of the papillæ beneath its "core," and when pressed upon gives rise to severe pain. It is generally produced by the pressure of a tight boot on the toes. When seated between the toes the maceration by retained moisture prevents it from assuming the horny character of the callosity, and hence this is the distinction between hard and soft corns.

Morbid Anatomy.—Tylosis consists of an undue thickening of the epithelium. The horny layers are increased in number and thickness, and the papillæ are somewhat enlarged and more vascular.

Sections through a corn show an epithelial accumulation and papillary hypertrophy identical with that in tylosis. In the centre of the patch, however, a conical epidermic plug is found, the layers of which are concave towards the free surface of the skin. The papillæ beneath it, at first enlarged, are gradually atrophied as the growth deepens, which causes wasting of the corium and glands, till the core finally lies in a pit in the corium.

Treatment.—Occasional rubbing down of the horny mass with a file is all that is needed in tylosis. When affecting the palm, dressing with lint soaked in liquor potassæ and covered with oiled silk, and subsequent scraping away of the softened epidermis, restores mobility to the parts.

Corns may be treated by placing a disk of felt plaster, with a hole in the centre, over them, so as to remove pressure. Dressing with liquor potassæ or with strong nitric acid will often, after a time, cause the disappearance of the affection, and in obstinate cases excision of the corn, with the papillæ from which it grows, may be necessary.

VERRUCA—WART.

Definition.—A wart is a small excrescence of the skin, or mucous membrane near the junction with the skin, consisting of a localized hypertrophy of the papillæ and the epidermis covering them.

Symptoms.—Warts may be *hard* when exposed to the air on cutaneous surfaces, or *soft* when seated on mucous membranes, kept constantly moist by secretions; they may also be simple or compound, the latter being made up of a bunch of filiform papillæ, usually pedunculate. Simple warts consist of a group of elongated papillæ, surrounded by a common epithelial envelope, the surface of which, however, usually presents fissures marking the extent of each papilla. Hard warts, on the hands, body, and head, may appear suddenly in great numbers, and grow rapidly, and as they are also liable to involution and spontaneous disappearance, various quack remedies, "charms," etc., have been able to acquire an easy but somewhat doubtful reputation.

Soft warts, or condylomata, are usually pointed, and are much softer and more vascular than the hard; they occur most often on the perinæum, round the anus, and on the genitals, owing to the irritation of the gonorrhœal discharge, syphilis, or decomposing sweat in persons of dirty habits. They have no tendency to spontaneous involution.

Morbid Anatomy.—In the flat warts vertical sections show merely an aggregation of hypertrophied, sometimes branched, papillæ, the vessels of which are enlarged, and the epidermis covering them is much thickened. The columnar cells of the rete are specially numerous, and fill up the interpapillary spaces. In the round, prominent, or conical warts the hypertrophied, much-elongated papillæ are still imbedded in a mass of thickened epithelium, which envelops them in a common sheath; but indications of the extent of each papilla are presented by numerous fine cracks, which split it up into polygonal areæ, each corresponding to a papilla and its envelope. In the filiform warts the papillæ, delicate and branched, have each a separate epidermic coat, and the little mass appears like a bundle of fine bristles.

Treatment.—Hard warts, not showing any tendency to disappear, may be snipped off with curved scissors, and some styptic or cautery may be applied to the seat of attachment if there is any bleeding. If sessile, the repeated application of glacial acetic acid, of chromic or nitric acids or liquor potassæ, will usually cause them to shrivel up.

Condylomata may also be treated by excision and styptics if few in number. If numerous, they should be removed with Paquelin's benzolin cautery.

CORNU—HORN.

Definition.—A cutaneous horn consists of a curved, conical-ridged, brownish mass, and may be considered as a wart, the epidermis over which has a columnar structure and is closely compressed like that of the nails.

Symptoms.—Horns usually occur on the head, but sometimes on the penis, and they may be several inches long and spirally twisted. Occasionally they arise within a sebaceous follicle. Their growth is attended with little or no pain.

Treatment.—Excision of the horn, with the portion of skin from which it grows, is the only effectual cure.

Of Connective Tissue.

   1. Keloid.   2. Fibroma.   3. Xanthoma.

KELOID—KELOID OF ALIBERT.

Definition.—Keloid is a rare affection of the skin, consisting in the formation, spontaneously or in the seat of former scars, of a firm nodular tumor, composed of hypertrophied fibrous tissue, tender on pressure and sometimes attended with itching and tingling.

Symptoms.—There is no essential difference between the "spontaneous" or "true" and the so-called "false" keloid, developed in cicatrices, and there is some doubt whether the "true" keloid of Alibert does not really arise in small, insignificant scars, the origin of which has been forgotten. The affection named keloid by Addison is identical with, and has been described under the head of, Morphœa.

Keloid grows slowly as a rounded, oval, fusiform, or nodular patch, raised one or more lines above the surface of the skin, in which it appears imbedded. Occasionally it presents the shape of a stellate or radiating, latticelike formation, and sends out processes like the claws of a crab, which gradually subside in the surrounding skin. It is firm and elastic to the touch, has a smooth surface, is white, or occasionally pinkish, shiny, and marked by ramifying vessels. The surface is never scaly, and the tumor has no tendency at any time to ulcerate or break down. Tenderness on pressure is usually present, and sometimes tingling, itching, or burning.

The growths occur as isolated patches on the sternum, mammæ, sides of the trunk, or back; they may be single, but are more frequently multiple, and sometimes are met with all over the body. The cicatricial variety may develop in scars, present in any situation, but it is said to be more common in the dark races in the scars left by flogging. It usually occurs in adults. Kaposi states that new patches arise as follows :

"They consist, at the commencement, of brownish-red streaks of skin, with a pale-red or whitish lustre, of the size of oats or barleycorns, flat or already slightly elevated, communicating a sense of resistance, and are for the most part slightly painful on pressure. In the course of many mouths, or of years, the linear or streaky keloid increases in one or other direction, or in every superficial dimension, and thus assumes one of the characteristic shapes mentioned above, with or without processes. At the same time it will have become somewhat thicker and more elevated."

Keloid, once fully developed, remains, as a rule, unaltered for life ; in only a few cases has spontaneous involution, or even complete disappearance of a single patch, been observed (Alibert and Hebra).

Clinically, keloid arising in or round about a scar is indistinguishable in its course and symptoms from the spontaneous variety.

Diagnosis.—A firm, whitish or pinkish, slightly elevated tumor in the skin, sending out clawlike processes, tender on pressure, growing slowly, and manifesting no tendency to degenerative changes, can only be a keloid or a hypertrophied scar. In course and symptoms there is no valid mark of separation between the two, and microscopic examination alone will complete the diagnosis.

Prognosis.—Keloid does not affect the general health, and causes only slight inconvenience by the tenderness and occasional tingling. When removed by operation, it almost invariably recurs, and is then larger than the previous growth.

Morbid Anatomy—Vertical sections of a " true " keloid tumor show a mass of dense white fibrous tissue, imbedded in the substance of the corium.

Under the microscope the bundles of tissue composing it are seen to run parallel to the surface of the skin and to the long axis of the tumor. The epidermis, and papillæ covering it, are normal, and the sebaceous and sweat glands, pushed aside at the margin, but not otherwise altered, may be strangulated and degenerated in the portion of corium above and below the nodule. Nuclei, spindle cells, and connective tissue corpuscles, almost wanting in the centre,

are more abundant in the periphery, especially round the
vessels which seem to form centres for the formation of the
growth.

In cicatricial keloid a nodule, of the same nature, is found
imbedded in ordinary scar tissue, which forms a sort of capsule round it, and is covered by a layer of pigmented epithelium without papillæ.

In a hypertrophied scar the pigmented rete layer of the
epidermis lies on a meshwork of irregularly interlacing
fibrous bundles, the papillæ being absent. Numerous round
spindle and stellate cells and bloodvessels—some pervious
while others are seen as fibrous, pigmented cord,—are
present throughout.

Treatment.—Any attempt to remove the tumor by excision, caustics, or the actual cautery should be discouraged,
on account of the speedy return and enlargement of· the
growth. The pain, if severe, should be mitigated by subcutaneous injection of morphia, or by an aconite ointment.

Fibroma—Molluscum Fibrosum.

Definition.—Small, sessile, pedunculate, usually multiple
growths, arising in the superficial layers of the corium and
of somewhat gelatinous structure.

Symptoms.—The disease begins by the appearance of
small, softish masses in the skin, most commonly on the
- chest, back, and neck, which grow slowly, and vary in size
from a small shot to a large nut. From being at first sessile, as they enlarge they become more or less pedunculated,
and sometimes even pendulous. They usually occur in
adults, are covered with normal skin, and cause no pain or
constitutional symptoms.

Diagnosis.—The little soft, usually multiple, tumors are
distinguished from molluscum contagiosum by the absence
of a central umbilicus, and by the fact that they consist

of solid tissue, and their contents cannot therefore be pressed out.

Prognosis.—Fibroma is troublesome only on account of the deformity it causes; it is, as a rule, unattended with pain, and is in no way dangerous to life.

Morbid Anatomy.—The little growths present a whitish centre and gelatinous margin, and on microscopic examination are found to consist, in the centre, of young connective tissue, the meshes of which contain abundant serous fluid with some spindle and round cells, while the periphery may be composed of more or less mucoid tissue, with numerous branched and spindle cells. The growth, according to Rindfleisch, begins in the papillary layer.

Treatment.—The only measure of any avail is the removal of the tumors by operation, which should only be undertaken if they cause considerable deformity, or if, by pressing on nerves, they give rise to pain or inconvenience. If pendulous, a ligature may be used, or they may be snipped off with scissors. As numerous vessels enter their base, sharp bleeding may follow their removal by operation, but this can be usually stopped by pressure.

XANTHOMA—XANTHELASMA—VITILIGOIDEA.

Definition.—Xanthoma consists in the formation of yellow or buff-colored, clearly defined patches in the skin, on a level with it or only slightly raised, and most frequently in association with prolonged jaundice.

Symptoms.—Xanthoma occurs in adults, and about twice as frequently in women as in men. It may be localized and limited to the eyelids only, where it usually begins, or patches may be found scattered all over the surface of the body, in the mucous membranes, and in the sheaths of tendons.

Two forms are described :

1. Xanthoma planum.   2. Xanthoma tuberosum.

1. *Xanthoma planum* begins, usually symmetrically, near the inner canthus, and extends slowly along both lids, especially the upper one, spreading then over the adjacent part of the cheek where the skin is thin. The patches, of different sizes, and varying in color from yellowish-white to a faded buff or a chamois-leather tint, have sharply defined margins, a smooth surface level with the skin or raised into little tubercles at the edges. There is no difference in consistence or thickness between the affected and the healthy skin, and usually no subjective symptoms are present.

2. *Xanthoma tuberosum* occurs as isolated nodules, or plaques, made up of aggregations of little tubercles, varying in size from a millet seed to a grain of wheat, just slightly raised above the level of the skin. They occur but rarely on the eyelids, more often on the cheeks and ears, hands and feet, and sometimes generally over the whole surface of the body. They can be pinched up with the skin, with which they are continuous, have a feeling of elasticity, and are attended with slight tenderness on pressure. On the palms and soles, however, they often cause severe pricking and burning pain, which interferes much with the use of the limb. Both forms of xanthoma not unfrequently occur in the same individual. The patches, growing slowly by extension or by the formation of new marginal spots, reach their full development, and remain unaltered for the rest of life, undergoing no degenerative changes and causing no impairment of the general health. They have been observed in various diseases, and even in healthy persons, but in a large number of cases—in 15 out 30 enumerated by Kaposi—persistent jaundice has preceded or accompanied them. Whether, however, the jaundice—produced most frequently, according to Charcot, by hypertrophic cirrhosis—is the cause of the skin affection, or whether both phenomena are due to some other factor, is as yet unsettled.

Diagnosis.—Xanthoma may be mistaken for confluent masses of milium, especially on the eyelids. A superficial cut over the mass enables the milium granules to be easily squeezed out, whereas xanthoma, being imbedded in and continuous with the healthy corium, cannot thus be enucleated.

Prognosis.—Xanthoma is in no way dangerous to life, exerts no influence on the general health, and is annoying only from its unsightliness and from the pain when on the palms or soles.

Morbid Anatomy.—Vertical sections show a pale-red surface, interspersed with yellow spots which cannot be squeezed out. Under the microscope the papillæ and epidermis are almost normal, the only change being the deposit of much yellowish pigment in the rete cells and throughout the corium. In the cutis the yellow spots are made up of densely fibrillated connective tissue, with more or less abundant stellate or roundish cells intermixed. The changes are most marked round the hair follicles and sebaceous glands. Pigment granules are scattered throughout, but the yellow color is due mainly to fat, which occurs as fine globules in the stellate cells, or as a coarsely granular mass with some large globules between and in the connective tissue bundles. The change differs from atheroma, which it much resembles, in being an infiltration, and not a degeneration, of the new-formed connective tissue.

Treatment.—The excision of the whole nodule down to the subcutaneous tissue, in such a place that the scar will not subsequently cause interference with the functions of the part, is the only remedy.

Granulation Tissue Growths.

1. Lupus vulgaris. 2. Lupus erythematosus. 3. Rhinoscleroma.

LUPUS.

Definition.—A chronic, non-infectious disease, consisting in the deposit of nests of small round cells, irregularly placed in the substance of the corium, or more specially round the vessels in the plexuses of sweat and sebaceous glands. The deposits terminate either in interstitial absorption or in breaking down and ulceration, and leave superficial scars.

Symptoms.—Though various forms of lupus have been described under separate names, and the distinctions laid down are sufficiently marked in typical instances, the occurrence, in practice, of various transitional forms, and the presence, occasionally, of two varieties in the same individual, tend to show that the different varieties of lupus are due, like those of eczema, merely to local peculiarities of site, and to degrees of development of one or other of the morbid phenomena met with in the disease. Thus in lupus vulgaris the cellular new growth is well marked, and may either be confined to the upper layer of the skin, or disseminated in nodules, or diffused through the whole thickness of the corium, while in lupus erythematosus the hyperæmia of the plexus round the sebaceous glands is the main feature, the new growth being but small.

Lupus vulgaris occurs at first as small reddish or yellowish-brown nodules—presenting an " apple-jelly " appearance—about the size of a pin's head or shot, either diffusely scattered or aggregated closely in groups in the substance of the skin. They are not raised, and get paler, but do not disappear on pressure, and are covered by smooth epidermis. They may be quite superficial or deep in the substance of the corium, and enlarge slowly, new nodules appearing as the old reach their full development. The firm, transparent masses thus formed are painless, and often, by confluence, form flattened plaques, the size of a sixpence or larger, raised about a line above the level of the surface, irregular or smooth, and covered by shiny desquamating epithelium. By continued growth of the nodules projecting tubercles may be formed, and persist without change for a long time.

As the disease progresses either involution or ulceration may take place. In the former the tubercle becomes flaccid, the skin over it shrunken and wrinkled, and covered with white scales or scabs, which on falling off leave a central white, glistening, cicatricial depression, that is firm and contracts but little. In the latter the tubercle softens, disintegrates, and secretes pus, which dries up, forming thin yellowish or greenish crusts, resting on a depressed ulcer, with soft, defined edges and a red, smooth, bleeding base. As time goes on the skin between the granulations is more or less thoroughly destroyed, the tendons, fasciæ, and other subcutaneous structures attacked, and an ulcer is formed with hard or undermined edges, and a base, covered with exuberant or friable granulations, which heals but slowly after it may be weeks, months, or even years. But while retrogression may be going on in one part, new nodules are constantly appearing in the margin of the patch, in skin previously free, or even in cicatrices left by the healing process, and thus the disease is constantly spreading. By the contact and fusion of two or more circular patches a gyrate appearance is produced, known as *lupus serpiginosus*. When the disease is superficial, and shrivels up without ulceration, it is called *lupus non-exedens*; when the growth forms prominent masses, *lupus tuberculatus*; *lupus exedens* and *lupus exulcerans* when ulceration has taken place ; and *lupus exfoliaceus* when it is undergoing absorption with desquamation, and not sloughing. Lupus vulgaris arises most commonly between the second and eighteenth years of life, and tends to disappear with advancing age, though relapses may occur at any period. It is rather more often met with in women than in men, is non-contagious, and though often and certainly associated with a strumous or phthisical diathesis, it does not appear to be hereditary. Lupus generally attacks the skin of the different parts of the body in the following order : the cheeks, the nose, the ears, the wrists, and the trunk. On the cheeks and nose it occurs usually as disseminated tubercles, which, after disappearance, leave the skin in a white, glistening, hairless condition, slightly pitted with scars. The mucous membrane of the mouth, nares, and fauces may be affected by extension of the disease from the nose and cheeks, in the nose the extension of the granulation tissue inwards to the mucous membrane eroding, and often replacing, the cartilage, and subsequently breaking down and giving rise to loss of substance and serious deformity. On the extremities lupus is usually serpiginous, though scattered spots may be found. The cicatrices which it produces may keep the elbows, knees, and fingers semiflexed and in a state of pseudo-anchylosis. In addition to this, lupus of the extremities is specially prone to erysipelas and lymphangitis, with occasional subcutaneous abscesses, and to the occurrence of periostitis, caries, and necrosis of the bones.

Lupus erythematosus begins usually as a reddish patch on the nose, with slightly irregular surface, followed soon by the development, on each cheek, of similar red patches. An erythematous spot, caused by heat or sunburn, or a small patch of eczema, may be the starting-point. On close examination the patches appear simply erythematous, and may come and go for some time before the disease becomes established, or they may be made up of an aggregation of slightly raised red spots, about the size of a pin's head, which become pale on pressure, and often present a light greasy scale in the centre. They constitute, according to Kaposi, the "primary eruptive spots" of the affection, and each corresponds with the opening of a sebaceous follicle, the little scale, made up of epidermis and sebum, sending a small conical plug down into the duct of the gland. In severe cases, where the spots are closely aggregated, the scales become rapidly confluent, and form an irregular, closely adherent crust. When this has been softened by oil and removed, numerous little processes, passing from its under surface into the follicles, can be seen, distinguishing it in the diagnosis from acute eczema.

When the spots remain discrete, they spread gradually at the margin, which is red, slightly raised, and covered with scales and comedones, while the centre becomes pale, depressed, and pitted.

In this way the patches join at the bridge of the nose, and the characteristic " butterfly " outline is produced, the portions on the cheeks representing the wings and that on the nose the body. Growing in this manner, the patches may spread to the scalp, or cover the whole side of the face, and new spots may develop on the ears, generally symmetrically, leaving a band of healthy skin between them and the cheek.

After persisting for a long time, often many years, the margins of the patch become paler, flatter, and gradually cease to grow, leaving a white superficial, slightly pitted scar, which may persist for the rest of life, or in process of time become almost imperceptible. Next to the cheeks, nose, and ears, the backs of the hands are most commonly affected, and it is rare for one hand only to suffer, the disease here, as elsewhere, preserving its tendency to symmetry.

In the disseminated and aggregated form (Kaposi) the individual spots do not spread at their margins as in the previously described or discoid variety, but run their course and cicatrize, leaving small pitted scars like those of acne or variola, and extension of the patches occurs by the development of new isolated spots in the adjacent tissue. Appearing first on the face, the patches may be confined to it or may spread thence to the scalp, neck, arms, and even the fingers and toes. At the onset the patch may be covered by an impetiginous scab, which, falling off after some days, exposes the primary eruptive spots. This form of lupus erythematosus is usually chronic, but may occur acutely, either primarily or supervening on the discoid or aggregated variety. Patches of densely aggregated spots appear first on the face, and in the course of a few days are followed by the eruption of hundreds of lupus spots all over the general surface. Other local and constitutional symptoms of some severity usually accompany the outburst. Of these Kaposi enumerates the following:

1. Subcutaneous, painful, and tender nodules, of doughy consistency, covered at first by normal skin, which in two or three days, as the swelling begins to subside, present a crop of primary eruptive spots.

2. Painful œdematous swellings of the skin and tissues round the joints of the hands and feet, and sometimes of the knee and elbow also, which, after some days, subside gradually with the development of spots of lupus erythematosus.

3. Large, hard, painful swellings of the submaxillary and axillary, and more rarely the inguinal and parotid glands, subsiding with the development of the eruption usually within a few weeks.

4. Erysipelas, or lymphangitis, only occurring chiefly in acute attacks in the parts affected by the painful subcutaneous swellings, and on the face and ears. It may also arise, in chronic cases, even if no operation have been performed, lupus erythematosus being more liable to it than lupus vulgaris. It is usually a grave complication, and is frequently fatal.

Diagnosis—Lupus Vulgaris.—The presence in the skin of the characteristic "apple-jelly" nodules is sufficient in itself for the diagnosis. Scabs, if present, should be removed by oiling, and if no spots are then discovered, waiting for a few weeks will usually enable the gradual development of new nodules to be seen.

From syphilis, in the form of serpiginous ulceration, lupus differs by its slower course, shallower and less painful ulcers, clean, soft, red base of granulatiou tissue, and by the presence in most cases of "apple-jelly" spots near the ulcerating surface. The failure of specific syphilitic treatment is also an important aid to diagnosis.

Epithelioma and rodent ulcer differ from it by reason of their greater hardness, by the induration of the margin, and by the fact that they never appear in childhood, and rarely till after thirty, whereas lupus, though it may recur later, usually appears for the first time in early life.

From lupus erythematosus lupus vulgaris differs so much in appearance, in typical cases, that no mistake can be made. When the two forms occur in combination in the same individual, the "apple-jelly" spots of vulgaris, and the hyperæmic follicles, with thin scales and sebaceous plugs of the erythematous variety, can usually be recognized.

Prognosis.—Lupus vulgaris affecting the skin is not in itself dangerous to life, although the attacks of erysipelas which occasionally complicate it may be serious. It sometimes disappears spontaneously and never recurs, and the diseased patches of tissue can be destroyed by energetic treatment. It is difficult, however, to do this effectually without damaging the skin so deeply as to cause subsequent cicatricial contraction, and hence, after all attempts to remove the diseased tissue alone, leaving the unaffected skin as little as possible damaged, the growth is prone to recur. Lupus erythematosus, except in the acute general form and when complicated with erysipelas, is also a benign disease.

The discoid is more amenable to treatment than the aggregated form, and the growth, when once destroyed, is less likely to recur than in lupus vulgaris.

Morbid Anatomy—Lupus Vulgaris.—According to Friedländer and Thoma, whose observations have been confirmed in this country by Dr. Thin, lupus vulgaris begins by an

21

aggregation of small round cells in the adventitia of the vessels of the corium. Local enlargements of the céllular deposit produce the little, scattered, roundish nodules, arranged like nests in fibrous loculi in the corium, composed of small young cells in a delicate fibrous network, permeated by a few dilated capillaries, and containing sometimes giant cells. The surrounding corium tissue remains at first free from infiltration, but the small-celled growth, extending along the vessels, reaches on one side the subpapillary layer and papillæ, and on the other the subcutaneous connective tissue and fat. The cellular infiltration next diffuses itself from these foci, till the whole corium, from the papillæ to the subcutaneous fat, is pervaded with small round cells, specially dense round the vessels, and hence accumulated thickly round the sweat glands, sebaceous and hair follicles. The cells of the glands and hair follicles, at first swollen and granular, soon degenerate and finally become atrophied and destroyed.

The rete Malpighii, at first normal, becomes later on thickened, and by the cellular infiltration, indistinguishable from the papillæ, its cells are swollen, more granular, and proliferating, and numerous round cells are scattered amongst them.

Fatty degeneration, breaking down of the cells, and ulceration of the growths next set in, but the process is a slow and superficial one, and the cells, in the deeper layers of an ulcerating spot, are frequently quite free from granules, and have distinct nuclei, while those on the surface are quite degenerated. Cicatrization finally occurs, and smooth scars result, from which the hair follicles and glands are absent.

Lupus Erythematosus.—In sections of the early "primary eruptive spots" of the disease, the first changes which have been observed are dilatation of the vessels round the sebaceous glands and hair follicles, with slight œdema, and, when the spots are superficial, similar appearances in the adjacent papillæ. In the next stage the connective tissue immediately around the glands is found thickly infiltrated with round cells, which extend into the corium and papillæ, obscuring the connective tissue bundles and the boundary between rete and papillæ; these, as atrophy begins, become cloudy, granular, and opaque, and begin to break down. The sweat glands are also sometimes affected.

Atrophy, or ulceration, with cicatrization being completed, the hairs and glands are found degenerated, the connective tissue thickened, indurated, and obscured by fatty globules, and the atrophied bloodvessels may be indicated only by pigmented strands. The rete is thinned, the papillæ absent, flattened, or wasted, and the whole corium is denser and has its meshes thickened.

Occasionally the granulation tissue, instead of spreading in lines along the meshes of the corium, becomes aggregated in nests, producing nodules identical with those of lupus vulgaris.

The painful nodes and swellings met with sometimes in acute outbreaks are due to inflammatory œdema of the skin and subcutaneous tissue.

Treatment.—Under the head of general treatment, applicable to both lupus erythematosus and lupus vulgaris, the chief indications are—first, if the general health is lowered, to restore and maintain it by means of a nutritious diet, with a moderate amount of stimulants and tonics, such as iron, quinine, etc.; and, secondly, to combat and remove, as far as possible, any morbid diathesis, such as the strumous or tubercular, with cod-liver oil, phosphate of lime, and iodide of iron. It should, however, be clearly understood that the administration of these remedies will not by itself remove the disease, for which purpose local treatment must be adopted.

In *lupus erythematosus* the local treatment consists in:

1. Removal of scales or crusts, if present.

2. Application of soothing remedies when the disease is in the acute stage.

3. Destruction of the new growth by mechanical or chemical means.

1. The removal of all crusts or scales, by careful oiling and washing with soap and water, is essential as a preliminary measure.

2. Simple ointments, such as vaseline ʒj with liq. plumbi ♏xxx, oleate of zinc or bismuth ʒiv to vaseline ʒj, zinc ointment, cold cream, cod-liver oil, sedative lotions containing calamine, or glycerin and prussic acid, will be found useful. Mr. Hutchinson has seen great improvement follow the steady use of an ointment of liq. carbonis detergens ʒss. to vaseline ʒj. All conditions that may irritate the skin, such as the heat of the sun, wind, or excessive cold, should be avoided.

3. For the destruction of the new growths, repeated multiple puncture, or linear scarification, as first recommended by Mr. Balmanno Squire, proves often of great service, destroying the dilated vessels and a portion of the new growth, which is still further removed by the subsequent inflammation. In very obstinate cases, where there is a more abundant formation of granulation tissue, scooping out the nodules with Volkmann's spoon may be necessary. Numerous caustics have been used, of which the spiritus saponatus alkalinus of Hebra is one of the best. It should be rubbed well into the patches with lint, removing all the scales. Crusts of dried-up blood and serum following the application should be removed by oiling, and the remedy used repeatedly till all traces of the disease have disappeared. Soft soap or liquor potassæ may be applied in the same way. Acids, such as the acid nitrate of mercury or nitric acid, may also be used, but are less effective than alkalies, as,

owing to the fatty crusts, they often operate less upon the diseased parts than upon adjacent healthy tissue. Hebra's arsenical paste is of value when other measures fail; its chief advantage is that it acts exclusively on the diseased tissue, and is not liable to cause toxic symptoms of absorption. It should be spread on lint and reapplied every twenty-four hours for two or three days. The severe pain and œdema of the skin, arising under its use, usually subside in a few days, and the destroyed patches of growth desquamate, leaving small cavities, which soon heal.

In *lupus vulgaris* the use of sedatives is also indicated, if there be much irritability or inflammation.

The nodules of growth may be destroyed by (1) mechanical means, (2) the actual cautery, (3) chemical caustics.

For the first purpose Squire's linear scarification is suitable, but only for the milder and more superficial forms of lupus, as it does not penetrate deep enough to destroy the little nests which lie in the substance of the corium. Multiple puncture, by making with a small sharp-pointed knife numerous little stabs close to one another in the diseased nodules, frequently yields good results, especially when the nodules are small, isolated, and penetrate deeply into the true skin. Where the growth occurs in the form of a large plaque, it is necessary to remove it by means of Volkmann's spoon. The scraping should be done vigorously, and, as there is a marked difference between the soft, friable lupus tissue and the dense, fibrous corium, even on the face there need be no fear of doing it to excess. The edges of the patch especially should be thoroughly well scraped, and, after wiping the surface dry, any little masses of growth, lying in "pockets" of the corium, should be scooped out or cauterized. When the crusts of dried blood and serum have separated, the patch will be found greatly diminished in size, and often entirely removed. The scrapings should be repeated from time to time till the growth is completely eradicated.

The actual cautery, as the galvanic wire or cone, the benzolin cautery, or hot iron, may be used to destroy the growth, preferably when it occurs in confluent patches on the trunk and parts where scars are of little importance, and on the mucous membranes. The growth should be thoroughly ploughed up by the wire or cone, the resistance of the healthy tissue indicating when all the soft lupus deposit has been traversed; oil should be subsequently applied, and should any reformation be observed after separation of the eschar and cicatrization, it should be again destroyed. Paquelin's thermocautère is a most useful instrument for this purpose.

Of chemical caustics, Hebra's arsenical paste, applied in the same way as in lupus erythematosus, and nitrate of silver in points bored into the nodules, are the best applications for disseminated patches. Potassa fusa, in stick or solution, or chloride of zinc paste, or acids, such as strong nitric acid, acid nitrate of mercury, or carbolic acid, are all valuable, and have been found efficacious in different cases.

RHINOSCLEROMA.

Definition.—A peculiar affection, of extremely chronic course, consisting in the formation, on the skin or mucous membrane around the anterior nares, of dense roundish tubercles, which have no tendency to ulcerate or undergo retrogression.

Symptoms.—An abstract of the description of Kaposi, based on fifteen cases, is as follows: The tubercles, isolated or conglomerate, are either smooth, supple, and the same color as the normal skin, or bright or brownish-red and glossy. The epidermis over them is cracked and fissured, and from the rhagades a viscid secretion, drying into yellowish scabs, exudes. The nodules are somewhat elastic, seem cartilaginous to the touch, and are painful on pressure; they are imbedded in the skin, which is normal at their margins.

The nodule, beginning slowly as a thickening and induration of the skin on the septum or edge of one of the alæ, extends gradually into the meatus, which it greatly narrows, to the cheek, and to the upper lip, and causes great deformity.

Diagnosis.—1. From a syphilitic gumma it is distinguished by the extremely chronic course, absence of degeneration or ulceration, obstinate resistance to treatment, and the peculiar localization and restriction of the disease.

2. If the tumor be prominent, glistening, and covered with dilated vessels, it can be diagnosed from keloid only by the history and by microscopical examination.

Prognosis.—Though rhinoscleroma absolutely resists treatment, it is not fatal to life, and is not liable to grow rapidly, affect the constitution, or undergo ulceration. The deformity and the obstruction to the nares are the chief inconveniences arising from it.

Morbid Anatomy.—According to Kaposi, who has described the disease at length, the nodule, which cuts easily, presents on section a pale-red, granular surface, bleeding moderately. Microscopically the epidermis is found normal, the papillæ somewhat longer and club-shaped, and their tissue and that of the corium replaced by a delicately fibrillated, small-meshed network, inclosing numerous small round cells and pervaded by a few small vessels. The growth, which somewhat resembles lymphoid tissue, is most abundant in the papillary layer, but extends to the deeper layers of the corium, and sometimes even to the cartilage. The hair follicles and root sheaths imbedded in the growth are normal.

Treatment.—Excision of the growth has hitherto been

followed by recurrence, and all internal or local applications fail to remove it.

Of Vessels.

1. Nævus.   2. Angioma.

NÆVUS.

Definition.—Is a spot limited to one or other region of the body, light bluish or dark red in color, composed usually of dilated capillaries and veins, congenital or appearing shortly after birth.

Symptoms.—Nævi may be smooth and level with, or only slightly raised above, the general surface, or tuberculated, with irregular prominences on the surface. They may affect merely the superficial layers of the skin, or extend throughout its whole thickness, and even into the subcutaneous tissue. They can be emptied of blood by pressure, the superficial varieties becoming pale and the nodular loose and flaccid, but the blood soon returns on removing the compression, and they resume their normal tint. They occur most commonly on the face, scalp, and neck, but they may be met with on the arms and trunk, and but rarely on the lower extremities.

Diagnosis.—Nævi can only be mistaken, immediately after birth, for the small bruises caused by forceps, but an interval of a week will decide the question.

Prognosis.—Nævi tend to grow slowly, and when composed of large vessels and ulceration takes place, serious hæmorrhage may be the result.

Morbid Anatomy.—A nævus consists of an aggregation of dilated bloodvessels, the walls of which are sometimes thickened, and the plexuses do not correspond with the normal meshwork of the part.

Treatment.—No satisfactory mode of treating the superficial nævi has been introduced, but those most usually employed are strong acids or the actual cautery. Both of these always leave a scar, but the latter is probably the best.

ANGIOMA.

Definition.—A new growth composed of dilated vessels, closely applied to one another, arising usually in the sub-cutaneous tissue, and sometimes in the skin, and not con-genital.

Symptoms.—Angiomata may arise as little slightly raised spots, of a bright-red color, resembling nævi, but differing from them in being developed in adult life instead of being congenital. When arising in the subcutaneous tissue, the skin, at first freely movable over them, becomes gradually involved, and they then appear as bluish-red tumors, much like nodular nævi. The growths may·be single or multiple, and often cause pain from pressure on nerves.

Morbid Anatomy.—Sections of the tumors show large roundish or oval spaces filled with blood, and limited by delicate connective-tissue trabeculæ lined by an endothe-lium. A kind of capsule frequently surrounds the growth.

Treatment.—If the size and situation be inconvenient, and hæmorrhage and pain result, it may be enucleated. It does not usually recur.

Lymphatic Tissue, New Growths.

LYMPHANGIOMA.

Tumors composed of dilated lymphatic vessels, or of lymphatic glands which have undergone cystic degenera-tion, are occasionally met with. As a rule they do not implicate the corium primarily, and belong to the domain of general surgery rather than to that of disease of the skin.

In a case described by Kaposi, under the name of lymph-angioma tuberosum multiplex, hundreds of small, rounded,

22

brownish, slightly raised nodules were found imbedded in the substance of the corium. They were about the size of lentils, became pale on pressure, and were slightly painful. On microscopic examination of an excised tubercle it was found to consist of circular or oval spaces, most numerous in the deeper layers of the corium, lined by endothelium, and identical in structure with dilated lymphatics. No changes were found in the bloodvessels or papillary layer, and, with the exception of pigmentation of the lower rete cells, the epidermis was normal.

The tumors exercised no influence on the general health, gave rise to no subjective symptoms, and extended but slowly; they showed no tendency to involution, and remained unaffected by treatment.

CHAPTER XX.

Sub-class B.—*Malignant.*

Lepra maculosa, tuberosa, anæsthetica—Carcinoma—Epithelioma—
Ulcus rodens—Sarcoma.

LEPRA—LEPROSY.

Definition.—A chronic constitutional disease, characterized by the development of small-celled nodular growths in
the skin, mucous membranes, and nerves.

Symptoms.—Leprosy, formerly prevalent throughout the
whole of Europe, and still occurring endemically on the
west coast of Norway and on the shores of the Mediterra-
nean, is now met with in this country only in sporadic cases.
The persons attacked, or their immediate progenitors, have
usually resided in countries where the disease is endemic,
and the tendency to its development is hereditary. Opinions
are still divided as to whether it is contagious; it is possible, however, that the secretions of a person affected with
the disease may at some period or other be capable of communicating it to others. Though no primary lesion, analogous to the hard chancre of syphilis, is known to occur in
leprosy, the disease frequently arises, and runs a typical
course several years after the person attacked has left an
infected locality, and though no morbid phenomena, resembling those of infantile syphilis, may be present at or soon
after birth, in the children they may develop leprosy after
an interval of many years, without ever having been exposed to the conditions supposed to give rise to it. Dr.

Liveing is of opinion that many instances in which the disease is thought to have arisen spontaneously in this country are possibly due to an untraceable hereditary taint. Mr. Hutchinson considers that a diet composed chiefly of fish favors the development of leprosy.

The disease usually begins by a *prodromal stage*, absent or very slight in some cases, during which no characteristic symptoms of leprosy are present. Malaise, languor and depression, gastric disturbance, and sometimes slight shivering and evening pyrexia, may last for months or even years. Finally, the phenomena peculiar to the disease make their appearance, and, according to the most prominent symptoms present, three varieties are described,—lepra maculosa, tuberosa, and anæsthetica. They differ in degree rather than in kind, and sometimes the characteristics of one variety are present together with those peculiar to another.

Leprosy affects both sexes equally, and though most frequent in early adult life, it is met with at all ages. The macular and tubercular forms are the most common in temperate climates, while the anæsthetic variety predominates in the tropics.

Lepra Maculosa.

After a prodromal stage of varying duration, maculæ, at first pale red and later dark brown or reddish-gray, appear on various parts of the surface. They are smooth, glistening, flat, or only slightly elevated, present defined or somewhat indistinct outlines, and vary from a half to three lines in diameter. The affected patches of skin, thickened, indurated, and somewhat tender on pressure, enlarge gradually at their margins, which are dark reddish-brown in color, while at their centre they become paler. They are largest and most numerous on the trunk, limbs, and sometimes on

the palms and soles also, but are less marked on the face.
Occasionally, in the earlier stages of the disease, the patches
undergo complete involution, leaving the skin normal in
color, or white, smooth, and glistening.   After existing in
this form for years, during which the patches appear and
disappear at intervals, with little or no constitutional disturbance, symptoms characteristic of the anæsthetic or tu-
berous varieties become superadded, and the disease assumes
graver features.

LEPRA TUBEROSA.

After a *prodromal* and a *macular* stage the smooth brownish infiltrated patches become more prominent, and cover a
larger surface.   Small round tubercles, varying in size from
a shot to a small nut, next make their appearance in the
centre of the macular elevations or in healthy skin.   They
are smooth or covered by fissured cuticle, reddish-brown in
color, with ramifying vessels on the surface, and are firm
and somewhat tender on pressure.   The natural prominences
of the skin and its furrows become exaggerated, and the face
presents a prematurely aged, a sad, and morose expression.
It is also broader and quadrangular in shape, brownish-red
and glazed in appearance.   The eyebrows are more prominent, and are bald except at their outer angles, and the
nose, cheeks, chin, and lips are affected with several tubercles, which give them a thickened, irregular appearance,
and produce a "pouting expression" of mouth, resembling
that of a mulatto.   This characteristic alteration of the
whole countenance is termed "facies leontina."

Similar large infiltrated patches and aggregations of
tubercles are met with on the body and extremities.   The
hands and feet become greatly deformed, the nails are
cracked and distorted, the hair and sebaceous glands on the
patches and tubercles atrophy and disappear, and, owing to
the pain and tenderness in the soles, walking becomes im-

possible. Chronic œdema of the legs, producing a condition
of elephantiasis, is usually met with in cases of long standing. After some time the mucous membrane of the mouth,
the pharynx, etc., are occupied by similar tubercles, which,
like the rest, may, at the commencement of the disease,
have undergone involution and atrophy, leaving roundish,
depressed, and deeply pigmented patches, and in the later
stages, becoming obstinate, may last, with little or no change,
for years. They may also give rise to abscesses, which
slowly discharge their contents, or on slight irritation undergo sloughing and ulceration, which, in the hands and
feet, may cause necrosis of the bones or openings in the
joints, and lead to the loss of fingers or toes.

At this stage more or less fever, with rigors and severe
depression, is usually present, and in acute cases the supervention of pneumonia, pleurisy, diarrhœa, or other internal
complications may rapidly prove fatal. In more chronic
cases the above symptoms gradually recede, and there may
be an interval of comparative comfort, during which the
disease remains stationary or progresses only slowly. Recurring periods of febrile exacerbations, with more extension
and rapid development and ulceration of the tubercles, pro-
gressively lower the general health, and may induce a condition of great prostration and marasmus, which ultimately
causes death. Very frequently, however, after the disease
in the tubercular form has lasted for some years, the symptoms of anæsthetic leprosy may set in and gradually become
predominant.

LEPRA ANÆSTHETICA.

After a prodromal stage, characterized frequently by the
periodic appearance of bullæ, resembling those of pemphigus, or sometimes of maculæ, during which the general
health presents little or no change, the anæsthetic variety
becomes developed. Patches of variable extent and situa-

tion on normal skin, as well as on that which is the seat of macular infiltration or has been previously attacked by bullæ, are found to be hyperæsthetic. Any attempt, therefore, to walk, grasp, or to use the hands excites painful or burning sensations or reflex spasmodic movements, and numbness and tingling in the extremities may also exist. Various subcutaneous nerves—the ulnar, radial, median, peroneal, etc.—present extremely painful nodular enlargements. After a variable period the hyperæsthetic parts gradually become less irritable, and anæsthesia commences in the previously sensitive patches or in places where some abnormal pigmentation has existed. A pinkish hyperæsthetic zone usually surrounds the anæsthetic area, in which sensibility to pain, to touch, to heat or cold, or to electricity, may be modified, and in the later stages wholly absent. During the course of the disease, as well as in the prodromal stage, bullæ may appear. Atrophy of the skin and of the muscles supplied by the affected nerves next sets in, and in consequence various paralytic deformities of the hands and feet are produced. Constant chilliness is complained of, and the temperature of the body is much diminished. Either spontaneously or on slight irritation, of which there is no consciousness on account of the loss of sensation, ulceration of the skin takes place at the extremities, opening the joints and leading to the separation of one or more fingers or toes; hence this variety has been called *lepra mutilans*. Necrosis and caries of the bones, and moist or dry gangrene of the extremities, attended with severe constitutional symptoms, are also liable to occur without obvious cause. Towards the termination of the disease marasmus, diarrhœa, or clonic and tetanic spasms set in, ultimately causing death.

Diagnosis.—A well-marked attack of leprosy, with the characteristic pigmentation and appearance of face, cannot be confused with any other disease. In milder forms, however, leprosy may be mistaken for pemphigus, leucoderma, lupus, or syphilis.

The bullous eruption of leprosy differs from pemphigus in that the blebs are solitary or few in number, and usually associated with the anæsthetic patches.

For diagnosis from leucoderma see p. 227.

When the tubercles of leprosy are arranged in aggregated patches or in small nodules round a cicatricial centre, there is much resemblance to lupus. The firmer, more persistent character of the nodules, which are not soft and like "apple-jelly," as in lupus, their tenderness on pressure, and the glistening, oily look of the infiltrated skin in leprosy are the chief points of diagnosis between them.

At an early stage of the disease, if the maculæ are small, pinkish, and fade on pressure, or present a small central tubercle, there is a resemblance to a papulo-macular syphilide. The spots of leprosy are, however, usually larger, even to the full size of the palm, an appearance never seen in syphilis; they are more infiltrated and tender on pressure, are more persistent, and change to a dark-brown or white color, remaining smooth and shining instead of acquiring scales, crusts, etc., or forming serpiginous ulcers. The "facies leontina" is also characteristic of leprosy.

Prognosis.—Leprosy, though usually chronic, is almost always a fatal disease, and only a few cases are recorded of complete recovery, most so-called cures being merely periods of remission, in which the symptoms remain in abeyance or undergo some retrogression, but after a longer or shorter period resume their former course. The tubercular form lasts a shorter time than the other varieties, its average duration being eight or ten years, while anæsthetic leprosy may be prolonged for twenty years. Occasionally tubercular leprosy, when once fully developed, runs an acute course, being attended with much fever and rapid evolution and disintegration of new tubercles, and then, the disease progresses in a few months to a stage which it would usually have reached only after years.

Morbid Anatomy.—Vertical sections through the cutaneous nodules show reddish granular masses, limited by a fibrous capsule or shading off gradually into the corium, which extend sometimes close to the epidermis and at other times invade the subcutaneous tissue. Under the microscope they are seen to consist of small round or spindle-shaped cells, which in young nodules are most abundant round the thick-walled vessels and the plexuses of the sweat and sebaceous glands and of the hair follicles, while in the older ones they are densely aggregated, and lie in the delicate meshwork derived from the fibres of the corium. Their central parts contain no vessels; the papillæ are obliterated, the cuticle thinned, and the glands and hairs atrophied or degenerated, but a rich vascular network is formed in the margins. The cells of the new growth have distinct nuclei, and their protoplasm presents a somewhat cloudy "ground-glass" appearance; globules are found here and there, and the arrectores pilorum are said to be hypertrophied. A very slight cellular infiltration has been found in parts which presented the appearance of discoloration or pinkish maculæ.

The morbid changes in the nerves—*neuritis leprosa*—are as follows: At points exposed to pressure, or where the nerve is near the surface, its trunk presents fusiform enlargements, grayish or yellowish, semi-translucent, sometimes even brown or blackish in appearance, and it is much firmer than when normal. Transverse sections show the general nerve sheath unaltered, except that its vessels are slightly thickened. Beneath the funicular sheaths, which are usually somewhat thickened and in old-standing cases sclerosed, aggregation of small cells of the same nature as those composing the cutaneous nodules are found, compressing the nerve fibrils and sending cords of cells in between them. More or less fatty degeneration and disintegration of the medullary sheaths, and in later stages complete atrophy of the nerve fibrils, next takes place, and the hyperæsthesia at first produced by the irritation of the nerves owing to the growth gives place to anæsthesia as they become destroyed. In the affected portions of nerves, as well as the skin in which they are distributed, Dr. Vandyke Carter has found roundish or oval brown pigmented bodies. Pigmentations and thickening of the vessels in the cerebral and spinal pia mater, as well as albuminous-looking deposits in the meninges and degenerative changes in the spinal cord, have been described by Danielssen and Boeck, but have not been met with by Dr. Carter in India.

Treatment.—This must be directed to the improvement of the general health by nutritious diet, tonics, good hygienic conditions, cleanliness, exercise, and removal from districts where the disease is endemic. Internal remedies, of which many have from time to time been vaunted as specifics, have little or no influence on the general malady. Cod-liver oil, internally and by inunction, chaulmoogra oil or gurjun balsam applied in the same way, and the local stimulation of the deposits by the inunction of cashew oil, iodine, etc., are sometimes attended with benefit. Ulcers should be treated on general principles, and the hyperæsthesia relieved by opiates.

In the quiescent intervals galvanism is often useful in the treatment of paralysis and muscular atrophy.

CARCINOMA CUTIS.

Definition.—A malignant growth in the skin, composed of nests of cells contained in an alveolar stroma, occurring in the form of nodules, which spread by infiltration of the surrounding tissues, affect the adjacent lymphatic glands, recur after removal, and prove fatal by ulceration, cachexia, and exhaustion.

Symptoms.—Carcinoma of the skin is usually secondary to the development of the disease in the organs; it affects the cutis by continuous extension from the deeper parts, or occurs in the form of isolated nodules, usually multiple, beginning either in the subcutaneous connective tissue and soon involving the corium or arising primarily in the latter. Structurally it presents sometimes the characters of scirrhus, sometimes those of encephaloid cancer.

In scirrhus of the breast, as the disease extends towards the surface, the skin becomes adherent to the tumor, drawn in at the centre, indurated, and infiltrated. The margin is often raised into reddish-brown, elastic nodules, and similar masses may develop in the vicinity of, but not in visible continuity with, the primary growth. Occasionally, when scirrhus affects the liver or stomach, numerous small roundish or oval, firm, and painful nodules may occur in the substance of the corium, which present the same structure as the original mass. If life be sufficiently prolonged, like the nodules in scirrhus mammæ, they gradually extend to the surface, break down, and form excavated ulcers with everted indurated edges, a sloughy firm base, and foul ichorous discharge.

Carcinoma encephaloides occurs sometimes primarily in the skin as a rare affection in old persons. Multiple nodular masses of various sizes, most numerous on the face and hands and of a dark-red color, are present over the whole surface. They soon break down and acquire a greenish, firm crust or slough, producing excavated ulcers like those of scirrhus, which tend to spread in all directions. The lymphatic glands and internal organs are less liable to secondary infection than in scirrhus.

Diagnosis.—Multiple scirrhus nodules may be mistaken for those of fibroma; their hard, painful nature, their rapid growth and tendency to break down if life lasts long enough, the presence usually of a primary spot of disease in some other organ, and the microscopical structure of one of the nodules, will be sufficient for diagnosis.

From gummata they are distinguished by the absence of a history or of other evidences of syphilis, by their great firmness, and by their structure. Encephaloid nodules, growing rapidly and forming ulcers with indurated everted edges, can hardly be mistaken for any other disease.

Prognosis.—Both forms of carcinoma are invariably fatal.

Morbid Anatomy.—Scirrhus of the skin presents the same structure as in other organs of the body, and consists of nests of small roundish or polygonal cells contained in alveoli, the walls of which are comparatively thick and firm. At the edges of the tumor, the alveolar structure gradually passes into that of the normal tissue, which is very thickly infiltrated with round cells. In encephaloid the cells are larger, contain large round nuclei with clear protoplasm surrounding them, and the alveoli are composed of thin septa of connective tissue. The bloodvessels are larger and more freely distributed than in scirrhus; their walls are thin and cavernous, and dilatations and hæmorrhages are frequent.

Treatment.—This can only be palliative. The strength should be supported by nutritious food and stimulants, the pain relieved by opiates, and the ulcers dressed with astringent and antiseptic lotions.

EPITHELIOMA CUTIS.

Definition.—A malignant new growth of the skin, infiltrating the tissues and spreading along the lymphatics to the glands, characterized by a tendency to local recurrence after removal and by slight liability to the formation of the secondary growths in distant parts.

Symptoms.—Epithelioma occurs but rarely under forty, and is most commonly met with on the lower lip, the external genitals, and the face. It begins as small rounded, isolated or aggregated nodules imbedded in the substance of the skin, which in the course of months or years enlarge and form a roundish, buttonlike mass, raised slightly above the surface of the skin, with defined sloping edges and a smooth or somewhat irregular warty-looking surface. The little tumor is yellowish or brownish in color, and covered with ramifying vessels, is extremely hard, usually somewhat painful, and, though at first freely movable, becomes at a later stage adherent to the deeper structures. The surface next desquamates, becomes excoriated, and is covered with a thin, adherent, brownish scab in its centre, under which is found a reddish ulcer with a granular base and slight sticky secretion. The edges are prominent, everted, indurated, irregular, and often present little translucent, rounded, vesicular-looking nodules towards their outer margin. Infiltration, followed by ulceration, goes on in all directions ; the neighboring lymphatic glands become enlarged, nodular, and indurated, and often break down to form malignant ulcers; and severe lancinating pains are usually present, with wasting and much prostration. On the scrotum the disease usually begins as an irregular, warty mass, frequently pigmented, which becomes excoriated on the surface, and then gives rise to sloughy ulcers. On the lip it often begins as a persistent fissure, covered by a thin scab, and at first without any induration of the surrounding tissues ; but the base gradually becomes hard, the margins prominent and infiltrated, till a typical ulcer is finally produced.

Diagnosis.—Epithelioma may be mistaken for syphilis, lupus, or a simple excoriated wart. The age, the previous history and course of the affection, the pain, which is usually greater than in syphilis, and occasionally the detection under the microscope of epithelial "globes" in the scrapings of the ulcers, will aid the diagnosis from syphilis, and when a hard, translucent edge or small, clear, marginal nodules are present the distinction is easy.

For diagnosis from lupus see p. 245.

An abraded wart cannot in many cases be distinguished from a commencing epithelioma, more especially since epithelioma not unfrequently attacks a wart which has lasted for some time. The persistence and the slowness of the ulcerated surface to heal point towards epithelioma.

Prognosis.—In the early stages epithelioma, if completely destroyed, may not recur, but if considerable infiltration of the tissue and glandular affection have set in, the disease will return after excision or cauterization, and will ultimately prove fatal.

Morbid Anatomy.—Vertical sections through a mass of epithelioma have a whitish, granular appearance, and are firm and friable. Under the microscope, at the margin of the growth the interpapillary processes of the rete are seen to be enlarged, much elongated, and pressing on the papillæ, which, towards the centre portion of the growth, are reduced to thin, fibrous septa. The epithelial cylinders, composed of spinous rete cells with a few scattered leucocytes, contain here and there rounded masses of flattened, laminated cells, resembling the transverse section of an onion, which are called the epidermic "globes" or "pearls." They extend into the corium, which is more vascular and infiltrated with numerous small cells, denser near the epithelium. The bloodvessels, at first numerous in the connective-tissue processes between the epithelial cylinders, become gradually pressed upon and obliterated by them, which causes the superficial and older portions of the nodule to break down and ulcerate. In sections parallel to surface epithelial growths, as was first shown by Köster, are seen filling the lymphatics, and in this way the glands become "infected" and the seats of secondary epithelial deposits. The sebaceous and sweat glands and the hair follicles involved in the growth show signs of epithelial proliferation, followed by degeneration, and are ultimately destroyed.

Treatment.—A thorough removal of the growth by free excision or its complete destruction by caustics are the only measures which give any hope of a cure.

As caustics, potassa fusa, Vienna paste, chloride of zinc, and Hebra's arsenical paste are the most suitable.

The disease in most cases recurs, and repeated operations or cauterizations, though they only temporarily check the progress of the disease, give some intervals of comparative comfort and prolong life.

Ulcus Rodens.

Rodent ulcer is considered by most Continental dermatologists to be merely a variety of epithelioma, and several English observers have found the growth to present the microscopic structure of the latter disease; it presents, however, certain clinical characters that require a separate description.

Symptoms.—It begins as a small, smooth, pale papule or tubercle, situated usually on the upper half of the face; it gradually increases in size, and, after lasting perhaps for many years, commences to ulcerate. An ulcer, with hard, sinuous edges, often irregular in outline, and attended with little or no pain, but extending gradually in depth and area, is thus produced. Its base is said to be not granulated, but smooth, glassy, and dull reddish-yellow in appearance, and as the margin extends cicatrization occasionally takes place in the centre. Slowly invading the deeper parts, ulceration may expose even the bones of the face, but there is never any secondary glandular infiltration, and the general health is little affected. It occurs in persons past middle age, and usually in those advanced in life.

Diagnosis.—The main differences from ordinary epithelioma consist in the extreme chronic, painless course, the absence of glandular infiltration and cachexia, the tendency in some cases to cicatrization, and the less marked liability to recurrence if the disease be once thoroughly destroyed.

Treatment.—Complete destruction of the growth at an early stage by excision, by scraping, or by caustics, will often cure, and in all cases much retard the progress of the disease.

Sarcoma Cutis.

Definition.—Sarcoma of the skin is a rare affection, occurring primarily in the corium and subsequently to the origin of the disease in some other situation.

Symptoms.—Small rounded reddish or bluish-brown nodules, varying in size from a small shot to a hazelnut, appear at first on the feet or hands, and then scattered over the whole surface of the body. They are isolated, smooth, and elastic to the touch, and in a late stage of the disease break down and slough. The disease occurs most frequently in males and in persons over forty years of age.

Diagnosis.—It differs from carcinoma in beginning most commonly in the feet, in the absence of alveolar structure, and in the general freedom from implication of the lymphatic glands.

Prognosis.—Death usually occurs within two or three years from the commencement, probably owing to the existence of similar tumors in the vital organs.

Morbid Anatomy.—The nodules, when examined under the microscope, are seen to consist of round or spindle-shaped pigmented cells, traversed by thin-walled, cavernous vessels, and often presenting patches of hæmorrhagic infiltration and degeneration.

Treatment.—As in carcinoma of the skin, this can be only palliative.

Division II.—DISEASES OF THE APPENDAGES OF THE SKIN.

CHAPTER XXI.

SUBDIVISION A.—*Of the Sebaceous Glands.*

Seborrhœa, oleosa sicca, Ichthyosis sebacea neonatorum—Acne punctata, comedo, milium—Acne vulgaris—Acne sycosis—Acne rosacea—Molluscum contagiosum.

SUBDIVISION B.—*Of the Sweat Glands.*

Hyperidrosis—Anidrosis—Bromidrosis—Chromidrosis—Sudamina.

―――――――――

SUBDIVISION A.—*Of the Sebaceous Glands.*

SEBORRHŒA—ACNE SEBACEA.

Definition.—Seborrhœa is a condition due to increased secretion of the sebaceous glands, in which the sebum mixed with dirt accumulates on otherwise healthy skin.

Before describing the different varieties of seborrhœa it will be well to discuss briefly the composition of sebum and how it is produced. Kölliker shows that the sebaceous glands are constantly giving off cells, which, when first formed at the bottom of the glands, are pale and only slightly granular, but which, when they are forced to the surface by the formation of fresh cells, become filled with a quantity of fat-granules. These granules at a later stage coalesce into a single globule, and the wall of the cell becomes stronger and more horny. Seborrhœa consists in the

23

increased production of these oil-globules, and may be divided into three varieties—S. oleosa, S. sicca, and ichthyosis sebacea neonatorum.

Symptoms.—*Seborrhœa oleosa* occurs usually between the ages of fifteen and twenty-five, and affects the cheeks, nose, and forehead. The exudation of oil from the sebaceous glands gives a greasy appearance to the skin, which next becomes dirty, owing to the liability of the oil to attract and absorb particles of dust and dirt floating in the air. When this condition has lasted for some time crusts are formed, which may vary greatly in color, and when they are raised small processes of sebum can be drawn from the follicles. When the disease occurs on hairy places the hair becomes matted, in consequence of which dirt adheres and vermin accumulate, constituting the condition known as *plica Polonica.*

S. oleosa also occurs on the genitals of both sexes, and is known as *smegma præputii et clitoridis.* When neglected it forms thin crusts, which in the male are situated on the glans penis beneath the prepuce, and in the female around the clitoris and in the neighboring grooves. If allowed to remain untouched for a long time, they cause severe local irritation and inflammation, a condition which may be mistaken for gonorrhœa. *Vernix caseosa* is a name given by Hebra to a similar deposit over the whole body of new-born infants.

Seborrhœa sicca is produced in a similar way to S. oleosa, but gives rise to the formation either of a dry, light-yellow crust or a branny coating to the skin. The regions most usually affected are the scalp and other hairy parts of the body. Scales of epidermis and dried sebum, which are constantly being formed and ought to be removed, are, owing to a want of cleanliness, allowed to accumulate in the hair, and are known as scurf. The affection does not last long without injuring the hair itself, which gradually falls off and is replaced by badly developed hair till partial baldness is the result. When the disease is of long standing further changes take place in the scalp, and itching, which is absent in the earlier stage of the disease, may eventually arise from an eczematous condition of the skin.

Ichthyosis sebacea neonatorum must not on account of its name be confused with true ichthyosis, but Hebra has thus termed the affection of new-born infants formerly known as ichthyosis congenita. The symptoms appear within a few hours of birth, when the skin presents a smooth, glossy, and somewhat purple appearance. It is also covered with a quantity of fissures, which are most numerous on the fingers and toes and over the flexures of the joints. The slightest movement causes pain, and in severe cases the child is unable to suck.

Diagnosis.—S. oleosa may be mistaken for lupus erythematosus, but greater swelling and redness, more adherent scales, and a tendency to scar are found in the latter.

S. sicca may be mistaken for three diseases when it attacks the scalp,—eczema, psoriasis, and ringworm. For the diagnosis from the two former see table, p. 161. From ringworm it may be distinguished by the history of the case, the absence of short broken hairs, the greater difficulty in extracting the hairs, and by aid of the microscope.

Ichthyosis sebacea neonatorum may be distinguished from genuine ichthyosis by the fact that the former is local and not general.

Prognosis.—This depends on the cause of the condition, for when it occurs in the course of a serious disease the prognosis is unfavorable, while under suitable treatment recovery is in ordinary cases usually rapid.

Treatment.—Both local and constitutional means are used, but the former are the most important. In all varieties thorough cleanliness is necessary, and if crusts are formed they should be removed with oil, soft soap, or lard. After removal of the crusts the part should be dressed with a slightly stimulating ointment, such as zinc, weak carbolic acid, or tar, and in S. sicca of the scalp a lotion of borax is useful.

Internally tonics, such as arsenic, iron, and the mineral acids, should be administered in full and repeated doses.

ACNE PUNCTATA.

Definition.—A disease of the skin caused by the retention of sebum in the ducts of the sebaceous glands and hair follicles.

Acne punctata occurs in two forms, differing in color, which are therefore respectively called *nigra* and *alba*, but are usually known as comedo and milium.

Symptoms.— *Comedones* usually occur between the ages of fourteen and twenty-five, and attack the face, chest, and back, in small black spots, which look, as Hebra suggests, like grains of gunpowder inserted into the skin. If one of these black spots be compressed between the nails, a long, wormlike body with a black head is forced out. The little mass thus ejected consists of retained sebum and the black head of dirt which has adhered to the cheesy material. The cavity from which the wormlike body is expressed is the neck of a hair follicle into which a sebaceous gland opens, and the wormlike appearance is caused by its shape. In the substance of the mass there is also, however, in some cases a living grub, which has nothing to do with the retention of the sebum and is quite as often found in normal glands. It is called the acarus folliculorum, and was first discovered by Henle in 1841.

Milium appears in the same situations as comedones, and at the same time of life, but often terminates in an inflammatory process, giving rise to acne vulgaris. It consists of a small swelling under the cuticle, which is caused by the retention of sebum in the sebaceous gland and not in the neck of the hair follicle, and is white in color, owing to the impossibility of accumulating dirt, as in the comedones.

Diagnosis.—These varieties of acne punctata can only be mistaken for acne vulgaris, but the absence of redness and other inflammatory signs in them is sufficiently characteristic.

Prognosis.—It is perfectly harmless and easy to cure, but is liable to recur.

Morbid Anatomy.—On incising the skin over one of the fine white granules in milium a small round body can be turned out with the point of a needle, which on compression breaks up into fine laminated scales. A thin vertical section examined with the microscope shows a mass of horny epithelial cells, surrounding frequently a central space filled with broken-down cells and fatty debris, and inclosed in a thin capsule of a finely fibrillated connective tissue. The whole mass consists of an altered sebaceous follicle, the cells of which, instead of undergoing fatty degeneration and alteration into sebum, have become cornified. It is covered by the papillary layer of the corium, which has to be cut through in order to remove it. Frequently the little epidermic globule is fixed by a fine pedicle, consisting of an atrophied hair follicle, to the corium.

Treatment.—For comedones thorough cleanliness and friction of the part affected is the best treatment. The plugs of sebum should be squeezed out by the finger nails or with a watch key, and a mild stimulating ointment containing a small quantity of sulphur or tar should be afterwards applied. The skin over the little tumors in milium should be carefully divided and the mass squeezed out. Constitutional remedies are necessary in both conditions if any functional irregularity can be discovered.

ACNE VULGARIS.

Definition.—Acne vulgaris is a disease of the skin characterized by the appearance of nodules or pustules, caused by inflammation of the hair follicles and sebaceous glands.

Symptoms.—It occurs in the same places as A. punctata and at the same time of life. It consists of comedones, which by their presence or by local irritation lead to an inflammatory condition of the gland, producing raised red pimples, varying in size from a small seed to a pea. The disease is termed *A. indurata* if the inflammation extends deeply into the skin, and *A. pustulosa* if pus is formed. In the latter, after the pustule bursts or the retained matter is expelled, the spot disappears, but a small shallow scar is left. If the disease attacks the forehead it is termed *A. frontalis,* and appears in the form of large papules, tubercles, or pustules, which leave scars when they are cured. At times, if the inflammation is severe, the disease resembles a boil. A severe form of A. vulgaris is produced by the local application of tar, and by the internal administration to susceptible persons of such drugs as iodide and bromide of potassium. The usual theories as to the cause of A. vulgaris— excessive venery, or the too free use of alcohol or highly seasoned food—are very doubtful, and its true cause is a matter of uncertainty. However, it is common in the scrofulous and tubercular diathesis.

Diagnosis.—Acne vulgaris is easily recognizable, but may be mistaken for small-pox in a certain stage (see p. 65) or for a syphilide. In the latter case some other syphilitic eruption at the same time is generally to be found (see A. syphilitica, p. 104).

Prognosis.—Acne vulgaris is never fatal, though it produces great annoyance to the individual, and in time the disease will disappear, for it rarely persists after twenty-five or twenty-six years of age.

Morbid Anatomy.—In A. vulgaris the sebaceous plug,

blocking the excretory duct of the gland, acts as a foreign body and excites inflammatory hyperæmia, followed by serous exudation into and round the hair follicles and glands. If the plug be not removed, the further inflammation it excites gives rise to pus formation in and round the sebaceous glands, surrounded by firm, painful, inflammatory induration of the adjacent connective tissue, which subsequently becomes hypertrophied. In this way the hard tubercles of A. indurata are produced. The formation of pus is usually slight, and being at the closed extremity of the gland, is not near the surface but in the substance of the corium, and is therefore not usually seen until the nodule is incised or contents evacuated. When the pus is in excess or obviously near the surface, the condition known as A. pustulosa is produced.

Treatment.—The treatment should be both local and constitutional. Thorough sponging with hot water and friction are of the greatest importance. The plugs of sebum should be removed by pressure, and the pus liberated by small incisions. Soaps containing free alkali are of value, and Hebra's spiritus saponatus alkalinus is one of the best forms. The part should be well rubbed with it, but its use should not be prolonged over more than a few days on account of the great irritation liable to be produced. It is well also to apply ointments containing a small quantity of sulphur and creasote, such as

Sublimed sulphur, ...	grs. xxx.
White precipitate, ...	grs. x.
Æthiops mineral, ...	grs. x.
Olive oil, ...	ʒij.
Creasote, ...	♏iv.
Lard, to	ʒix.

—*Skin Hospital;*

or lotions containing perchloride of mercury gr. $\frac{1}{4}$ or $\frac{1}{2}$ to the ʒj. While the pustules are forming it is well to touch

them lightly with acid nitrate of mercury, taking care that
the first does not run in to the sound skin.

The constitutional treatment should consist of such remedies as are calculated to maintain the general health by
regulating the various functions of the body. The diet
should be carefully attended to, and stimulants should be
prohibited.

ACNE SYCOSIS—ACNE MENTAGRA.

Definition.—Hebra's definition is "a disease of chronic
course, non-contagious, attacking the hairy parts of the cutaneous surface, and characterized by the development of
papules and tubercles, continuous thickenings, and pustules
of various sizes, all of these having invariably hairs passing
through them."

Symptoms.—Acne sycosis consists of a chronic inflammation and suppuration of the hair follicles, and therefore attacks only the hairy parts of the body, but the most usual
site is the beard. The cause often suggested for A. sycosis
is the use of blunt razors, but this is doubtful, since persons
who never shave are liable to it. The pimples first appear
like those of A. vulgaris, but with a hair passing through
each of them, and as they get larger and assume the character
of tubercles they may coalesce and form a thick, indurated
mass, limited entirely to the hairy region and through
which the hairs protrude. These hairs are easily extracted
on account of the inflammation at their root, which itself appears swollen. From the indurated mass pus oozes, which
dries and forms thin yellow scabs, and when the eruption
disappears cicatrices are left and the place remains bald.
The disease is specially liable to follow attacks of eczema.

Diagnosis.—A. sycosis may be mistaken for A. vulgaris,
eczema, or a syphilide. From them it may be distinguished
because it always attacks the hairy parts alone, and does
not spread beyond them, because the hairs pierce the pus-

tules or tubercles, and no similar eruptions are seen elsewhere.

Prognosis.—The course is always tedious and the disease is difficult to cure, but it rarely terminates fatally unless erysipelas occurs as well.

Morbid Anatomy.—This is very much the same as in A. indurata, but differs in the greater length of the hairs and their follicles, and in the greater depth to which they penetrate the corium. The purulent foci, therefore, lie at a greater distance from the surface, and excite more severe inflammatory exudation into and hypertrophy of the tissues surrounding the follicles. Pus is also found outside the follicles and sebaceous glands and at the roots of the hairs, which are thus more or less completely destroyed. There is, however, no obstructing plug of sebum acting as a mechanical irritant, as in A. vulgaris.

Treatment.—This consists, in the first place, in epilating the hairs of the diseased parts and in shaving the rest of the patch, but to be of real service epilation should be commenced as early as possible in the attack and should be continued as it spreads. The pustules should be pricked and the pus let out, and if the part is not very painful or inflamed they should be lightly touched with acid nitrate of mercury, but if it is tender cold-water rags covered with oil silk should be applied. As the disease becomes more chronic ointments and lotions similar to those recommended in A. vulgaris should be tried. Hebra strongly insists on the importance of regular shaving after the disease has been cured, to prevent its recurrence.

ACNE ROSACEA.

Definition.—A disease of the skin occurring on the face, and characterized by great hyperæmia of the part and dila-

24

tation of the vessels, accompanied by hypertrophy of the fibrous elements and of the glands, which sometimes leads to the production of tumors.

Symptoms.—A. rosacea is believed to be to some extent hereditary, and is certainly due to some condition affecting the general health. Indigestion, produced by excess of food or strong drinks, causes flushing of the face, which often terminates in this disease, and in women irregularities of menstruation must also be mentioned. It may appear at any time except during childhood, but generally in middle or advanced life.

A. rosacea is not in itself a disease of the sebaceous glands, although they are frequently among the tissues affected. It is always limited to the face, and attacks in preference the nose, cheeks, forehead, and chin. It commences by an injection of the bloodvessels, leading to a reddening of the skin, which fades on pressure, and is increased greatly after a meal or on exposure to cold. This hyperæmia of the part produces a burning or tingling sensation. The disease may stop at this stage or may be associated with other morbid changes, but when these are absent the nose is usually alone affected. With the reddening there may be a considerable increase in the amount of sebum secreted, which gives the part a very greasy appearance, or the sebaceous glands may be inflamed and filled with secretion and their ducts remain open. At a later stage round nodules form, and great hypertrophy of the part takes place, which, when the nose is attacked, causes great deformity. The nodules may be of varying shape and size, and sometimes hang from the nose in pendulous masses.

The disease may persist or the redness may fade, and the tubercles either become absorbed or drop off, but extensive suppuration and ulceration never occurs.

Diagnosis.—A. rosacea has to be distinguished from A.

vulgaris, lupus erythematosus, and on the nose from frost-bite.

From the first it may be recognized by the limitation of A. rosacea to the face, while A. vulgaris attacks the chest and back, and also because the inflammation in the former affects the skin between the acne spots and causes a tingling sensation.

From lupus erythematosus A. rosacea can be distinguished by the absence of ulceration and of the scabs which are present in the former.

From frostbite the early stage of A. rosacea is also distinguished by the amount of swelling, and the dark-purple, shining appearance in frostbite contrasts with the bright-red and greasy appearance in A. rosacea.

Prognosis.—It is never fatal, but is very obstinate, lasting sometimes for life.

Morbid Anatomy.—The anatomy of A. rosacea cannot be clearly described, but there is no doubt that the disease begins with hyperæmia of the part and increased growth of the fibrous and connective tissue, and that hypertrophy of the glands also takes place.

Treatment.—Regulation of the diet, and, when necessary, of the menses, should be attended to before any good result can be expected from local treatment. The inunction of sulphur or iodide of sulphur ointment, the application of a weak solution of perchloride of mercury, or lightly touching the spots with acid nitrate of mercury, are the best forms of local treatment, but three or four days must frequently be allowed to intervene in order that the inflammation excited by this treatment may have time to subside.

In the more severe form the local hyperæmia is relieved by frequent multiple linear scarifications, and when any great deformity exists the complete removal of the tubercular excrescence is desirable.

MOLLUSCUM CONTAGIOSUM.

Definition.—A contagious disease of the skin, affecting the sebaceous glands, leading to the blocking up of the duct and an increased growth of the gland, which becomes filled with a white, fatty, and granular substance.

Symptoms.—The cause of the disease is unknown, but there is no doubt that it can be communicated from one person to another, although the mode has not been yet discovered. The disease appears first as a minute hard, white, shiny swelling, which gradually grows until it becomes as large as a hazelnut, but it is usually about the size of a pea. This little tumor, which may be sessile or pedunculated, is circular in form, with a flat top, having in its centre a small depression, which is the mouth of a sebaceous gland, and from which, when the tumor is squeezed, a soft, white, milky substance is forced. The tumors may occur singly or in scattered groups on the face, especially the eyelids, chest, arms, genitals, and on the breasts in women, and cause no pain, tenderness, or irritation, but occasionally producing, when inflamed, an ecthymatous pustule. As the tumors dry up, small horns or warts are sometimes left. The disease is more common in children than in adults.

Diagnosis.—It is easily recognized by the umbilication and ease with which the tumor can be emptied, and is not liable to be mistaken for any other disease.

Morbid Anatomy.—The white material of which the tumor is composed is found to consist of granular and fatty matter with altered epithelium cells. On examining vertical sections some of the tumors are seen to be composed of cystlike dilatations of sebaceous glands, filled with the products of the broken-down epithelial lining. Others present a lobulated structure, and microscopically are seen to be inclosed in fibrous capsules, which send delicate septa between the lobules. In each lobule there is first a layer of columnar cells next the fibrous wall, and then two or three layers of polygonal cells more or less infiltrated with fat-globules, whilst the centre is occupied by roundish or oval bodies, the so-called "molluscum corpuscles," mixed with some fatty debris. These oval bodies, which were formerly supposed to be peculiar to molluscum, are merely epithelial cells that have undergone lardaceous or albuminoid degeneration.

The whole tumor is covered by the superficial portion of the corium, which is somewhat thinned and has its papillæ flattened by the pressure of the subjacent growth. Its walls and base are surrounded by a network of fine vessels, which bleed when the tumor is snipped off.

Treatment. — Treatment consists in making an incision across the tumor with a sharp knife and then squeezing out the contents.

SUBDIVISION B.—*Of the Sweat Glands.*

HYPERIDROSIS.

Definition.—A condition characterized by excessive sweating, which may be general or local.

Symptoms.—General sweating may occur in the course of any of the acute constitutional diseases, such as acute rheumatism, when the whole surface of the body may be bathed in perspiration.

Local sweating may affect the hands or feet, or one hand or foot, or even one-half of the body, and produces a sodden appearance, such as is seen after prolonged immersion in water. From the constant irritation of the sweat eczema may result.

Treatment.—This should depend on the cause, internal remedies, such as belladonna, being required if the sweating is general. Sponging with vinegar and water is useful to check the nightsweats in phthisis. Locally the part should be constantly washed with yellow soap and water, and bathed with a lead or tannic acid lotion.

ANIDROSIS.

Definition.—A condition characterized by a deficiency of perspiration, and occurring as a result either of a constitutional disease or of an altered state of the skin, as in ichthyosis.

BROMIDROSIS.

Definition.—A condition characterized by the odor of the perspiration.

Symptoms.—This disease may be general or local. The former occurs usually in the course of some constitutional disease, when the smell differs according to the variety. Local bromidrosis is normally present in certain regions of the body, such as the axillæ, perinæum, and feet, and it can therefore only be considered a disease when the smell is excessive. When the feet are affected the odor is at times so offensive that the person is unable to attend to his duties, though his general health is perfectly good. The perspiration is greatly increased above the normal, and is quickly absorbed by the socks, from which the smell arises, owing to rapid decomposition.

Treatment.—Local bromidrosis is often very difficult to cure. Thorough cleanliness is essential; the part should be washed at least twice daily with plenty of soap, then dried and powdered with starch or flour. Sea-water baths at night are of value in some cases, and so also is painting the whole part occasionally with iodine. In severe cases, when other measures fail, Hebra recommends the following plan, which he says "will invariably be attended with success:"

"A certain quantity of the simple diachylon plaster (emp. plumbi, emp. lithargyri) is to be melted over a gentle fire, and an equal weight of linseed oil is then to be incorporated with it, the product being stirred till a homogeneous mass is produced, sufficiently adhesive not to crumble readily to pieces. This is then to be spread over a piece of linen measuring about a square foot. The foot of the patient, having been first well washed and thoroughly dried, is now to be wrapped in the dressing thus prepared. Pledgets of lint on which the same ointment has been spread are also to be introduced into the space between each pair of toes, to prevent their touching one another; and care must be taken that the foot is completely covered, and that the dressing is accurately in contact with the skin. When this has been done an ordinary sock or stocking may be put on the foot, and outside this a new shoe, which must be light and should not cover the dorsum of the foot. After twelve hours the dressing is to be removed; the foot is then not to be washed, but must be rubbed with a dry cloth. The dressing is then to be renewed in the same way as before, and its application is afterwards to be repeated twice a day. This procedure must be continued for eight to twelve days, according to the severity of the case. . . . In the course of a few days it will be found that a brownish-yellow cuticle, about $\frac{1}{2}'''$ thick, is beginning to peel off from all those parts of the skin which were before affected with the disease, and that a healthy, clean, white surface of epidermis is exposed as this substance separates."

CHROMIDROSIS.

Definition.—A very rare condition in which the sweat is said to be colored.

SUDAMINA—MILIARIA.

Definition.—An eruption of small transparent vesicles, chiefly on the abdomen, which contain sweat.

Symptoms.—In the course of an acute disease, in which excessive sweating is a prominent feature, small transparent vesicles suddenly appear. At first sight they look like drops of water on the surface, but they are hard to the touch. The vesicles contain sweat, which is proved by analysis. When they burst an eczema may result from the irritation of the sweat.

Treatment.—None is required, unless the disease is accompanied by eczema, which should be treated accordingly.

CHAPTER XXII.

SUBDIVISION C.—*Of the Hair.*

Hirsuties — Lichen pilaris — Nævus pilosus — Canities—Alopecia—
Alopecia areata—Trichorexis nodosa.

SUBDIVISION D.—*Of the Nails.*

Onychia — Onychogryphosis — Onychauxis — Onychatrophia — In
General Diseases.

———

SUBDIVISION C.—*Of the Hair.*

HIRSUTIES.

HIRSUTIES, or an excessive growth of hair on parts where
normally only fine down occurs, may be either congenital or
acquired.

In the congenital variety the excessive growth may be
either diffuse, covering the whole surface or a large portion
of it, as in the so-called " hairy men," or localized to certain smaller areæ, as in moles or nævi.

In the acquired variety large hairs, more or less numerous, develop in places generally covered only with lanuginous hairs, such as the upper lip or chin of women, the areola
of the nipple, or on warts. The irritation of the skin by
blisters or stimulating applications produces in some individuals an abundant growth of long downy or bristly hairs.

The process consists usually of an increase in number
and a closer aggregation of the hairs, which are occasionally thick and bristly. The condition does not affect- the

general health, and is only troublesome in consequence of the disfigurement it produces.

Treatment.—When the hairs are scanty and long, epilation is the best mode of removing them; but when they are numerous, and are situated on the lip or chin of women, a depilatory paste, containing orpiment and slaked lime or sulphide of calcium, may be applied every three or four days.

LICHEN PILARIS.

Lichen pilaris consists in the development of small papular swellings around the hair follicles, and affects the extensor surfaces of the limbs. On the outer side of the thighs, where they are most frequently observed, the skin feels rough and harsh to the touch. The papules, which are about the size of a pin's head, are pale, or only slightly hyperæmic, and do not itch or cause any other subjective sensation.

Morbid Anatomy.—The papules are due to epithelial debris accumulating in and blocking up the mouth of a hair follicle, with usually some exudation into and hypertrophy of the connective tissue around the neck of the follicle.

Treatment.—This consists in washing the skin thoroughly with soap and water, frequent warm baths, and in the inunction of vaseline or some simple ointment.

NÆVUS PILOSUS—HAIRY MOLE.

Nævus pilosus is the term applied to the brown pigmented patches, covered usually with long hairs, which are usually congenital.

They are smooth and level with the surface, or only slightly raised, and consist of slight hypertrophy of the papillary layer, in which and in the rete much brown or black pigment is deposited, while the hairs are considerably hypertrophied. The patches are sometimes the starting-points of melanotic sarcomatous growths.

Treatment.—They can be destroyed by blistering or with potassa fusa or other caustics, or by scraping with Volkmann's spoon.

CANITIES.

Canities is the term applied to the blanching of the hair, occurring normally as a gradual senile change or suddenly under the influence of severe mental emotions. The change begins at the root of the hair by a diminished formation of pigment, and a papilla which has once produced a gray hair does not usually form colored ones. The sudden alteration is ascribed to a development of air-bubbles in the substance of the hair shaft, which obscure the pigment present in the medullary portion. Sometimes canities occurs as a result of disease of the hair follicles, but after a time the hairs may become recolored.

ALOPECIA—BALDNESS.

Deficient growth of hair may be either congenital or acquired. The former is rare, and in it the hair is scanty and downy, or entirely absent from the scalp, but usually after a time the growth may become normal. Acquired baldness may result either as a senile change, when it is often preceded by grayness of the hair with more or less atrophy of the skin, sebaceous glands, and hair follicles, or at a comparatively early period as a sequel of one of the acute diseases, such as scarlatina, erysipelas, etc., or as a result of a local inflammatory process which affects the hair follicles and papillæ, as in acute or chronic eczema, psoriasis, syphilis, favus, ringworm, etc.

In *alopecia senilis* the skin, hair follicles, and glands are diminished in size and wasted, and only fine lanuginous hairs are produced. The change is a permanent one and not amenable to treatment.

In *premature alopecia*, resulting from acute diseases, the baldness is usually temporary. In eczema, psoriasis, and other affections the shedding of the hair is analogous to the desquamation of the cuticle from the inflamed skin, and unless the inflammation has been sufficiently severe to destroy the hair papillæ, new hair, at first downy and afterwards normal, is reproduced. But where the follicles and papillæ have been destroyed by suppuration and ulceration the baldness is permanent, and no treatment is of any avail. For the loss of hair after fevers tonics, generous diet, and a local stimulating lotion containing cantharides are the proper measures to be relied upon.

ALOPECIA AREATA.

Definition.—An atrophic disease characterized by the sudden loss of hair in small roundish limited patches, which have a tendency to enlarge slowly.

Symptoms.—The disease begins on the head or beard by the sudden loss of hair on a limited area. The hair comes out easily, and shows no signs of brittleness or any morbid change. Usually there is no sensation to indicate the position of the disease. The patches from which the hair has fallen are extremely smooth, white, and glistening, or polished like a billiard ball, and on the same level with or slightly more depressed than the adjacent skin. The patches are most common on the scalp, but may occur on the eyebrows, cheeks, or other hairy parts of the body ; they are sharply limited and surrounded by healthy hair, growing luxuriantly. As the disease spreads the hairs at the margin of the patch become loose and easily fall out, and thus by the confluence of patches large irregular areæ are formed. After a time the disease becomes spontaneously arrested, the smooth shiny

skin becomes marked by little prominences corresponding
to the hair follicles, and thin hairs, at first white and downy,
but afterwards stronger and darker, are slowly reproduced.
In rare instances the hair never grows again, or only as fine,
pale, or downy threads.

Diagnosis.—The patches of alopecia areata are sometimes
mistaken for tinea tonsurans, but the differences between the
two diseases are so marked that the diagnosis is easy.   In
tinea tonsurans the patches are rarely bald, but are covered
with short stubby hair, which comes out easily and under
the microscope shows the fungoid character of the disease.
The patches are also scaly, contrasting strongly with the
perfectly smooth shiny patches of alopecia areata.

Prognosis.—The disease, arising suddenly, like zoster and
morphœa, runs a definite though prolonged course, and tends
to spontaneous recovery. It is probably a neurosis, and due
to some nutritive lesion affecting the formation and growth
of the hair. The occasional occurrence of alopecia areata on
neuralgic patches is a fact somewhat in favor of this view.

Morbid Anatomy.—No visible changes have been discovered in the cutis. The bulbs of the affected hairs are atrophied, and a nodular swelling, due to the inversion of the
root sheath on them, is sometimes seen near the end.   The
fungus described by Gruby, Bazin, and some others, and
named microsporon Audouinii, has not been found by the
majority of modern observers, and the cases described as
alopecia areata by the first-named observers were probably
only old-standing and severe forms of ringworm in which
the hair had been completely destroyed. Inoculations from
true alopecia areata have not produced any result (Dyce
Duckworth).

Treatment.—The spreading of the disease can sometimes
be arrested, and the new growth of hair encouraged by severe blistering with acetum cantharidis or Burt's vesicating
fluid. The blistering should be repeated every fortnight.

Internally iron, strychine, arsenic, and other nervine tonics are said to be of value; at all events they should be tried in conjunction with local stimulation.

TRICHOREXIS NODOSA.

Trichorexis nodosa consists in the formation of little oval or round swellings on the hairs of the beard and mustache. The little nodes look like nits, but are seen under the microscope to be formed by a localized splitting and bulging of the hair itself, which presents somewhat the appearance of two brooms thrust into one another. No parasite is present, and the condition is ascribed by Beigel, who first described it, to the generation of gas in the medulla bursting the cortical substance of the hair. The affected hairs are not more easily extracted than normal hairs, but they break very readily at the nodes, leaving a frayed, brushlike extremity. The disease is very common and of little consequence. The treatment usually recommended is shaving, though the hairs are apt to split again when allowed to grow.

SUBDIVISION D.—Of the Nails.

ONYCHIA.

Inflammation of the nails occurs after mechanical injuries to the matrix, such, for instance, as pressure on the edges of an hypertrophied toe nail (paronychia lateralis), or spontaneously after a slight scratch or tear of the skin about the fold round the nail.

There is redness and swelling of the fold round the nail, most marked at the sides near each angle in "ingrowing toe nail," together with a deep-red discoloration of the matrix, attended with great tenderness on pressure and a sensation of heat and throbbing. The nail on its margin in idiopathic onychia becomes opaque, pus collects under it and under the cuticle of the fold, and the nail, becoming loosened in places, covers a sloughy, raw, tender surface, from which a brownish-red fluid exudes. Frequently the whole nail is shed, and after a slow process of healing a new nail forms, which is thin, rough, and brittle. In "ingrowing toe nail" the inflammation and subsequent suppuration is limited to one or other angle of the nail and to the adjacent nail fold, from which exuberant tender granulations protrude.

In acute onychia, or "whitlow," there is often pyrexia and constitutional disturbance, and necrosis of the terminal phalanx, suppuration in the synovial sheaths, and cellulitis of the hand and arm may occur.

Treatment.—"Ingrowing toe nail" in its milder forms may be well treated, as suggested by Dr. Tilbury Fox, by scraping the centre of the nail quite thin with a piece of glass and softening it with liquor potassæ. The granulations should be touched with nitrate of silver from time to time. Should the disease be more advanced, the nail should be completely removed by operation. In acute onychia, or "whitlow," poultices should be applied to the part, to promote suppuration; dead skin or nail must be removed, and subsequently it should be dressed with astringent lotions. Internally tonics and stimulants should be prescribed.

ONYCHOGRYPHOSIS.

This is the term applied to a condition observed most frequently in the little and great toes, in which the central portion of the nail becomes converted into an irregular clawlike or horny growth, ridged and more opaque and brittle than the normal nail. It is due to the local hypertrophy of the papillæ of the matrix and of the nail bed in front of it, as a result of continued pressure.

The papillæ, sometimes two or three lines in length, project into the horny mass and form a tender, vascular core imbedded in greatly thickened epithelial layers, as seen in ichthyosis.

ONYCHAUXIS.

Onychauxis, or hypertrophy of the nail, assumes either the form of a lateral outgrowth which may press upon and irritate the adjacent folds of skin, causing the so-called "ingrowing toe nail," or in the form of a somewhat chisel-shaped thickening of the nail, with the thick, broad part at the free border produced by hypertrophy of the papillæ in the anterior part of the nail bed.

The condition is analogous to tyloma, as onychogryphosis is to clavus.

Treatment.—Both these forms of undue growth of nail substance can be treated by paring away the excess of horny substance by means of the knife, scissors, or pliers. Should the soft, vascular part be exposed, it should be divided and the bleeding spot rapidly cauterized.

ONYCHATROPHIA.

Absence or defective development of the nails occurs sometimes as a congenital condition, and frequently in association with absence of hair. The more common variety results from disease or destruction of the matrix or bed of the nail in the course of various local or general diseases, but most usually from injury.

IN GENERAL DISEASES.

The changes met with in the nails as a result of general or local disease may be classed under the following heads:

1. *Acute.*—Desquamative, in erysipelas, scarlatina, pityriasis rubra, and acute eczema.
2. *Chronic.*—From severe diseases, such as enteric fever, pneumonia, peritonitis, etc.

3. In chronic eczema, psoriasis, and lichen ruber.
4. As a result of parasitic growths in favus and tinea
circinata.

1. In acute eczema, erysipelas, scarlatina, and pityriasis
rubra, the nails are sometimes shed as a consequence of the
local hyperæmia and exudation, the process being of the
same nature as the desquamation of the cuticle.

2. After severe diseases, such as enteric fever, pneumonia,
and acute rheumatism, depressed transverse lines are often
found on the nails during convalescence. The nail at these
places is much thinner than normal, and often somewhat
opaque and brittle.

3. In chronic eczema, when the disease attacks the hands
or feet, it may spread to the nails, causing them at first to
become pitted like the rind of an orange. Later they split
longitudinally, at first slightly, when the dirt which fills
the cracks makes them look like black lines, but widening
as the disease progresses until the whole nail splits from
end to end and finally is shed.

In psoriasis the nails may become thickened, opaque,
irregular, and darker in color. They are very brittle, short,
fissured at their extremities, and present transverse cracks.
In the bed and under the margin small spots of psoriasis
may be seen in the early stages of the disease.

In lichen ruber, in severe cases, the nails are opaque,
rough, and brittle, sometimes thickened, and at other times
thin and atrophied.

4. In some cases of tinea tonsurans and of favus the nails
become affected with the fungous growth. They are irregular, thickened, and brittle, and in places are marked with
yellowish spots and lines, in which the nail is more friable
than normal and appears rotten. Under the microscope,
after soaking in liquor potassæ, scrapings show mycelium
filaments and the spores of trichophyton or achorion.

25

CHAPTER XXIII.

Class A.—PARASITIC AFFECTIONS.

Sub-class A.—*Animal.*
Pediculosis—Scabies—Eruptions produced by Fleas, Bugs, etc.

Sub-class B.—*Vegetable.*
Tinea tonsurans—Kerion—Tinea sycosis—Tinea circinata—Eczema
marginatum—Tinea versicolor—Tinea favosa.

Sub-class A.—*Animal.*

PEDICULOSIS—PHTHIRIASIS.

Definition.—A diseased condition of the skin produced
by the attacks of lice.

Symptoms.—Three species of lice infest the human body,—
pediculus capitis, restricted to the hairy scalp; *pediculus
pubis*, found about the genitals, and occasionally on the
margins of the eyelids, beard, and axillæ; and *pediculus
corporis*, or vestimenti, chiefly affecting the trunk.

In *pediculosis capitis*, produced by the presence of pediculi
capitis, the lice are found wandering about the roots of the
hair, most abundantly on the occipital and temporal regions,
and more frequently in women and children than in male
adults. They excite intense itching by thrusting their pro-
bosces into the hair follicles and sucking blood from the
capillaries, and soon, owing to the scratching which results,
excoriations, eczematous eruptions, and crusts appear. The

hair becomes matted, foul-smelling, and covered with adherent "nits" or ova; the glands in the anterior triangle and
at the back of the neck frequently swell and even suppurate, and excoriated spots and boils often appear on the
nape of the neck.

In *pediculosis pubis*, the *crab lice*, as they are termed from
their shape, anchor themselves firmly to the roots of the
pubic hairs, and by their sucking produce itching and follicular irritation, which excites scratching and thereby
causes excoriations and eczema. The lice are seen as little
grayish specks adhering to the bases of the hairs, and are
mostly found in adults.

Pediculosis corporis, occurring mostly in elderly persons,
like the previous affection, is excited by lice, which, however, are rarely visible on stripping the patient, as they in-
habit and deposit their ova in the folds of the under-clothing and the interstices of flannel garments worn next the
skin. Thrusting their proboses into the hair follicles, they
wound the capillaries and produce minute hæmorrhagic
specks, surrounded at first, like fleabites, by a hyperæmic
zone. These spots are the seats of intense itching or creep-
ing sensations. Violent scratching ensues; the cuticle is
torn off over the parts affected, and excoriations are produced, covered by scabs of dried blood. Papular, urticarial, eczematous, and furuncular or pustular eruptions are
usually excited in the same way, and in old-standing cases
the skin becomes deeply pigmented and covered with scabs,
which are most numerous about the shoulders and the front
of the chest beneath the clavicles. This eruption was
formerly named prurigo senilis, and is not pathognomonic
of pediculi in itself, being capable of production by any
intense itching, but its restriction to certain sites and the
presence of hæmorrhagic puncta determine the diagnosis.

Diagnosis.—In *pediculosis capitis* the presence of the
"nits" or ova—small whitish, semi-translucent bodies—

firmly adherent to the hairs, and the discovery of the parasites near their roots or attaching to the comb, settles the question.

In *pediculosis pubis* the parasites adhere to the roots of the hairs, and have the appearance of little grayish or brownish scales, which when pulled off with forceps often tear out the hair to which they cling.

In *pediculosis corporis* the lice must be looked for on the folds of the under-clothing, about the junctions of the sleeves with the body, and under the collar of the shirt. The restriction of the " pruritic rash " to the shoulders and infraclavicular region, and the presence of hæmorrhagic puncta, may occasionally, when, from the under-clothing having recently been changed, no pediculi can be found thereon, lead to an accurate diagnosis.

Prognosis.—Pediculi, if untreated, may increase and multiply for years, causing eczema, pruritic eruptions, glandular enlargements, abscesses, etc. Under appropriate measures, however, they are readily exterminated, and the eruptions excited by them subside either spontaneously or under ordinary treatment in a short time.

Anatomy.—The pediculus belong to the class Insecta. Its head, which is small, is furnished with a delicate retractile proboscis, not usually discernible after death; and it has a compressed thorax, six legs, and a somewhat flattened abdomen.

The pediculus capitis has a slender shape, and is generally smaller than the other varieties; its abdomen is ovoid and terminates in a blunt cone.

The pediculus corporis is much larger, averaging $\frac{1}{24}$th to $\frac{1}{8}$th inch in length; its abdomen presents a terminal triangular notch.

The pediculus pubis, the crab louse, is relatively much broader and shorter than the other kinds; its abdomen is nodulated, and the anterior pairs of its short stout legs are provided with strong claws, with which it anchors itself firmly to the skin.

Treatment.—The full-grown lice are easily destroyed by a carbolic lotion (1 to 20), or by the inunction of dilute ammonio-chloride, red precipitate ointment, oleate of mercury 5 per cent., or ung. hyd. c. sulph. As the ova are not readily attacked by these remedies, they must be applied for a week or ten days, so as to destroy the young lice as they become hatched.

For pediculus pubis, ung. staphisagriæ, scented with oil of lavender or roses, is a very valuable application.

Pediculus corporis should be treated by warm baths, thorough change of clothing, and baking the old garments in a disinfecting oven at a temperature of 250°–300° Fahr., so as to destroy the lice or their ova.

Itching may be mitigated by soothing alkaline or prussic acid and glycerin lotions, and any eczematous or other eruptions treated on general principles.

Scabies—Itch.

Definition.—A contagious disease of the skin, produced by the presence of the acarus scabiei in the epidermis.

Symptoms.—Following the arrangement of Hebra, we may class the phenomena of scabies under three headings, viz. :

1. Those arising directly from the presence of acari in the skin.
2. Those which are the result of scratching.
3. Those which are produced by the action of other irritants upon portions of skin affected by acari.

1. Those directly due to the presence of acari in the skin.

The full-grown female acarus after impregnation begins at once to work her way into the epidermis, and burrows

somewhat obliquely under the surface into the soft cells of
the stratum lucidum or the rete, giving rise to a narrow,
somewhat sinuous tunnel or cuniculus. The tunnel, whitish,
and dotted here and there with darkish spots,—six or eight
in number, which are the deposited ova,—is somewhat dilated
at its terminal extremity into a small roundish chamber, in
which the acarus lies. At times the burrow is seen as a
whitish line on the summit of a reddish ridge, and occasionally vesicles or pustules form near to or along the course
of the cuniculus, but never involve its terminal chamber.
At the extremities the burrows, which average $\frac{1}{8}$th of an
inch in length, but which may vary from $\frac{1}{25}$th of an inch
to two or three inches, are usually blackened by contact
with staining materials, dirt, etc., on the trunk, penis, buttocks, elbows, and knees, and in the skin of children; while
upon the hands of very cleanly people they are pale and
not easily detected. In adults the disease most frequently
attacks the interdigital webs and the thin skin on the flexor
surface of the wrist; it also attacks the penis, hypogastrium,
the buttocks, axillæ or flexures of the elbows, mammæ, and
inner ankles. In children the buttocks and feet are the
chief seats of the disease, but any part of the body may
become inoculated. The scalp and face are never implicated in adults, and only very rarely in children. The
burrowing of the acarus is accompanied by itching, which
is worse at night; and by the irritation of the parasite
alone, as well as by the scratching it excites, urticarial,
eczematous, pustular, or ecthymatous eruptions may be
produced.

2. As a result of scratching linear wheals, excoriated
papules covered with black crusts of dried blood, vesicles,
pustules, etc., are usually developed, forming a "pruritic
rash" similar to that of pediculosis. It is always most
marked on the front of the trunk and thighs, being limited
to, or at all events most intense on, a space bounded by the

mammary line above and the knees below. The face is very seldom scratched, and the back to a less extent than the front of the trunk.

3. If the skin affected with itch be exposed to pressure or friction, papules, tubercles, pustules, or crusts appear over the tubera ischii,—e. g., when persons sit on hard benches,—or they may present themselves on the tracts of skin indurated by crutches, trusses, belts, garters, or tight clothes. These nodules may or may not exhibit burrows on their summits.

Diagnosis.—The diagnosis of scabies is based upon the history of contagion, usually to be elicited, the steady progress of the affection, the presence of itching, aggravated at night, the particular site of the eruption, on the wrists and between the fingers most frequently in adults (unless parasiticide soaps be used), on the penis, hypogastrium, and mammæ, or on the buttocks and feet, in infants, and by the discovery of cuniculi, from the terminal dilatations of which the acari can be extracted and examined microscopically.

When, as in infants, the burrows cannot be easily distinguished and crusts are abundant, the maceration of these with liquor potassæ will often assist the discovery of full-grown or embryonic acari.

Attention to these distinctive features will simplify the diagnosis of scabies, even though it should be complicated with pruritic, eczematous, or ecthymatous eruptions. Prurigo of Hebra differs from scabies by the presence of hard, solid, fleshy papules, by its history, and by the greater severity of the itching.

In pediculosis corporis, as in scabies, a "pruritic rash" may be present upon the trunk, but the absence of cuniculi in the skin will sufficiently distinguish the former from the latter.

Prognosis.—Scabies is merely a local trouble; exerts no deteriorating influence on the constitution even in inveterate

ing seve`ral days, and known as the
in some persons urticarial wheals or

ia lectularia, causes erythematous or
a itch much and are more persistent
_n the redness fades in a day or so,
l papule with central hæmorrhagic
r three days more.

ans autumnalis, a minute reddish
the itch insect, to the class Arach-
skin, and causes a papular erup-
lied at night as the temperature
The appearance lasts a week or ten

belonging to the genus Culex, and
cause erythematous or urticarial
ntions, which itch intensely, are
by the hairs of a certain class of

may be allayed by the applica-
mat., of lot. carbonis detergens
perchlor. grs. ij to ʒj with the
dilute prussic acid in the ounce.

" — *Vegetable.*

Hebra and Neumann, are of
caused by the growth of fungi
es are due to one species of
differences according to the
ich it is found. It is more
different varieties of fungi,

n tonsurans.
furfur.
hoenleinii.

cases. It usually yields to parasiticides, and the eczematous eruptions excited by it and by the scratching subside under suitable treatment.

Anatomy.—The adult female acarus scabiei is oval, about $\frac{1}{80}$th to $\frac{1}{87}$th of an inch long by $\frac{1}{160}$th to $\frac{1}{80}$th of an inch broad; the dorsal surface is convex and armed with angular spines, while the ventral presents four pairs of legs, the two anterior of which have stalked suckers. In the male the third pair are furnished with fine setæ, and the fourth with suckers. In the female both hinder pairs are provided with setæ only, and, whereas the male wanders upon the surface, she burrows into the cuticle and deposits from twelve to twenty ova, from which are hatched six-legged embryos. These undergo several changes of skin, and acquire their fourth pair of legs after the first moulting.

Treatment.—Give a warm bath, wash well with soap, thoroughly rub in some parasiticide ointment, containing as the essential ingredient grs. xx to ℥ss. of sulphur to ℥j of lard, scented with various aromatic oils; put on close-fitting flannel drawers and jerseys, so as to keep the ointment acting upon the skin; and repeat the bath and the washing at the end of forty-eight hours. If itching continues after this, the same plan must be adopted again. Care must be taken not to use too strong preparations of sulphur, as they are apt to produce a severe eczematous condition. As a substitute balsam of Peru, or storax in the form of an ointment, may be tried. Sulphur vapor baths have been recommended, but they are not so efficacious as the other modes of treatment.

ERUPTIONS PRODUCED BY FLEAS, BUGS, ETC.

The common flea, *pulex irritans*, gives rise to a roseolar spot, sometimes slightly raised, with a central red punctum, and as the redness fades the centre remains as a red or dark-colored petechia, lasting several days, and known as the purpura pulicosa. In some persons urticarial wheals or vesicles may result.

The bed bug, *acanthia lectularia*, causes erythematous or urticarial spots, which itch much and are more persistent than fleabites. Though the redness fades in a day or so, a small itchy, indurated papule with central hæmorrhagic punctum may last two or three days more.

The harvest mite, *leptus autumnalis*, a minute reddish parasite, belonging, like the itch insect, to the class Arachnida, imbeds itself in the skin, and causes a papular eruption with itching, intensified at night as the temperature of the body increases. The appearance lasts a week or ten days and then subsides.

Gnats and mosquitoes, belonging to the genus Culex, and some kinds of midges also, cause erythematous or urticarial papules, and similar eruptions, which itch intensely, are excited in some persons by the hairs of a certain class of caterpillars.

Treatment.—The itching may be allayed by the application of diluted sp. amm. aromat., of lot. carbonis detergens (ʒj to ʒj), or lot. hydrarg. perchlor. grs. ij to ʒj with the addition of ℞ x to ℞ xij of dilute prussic acid in the ounce.

Sub-class B. — *Vegetable.*

Some authors, among them Hebra and Neumann, are of opinion that all skin diseases caused by the growth of fungi in the epidermis or appendages are due to one species of parasite, which present certain differences according to the conditions of the nidus in which it is found. It is more usual, however, to describe three different varieties of fungi, viz.:

a. Trichophyton tonsurans.
b. Microsporon furfur.
c. Achorion Schoenleinii.

Trichophyton tonsurans, occurring in various parts of the body, gives rise to cutaneous affections, to which the term tinea with some qualifying adjective has usually been applied. In the scalp it causes *tinea tonsurans*, the common ringworm, and *kerion* where prominent, boggy, honeycombed patches are present. On the hairy parts of the face it produces *tinea sycosis*, on the body *tinea circinata* (herpes circinatus, etc.), and the so-called *eczema marginatum*. The nails also occasionally become affected. The disease attacks all classes, the healthy and prosperous as well as the poor and debilitated.

TINEA TONSURANS—RINGWORM OF THE HEAD.

Definition.—A contagious disease of the scalp, caused by the presence of trichophyton tonsurans in the epidermis, the hairs, and their follicles.

Symptoms.—Tinea tonsurans is met with most frequently in children, but is occasionally seen in adults. From the fact that persons who have suffered long from ringworm of the scalp in childhood frequently present patches of tinea versicolor when grown up, it has been supposed that the latter affection is due to a modification of the trichophyton, produced by the difference between the skin of an adult and that of a child. In the early stage, which rarely comes under observation, a small red, erythematous or slightly raised patch arises on some part of the hairy scalp, accompanied by considerable itching. As the patch gradually enlarges, the redness and elevation of the centre subside, and a roundish ring with a bright-red raised margin, often presenting a crop of small vesicles (herpes circinatus), and a paler, rough, or scurfy-looking centre, is produced. If . the rings be concentric, an eruption simulating erythema or herpes iris is produced.

In the fully developed condition ringworm appears as a pale-brown or slaty-looking, roundish patch ($\frac{1}{2}$ inch to 3 or

4 inches in diameter), slightly elevated above the adjacent healthy scalp, and covered with short stubbly hairs ⅛ inch long and small opaque branny scales. The hairs are thick, twisted, or bent, frayed at their extremities, have a dull-grayish look, and break off or fall out easily from their follicles, which are somewhat prominent. At this stage the brittleness, loss of color, and deformity of the stubbly hairs are marked features, and should always be looked for. In some instances the parasite excites an acute inflammation of the hair follicles, which become pustular, and as a consequence destruction of the papillæ of the hairs and permanent alopecia may follow.

Eczema is sometimes produced, and the yellowish-green, brittle crusts which then form conceal the appearances of ringworm.

Occasionally ringworm of the scalp becomes *diffuse,* and much resembles eczema capitis in the scaly stage. After lasting for a variable time ringworm begins to subside, and the patch is covered with fine scales and young hairs, which are apparently normal; or both skin and hairs may, on superficial observation, appear quite natural. Here and there, however, and chiefly at the margins of the patch, short, stubbly, discolored hairs can be found on careful examination, and unless these are eradicated the disease is liable to relapse and to affect other persons.

In a few cases smooth, hairless patches, resembling those of alopecia areata, are produced, which, according to Dr. Liveing, has led to the erroneous belief that there is a parasitic disease (which has been called *tinea decalvans*) distinct, on the one hand, from tinea tonsurans, and on the other from alopecia areata.

KERION.

This is a rare condition, in which one or more of the patches of ordinary ringworm becomes raised, tender, and

uneven; small prominences, resembling inflamed hair follicles, soon appear, from which a viscid, honeylike secretion
exudes, and the whole mass becomes what may be termed
"boggy" to the touch. As a rule no pus is formed, but
the hairs and their follicles are gradually destroyed, the
result being permanent baldness.

Tinea Sycosis.

This variation is produced when the parasite attacks the
hair of the beard and mustache, and extends into their
deepseated follicles. The primary symptom, as in tinea
tonsurans, is a red, scaly, and itching patch; the follicles
next become indurated and tender, forming reddish, prominent tubercles, which suppurate; the hairs become dull and
brittle, and are easily extracted. When the pustules and
small abscesses round the follicles burst, crusting takes
place, but to a less extent than in eczema of the face.

Tinea Circinata.

This results from the development of trichophyton on the
non-hairy parts of the body; it appears most commonly on
the face, neck, and trunk, and may or may not be accompanied by patches of tinea tonsurans; it also shows itself on
the hands and arms of those attending to cases of ringworm
of the scalp. Small reddish, somewhat raised, circular
patches, covered with branny scales, and usually presenting
a ring of minute vesicles at their margins, make their appearance, and are commonly attended by marked itching.
Fading in the centre, the patch gradually extends at the
margins, which are usually vesicular (hence the name herpes
circinatus), and forms "fairy rings," like those of other
fungi. By the coalescence of these rings irregular circinate
or gyrate bands are produced, the rings ceasing to extend
and overlap where they blend, as if the material for their

further growth had been exhausted in spots already affected with the disease. T. circinata, when it reaches the scalp or hairy parts of the face, gives rise to T. tonsurans or T. sycosis, and is often found in isolated patches in persons affected with those diseases, or in those who have come in contact with them.

ECZEMA MARGINATUM.

Affecting the genitals, the inner sides of the thighs, and the buttocks, is merely a variety of tinea circinata occurring in parts where the abundant perspiration, warmth, and friction predispose the skin to inflammatory action. The red, elevated, and itching patches fade in the centre, leaving it deeply pigmented, and at the raised margins vesicles, pustules, excoriations, or crusts are met with. It spreads in the same way and presents the same fungus as T. circinata. In some cases the parasite may not be found, though the eczema which it has started persists.

Diagnosis.—In T. tonsurans the round, scaly, itching patches on the scalp, the dull, brittle, or stubbly hairs, which are easily pulled out, and the reddish, spreading margin, while the centre is pale, are features which are diagnostic of the disease. When impetiginous crusts hide the whole patch, when smooth bald patches occur, when new hairs are growing and the disease is receding, or when it is in the early stage and appears as an erythematous or vesicular patch, ringworm may be mistaken for eczema of the scalp, alopecia areata, or erythema vesicans. When the entire scalp is affected, it is almost impossible to distinguish it from scaly eczema of the scalp. In all these cases, however, the detection of the parasite in the stubbly hairs, crusts, or scales, after maceration in liq. potassæ, will clear up the difficulty. The frequent occurrence of T. circinata on other parts of the body, or the detection of dull, brittle, broken-off or distorted, easily extracted hairs, will also help the diagnosis.

Even to the naked eye the appearances of T. kerion are so peculiar that the nature of the affection can hardly be mistaken. In the early stages, where the puffy swelling may simulate a subcutaneous abscess, microscopical examination of the loosened hairs settles the question.

T. sycosis differs from eczema of the beard in the development of indurated tubercles and abscesses, the dull, brittle character of the hairs, which are readily extracted, the presence usually of T. circinata on other parts, and in the presence of trichophyton on microscopic examination. *T. circinata* and *eczema marginatum* may resemble some forms of erythema multiforme and of eczema respectively, but the spreading in "fairy rings" and the presence of the parasite are diagnostic.

Prognosis.—Ringworm of the body is usually easily amenable to appropriate treatment, but on the hairy parts, on the other hand, it is extremely obstinate, persisting for months, and sometimes for years, in spite of all remedies, and being liable to recur if the treatment have been left off too soon. The parasite does not endanger life, but is troublesome on account of the loss of hair it causes, the secondary inflammations it sometimes excites, and the marked contagiousness of the affection.

Morbid Anatomy.—Examining under the microscope, after maceration for twenty-four hours in dilute liq. potassæ, the dull, brittle hairs or the epidermic scales obtained by scraping with a blunt knife a patch of tinea, fine mycelium filaments, made up of roundish or cylindrical segments, are seen running longitudinally throughout the hair, or forming a feltwork in and between the epidermic scales. Where the filaments reach the surface of the hair they give rise to globular aggregations (conidia), made up of minute round refracting bodies, the spores of the fungus, which measure about $\frac{1}{8000}$ inch in diameter. Occasionally no filaments are met with, the hair presenting only collections of conidia and scattered spores on the surface and in its substance.

Dr. F. Taylor, in examining vertical sections of a scalp affected with ringworm, found the following changes: In hairs slightly affected mycelium filaments only were found, running along the length of the hair, which was not altered in shape. The hair was in later stages obscured by a dense aggregation of spores in its follicle, and its substance, as far down as the upper part of the bulb, was destroyed, or replaced by mycelium threads. The hair papillæ were never affected, and laterally the internal root sheath formed the outer boundary of the fungus growth, no traces of it being found in the outer root sheath, follicle walls, cutis, or epidermis. Only slight traces of inflammation were found round the hairs.

Treatment.—In the different varieties of tinea produced by trichophyton attention must be directed to:

1. The destruction of the parasite.

2. The removal of any secondary inflammation which may have been caused by the parasite or the remedies employed for its destruction.

Where the disease is superficial, as in T. circinata and eczema marginatum, there is little or no difficulty in carrying out the first indication. Lotions containing bichloride of mercury (grs. ij ad ℥j), sulphurous acid, or hyposulphite of soda (℥j ad ℥j), or the persistent inunction of dilute ammonio-chloride or nitrate of mercury ointments, or of oleate of mercury 5 per cent., are usually curative in a few weeks. Vaseline, oleate of zinc, or bismuth, etc., should be used subsequently if there is any eczema.

In ringworm of the scalp or of the beard (T. sycosis) the main difficulty is to get the parasiticide brought into contact with *all* the mycelial filaments and spores, many of which lie deep down in the hair follicles. Hence, though the superficial fungus growth is easily destroyed, and the disease appears to be eradicated, much annoyance is caused by the recurrence of the affection, a few conidia which have eluded the poison being sufficient to start a fresh growth, and subsequently to infect other persons.

The indications, therefore, for treatment are to:

1. Remove as much as possible of the diseased hairs and epidermis.

2. Use a parasiticide which will penetrate readily and deeply into the cuticle and hair follicles.

3. Continue the treatment, more or less modified, for at least a month after all signs of the disease are gone.

1. The hair over the diseased patch, and for ⅓ to ½ inch round, or of the whole scalp, beard, etc., should be cut short with scissors, all crusts removed by oiling or poulticing, and the surface washed well with soft soap and water. Loose hairs and scales should be removed by rubbing, and in the case of T. sycosis by epilation, which, owing to the loosening of the hairs, is here less painful than in eczema of the beard. Blistering by liq. epispasticus, acetum cantharidis glaciale, or Coster's paint of iodine and oil of wood tar, is also useful for this purpose.

2. A solution of bichloride of mercury in acetic acid (grs. vj to ℥iv), which has the combined advantages of penetrating deeply, of macerating the hair and epidermic tissues, and of blistering, is one of the best. It should be repeated from time to time, and weak acid nitrate or ammonio-chloride of mercury ointments applied in the intervals to the irritated skin.

3. After removing all the stubbly hairs, and when no further reproduction of the disease has appeared for some time after the last application of vesicants or of the mercury and acetic acid paint, weak ammonio-chloride of mer-

cury ointment should be rubbed in twice a day for some time further, to guard against the possibility of some overlooked portion of fungus starting into fresh growth.

Any eczema of the scalp thus excited should be treated in the usual way.

Goa powder, or its active principle, chrysophanic acid, are useful only as irritants, and do not cure tinea tonsurans, though, like simple blistering, they may suffice to remove T. circinata.

Any constitutional debility, strumous condition, etc., should be treated with cod-liver oil, tonics, and good food and hygiene, which, though unable to cure the disease, by improving the general health lessen the risk of eczema, etc.

Cases of ringworm of the scalp are rarely cured within less than four to six months, and even with the most efficient and thorough treatment they may last for years. In public institutions and schools the separation of the patients and of their clothing, towels, etc., is necessary to check further spread of the disease.

TINEA VERSICOLOR—CHLOASMA—PITYRIASIS VERSICOLOR.

Definition.—A parasitic contagious disease, excited by the presence of microsporon furfur in the epidermis, usually occurring on the trunk as yellowish or pale buff-colored patches.

Symptoms.—Tinea versicolor does not occur in childhood, and is hardly ever seen after fifty; it is met with most frequently between the ages of puberty and forty. It is far less communicable than T. circinata, and usually attacks only those who have warm, easily-perspiring skins. Occurring chiefly on the front of the chest and abdomen, on parts covered by flannel garments, it may extend to the upper arm or thigh, rarely affecting the face, scalp or leg, and never developing on the palmar and plantar surfaces.

Small, roundish, slightly-reddened patches appear usually symmetrically on the trunk, extending by a slightly raised and somewhat scaly margin. The patch soon becomes pale yellow, fawn-colored, buff, or brownish in color, and unites with neighboring spots, forming irregular areæ with detached roundish patches at the margin. Itching, slight or absent in most cases, may sometimes be severe, and give rise to scratching and pruritic rashes. Occasionally the hair follicles become hyperæmic, giving the patch an irregular, punctuated appearance; the pigmentary deposit may be excessive, almost sooty black, the so-called *pityriasis nigra;* or urticarial or eczematous eruptions may be excited by the parasite.

Diagnosis.—Tinea versicolor may be mistaken for a macular syphilide, or for ordinary non-parasitic chloasma (melanoderma).

The syphilide is usually accompanied by other specific eruptions, is preceded by roseola, sore throat, alopecia, etc., does not usually itch, occurs on the trunk, face, arms, and legs indiscriminately, and is of a brownish or coppery color. T. versicolor, though it may be met with in a syphilitic person, usually occurs *per se;* the patches frequently itch, occur most frequently on the front of the trunk, and are of a pale-yellow or buff color.

Spots of melanoderma are seen most often on exposed parts, rarely on the trunk; they are perfectly smooth, not rough or branny, and itching is not met with.

In all doubtful cases the discovery of the parasite (see morbid anatomy), on microscopic examination of the scales, will clear up the diagnosis.

Prognosis.—In those who perspire freely and do not wash the body the disease is usually chronic, and may last for years. The parasite, affecting as a rule only the superficial layers of the cuticle, can easily be got rid of by treatment.

Morbid Anatomy.—Microscopic examination of the scales scraped off from a patch of T. versicolor, and macerated in liq. potassæ, shows a network of mycelium made up of branching filaments, the segments of which are usually long and cylindrical, interspersed with roundish aggregations of large round spores, which look like bunches of grapes. The little hairs are more or less infiltrated and split up by the fungus, but the disease does not extend deeply into the epidermis or hair follicles.

Treatment.—Cleanliness, frequent washing with soft soap, and the subsequent application of sulphurous acid (1 to 4) or hyposulphite of soda lotion (℥j ad ℥j), or the inunction of a mild mercurial ointment, easily cure the disease. No internal treatment is necessary.

Tinea Favosa—Favus.

Definition.—A contagious, chronic disease, excited by the presence of achorion Schoenleinii in the epidermis, hairs, and corium; met with most frequently on the scalp.

Symptoms.—Favus, met with rarely in England, is much more common on the Continent, in Scotland, and in some parts of the United States, and, though contagious, attacks chiefly poor and dirty children. It begins on the scalp as an itching, reddish, scaly patch, resembling that of tinea tonsurans, the hairs on which are dull, but not so brittle as in ringworm. Small yellowish crusts, about the size of pins' heads, next appear round isolated hairs, which pull out more easily with their bulbs entire, not broken off; the crusts (favi), convex at first, become, as they gradually enlarge, depressed and cup-shaped in the centre, and of a bright sulphur-yellow color. Solitary favi may enlarge till they measure ½ inch or more in diameter, or may become confluent, and by admixture with epidermis, eczematous secretions, etc., form irregular crusts. The favi have a disagreeable, mousy odor, and when removed leave a depressed pit, which is excoriated or covered with smooth epithelium. In the later stages the typical cups disappear, and the surface resembles a scaly eczema capitis. Destruction of the hair follicles and permanent alopecia are frequent results of the disease.

On the body erythematous patches or rings, resembling those of T. circinata, are occasionally met with; they seldom exceed ½ inch in diameter, and have not the tendency to rapid extension seen in ringworm.

It is essentially a chronic disease, lasting for many years, and, though contagious, does not seem so easily communicable as ringworm.

It is more prone to excite secondary inflammatory affections than ringworm.

In America domestic animals (cats, mice, etc.) are said frequently to transmit the disease to man.

Diagnosis.—Favus, in the early erythematous stage, resembles ringworm, but the hairs are not so brittle, are not stubbly, and pull out with their bulb entire, instead of breaking off sharply. In the developed condition the mousy-smelling sulphur-yellow cups adherent to a hair in their centre are quite typical. In the later stages, when the cups have given way to whitish scales and flakes, or are covered over by impetiginous crusts, the discovery of the fungus under the microscope will distinguish favus from eczema in the scaly or moist and crusting stage.

Prognosis.—The disease is very chronic, and, on account of its tendency to invade the deeper tissues, resists treatment even more obstinately than ringworm of the hairy parts. Permanent alopecia is frequently caused by it, and some observers believe that it exerts a lowering influence on the general health.

Morbid Anatomy.—Microscopic examination of a portion of favus crust macerated in liq. potassæ, and subsequently tinted with iodine solution, shows a mycelium made up of ovoidal segments, averaging $\frac{1}{8000}$ inch in diameter, containing granules in their interior, and terminating in large rounded spores $\frac{1}{3500}$ inch in diameter with a distinct double contour.

Vertical sections through a favus cup show the epidermis infiltrated with spores, micrococci, and fatty granules, most numerous at the margin. In the centre of the cup the diseased hairs, which have a mycelium running longitudinally and numerous collections of spores in their substance, are met with extending down to the bulbs. Beneath them, in favi $\frac{1}{4}$ to $\frac{1}{2}$ inch in diameter, mycelial filaments are found running into the corium substance at right angles to the surface for a more or less considerable distance; they terminate in chaplets of spores, which, with numerous leucocytes, are found in abundance between them. The chronic exudation, and in some cases the suppuration excited by this mycelial invasion, leads to gradual wasting of the affected corium, and is perhaps the cause of the depression and loss of hair.

Treatment.—Epilation, advisable in ringworm, is here almost indispensable. The removal of crusts, blistering, and the application of the mercury and acetic acid paint, followed by hyposulphite of soda lotion or the inunction of ammonio-chloride of mercury, ung. sulph. co. (see p. 275), etc., must be persevered in for a long time. Tonics, cod-liver oil, good food, and hygiene are usually necessary.

ings, resembling acne, round the sebaceous and hair follicles, which occasionally run on into pustules, or definite
furuncles are produced.   The cessation of the drugs, and
the application of local sedatives, with purgatives internally,
is usually followed by the subsidence of the eruptions.

INDEX.

Acarus folliculorum, 272
  scabiei, 297
Acne frontalis, 274
  indurata, 274
  mentagra, 276
  punctata, 272
  pustulosa, 274
  rosacea, 277
  sebacea, 269
  sycosis, 276
  syphilitica, 104
  vulgaris, 274
    treatment of, 275
Active hyperæmia, 188
Acute bedsore, 207
  eczema, 151
  infectious diseases, remarks on, 46
Addison's disease, 210
  keloid, 213
Adipose tissue, anatomy of, 18
Albinismus, 226
Alibert's keloid, 233
Alopecia, 287
  areata, 288
  senilis, 287
Anatomy of the skin, 13–29
Anæmia, 190
Anidrosis, 282
Angioma, 253
Anthrax, 178
Atrophia cutis, 228

Baldness, 287
Bedsore, acute, 207
Bloodvessels, anatomy of, 26
Boil, 177
  treatment of, 178
Bromidrosis, 283
Bug, eruption from, 301
Bulla, definition of, 31, 33, 38

Canities, 287
Carbuncle, 178
  treatment of, 180
Carcinoma cutis, 262
Chancre, 99
Cheiro-pompholyx, 203
Chicken-pox, 68
Chilblain, 189
Chloasma, 309
  uterinum, 210
Chromidrosis, 283
Chronic eczema, 152
Cicatrix, definition of, 36
Clavus, 230
Classification 40–45
Comedones 272
Condylomata, 103–113
Corium, anatomy of, 17
Corn, 233
Cornu, 230
Crab lice, 295
Crust, definition of, 35

Delhi boil, 181
Dermatolysis, 224
Diphtheria, 81
Drugs, eruptions from, 314
Dystrophia cutis, 206

Ecchymoses, 191
Ecthyma syphilitica, 104
Eczema, 150–165
  articulorum, 156
  capillitii, 154
  chronic, 152
  corporis, 157
  crurale, 156
  of the ears, 155
  erythematosum, 153
  of the eyelashes, 155
  faciei, 155

27

Sudamina, 283
Surgical rash, 96
Sweat, composition of, 29
Sweat glands, anatomy of, 19
Sycosis (acne), 276
　　(tinea), 304
Syphilis, 97
Syphilides, general characters of, 107
Syphilis of the tongue, 108
Syphilitic iritis, 108

Tactile corpuscles, anatomy of, 28
Tertiary syphilis, 105
Tinea circinata, 304
　　favosa, 311
　　tarsi, 155
　　tonsurans, 302
　　versicolor, 309
Traumatic hæmorrhages, 191
Trichorexis nodosa, 290
Tubercles, definition of, 31, 32, 38
Tubercular syphilide, 105
Tylosis, 230
Typhus fever, 74

Ulcers, 182
Ulcus rodens, 267
Universal acute eczema, 152
Urticaria, 124
　　bullosa, 125
　　conferta, 125
　　evanida, 125
　　febrilis, 124
　　miliaris, 125
　　papulosa, 125
　　perstans, 125
　　pigmentosa, 125
　　tuberosa, 125
　　vesicularis, 125

Vaccination, 70
Vaccinia, 70
Vaccino-syphilis, 114
Varicella, 68
Variola, 61
　　confluens, 63
　　corymbosa, 63
　　discreta, 63
　　hæmorrhagica, 63
　　semiconfluens, 63
Verruca, 232
　　necrogenica, 90
Vesicle, definition of, 31, 33, 39
Vibices, 191
Vitiligoidea, 237

Wart, 232
Warts, treatment of, 233
Wheal, definition of, 31, 33
White leprosy, 227

Xanthelasma, 237
Xanthoma, 237
　　planum, 238
　　tuberosum, 238
Xeroderma, 211

Yaws, 90

Zoster, 197
　　capillitii, 199
　　cervico-brachialis, 200
　　faciei, 200
　　femoralis, 201
　　nuchæ et colli, 200
　　pectoralis, 201
　　pudentalis, 201
　　treatment of, 202

Lightning Source UK Ltd.
Milton Keynes UK
UKHW011843271118
333053UK00011B/851/P